Evidence-Based
Physical Diagnosis

T0195535

EDITION

Evidence-Based Physical Diagnosis

STEVEN McGEE, M.D.

Professor Emeritus, Medicine
University of Washington School of Medicine

ELSEVIER

ohn F. Kennedy Blvd.
300
adelphia, PA 19103-2899

EVIDENCE-BASED PHYSICAL DIAGNOSIS,
FIFTH EDITION

ISBN: 9780323754835

Previous editions copyrighted 2018, 2012, and 2007.

Library of Congress Control Number: 2021941821

Content Strategist: Charlotta Kryhl
Content Development Specialist: Kathryn DeFrancesco
Publishing Services Manager: Deepthi Unni
Project Manager: Radjan Lourde Selvanadin
Design Direction: Renee Duenow

Printed in the United States of America.

Last digit is the print number: 9   8   7   6   5   4   3   2

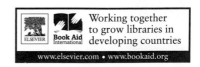

Working together
to grow libraries in
developing countries

www.elsevier.com • www.bookaid.org

To Rosalie, Connor, and Matt

Since the appearance of the fourth edition of this work, hundreds of new studies on physical diagnosis have appeared, and research has further defined how physical findings help identify disease, solve clinical problems, and forecast patient outcomes. In this fifth edition of *Evidence-Based Physical Diagnosis*, 203 of these new studies have been added to the *Evidence-Based Medicine (EBM) Boxes*, thus providing the most up-to-date summary of physical examination and its diagnostic accuracy. New references have replaced outworn ones, although classic articles and original descriptions remain. Every chapter has been updated. Many findings not previously addressed in prior editions appear here, along with their diagnostic accuracy and likelihood ratios. These findings include the Romberg test (spinal stenosis); oximeter paradoxus (cardiac tamponade); platypnea (liver disease); relative afferent pupil defect (unilateral visual loss); pupil size in red eye (acute glaucoma); hum test (hearing loss); jolt accentuation headache (meningitis); nasal flaring, intercostal retractions, and suprasternal retractions (dyspnea); diastolic rumble (mitral stenosis); bendopnea test (congestive heart failure); hand vein estimates of central venous pressure; adenopathy (infectious mononucleosis); abnormal bowel tones (recovery from postoperative ileus); Ipswich touch test (diabetic foot); the Edinburgh algorithm for diplopia; and the bedside diagnosis of orbital fractures. As in the last edition, each chapter begins with a list of *Key Teaching Points*, intended for individuals desiring quick summaries and for teachers constructing concise bedside lessons. Each EBM Box remains linked to the Elsevier *online EBM* calculator to quickly estimate post-test probability using the likelihood ratios in each chapter.

I am grateful to many investigators who supplied me with unpublished information from their original work: Bastiaan Bloem, Jorik Nonnekes, and W.F. Abdo (tandem gait in atypical parkinsonism); Loris Bonetti, Ivana Maria Rosi, Rossella Guastaferro, Alessandra Cerra, Roberto Milos, and Enrico Messina (dehydration in the elderly); Takashi Matono (relative bradycardia in enteric fever); Mark Wright (unilateral visual loss and Marcus Gunn pupil); Alex Butskiy (Rinne test, conductive hearing loss; orientation of tines); William Strawbridge (hearing tests); Vincent Quagliarello (meningeal signs); Johann Steurer (pneumonia); Jason Weatherald (diagnosis of pulmonary hypertension); Gerben ter Riet (red eye); Anikar Chhabra, Keith Jarbo, David E. Hartigan, Kelly Scott, and Karan Patel (tests of anterior cruciate ligament tears); and Kenneth Arinze Ohagwu and Innocent Ijezie Chukwuonye (Siriraj Stroke scale). I greatly appreciate their promptness in responding to my questions and their generosity in sharing data from their research.

Insights into physical signs continue to evolve and progress. This textbook presents the most recent evidence supporting this fundamental clinical skill. By applying this evidence-based approach, clinicians will glean the most from what they hear, see, and feel at the bedside, information that, combined with modern technological testing, will grant clinicians the keys to outstanding patient care.

Steven McGee, M.D.
February 2021

The purpose of this book is to explore the origins, pathophysiology, and diagnostic accuracy of many of the physical signs used today in adult patients. We have a wonderfully rich tradition of physical diagnosis, and my hope is that this book will help square this tradition, now almost two centuries old, with the realities of modern diagnosis, which often rely more on technologic tests such as clinical imaging and laboratory testing. The tension between physical diagnosis and technologic tests has never been greater. Having taught physical diagnosis for 20 years, I frequently observe medical students purchasing textbooks of physical diagnosis during their preclinical years to study and master traditional physical signs, but then neglecting or even discarding this knowledge during their clinical years, after observing that modern diagnosis often takes place at a distance from the bedside. One can hardly fault a student who, caring for a patient with pneumonia, does not talk seriously about crackles and diminished breath sounds when all of his or her teachers are focused on the subtleties of the patient's chest radiograph. Disregard for physical diagnosis also pervades our residency programs, most of which have formal X-ray rounds, pathology rounds, microbiology rounds, and clinical conferences addressing the nuances of laboratory tests. Very few have formal physical diagnosis rounds.

Reconciling traditional physical diagnosis with contemporary diagnostic standards has been a continuous process throughout the history of physical diagnosis. In the 1830s, Professor Pierre Adolphe Piorry, the inventor of topographic percussion taught that there were nine distinct percussion sounds, which he used to outline the patient's liver, heart, lungs, stomach, and even individual heart chambers or lung cavities. Piorry's methods flourished for over a century and once filled 200-page manuals,[1] although today, thanks to the introduction of clinical imaging in the early 1900s, the only vestige of his methods is percussion of the liver span. In his 1819 *A Treatise on Diseases of the Chest*,[2] Laennec wrote that lung auscultation could detect "every possible case" of pneumonia. It was only a matter of 20 years before other careful physical diagnosticians tempered Laennec's enthusiasm and pointed out that the stethoscope had diagnostic limitations.[3] For most of the 20th century, expert clinicians believed that all late systolic murmurs were benign, until Barlow in 1963 showed that they often represented mitral regurgitation, sometimes of significant severity.[4]

There are two contemporary polar opinions regarding physical diagnosis. Holding the less common position are clinicians who believe that all traditional physical signs remain accurate, and these clinicians continue to quiz students about Krönig's isthmus and splenic percussion signs. A more common position is that physical diagnosis has little to offer the modern clinician and that traditional signs, though interesting, cannot compete with the accuracy of our more technologic diagnostic tools. Of course, neither position is completely correct. I hope this book, by examining the best evidence comparing physical signs to current diagnostic standards, will bring clinicians to a more appropriate middle ground: that physical diagnosis is a reliable diagnostic tool that can still help clinicians with many, but not all, clinical problems.

Although some regard evidence-based medicine as "cookbook medicine," this is incorrect, because there are immeasurable subtleties in our interaction with patients that clinical studies cannot address (at least, not as yet) and because the diagnostic power of any physical sign (or any test, for that matter) depends in part on our ideas about disease prevalence, which in turn depend on our own personal interviewing skills and clinical experience.* Instead, evidence-based physical diagnosis simply summarizes the best evidence available on whether a physical sign is accurate

---

*These subjects are discussed fully in Chapters 2 and 5.

or not. The clinician who understands this evidence can then approach his or her own patients with the confidence and wisdom that would have developed had he or she personally examined and learned from the thousands of patients reviewed in the studies of this book.

Sometimes, comparing physical signs with modern diagnostic standards reveals that the physical sign is outdated and perhaps best discarded (e.g., topographic percussion of diaphragm excursion). Other times the comparison reveals that physical signs are extremely accurate and probably underused (e.g., early diastolic murmur at the left lower sternal area for aortic regurgitation, conjunctival rim pallor for anemia, or a palpable gallbladder for extrahepatic obstruction of the biliary ducts). At other times, the comparison reveals that the physical sign *is* the diagnostic standard, just as most of the physical examination was a century ago (e.g., systolic murmur and click of mitral valve prolapse, hemiparesis for stroke, neovascularization for proliferative diabetic retinopathy). For some diagnoses, conflict remains between physical signs and technologic tests, making it still unclear which should be the diagnostic standard (e.g., the diagnoses of cardiac tamponade and carpal tunnel syndrome). And for still others, the comparison is impossible because clinical studies comparing physical signs to traditional diagnostic standards do not exist.

My hope is that the material in this book will allow clinicians at all levels—students, house officers, and seasoned clinicians alike—to examine patients more confidently and accurately, thus restoring physical diagnosis to its appropriate, and often pivotal, diagnostic role. Once well-versed in evidence-based physical diagnosis, clinicians can then settle the most important clinical questions at the time and place they should be first addressed—the patient's bedside.

Steven McGee, M.D.
July 2000

References

1. Weil A. *Handbuch und Atlas der topographischen Perkussion.* Leipzig: F.C.W. Vogel; 1880.
2. Laennec RTH. *A Treatise on the Diseases of the Chest (Facsimile Edition by Classics of Medicine Library).* London: T. and G. Underwood; 1821.
3. Addison T. The difficulties and fallacies attending physical diagnosis of diseases of the chest. In: Wilks, Daldy, ed. *A Collection of the Published Writings of the Late Thomas Addison (Facsimile Edition by Classics of Medicine Library).* London: The New Sydenham society; 1846:242.
4. Barlow JB, Pocock WA, Marchand P, Denny M. The significance of late systolic murmurs. *Am. Heart J.* 1963;66(4):443–452.

CONTENTS

PART 1

Introduction

CHAPTER 1

What is Evidence-Based Physical Diagnosis?

When clinicians diagnose disease, their intent is to place the patient's experience into a particular category (or diagnosis), a process implying specific pathogenesis, prognosis, and treatment. This procedure allows clinicians to explain to patients what is happening and to identify the best way to restore the patient's health. A century ago, such categorization of disease rested almost entirely on empiric observation—what clinicians saw, heard, and felt at the patient's bedside. Although some technologic testing was available then (e.g., microscopic examination of sputum and urine), its role in diagnosis was meager, and almost all diagnoses were based on traditional examination (Fig. 1.1). For example, if patients presented a century ago with complaints of fever and cough, the diagnosis of lobar pneumonia rested on the presence of the characteristic findings of pneumonia—fever, tachycardia, tachypnea, grunting respirations, cyanosis, diminished excursion of the affected side, dullness to percussion, increased tactile fremitus, diminished breath sounds (and later bronchial breath sounds), abnormalities of vocal resonance (bronchophony, pectoriloquy, and egophony), and crackles. If these findings were absent, the patient did not have pneumonia. Chest radiography played no role in diagnosis because it was not widely available until the early 1900s.

Modern medicine, of course, relies on technology much more than medicine did a century ago (to our patients' advantage), and for many modern categories of disease the diagnostic standard is a technologic test (Fig. 1.1). For example, if patients present today with fever and cough, the diagnosis of pneumonia is based on the presence of an infiltrate on the chest radiograph. Similarly, the diagnosis of systolic murmurs depends on echocardiography and that of ascites on abdominal ultrasonography. In these disorders, the clinician's principal interest is the result of the technologic test, and decisions about treatment depend much more on that result than on whether the patient has egophony, radiation of the murmur into the neck, or shifting dullness. This reliance on technology creates tension for medical students, who spend hours mastering the traditional examination yet later learn (when first appearing on hospital wards) that the traditional examination pales in importance compared to technology, a realization prompting a fundamental question: What is the diagnostic value of the traditional physical examination? Is it outdated and best discarded? Is it completely accurate and underutilized? Is the truth somewhere between these two extremes?

Examination of Fig. 1.1 indicates that diagnosis today is split into two parts. For some categories of disease, the diagnostic standard still remains empiric observation— what the clinician sees, hears, and feels—just as it was for all diagnosis a century ago. For example, how does a clinician know the patient has cellulitis? The only way is to go to the patient's bedside and observe fever and localized bright erythema, warmth, swelling, and tenderness on the leg. There is no other way to make this diagnosis (technologic or not). Similarly, there is no technologic standard for Parkinson disease (during the patient's life), Bell palsy, or pericarditis. All of these diagnoses—and many

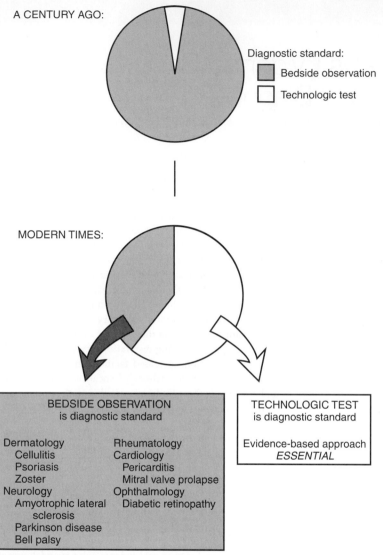

Fig. 1.1 Evolution of Diagnostic Standard. The figure compares the diagnostic process one century ago (*top*, before introduction of clinical imaging and modern laboratory testing) to modern times (*bottom*), illustrating the relative contributions of bedside examination (*grey shade*) and technologic tests (*white shade*) to the diagnostic standard. One century ago, most diagnoses were defined by bedside observation, whereas today technologic standards have a much greater diagnostic role. Nonetheless, there are many examples today of diagnoses based solely on bedside findings (examples appear in *large grey shaded box*). Evidence-based physical diagnosis, on the other hand, principally addresses those diagnoses *defined by technologic standards*, because it identifies those traditional findings that accurately predict the result of the technologic test, as discussed throughout the book.

others in the fields of dermatology, neurology, musculoskeletal medicine, and ophthalmology—are based entirely on empiric observation by experienced clinicians; technology has a subordinate diagnostic role. In fact, the principal reasons medical students still must study and master the traditional examination is the dependence of many diagnoses on bedside findings.

The principal role of evidence-based physical examination, in contrast, is the second category of diseases—that is, those whose categorization today is based on technologic studies. Clinicians want to know the results of the chest radiograph when diagnosing pneumonia, the echocardiogram when diagnosing systolic murmurs, and the ultrasound when diagnosing ascites. For each of these problems, the evidence-based approach compares traditional findings to the technologic standard and then identifies those findings that increase or decrease probability of disease (as defined by the technologic standard), distinguishing them from unhelpful findings that fail to change probability. Using this approach, the clinician will calculate the Heckerling score* to predict the findings on the chest radiograph (Chapter 32), define the topographic distribution of the murmur on the chest wall to predict the findings on the echocardiogram (Chapter 43), and look for a fluid wave or edema to predict the findings on the abdominal ultrasound examination (Chapter 51).

There are thus two distinct ways physical examination is applied at the bedside. For many disorders—those still lacking a technologic standard—the clinician's observations define diagnosis. For other disorders—those based on technologic tests—the clinician's application of an evidence-based approach quickly identifies the relatively few findings that predict the results of technologic standard. Both approaches to bedside examination make physical examination more efficient and accurate, and ultimately more relevant to the care of patients.

---

*The Heckerling score assigns one point to each of five independent predictors of pneumonia that are present: temperature > 37.8°C; heart rate > 100/min; crackles; diminished breath sounds; and absence of asthma (see Chapter 32).

PART 2

Understanding the Evidence

CHAPTER 2

Diagnostic Accuracy of Physical Findings

KEY TEACHING POINTS

- Likelihood ratios (LRs) are nothing more than *diagnostic weights*, numbers that quickly convey to clinicians how much a physical sign argues for or against disease.
- LRs have possible values between 0 to ∞. Values greater than 1 *increase* probability of disease. (The greater the value of the LR, the greater the increase in probability.) LRs less than 1 *decrease* probability of disease. (The closer the number is to zero, the more the probability of disease decreases.) LRs that equal 1 do not change probability of disease at all.
- LRs of 2, 5, and 10 increase probability of disease about 15%, 30%, and 45%, respectively (in absolute terms). LRs of 0.5, 0.2, and 0.1 (i.e., the reciprocals of 2, 5, and 10) decrease probability 15%, 30%, and 45%, respectively.
- EBM Boxes comparing LRs of different physical signs quickly inform clinicians about which findings have the greatest diagnostic value.

I. Introduction

If a physical sign characteristic of a suspected diagnosis is present (i.e., **positive finding**), that diagnosis becomes more likely; if the characteristic finding is absent (i.e., **negative finding**), the suspected diagnosis becomes less likely. How much these positive and negative results modify probability, however, is distinct for each physical sign. Some findings, when positive, shift probability upward greatly, but they change it little when negative. Other signs are more useful if they are absent, because the negative finding practically excludes disease, although the positive one changes probability very little.

Much of this book consists of EBM Boxes that specifically describe how positive or negative findings change the probability of disease, a property called **diagnostic accuracy**. Understanding these tables first requires review of four concepts: pre-test probability, sensitivity, specificity, and LRs.

II. Pre-Test Probability

Pre-test probability is the probability of disease (i.e., prevalence) before application of the results of a physical finding. Pre-test probability is the starting point for all clinical decisions. For example, the clinician may know that a certain physical finding shifts the probability of disease upward 40%, but this information alone is unhelpful unless the clinician also knows the starting point: if the pre-test probability for the particular diagnosis was 50%, the finding is diagnostic (i.e., post-test probability

TABLE 2.1 ■ Pre-Test Probability

Setting (Reference)	Diagnosis	Probability (%)
Acute abdominal pain [1-3]	Small bowel obstruction	4–8
Ankle injury[4,5]	Ankle fracture	10–14
Cough and fever[6]	Pneumonia	15–35
Acute calf pain or swelling[7-19]	Proximal deep vein thrombosis	6–43
Pleuritic chest pain, dyspnea, or hemoptysis[20-31]	Pulmonary embolism	9–43
Diabetic foot ulcer[32-34]	Osteomyelitis	52–68

50% + 40% = 90%); if the pre-test probability was only 10%, the finding is less helpful, because the probability of disease is still akin to a coin toss (i.e., post-test probability 10% + 40% = 50%).

Published estimates of disease prevalence, given a particular clinical setting, are summarized in the Appendix for all the clinical problems discussed in this book (these estimates derive from clinical studies reviewed in all the EBM Boxes); Table 2.1 provides a small sample of these pre-test probabilities. Even so, clinicians must adjust these estimates with information from their own practice. For example, large studies based in emergency departments show that 15% to 35% of patients presenting with cough and fever have pneumonia (Table 2.1). The probability of pneumonia, however, is certainly lower in patients presenting with cough and fever to an office-based practice in the community, and it may be higher if cough and fever develop in patients with cancer or chronic lung disease. In fact, because the best estimate of pre-test probability incorporates information from the clinician's own practice—how specific underlying diseases, risks, and exposures make disease more or less likely—the practice of evidence-based medicine is never "cookbook" medicine, but instead consists of decisions based on the unique characteristics of the patients the clinician sees.

III. Sensitivity and Specificity

A. DEFINITIONS

The terms *sensitivity* and *specificity* describe the discriminatory power of physical signs. **Sensitivity** is the proportion of patients *with* the diagnosis who *have* the physical sign (i.e., have the *positive* result). **Specificity** is the proportion of patients *without* the diagnosis who *lack* the physical sign (i.e., have the *negative* result).

Calculation of sensitivity and specificity requires construction of a 2 × 2 table (Fig. 2.1) that has two columns (one for "diagnosis present" and another for "diagnosis absent") and two rows (one for "physical sign present" and another for "physical sign absent"). These rows and columns create four boxes: one for the "true positives" (cell a, sign and diagnosis present), one for "false positives" (cell b, sign present but disease absent), one for the "false negatives" (cell c, sign absent but disease present), and one for the "true negatives" (cell d, sign and disease absent).

Fig. 2.1 presents data from a hypothetical study of 100 patients presenting with pulmonary hypertension. The clinician knows that tricuspid regurgitation is a complication of pulmonary hypertension and wonders how accurately a single physical sign—the presence of a holosystolic murmur at the left lower sternal border—detects this complication*.[35] Forty-two patients have significant tricuspid regurgitation (the sum of column 1), and 58 patients do not (the sum of column 2). The **sensitivity** of the holosystolic murmur is the proportion of patients with disease

---

*The numbers used in this example are very close to those in reference 35. See also Chapter 46.

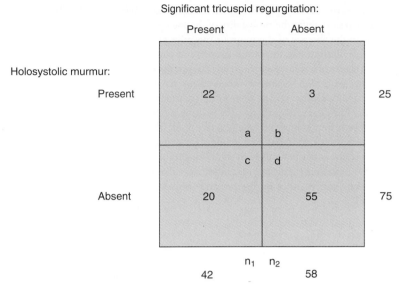

Fig. 2.1 **2 × 2 table.** The total number of patients with disease (tricuspid regurgitation in this example) is the sum of the first column, or $n_1 = a + c$. The total number of patients without disease is the sum of the second column, or $n_2 = b + d$. The *sensitivity* of a physical finding (holosystolic murmur at the left lower sternal edge, in this example) is the proportion of patients with disease who have the finding [i.e., a/(a + c) or a/n_1]. The *specificity* of a physical finding is the proportion of patients without disease who lack the finding [i.e., d/(b + d) or d/n_2]. The *positive likelihood ratio (LR)* is proportion of patients with disease who have a positive finding (a/n_1) divided by the proportion of patients without disease who have a positive finding (b/n_2), or sensitivity/(1−specificity). The *negative LR* is the proportion of patients with disease who lack the finding (c/n_1) divided by the proportion of patients without disease who lack the finding (d/n_2), or (1−sensitivity)/specificity. In this example, the sensitivity is 0.52 (22/42), the specificity is 0.95 (55/58), the positive LR is 10.1 [(22/42)/(3/58)], and the negative LR is 0.5 [(20/42)/(55/58)].

(i.e., tricuspid regurgitation, 42 patients) who have the characteristic murmur (i.e., the *positive* result, 22 patients), which is 22/42 = 0.52 or 52%. The **specificity** of the holosystolic murmur is the proportion of patients *without* disease (i.e., no tricuspid regurgitation, 58 patients) who *lack* the murmur (i.e., the *negative* result, 55 patients), which is 55/58 = 0.95 or 95%. To recall how to calculate sensitivity and specificity, Sackett and others have suggested helpful mnemonics: Sensitivity is represented as "PID" for "positivity in disease" (an abbreviation normally associated with "pelvic inflammatory disease"), and specificity is represented as "NIH" for "negativity in health" (an abbreviation normally associated with the "National Institutes of Health").[36,37]

B. USING SENSITIVITY AND SPECIFICITY TO DETERMINE PROBABILITY OF DISEASE

The completed 2 × 2 table can be used to determine the accuracy of the holosystolic murmur, which is how well its presence or absence discriminates between those with tricuspid regurgitation and those without it. In Fig. 2.1, the first row includes all 25 patients with the murmur (i.e. the positive results). Of these 25 patients, 22 have tricuspid regurgitation; therefore, the probability of tricuspid regurgitation, if the murmur is present (*positive* finding), is 22/25 or 88% (i.e., the "post-test probability" if the murmur is present). The second row includes all 75 patients without the murmur. Of these 75 patients, 20 have tricuspid regurgitation; therefore, the post-test probability of tricuspid regurgitation, if the murmur is absent (i.e., *negative* finding), is 20/75 or 27%.

In this example, the pre-test probability of tricuspid regurgitation is 42%. The presence of the murmur (positive result) shifts the probability of disease upward considerably more (i.e., 46%, from 42% to 88%) than the absence of the murmur (negative result) shifts it downward (i.e., 15%, from 42% to 27%). This illustrates an important property of physical signs with a high specificity: when present, physical signs with *high specificity* greatly *increase* the probability of disease. A corollary to this applies to findings with high sensitivity: when *absent*, physical signs with a high *sensitivity* greatly *decrease* the probability of disease. The holosystolic murmur has a high specificity (95%) but only a meager sensitivity (52%), meaning that, at the bedside, a positive result (the presence of a murmur) has greater diagnostic importance than the negative result (the absence of the murmur). The presence of the characteristic murmur argues compellingly for tricuspid regurgitation, but its absence is less helpful, simply because many patients with significant regurgitation lack the characteristic murmur.

Sackett and others have suggested mnemonics for these characteristics as well: "SpPin" (i.e., a *Sp*ecific test, when *P*ositive, rules *in* disease) and "SnNout" (i.e., a *Sn*sitive test, when *N*egative, rules *out* disease).[37]

IV. Likelihood Ratios

LRs, like sensitivity and specificity, describe the discriminatory power of physical signs. Although they have many advantages, the most important is how simply and quickly they can be used to estimate post-test probability.

A. DEFINITION

The LR of a physical sign is the proportion of patients *with* disease who have a particular finding divided by the proportion of patients *without* disease who also have the same finding.

$$LR = \frac{\text{Probability of a finding in patients } \textit{with} \text{ disease}}{\text{Probability of the same finding in patients } \textit{without} \text{ disease}}$$

The adjectives *positive* or *negative* indicate whether that LR refers to the presence of the physical sign (i.e., positive result) or to the absence of the physical sign (i.e., the negative result).

A **positive LR**, therefore, is the proportion of patients *with* disease who *have* a physical sign divided by the proportion of patients *without* disease who also *have* the same sign. The numerator of this equation—proportion of patients with disease who have the physical sign—is the sign's sensitivity. The denominator—proportion of patients without disease who have the sign—is the complement of specificity, or (1 − specificity). Therefore,

$$\text{Positive LR} = \frac{(\text{sens})}{(1 - \text{spec})}$$

In our hypothetical study (Fig. 2.1), the proportion of patients with tricuspid regurgitation who have the murmur 22/42 or 52.4% (i.e., the finding's sensitivity) and the proportion of patients without tricuspid regurgitation who also have the murmur is 3/58 or 5.2% (i.e., 1 − specificity). The ratio of these proportions [i.e., (sensitivity)/(1−specificity)] is 10.1, which is the positive LR for a holosystolic murmur at the lower sternal border. This number means that patients *with* tricuspid regurgitation are 10.1 times more likely to have the holosystolic murmur than those *without* tricuspid regurgitation.

Similarly, the **negative LR** is the proportion of patients *with* disease *lacking* a physical sign divided by the proportion of patients *without* disease also *lacking* the sign. The numerator of this equation—proportion of patients with disease *lacking* the finding—is the complement of sensitivity, or (1 − sensitivity). The denominator of the equation—proportion of patients without disease *lacking* the finding—is the specificity. Therefore,

$$\text{Negative LR} = \frac{(1 - \text{sens})}{(\text{spec})}$$

In our hypothetical study, the proportion of patients with tricuspid regurgitation lacking the murmur is 20/42 or 47.6% (i.e., 1- sensitivity) and the proportion of patients without tricuspid regurgitation lacking the murmur is 55/58 or 94.8% (i.e., the specificity). The ratio of these proportions [i.e., (1-sensitivity)/(specificity)] is 0.5, which is the negative LR for the holosystolic murmur. This number means that patients *with* tricuspid regurgitation are 0.5 times less likely to lack the murmur than those *without* tricuspid regurgitation (the inverse statement is less confusing: patients *without* tricuspid regurgitation are 2 times more likely to lack a murmur than those *with* tricuspid regurgitation).

Although these formulae are difficult to recall, the interpretation of LRs is straightforward. Findings with LRs greater than 1 increase the probability of disease; the greater the LR, the more compelling the argument *for* disease. Findings whose LRs lie between between 0 and 1 decrease the probability of disease; the closer the LR is to zero, the more convincing the finding argues *against* disease. Findings whose LRs equal 1 lack diagnostic value because they do not change probability at all. "Positive LR" describes how probability changes when the finding is *present*. "Negative LR" describes how probability changes when the finding is *absent*.

LRs, therefore, are nothing more than diagnostic weights, whose possible values range from 0 (i.e., excluding disease) to infinity (i.e., pathognomonic for disease, Fig. 2.2).

B. USING LRS TO DETERMINE PROBABILITY

The clinician can use the LR of a physical finding to estimate probability of disease in three ways: (1) by using graphs or other easy-to-use nomograms,[38,39] (2) by using bedside approximations, or (3) by using formulae.

1. Using Graphs

a. Parts of the graph

Fig. 2.3 is an easy-to-use graph that illustrates the relationship between pre-test probability (x-axis) and post-test probability (y-axis), given the finding's LR. The straight line bisecting the

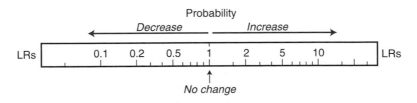

Fig. 2.2 Likelihood ratios as diagnostic weights. The relationship between a specific physical sign and a specific disease is described by a unique number—its likelihood ratio—which is nothing more than a diagnostic weight describing how much that sign argues for or against that specific disease. The possible values of LRs range from zero to infinity (∞). Findings with LRs greater than 1 argue *for* the specific disease (the greater the value of the LR, the more the probability of disease increases). Findings with LRs less than 1 argue *against* the disease (the closer the number is to zero, the more the probability of disease decreases). LRs that equal 1 do not change probability of disease at all.

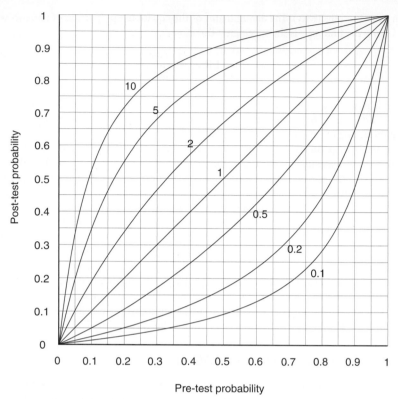

Fig. 2.3 **Probability and likelihood ratios.** The curves describe how pre-test probability (x-axis) relates to post-test probability (y-axis), given the likelihood ratio (LR) for the physical finding. Only the curves for seven likelihood ratios are depicted (from LR = 0.1 to LR = 10).

graph into an upper left half and lower right half describes the LR of 1, which has no discrimina-tory value because, for findings with this LR, post-test probability always equals pre-test prob-ability. Physical findings that argue *for* disease (i.e., LRs >1) appear in the upper left half of the graph; the larger the value of the LR, the more the curve approaches the upper left corner. Physical findings that argue *against* disease (i.e., LRs <1) appear in the lower the lower right half of the graph: the closer the LR is to zero, the more the curve approaches the lower right corner.

In Fig. 2.3, the three depicted curves with LRs greater than 1 (i.e., LR = 2, 5, and 10) are mir-ror images of the three curves with LRs less than 1 (i.e., LR = 0.5, 0.2, and 0.1). (This assumes the "mirror" is the line LR = 1.) This symmetry indicates that findings with an LR of 10 argue as much *for* disease as those with an LR = 0.1 argue *against* disease (although this is true only for the intermediate pre-test probabilities). Similarly, LR = 5 argues as much for disease as LR = 0.2 argues against it, and LR = 2 mirrors LR = 0.5. Keeping these companion curves in mind will help the clinician interpret the LRs throughout this book.[†] If a finding has an LR other than one of these depicted seven curves, its position can be estimated with little loss in accuracy. For example, the curve for LR = 4 lies between LR = 5 and LR = 2, though closer to LR = 5 than to LR = 2.

[†]These companion pairs are easy to recall because they are the inverse of each other: the inverse of 10 is 1/10 = 0.1; the inverse of 5 is 1/5 = 0.2; the inverse of 2 is 1/2 = 0.5.

b. Using the Graph to Determine Probability

To use this graph, the clinician identifies on the x-axis the patient's pre-test probability, derived from published estimates and clinical experience, and extends a line upward from that point to meet the LR curve for the physical finding. The clinician then extends a horizontal line from this point to the y-axis to identify post-test probability.

Figure 2.4 depicts this process for the lower sternal holosystolic murmur and tricuspid regurgitation. The pre-test probability of tricuspid regurgitation is 42%. If the characteristic murmur is present (positive LR = 10), a line is drawn upward from 0.42 on the x-axis to the LR = 10 curve; from this point, a horizontal line is drawn to the y-axis to find the post-test probability (88%). If the murmur is absent (negative LR = 0.5), the post-test probability is the y-value where the vertical line intersects the LR = 0.5 curve (i.e., post-test probability of 27%).

These curves illustrate an additional important point: physical signs are diagnostically most useful when they are applied to patients who have pre-test probabilities in the intermediate range (i.e. 20% to 80%), because in this range the different LR curves diverge the most from the LR = 1 curve (thus, shifting probability up or down a large amount). If instead the pre-test probability is already very low or very high, all the LR curves cluster close to the line LR = 1 curve in either the bottom left or upper right corners, thus with only a relatively small impact on probability.

2. Approximating Probability

The clinician can avoid using graphs and instead approximate post-test probability by remembering the following two points: (1) The companion LR curves in Fig. 2.3 are LR = 2 and LR = 0.5, LR = 5 and LR = 0.2, and LR = 10 and LR = 0.1. (2) The first three multiples of "15" are 15, 30, and 45. Using this rule, the LRs of 2, 5, and 10 *increase* probability about 15%, 30%, and 45%, respectively (see Fig. 2.5). The LRs of 0.5, 0.2, and 0.1 *decrease* probability about 15%, 30%, and 45%, respectively.[40] These estimates are accurate to within 5% to 10% of the actual value, as long as the clinician rounds estimates over 100 to an even 100% and estimates below zero to an even 0%.

Therefore, in our hypothetical patient with pulmonary hypertension, the finding of a holosystolic murmur (LR = 10) increases the probability of tricuspid regurgitation from 42% to 87% (i.e., 42% + 45% = 87%, which is only 1% lower than the actual value). The absence of the murmur (LR = 0.5) decreases the probability of tricuspid regurgitation from 42% to 27% (i.e., 42% − 15% = 27%, which is identical to actual value).

Table 2.2 summarizes similar bedside estimates for all LRs between 0.1 and 10.0.

3. Calculating Probability

The post-test probability also can be calculated by first converting pre-test probability (P_{pre}) into pre-test odds (O_{pre}):

$$O_{pre} = \frac{P_{pre}}{\left(1 - P_{pre}\right)}$$

The pre-test odds (O_{pre}) is multiplied times the LR of the physical sign to determine the post-test odds (O_{post}):

$$O_{post} = O_{pre} \times LR$$

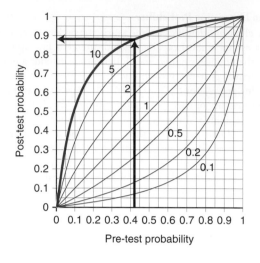

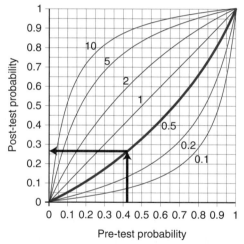

Fig. 2.4 Probability and likelihood ratios: patients with pulmonary hypertension. In our hypothetical clinician's practice, 42% of patients with pulmonary hypertension have the complication of tricuspid regurgitation (i.e., pre-test probability is 42%). To use the curves, the clinician finds 0.42 on the x-axis and extends a line upward. The post-test probability of tricuspid regurgitation is read off the y-axis where the vertical line intersects the curve of the appropriate LR. The probability of tricuspid regurgitation if a holosystolic murmur is present at the left lower sternal edge (LR = 10.1) is 88%; the probability if the finding is absent (LR = 0.5) is 27%.

The post-test odds (O_{post}) converts back to post-test probability (P_{post}), using:

$$P_{post} = \frac{O_{post}}{\left(1 + O_{post}\right)}$$

Therefore, in our hypothetical example of the patients with pulmonary hypertension, the pre-test odds for tricuspid regurgitation would be [(0.42)/(1−0.42)] or 0.72. If the murmur is present (LR = 10), the post-test odds would be [0.72 × 10] or 7.2, which translates to a post-test probability of [(7.2)/(1 + 7.2)] or 0.88 (i.e., 88%). If the murmur wave is absent (LR = 0.5), the post-test odds would be [0.72 × 0.5] or 0.36, which translates to a post-test probability of [(0.36)/(1 + 0.36)] or 0.27 (i.e., 27%).

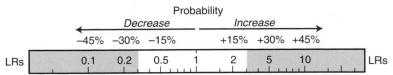

Fig. 2.5 **Approximating probability.** Clinicians can estimate changes in probability by recalling the LRs 2, 5, and 10 and the first 3 multiples of 15 (i.e., 15, 30, 45). A finding whose LR is 2 increases probability about 15%, one of 5 increases it 30% and one of 10 increases it 45% (these changes are *absolute* increases in probability). LRs whose values are 0.5, 0.2, and 0.1 (i.e., the reciprocals of 2, 5, and 10) decrease probability 15%, 30%, and 45%, respectively. Throughout this book, LRs with values ≥3 or ≤0.3 (represented by the *shaded part* of the diagnostic weight "ruler") are presented in boldface type to indicate those physical findings that change probability sufficiently to be clinically meaningful (i.e., they increase or decrease probability at least 20% to 25%).

TABLE 2.2 ■ **Likelihood Ratios and Bedside Estimates**

Likelihood Ratio	Approximate Change in Probability*
0.1	−45%
0.2	−30%
0.3	−25%
0.4	−20%
0.5	−15%
1	No change
2	+15%
3	+20%
4	+25%
5	+30%
6	+35%
7	
8	+40%
9	
10	+45%

From McGee S. Simplifying likelihood ratios. *J Gen Intern Med*. 2002;17(8):646–649.
*These changes describe *absolute* increases or decreases in probability. For example, a patient with pre-test probability of 20% and physical finding whose LR is 5 would have a post-test probability of 20% + 30% = 50%. The text describes how to easily recall these estimates.

Clinical medicine, however, is rarely as precise as these calculations suggest, and for most decisions at the bedside, the approximations described earlier are more than adequate.

C. ADVANTAGES OF LIKELIHOOD RATIOS

1. Simplicity

In a single number, the LR conveys to clinicians how convincingly a physical sign argues for or against disease. If the LR of a finding is a large number, disease is likely; and if the LR of a finding is close to zero, disease is doubtful. This advantage allows clinicians to quickly compare different diagnostic strategies and thus refine clinical judgment.[40]

2. Accuracy

Using LRs to describe diagnostic accuracy is superior to sensitivity and specificity, because the earlier described mnemonics, SpPin and SnNout, are sometimes misleading. For example, according to the mnemonic SpPin, a finding with a specificity of 95% should argue conclusively for disease, but it does so only if the positive LR for the finding is a high number. If the finding's sensitivity is 60%, the positive LR is 12 and the finding does argue convincingly for disease (i.e., consistent with the SpPin mnemonic); if the finding's sensitivity is only 10%, however, the positive LR is 2 and post-test probability changes only slightly (i.e., inconsistent with SpPin mnemonic). Similarly, a highly sensitive finding argues convincingly against disease (i.e., SnNout) only when its calculated negative LR is a number close to zero.

3. Levels of Findings

Another advantage of LRs is that a physical sign measured on an ordinal scale (e.g., 0, 1+, 2+, 3+) or continuous scale (e.g., blood pressure) can be categorized into different levels to determine the LR for each level, thereby increasing the accuracy of the finding. Other examples include continuous findings such as heart rate, respiratory rate, temperature, and percussed span of the liver, and ordinal findings such as intensity of murmurs and degree of edema.

For example, in patients with chronic obstructive lung disease (i.e., emphysema, chronic bronchitis), breath sounds are typically faint. If the clinician grades the intensity of breath sounds on a scale from 0 (absent) to 24 (very loud), based on the methods discussed in Chapter 30,[41,42] he or she can classify the patient's breath sounds into one of four groups: scores of 9 or less (very faint), 10 to 12, 13 to 15, or greater than 15 (loud). Each category then has its own LR (Table 2.3): scores of 9 or less significantly increase probability of obstructive disease (LR = 10.2), whereas scores greater than 15 significantly decrease it (LR = 0.1). Scores from 10 to 12 argue somewhat for disease (LR = 3.6), and scores from 13 to 15 provide no diagnostic information (LR not significantly different from 1). If the clinician had instead identified breath sounds as simply "faint" or "normal/increased" (i.e., the traditional positive or negative finding), the finding may still discriminate between patients with and without obstructive disease, but it misses the point that the discriminatory power of the sign resides mostly with scores less than 10 and greater than 15.

When findings are categorized into levels, the term *specificity* becomes meaningless. For example, the specificity of a breath sound score of 13 to 15 is 80%, which means that 80% of patients without chronic airflow limitation have values other than 13 to 15, though the "80%" does not convey whether most of these other values are greater than 15 or less than 13. Similarly, when findings are put in more than 2 categories, the LR descriptor *negative* is no longer necessary, because all LRs are *positive* ones for their respective category.

TABLE 2.3 ■ Breath Sound Intensity and Chronic Airflow Limitation

Breath sound score	Likelihood ratio
9 or less	10.2
10–12	3.6
13–15	NS
>15	0.1

Data from Bohadana AB, Peslin R, Uffholtz H. Breath sounds in the clinical assessment of airflow obstruction. *Thorax.* 1978;33:345–351; Pardee NE, Martin CJ, Morgan EH. A test of the practical value of estimating breath sound intensity: breath sounds related to measured ventilatory function. *Chest.* 1976;70(3):341–344.
NS, Not significant.

4. Combining Findings

A final advantage of LRs is that clinicians can use them to combine findings, which is particularly important for those physical signs with positive LRs around 2 or negative LRs around 0.5, signs that by themselves change probability little but when combined have significant effects on probability. Individual LRs can be combined, however, only if the findings are "independent."

a. Independence of Findings

Independence means that the LR for second finding does not change once the clinician determines whether the first finding is present or absent. For a few diagnostic problems, investigators have identified which findings are independent of each other. These findings appear as components of "diagnostic scoring schemes" in the EBM Boxes throughout this book (e.g., Wells score for deep venous thrombosis). For most physical findings, however, very little information is available about independence, and the clinician must judge whether combining findings is appropriate.

One important clue is that most independent findings have unique pathophysiology. For example, when considering pneumonia in patients with cough and fever, the clinician could combine the findings of abnormal mental status and diminished breath sounds, using the individual LR of each finding because abnormal mental status and diminished breath sounds probably have separate pathophysiology. Similarly, when considering heart failure in patients with dyspnea, the clinician could combine the findings of elevated neck veins and third heart sound because these findings also have different pathophysiology.

Examples of findings whose individual LRs should not be combined (because the findings share the same pathophysiology) are flank dullness and shifting dullness in the diagnosis of ascites (both depend on intraabdominal contents dampening the vibrations of the abdominal wall during percussion), neck stiffness and Kernig sign in the diagnosis of meningitis (both are caused by meningeal irritation), and edema and elevated neck veins in the diagnosis of heart failure (both depend on elevated right atrial pressure).

Until more information is available, the safest policy for the clinician to follow, when combining LRs of individual findings, is to combine no more than three findings, all of which have distinct pathophysiology.

b. How to Combine Findings

The clinician can use any of the methods previously described to combine findings, simply by making the post-test probability from the first finding the pre-test probability for the second finding. For example, a hypothetical patient with acute fever and cough has two positive findings that we believe have separate pathophysiology and therefore are independent: abnormal mental status (LR = 1.9 for pneumonia) and diminished breath sounds (LR = 2.4 for pneumonia). The pre-test probability of pneumonia, derived from published estimates and clinical experience, is estimated to be 20%. Using the graph, the finding of abnormal mental status increases the probability from 20% to 32%; this post-test probability then becomes the pre-test probability for the second finding, diminished breath sounds, which increases probability from 32% to 53%—the overall probability after application of the two findings. Using the approximating rules, both findings (LRs ≈ 2.0) increase the probability about 15%; the post-test probability is thus 20% + 15% + 15% = 50% (an error of only 3%). Using formulas to calculate probability, the LRs of the separate findings are multiplied together and the product is used to convert pre-test into post-test odds. The product of the two LRs is 4.56 (1.9 × 2.4); the pre-test odds would be 0.2/0.8 = 0.25; the post-test odds would be 0.25 × 4.56 = 1.14, which equals a probability of 1.14/2.14 = 53%.

References may be accessed online at *Elsevier eBooks for Practicing Clinicians*.

Using the Tables in This Book

- **Frequency of findings** tables present only the sensitivity of findings (derived from studies of large numbers of patients with a confirmed diagnosis). In these tables, only those findings with *high* sensitivity are clinically useful: if these key findings are *absent* in symptomatic patients, diagnosis of disease is *unlikely*.
- **EBM Boxes**, derived from large numbers of patients presenting with similar symptoms but different final diagnoses, quickly convey to clinicians which physical signs are most accurate for a particular diagnosis. Those findings with likelihood ratios (LRs) having the greatest value *increase* probability of disease the most (i.e., LRs function like diagnostic weights). Those findings with LRs closest to the value of 0 *decrease* probability of disease the most.

I. Introduction

Information about the diagnostic accuracy of physical findings is presented in two types of tables in this book: (1) "frequency of findings" tables, which display only the sensitivity of physical signs, and (2) evidence-based medicine (EBM) boxes, or "diagnostic accuracy" tables, which present the sensitivity, specificity, and LRs of various physical signs.

II. Frequency of Findings Tables

A. DEFINITION

Frequency of findings tables summarize multiple studies of patients with a specific diagnosis and present the sensitivity of physical signs found in that disorder. These tables provide no information about a sign's specificity. An example is Table 3.1, listing the frequency of findings in constrictive pericarditis, a disorder in which a diseased and unyielding pericardium interferes with diastolic filling of the heart.

B. PARTS OF THE TABLE

1. Finding

The first column lists the various physical signs, organized by organ system, with the findings of each organ system listed from most to least frequent.

TABLE 3.1 ■ Constrictive Pericarditis*

Physical Finding	Frequency (%)†
Neck veins	
Elevated neck veins	94
Prominent y descent (Friedreich sign)	57–100
Kussmaul sign	14–50
Arterial pulse	
Irregularly irregular (atrial fibrillation)	36–70
Blood pressure	
Pulsus paradoxus >10 mm Hg	13–64
Auscultation of heart	
Pericardial knock	20–94
Pericardial rub	3–16
Other	
Hepatomegaly	53–100
Edema	58–100
Ascites	37–89

Data from 780 patients from references 1–13.
*Diagnostic standard: for *constrictive pericarditis*, surgical and postmortem findings,[1-5] sometimes in combination with hemodynamic findings.[6-12]
†Results are overall mean frequency or, if statistically heterogeneous, the range of values.

2. Frequency

The second column lists the sensitivity (or frequency) of the physical signs. If the sensitivity from every study is statistically similar, the overall mean frequency is presented (e.g., in Table 3.1, 94% of patients with constrictive pericarditis have elevated neck veins). If the sensitivities from the different studies are statistically diverse (p <0.05 by the chi-squared test), the range of values is instead presented (e.g., in Table 3.1, 20% to 94% have a pericardial knock—a loud heart sound heard near the apex during early diastole).

3. Footnotes

The footnotes to these tables present the source of the information and the diagnostic standards used. For example, the information in Table 3.1 is based on 780 patients from 13 different studies, which based the diagnosis of constrictive pericarditis on surgical, postmortem, or hemodynamic findings.

C. Interpretation

Because the frequency of findings tables provide just information about a sign's sensitivity, they can only be used to support a statement that a physical sign, when *absent*, argues *against* disease. The absence of any finding whose sensitivity (or frequency) is 94% or more is a compelling argument against that diagnosis (i.e., the negative LR is 0.1 or less, even if the specificity of the finding, which is unknown, is as low as 50%). In Table 3.1, elevated venous pressure is such a finding (sensitivity = 94%): if the clinician is considering the diagnosis of constrictive pericarditis, but the patient's bedside estimate of venous pressure is normal, the diagnosis is unlikely.

Similarly, the absence of two or three independent findings having sensitivities greater than 80% is also a compelling argument against disease* (see Chapter 2 for a definition of *independent findings*).

---

*This statement assumes that the product of the LRs being combined is less than 0.1. Therefore,

$$\text{LR}^n = \left|\frac{(1-\text{sens})}{(\text{spec})}\right|^n \leq 0.1$$ where n is the number of findings being combined. If the specificity of the findings

is as low as 50%, each of two findings being combined must have a sensitivity greater than 84%, and each of three findings being combined must have a sensitivity greater than 77%.

III. Diagnostic Accuracy Tables (EBM Boxes)

A. DEFINITION

Diagnostic accuracy tables summarize information from large numbers of patients who present with similar symptoms but different diagnoses. These EBM Boxes present the physical sign's sensitivity, specificity, and positive and negative LRs, which then indicate how well that physical sign discriminates between patients with the particular diagnosis of interest and those without it.

EBM Box 3.1 presents an example summarizing the diagnostic accuracy of physical signs for pneumonia, as applied to large numbers of patients with cough and fever (see Chapter 32 for the complete EBM Box). In these studies, only about 20% of patients had pneumonia; the remainder had other causes of cough and fever such as sinusitis, bronchitis, or rhinitis.

B. PARTS OF THE EBM BOX

1. Finding

The first column presents the physical signs, organized by organ system, and the source of the information. Validated scoring schemes that combine findings appear in the bottom rows of EBM Boxes.

2. Sensitivity and Specificity

The second and third columns present the range of a physical sign's sensitivity and specificity observed in these studies.

3. Likelihood Ratios

The third and fourth columns present the physical sign's positive and negative LR (for clarity, "likelihood ratio if finding *present*" refers to the positive LR, and "likelihood ratio if finding *absent*" refers to the negative LR). In contrast to sensitivity and specificity, which are presented as a range of values, LRs are described by a single number, derived by using a statistical technique called the random effects model (see the section on Summarizing LRs in this chapter).[29] Only statistically significant LRs are presented in the EBM Boxes. If the 95% confidence interval (CI) for an LR, positive or negative, includes the value of 1, that result of the physical finding fails to statistically discriminate between patients with disease and those without it, and the notation "NS" (for "not significant") is recorded in the EBM Box.

4. Footnote

The footnotes to EBM Boxes describe the diagnostic standards used in the studies and, if necessary, definitions of findings. The footnote for EBM Box 3.1, for example, indicates that the diagnostic standard for pneumonia was the chest radiograph; it also describes the components of Heckerling diagnostic scoring scheme presented in the bottom rows of the EBM Box.

C. Interpretation of EBM Box

To use these EBM Boxes, the clinician needs to only glance at the LR columns to appreciate the discriminatory power of different findings. LRs with the greatest value increase probability of disease the most; LRs with the value closest to zero decrease probability the most. Boldface type highlights all findings with an LR of 3 or more or of 0.3 or less, thus allowing quick identification of those physical signs that increase probability more that 20% to 25% (LR $\geq$3) and those that decrease it more that 20% to 25% (LR $\leq$0.3; see also Chapter 2).

In patients with cough and fever (EBM Box 3.1), the individual findings increasing probability of pneumonia the most are egophony (LR = 4.1), cachexia (LR = 4), percussion dullness (LR = 3.6), and bronchial breath sounds (LR = 3.3). In contrast, no *individual* finding in this EBM box, whether present or absent, significantly *decreases* probability of pneumonia. (No LR has a value $\leq$0.3.)

EBM BOX 3.1	Pneumonia*				

| Finding (Reference)[†] | Sensitivity (%) | Specificity (%) | Likelihood Ratio[‡] if Finding Is | |
			Present	Absent
General appearance				
Cachexia[14]	10	97	**4.0**	NS
Abnormal mental status[15–17]	12–14	92–95	1.9	NS
Lung findings				
Percussion dullness[14–16,18–21]	4–26	82–99	**3.6**	NS
Diminished breath sounds[15,16,18–20,22–26]	7–60	73–98	2.4	0.8
Bronchial breath sounds[15,20]	14–19	94–96	**3.3**	0.9
Egophony[14–16]	4–16	96–99	**4.1**	NS
Crackles[14–19,22–27]	19–67	36–97	2.8	0.8
Wheezing[15–19,22,24,26,27]	4–36	50–96	0.8	NS
Diagnostic score (Heckerling et al.)[15,28]				
0 or 1 findings	7–29	33–65	**0.3**	…
2 or 3 findings	48–55	…	NS	…
4 or 5 findings	38–41	92–97	**8.2**	…

*Diagnostic standard: for *pneumonia*, infiltrate on chest radiograph.
†Definition of findings: for *Heckerling diagnostic score*, the clinician scores 1 point for each of the following 5 findings that are present: temperature >37.8°C, heart rate >100/min, crackles, diminished breath sounds, and *absence* of asthma.
‡Likelihood ratio (LR) if finding present = positive LR; LR if finding absent = negative LR.
NS, Not significant.

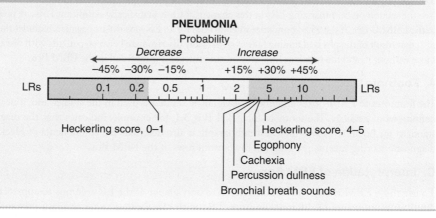

EBM Box 3.1 also shows that 4 or more points using Heckerling's diagnostic scheme significantly *increases* probability of pneumonia (LR = 8.2), whereas the presence of 0 or 1 point significant *decreases* it (LR = 0.3).

IV. Criteria for Selecting Studies Used in Diagnostic Accuracy Tables

All studies of adult patients that meet the following four criteria are included in the EBM Boxes of this book.

A. PATIENTS WERE SYMPTOMATIC

The study must have enrolled patients presenting to clinicians with symptoms or other problems. Therefore, studies using asymptomatic controls, which tend to inflate the specificity of physical signs, are excluded. Clinicians do not need a physical sign to help them distinguish patients with pneumonia from healthy persons (who would not be consulting the doctor); instead, they are interested in those physical signs distinguishing pneumonia from other causes of cough and fever.

B. DEFINITION OF PHYSICAL SIGN

The physical sign in the study must be clearly defined.

C. INDEPENDENT COMPARISON TO A DIAGNOSTIC STANDARD

There must be an independent comparison to an acceptable diagnostic standard. *Independent comparison* means that the physical sign was not used to select patients for testing with the diagnostic standard. Acceptable diagnostic standards include laboratory testing, clinical imaging, surgical findings, or postmortem analysis.

D. 2 × 2 TABLE COULD BE CONSTRUCTED

The studies must provide figures or tables from which numbers could be extracted to construct 2 × 2 tables and calculate sensitivity, specificity, and LRs. If any cell of the 2 × 2 table contained the value of zero, 0.5 was added to all cells, to avoid creating the unlikely LRs of 0 or infinity.

V. Summarizing Likelihood Ratios

The random effects model by Dersimonian and Laird,[29] which considers both within study and between study variance to calculate a pooled LR, was used to summarize the LRs from the various studies. Table 3.2 illustrates how this model works. In the top rows of this table are the individual data from all studies of egophony that appear in EBM Box 3.1, including the finding's sensitivity, specificity, the positive and negative LRs, and the LRs 95% confidence intervals (CIs). The bottom row of Table 3.2 shows how all of this information is summarized throughout the book.

In each of the studies, egophony is specific (96% to 99%) but not sensitive (4% to 16%). The positive LRs are all greater than 1, indicating that the finding of egophony increases probability of pneumonia. For one of the three studies (i.e. Gennis and others[16]), the positive LR lacks statistical significance because its 95% CI includes the value of 1 (i.e., a LR value of 1 has no discriminatory value). For the other two studies, the 95% confidence interval of the positive LR excludes the value of 1, thus making them statistically significant. The summary measure for the positive LR (fourth row of this table) is both clinically significant (4.08, a large positive number) and statistically significant (its 95% CI excludes 1.0). All of this information is summarized, in the notation used in this book (last row), by simply presenting the pooled LR of 4.1. (Interested readers may consult the Appendix for the 95% CIs of all LRs in this book.)

In contrast, the negative LRs from each study have both meager clinical significance (i.e., 0.87 to 0.96, values close to 1) and, for two of the three studies, no statistical significance (i.e., the 95% CI includes 1). The pooled negative LR also lacks clinical and statistical significance. Because it is statistically no different from 1.0 (i.e., the 95% CI of the pooled value, 0.88 to 1.01, includes 1), it is summarized using the notation "NS" for "*not significant.*"

TABLE 3.2 ■ Egophony and Pneumonia - Individual Studies

Reference	Sensitivity (%)	Specificity (%)	Positive LR (95% CI)	Negative LR (95% CI)
Heckerling[15]	16	97	4.91 (2.88, 8.37)	0.87 (0.81, 0.94)
Gennis[16]	8	96	2.07 (0.79, 5.41)	0.96 (0.90, 1.02)
Diehr[14]	4	99	7.97 (1.77, 35.91)	0.96 (0.91, 1.02)
Pooled result			4.08 (2.14, 7.79)	0.93 (0.88, 1.01)
Notation used in book	4–16	96–99	4.1	NS

CI, Confidence interval; *LR*, likelihood ratio; *NS*, not significant.

Presenting the single pooled result for statistically significant LRs and NS for the statistically insignificant ones simplifies the EBM Boxes and makes it much simpler to grasp the point that the finding of egophony in patients with cough and fever increases probability of pneumonia (LR = 4.1), but the absence of egophony changes probability very little or not at all.

References may be accessed online at *Elsevier eBooks for Practicing Clinicians*.

CHAPTER 4

Using the Online EBM Calculator

I. The Evidence-Based Medicine Calculator

An easy-to-use online calculator is provided on the *Elsevier eBooks for Practicing Clinicians* platform, allowing clinicians to quickly calculate post-test probabilities when applying the likelihood ratios (LRs) in this book.

II. Using the Calculator

A. BLANK CALCULATOR

After opening the evidence-based medicine (EBM) calculator, the **Blank Calculator** appears (see Fig. 4.1). The blank calculator has three horizontal rules: **Pre-test probability, Likelihood ratio (LR),** and **Post-test probability**, each with its own arrow. The clinician can move the arrows under the first two rules to indicate the appropriate pre-test probability and LR. Then, the third arrow (post-test probability) automatically displays the corresponding post-test probability. For example, dragging the pre-test probability arrow to 32% and LR arrow to 5 reveals the post-test probability to be approximately 70% (Fig. 4.1).

B. CALCULATING PROBABILITY FOR SPECIFIC CONDITIONS

If the clinician taps the arrow to the right of the box titled **Problem** (at the top of the calculator), a drop-down list of over 70 clinical problems will appear. By selecting any problem from this list, 2 additional items of information appear: (1) the pre-test probability for that particular clinical problem derived from the actual studies used in this book, with both the range and median pre-test probabilities displayed automatically on the first rule, and (2) a **View LR Value** button located in the upper right corner of the calculator (Fig. 4.2).

As an example, the clinician discovers the physical finding of *clubbing* in a patient with cirrhosis, a finding raising the possibility of hepatopulmonary syndrome (see Chapter 8). To use the calculator, the clinician first selects *Hepatopulmonary syndrome* from the drop-down list (Fig. 4.2), which changes the appearance of the **Pre-test probability** rule to display both the range and median pre-test probabilities (or prevalence) of hepatopulmonary syndrome in patients with cirrhosis derived from the studies in this book (i.e., range, 14% to 37%; median, 26%). In our example, however, the clinician using the calculator believes that the prevalence of hepatopulmonary syndrome in his or her own practice is slightly higher than the median (i.e., he or she believes it is about 30%). Therefore, the clinician sets the **Pre-test probability** arrow to 30%. Next, the clinician clicks on the **View LR Value** button (at the upper right) to reveal the EBM Box for Hepatopulmonary syndrome (from Chapter 8). This EBM Box reveals that the LR for clubbing

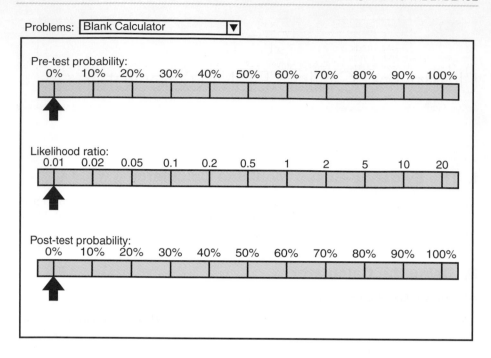

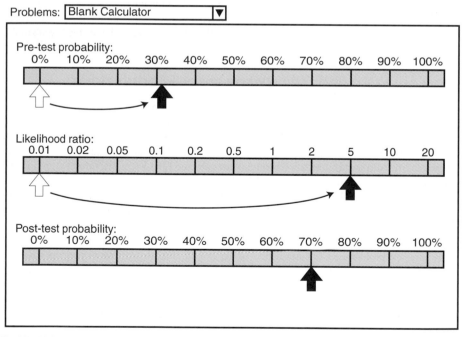

Fig. 4.1   Using the blank calculator. In this example, the clinician knows the pre-test probability is 32% and the finding's LR is 5. Therefore, the clinician drags the arrow under the first rule (*pre-test probability*) to 32% and the arrow under the second rule (*likelihood ratio*) to 5; the arrow under the third rule (*post-test probability*) automatically displays the corresponding post-test probability (70%).

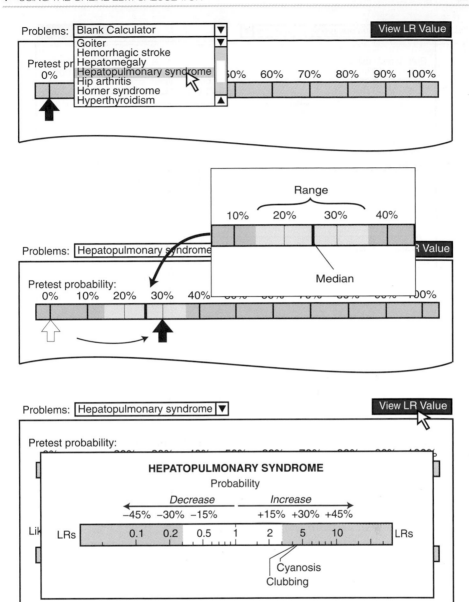

A

Fig. 4.2 Diagnosing hepatopulmonary syndrome with the EBM Calculator. The clinician is evaluating a patient with cirrhosis and clubbing and wonders about the likelihood of hepatopulmonary syndrome. Selecting *hepatopulmonary syndrome* (*top left*) reveals the pre-test probability in clinical studies ranges from 14% to 37%, with a median probability of 26% (*middle left*). Believing hepatopulmonary syndrome to be more prevalent in his own practice than 26%, the clinician drags the **pre-test probability arrow** to 30% (*middle left*), clicks *view LR value* (*bottom left*) to reveal the LR for clubbing (LR = 4.3). Dragging the **LR arrow** to 4.3 demonstrates the post-test probability of hepatopulmonary to be approximately 65% (*right*).

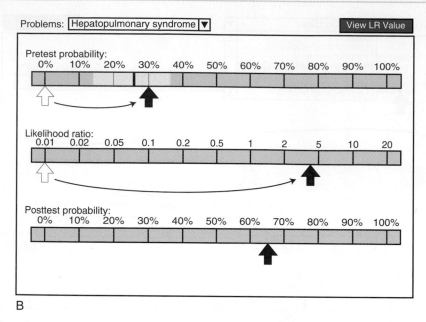

B

Fig. 4.2 *Continued*

is 4.3. After dragging the **LR arrow** to 4.3, the calculator indicates that the post-test probability of hepatopulmonary syndrome (in this clinician's patient with cirrhosis and clubbing) is 65% (Fig. 4.2).

Following the rules discussed in Chapter 2, the clinician may combine findings using this calculator by simply transferring the post-test probability from the first finding to the pre-test probability rule of the second finding. (See the section on Combining Findings in Chapter 2.)

CHAPTER 5

Reliability of Physical Findings

KEY TEACHING POINTS

- Reliability refers to how often two clinicians examining the same patient agree about the presence or absence of a particular physical finding. Commonly used measurements of reliability are *simple agreement* or the *kappa (κ-) statistic*.
- About 60% of physical findings have κ-statistics of 0.4 or more, indicating that observed agreement is moderately good or better.
- Despite the common belief that technologic tests are more precise than bedside observation, the κ-statistics observed for most diagnostic standards (e.g., chest radiography, computed tomography, angiography, magnetic resonance imaging, endoscopy, and pathology) are similar to those observed for physical signs.
- Some causes of interobserver disagreement can be eliminated, but because clinical medicine is inherently a human enterprise (even when interpreting technologic tests), subjectivity and a certain level of clinical disagreement will always be present.

Reliability refers to how often multiple clinicians, examining the same patients, agree that a particular physical sign is present or absent. As characteristics of a physical sign, reliability and accuracy are distinct qualities, although significant interobserver disagreement tends to undermine the finding's accuracy and prevents clinicians from applying it confidently to their own practice. Disagreement about physical signs also contributes to the growing sense among clinicians, not necessarily justified, that physical examination is less scientific than more technologic tests, such as clinical imaging and laboratory testing, and that physical examination lacks their diagnostic authority.

The most straightforward way to express reliability, or interobserver agreement, is **simple agreement**, which is the proportion of total observations in which clinicians agree about the finding. For example, if two clinicians examining 100 patients with dyspnea agree that a third heart sound is present in 5 patients and is absent in 75 patients, simple agreement would be 80% [i.e., $(5 + 75)/100 = 0.80$]; in the remaining 20 patients, only one of the two clinicians heard a third heart sound. Simple agreement has advantages, including being easy to calculate and understand, but a significant disadvantage is that agreement may be quite high by chance alone. For example, if one of the clinicians in our hypothetical study heard a third heart sound in 10 of the 100 dyspneic patients and the other heard it in 20 of the patients (even though they agreed about the presence of the heart sound in only 5 patients), simple agreement by chance *alone* would be 74%.* With chance agreement this high, the observed 80% agreement no longer seems so impressive.

To address this problem, most clinical studies now express interobserver agreement using the kappa (κ) statistic, which usually has values between 0 and 1 (the Appendix at the end of this

---

*Agreement by chance approaches 100% as the percentage of positive observations for both clinicians approaches 0% or 100% (i.e., both clinicians agree that a finding is very uncommon or very common). The Appendix at the end of this chapter shows how to calculate chance agreement.

chapter shows how to calculate the κ-statistic). A κ-value of 0 indicates that observed agreement is the same as that expected by chance, and a κ-value of 1 indicates perfect agreement. According to convention, a κ-value of 0 to 0.2 indicates *slight* agreement; 0.2 to 0.4 *fair* agreement; 0.4 to 0.6 *moderate* agreement; 0.6 to 0.8 *substantial* agreement; and 0.8 to 1.0 almost *perfect* agreement.[†]

TABLE 5.1 ■ Interobserver Agreement and Physical Signs

Finding (ref)	κ-statistic*
General Appearance	
Mental status examination	
Mini-Mental Status Examination[1]	0.28–0.80
Clock-drawing test (Wolf-Klein Method)[2]	0.73
Confusion Assessment Method for delirium[3–6]	0.70–0.91
Altered mental status[7]	0.71
Stance and gait	
Abnormal gait[8,9]	0.11–0.71
Skin	
Patient appears anemic[10,11]	0.23–0.48
Nailbed pallor[12]	0.19–0.34
Conjunctival pallor (rim method)[13,14]	0.54–0.77
Palmar crease pallor[14]	0.44
Ashen or pale skin[7]	0.34
Cyanosis[10,15]	0.36–0.70
Jaundice[16]	0.65
Loss of hair[17]	0.51
Vascular spiders[16–18]	0.64–0.92
Palmar erythema[16–18]	0.37–1.00
Hydration status	
Patient appears dehydrated[10]	0.44–0.53
Axillary dryness[19]	0.50
Increased moisture on skin[10]	0.31–0.53
Capillary refill > 3 seconds[7]	0.29
Capillary refill > 5 seconds[20]	0.74–0.91
Nutritional assessment	
Abnormal nutritional state[10]	0.27–0.36
Other	
Consciousness impaired[10]	0.65–0.88
Patient appears older than age[10]	0.38–0.42
Patient appears in pain[10]	0.43–0.75
Generally unwell in appearance[10]	0.52–0.64
Vital Signs	
Tachycardia (heart rate >100/min)[21]	0.85
Bradycardia (heart rate <60/min)[21]	0.87
Systolic hypertension (SBP>160 mm Hg)[21]	0.75
Hypotension (SBP <90 mm Hg)[21,22]	0.27–0.90
Osler sign[23–25]	0.26–0.72
Rumpel-Leede ("tourniquet") test[26,27]	0.76–0.88
Elevated body temperature, palpating the skin[10]	0.09–0.23
Tachypnea[7,15,21]	0.25–0.60

[†]No measure of reliability is perfect, especially for findings whose prevalence clinicians agree approaches 0% or 100%. For these findings, simple agreement tends to overestimate reliability, and the κ-statistic tends to underestimate the reliability.

Continued

TABLE 5.1 ■ Interobserver Agreement and Physical Signs—Cont'd

Finding (ref)	κ-statistic*
Head and Neck	
Pupils	
Swinging flashlight test (relative afferent pupil defect)[28]	0.63
Diabetic retinopathy	
Microaneurysms[29,30]	0.58–0.66
Intraretinal hemorrhages[29,30]	0.89
Hard exudates[29,30]	0.66–0.74
Cotton wool spots[29,30]	0.56–0.67
Intraretinal microvascular abnormalities ("IRMA")[29,30]	0.46
Neovascularization near disc[29,30]	0.21–0.48
Macular edema[29,30]	0.21–0.67
Overall grade[29,30]	0.65
Hearing	
Whispered voice test[31,32]	0.16–1.0
Finger rub test[33]	0.83
Thyroid	
Thyroid gland diffuse, multinodular or solitary nodule[34]	0.25–0.70
Goiter[35,36]	0.38–0.77
Meninges	
Nuchal rigidity, present or absent[37–39]	0.24–0.76
Lungs	
Inspection	
Clubbing (general impression)[15,40]	0.33–0.45
Clubbing (interphalangeal depth ratio)[41]	0.98
Clubbing (Schamroth sign)[41]	0.64
Breathing difficulties[10]	0.54–0.69
Gasping respirations[7]	0.63
Reduced chest movement[15,42,43]	0.14–0.38
Kussmaul respirations[44]	0.70
Pursed lip breathing[43]	0.45
Asymmetric chest expansion[45]	0.85
Scalene or sternocleidomastoid muscle contraction[7,43,46]	0.52–0.57
Kyphosis[40]	0.37
Barrel chest[43]	0.62
Thoracic ratio ≥0.9[43]	0.32
Displaced trachea[15]	0.01
Palpation	
Tracheal descent during inspiration[46]	0.62
Laryngeal height ≤5.5 cm[43]	0.59
Impalpable apex beat[15,40]	0.33–0.44
Decreased tactile fremitus[15,45]	0.24–0.86
Increased tactile fremitus[15]	0.01
Subxiphoid point of maximal cardiac impulse[47]	0.30
Paradoxical costal margin movement[46,48]	0.56–0.82
Percussion	
Hyperresonant percussion note[15,42,47]	0.26–0.50
Dull percussion note[15,42,45,49]	0.16–0.84
Diaphragm excursion more or less than 2 cm by percussion[47]	−0.04
Diminished cardiac dullness[47]	0.49
Auscultatory percussion abnormal[45,50]	0.18–0.76

Continued

TABLE 5.1 ■ Interobserver Agreement and Physical Signs—Cont'd

Finding (ref)	κ-statistic*
Auscultation	
Reduced breath sound intensity[15,42,43,45,47,49,51,52]	0.16–0.89
Bronchial breathing[15,42]	0.19–0.32
Whispering pectoriloquy[15]	0.11
Reduced vocal resonance[45]	0.78
Crackles[15,49,51,53–56]	0.21–0.65
Wheezes[15,47,49,51,52]	0.43–0.93
Rhonchi[42,52]	0.38–0.55
Pleural rub[15,45]	−0.02–0.51
Special tests	
Snider test <10 cm[47]	0.39
Forced expiratory time[43,47,57,58]	0.27–0.70
Hoover sign[52]	0.74
Wells simplified rule for pulmonary embolism[59]	0.54–0.62
Heart	
Neck veins	
Neck veins, elevated or normal[53–55,60,61]	0.08–0.71
Abdominojugular test[60]	0.92
Palpation	
Palpable apical impulse present[62–64]	0.68–0.82
Palpable apical impulse measureable[65]	0.56
Palpable apical impulse displaced lateral to midclavicular line[53,62,63,66]	0.43–0.86
Apical beat normal, sustained, double, or absent[66]	0.88
Palpable right ventricular heave[61]	0.18–0.23
Percussion	
Cardiac dullness >10.5 cm from midsternal line[67,68]	0.57
Auscultation	
S2 diminished or absent, vs. normal[69]	0.54
Third heart sound[53–55,60,70–72]	−0.17–0.84
Fourth heart sound[71,73]	0.15–0.71
Systolic murmur, present or absent[69]	0.19
Systolic murmur radiates to right carotid[69]	0.33
Systolic murmur, long systolic or early systolic[74]	0.78
Murmur intensity (Levine grade)[75]	0.43–0.60
Systolic murmur grade >2/6[76]	0.59
Carotid pulsation	
Delayed carotid upstroke[69]	0.26
Reduced carotid volume[69]	0.24
Abdomen	
Inspection	
Abdominal distention[77,78]	0.35–0.42
Abdominal wall collateral veins, present vs. absent[16]	0.47
Palpation and percussion	
Ascites[16,18,55]	0.47–0.75
Abdominal tenderness[77–79]	0.31–0.68
Surgical abdomen[78]	0.27
Abdominal wall tenderness test[80,81]	0.52–0.81
Rebound tenderness[77]	0.25
Guarding[77,78]	0.36–0.49
Rigidity[77]	0.14
Abdominal mass palpated[78]	0.82

TABLE 5.1 ■ Interobserver Agreement and Physical Signs—Cont'd

Finding (ref)	κ-statistic*
Palpable spleen[16,18,82]	0.33–0.75
Palpable liver edge[83]	0.44–0.53
Liver consistency, normal or abnormal[16]	0.4
Liver firm to palpation[84]	0.72
Liver, nodular or not[16]	0.29
Liver, tender or not[18]	0.49
Liver, span >9 cm by percussion[53]	0.11
Spleen palpable or not[85]	0.56–0.70
Spleen percussion sign (Traube), positive or not[86]	0.19–0.41
Spleen percussion sign (Castell), positive or not[82]	0.45
Abdominal aortic aneurysm, present vs. absent[87]	0.53
Auscultation	
Normal bowel sounds[78]	0.36
Extremities	
Peripheral vascular disease	
Peripheral pulse, present vs. absent[88–91]	0.52–0.92
Peripheral pulse, normal or diminished[88]	0.01–0.15
Cool extremities[55]	0.46
Severity of skin mottling over leg[92,93]	0.87
Diabetic foot	
Monofilament sensation, normal or abnormal[94–96]	0.48–0.83
Probe-to-bone test[97–99]	0.59–0.84
Edema and deep venous thrombosis	
Dependent edema[53–55]	0.39–0.73
Wells pretest probability for deep vein thrombosis[100,101]	0.74–0.75
Musculoskeletal system-shoulder	
Shoulder tenderness[102]	0.32
Painful arc[102–105]	0.45–0.64
Neer impingement sign[106]	0.64
Hawkins impingement sign[106]	0.54
External rotation of shoulder <45 degrees[102]	0.68
Supraspinatus test (empty can)[102,105,107]	0.44–0.94
Infraspinatus test (resisted external rotation)[102,103]	0.49–0.67
Impingement sign (Hawkins-Kennedy)[102,103,105,107]	0.29–1.0
Drop arm test[102,105]	0.28–0.35
Musculoskeletal system-hip	
Patrick test[108]	0.47
Passive internal rotation ≤25 degrees[108]	0.51
Musculoskeletal system-knee	
Ottawa knee rules[109,110]	0.51–0.77
Knee effusion visible[109,111–113]	0.28–0.78
Knee flexion <90 degrees[109]	0.74
Patellar tenderness[109,111]	0.69–0.76
Head of fibula tenderness[109]	0.64
Inability to bear weight immediately and emergency room after knee injury[109,111]	0.75–0.81
Bony swelling of knee[113,114]	0.55–0.66
Joint line tenderness[112,114–116]	0.11–0.43
Patellofemoral crepitus[114]	0.24
Mediolateral instability of knee[114]	0.23
McMurray sign[112,116,117]	0.16–0.35
Lachman test[118]	0.72

Continued

TABLE 5.1 ▪ Interobserver Agreement and Physical Signs—Cont'd

Finding (ref)	κ-statistic*
Musculoskeletal system-ankle	
Inability to walk 4 steps immediately and in emergency room after ankle injury[119,120]	0.71–0.97
Medial malleolar tenderness[120]	0.82
Lateral malleolar tenderness[120]	0.80
Navicular tenderness[120]	0.91
Base of 5th metatarsal tenderness[120]	0.94
Ottawa ankle rule[121,122]	0.41–0.45
Ottawa midfoot rule[121]	0.77
Neurologic Examination	
Visual fields	
Visual fields by confrontation[123]	0.63–0.81
Cranial nerves	
Pharyngeal sensation, present or absent[124]	1.0
Facial palsy, present or absent[125,126]	0.57
Dysarthria, present or absent[127,128]	0.41–0.77
Water swallow test (50 mL)[129]	0.60
Oxygen desaturation test (for aspiration risk)[129]	0.60
Abnormal tongue strength[127]	0.55–0.63
Motor examination	
Muscle strength, MRC scale[130–133]	0.69–0.93
Foot tapping test[134,135]	0.73–0.83
Muscle atrophy[136,137]	0.32–0.82
Spasticity, 6 point scale[138]	0.21–0.61
Rigidity, 4 point scale[139]	0.64
Asterixis[16]	0.42
Tremor[137]	0.74
Pronator drift[140]	0.39
Forearm rolling test[140]	0.73
Sensory examination	
Light touch sensation, normal, diminished, or increased[136,137]	0.22–0.63
Pain sensation, normal, diminished, or increased[131,136,137]	0.41–0.57
Vibratory sensation, normal or diminished[136,137]	0.28–0.54
Romberg test[137]	0.64
Reflex examination	
Reflex amplitude, NINDS scale[141]	0.51–0.61
Ankle jerk, present or absent[131,142,143]	0.34–0.94
Asymmetric knee jerk[131]	0.42
Babinski response[125,126,134,135,137,144,145]	0.17–0.60
Finger flexion reflex[146]	0.65
Palmomental reflex[147]	0.53
Primitive reflexes, amplitude and persistence[148]	0.46–1.0
Coordination	
Finger-nose test[125,126,137,140]	0.14–0.65
Heel-shin test[137]	0.58
Peripheral nerve	
Spurling test[149]	0.60
Katz hand diagram[150]	0.86
Flick sign[151]	0.90
Hypalgesia index finger[151]	0.50
Tinel sign[151]	0.47
Phalen sign[151]	0.79

TABLE 5.1 ■ Interobserver Agreement and Physical Signs—Cont'd

Finding (ref)	κ-statistic*
Straight leg raising test[131,152–156]	0.21–0.80
Crossed leg raising test[131]	0.49
Other	
Head impulse test[157]	0.86
Knee lift test (for nonorganic weakness)[158]	0.91

*Interpretation of the κ-statistic: 0 to 0.2 slight agreement, 0.2 to 0.4 fair agreement, 0.4 to 0.6 moderate agreement, 0.6 to 0.8 substantial agreement, 0.8 to 1.0 almost perfect agreement.
MRC, Medical Research Council; *NINDS*, National Institute of Neurological Disorders and Stroke.

Rarely, physical signs have κ-values less than 0 (theoretically as low as −1), indicating the observed agreement was worse than chance agreement.

Table 5.1 presents the κ-statistic for most of the physical signs discussed in this book, demonstrating that, with rare exceptions, observed agreement is better than chance agreement (i.e., κ-statistic exceeds 0). About 60% of findings have a κ-statistic of 0.4 or more, indicating that observed agreement is moderate or better.

Clinical disagreement occurs for many reasons—some causes clinicians can control, but others are inextricably linked to the very nature of clinical medicine and human observation in general. The most prominent reasons include the following: (1) The physical sign's definition can be vague or ambiguous. For example, experts recommend about a dozen different ways to perform auscultatory percussion of the liver, thus making the sign so nebulous that significant interobserver disagreement is guaranteed. Ambiguity also results if signs are defined with terms that are not easily measurable. For example, clinicians assessing whether a peripheral pulse is present or absent demonstrate moderate-to-almost perfect agreement (κ = 0.52–0.92, Table 5.1), but when the same clinicians are asked to record whether the palpable pulse is normal or diminished, they have great difficulty agreeing about the sign (κ = 0.01–0.15) simply because they have no idea what the next clinician means by "diminished." (2) The clinician's technique is flawed. For example, common mistakes are using the diaphragm instead of the bell of the stethoscope to detect the third heart sound, or stating a muscle stretch reflex is absent without first trying to elicit it using a reinforcing maneuver (e.g., Jendrassik maneuver). (3) Biologic variation of the physical sign. The pericardial friction rub, pulsus alternans, cannon A waves, Cheyne-Stokes respirations, and many other signs are notoriously evanescent, tending to come and go over time. (4) The clinician could be careless or inattentive. The bustle of an active practice may lead clinicians to listen to the lungs while conducting the patient interview, or to search for a subtle murmur in a noisy emergency room. Reliable observations require undistracted attention and an alert mind. (5) The clinician's biases can influence the observation. When findings are equivocal, expectations influence perceptions. For example, in a patient who just started blood pressure medications, borderline hypertension may become normal blood pressure; in a patient with increasing bilateral edema, borderline distended neck veins may become clearly elevated venous pressure; or in a patient with new weakness, the equivocal Babinski sign may become clearly positive. Sometimes, biases actually create the finding: if the clinician holds a flashlight too long over an eye with suspected optic nerve disease, he or she may temporarily bleach the retina of that eye and produce the Marcus Gunn pupil, thus confirming the original suspicion.

The lack of perfect reliability with physical diagnosis is sometimes regarded as a significant weakness, leading to the charge that physical diagnosis is less reliable and scientific than clinical imaging and laboratory testing. Nonetheless, Table 5.2 shows that, for most of our **diagnostic standards**—chest radiography, computed tomography, screening mammography, angiography, magnetic resonance imaging, ultrasonography, endoscopy, and pathology—interobserver

TABLE 5.2 ■ Interobserver Agreement – Diagnostic Standards

Finding (ref)	κ-statistic*
Chest radiography	
Cardiomegaly[60]	0.48
Pulmonary infiltrate[159,160]	0.38–0.58
Pneumonia[161]	0.45
Interstitial edema[60]	0.83
Pulmonary vascular redistribution[60]	0.50
Grading pulmonary fibrosis, 4 point scale[162]	0.45
Contrast venography	
Deep vein thrombosis in leg[163]	0.53
Screening mammography	
Suspicious lesion, present vs. absent[164]	0.47
Digital subtraction angiography	
Renal artery stenosis[165]	0.65
Coronary arteriography	
Classification of coronary artery lesions[166]	0.33
Arthroscopy	
Inflamed or torn supraspinatus tendon[167]	0.47
Computed tomography of head	
Normal or abnormal, patient with stroke[168]	0.60
Lesion on right or left side, patient with stroke[168]	0.65
Mass effect, present or absent[168]	0.52
Computed tomography of the chest	
Lung cancer staging[169]	0.40–0.60
Submassive pulmonary embolism present (angiography)[170]	0.47
Coronary lesion on CT coronary angiography[171]	0.57
Magnetic resonance imaging of head	
Compatible with multiple sclerosis[172]	0.57–0.87
Pituitary microadenoma present[173]	0.30
Magnetic resonance imaging of lumbar spine	
Intervertebral disc extrusion, protrusion, bulge, or normal[174,175]	0.59
Lumbar nerve root compression[175,176]	0.63–0.83
Ultrasonography	
Calf deep vein thrombosis, present or absent[177]	0.69
Thyroid nodule, present or absent[178,179]	0.57–0.66
Thyroid nodule, cystic or solid[180]	0.64
Goiter is present[36]	0.63
Electrocardiography	
Diagnosis of narrow-complex tachycardia[181]	0.70
Echocardiography	
Severity of valvular regurgitation[182,183]	0.32–0.55
Endoscopy	
Grade of reflux esophagitis[184]	0.55
Pathologic examination of liver biopsy	
Cholestasis[185]	0.40
Alcoholic liver disease[185]	0.49
Cirrhosis[185]	0.59

*Interpretation of the κ-statistic: 0 to 0.2 slight agreement, 0.2 to 0.4 fair agreement, 0.4 to 0.6 moderate agreement, 0.6 to 0.8 substantial agreement, 0.8 to 1.0 almost perfect agreement.

agreement is also less than perfect, with κ-statistics similar to those observed with physical signs. Even with laboratory tests, which present the clinician with a single, indisputable number, interobserver disagreement is still possible and even common, simply because the clinician has to interpret the laboratory test's **significance**. For example, in one study of three endocrinologists reviewing the same thyroid function tests and other clinical data of 55 consecutive outpatients with suspected thyroid disease, the endocrinologists disagreed about the final diagnosis 40% of the time.[34] Computerized interpretation of test results performs no better: in a study of pairs of electrocardiograms taken only 1 minute apart from 92 patients, the computer interpretation was significantly different 40% of the time, even though the tracings showed no change.[186]

By defining abnormal findings precisely, by studying and mastering examination technique, and by observing every detail at the bedside attentively and without bias or distraction, we can minimize interobserver disagreement and make physical diagnosis more precise. It is simply impossible, however, to abstract every detail of clinicians' observations of patients into exact physical signs, and, in this way, physical diagnosis is no different than any of the other tools we use to categorize disease. So long as both the material and the observers of clinical medicine are human beings, a certain amount of subjectivity always will be with us.

Appendix. Calculation of the κ-statistic

The observations of two observers who are examining the same N patients independently are customarily displayed in a 2 × 2 table, similar to that in Fig. 5.1. Observer A finds the sign to be present in w_1 patients and absent in w_2 patients; observer B finds the sign to be present in y_1

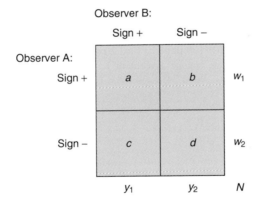

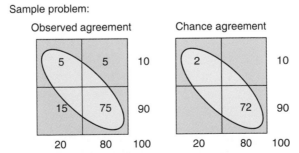

Fig. 5.1 Interobserver agreement and the κ-statistic. *Top half:* Conventional 2 × 2 table displaying data for calculation of κ-statistic. *Bottom half:* A sample case, in which observed agreement is 80%, chance agreement is 74%, and the κ-statistic is 0.23 (see Appendix for discussion).

patients and absent in y_2 patients. The 2 observers agree the sign is present in a patients and absent in d patients. Therefore, the observed agreement (P_O) is:

$$P_O = (a + d)/N$$

Calculation of the κ-statistic first requires calculation of the agreement that would have occurred by chance alone. Among all the patients, observer A found the fraction w_1/N to have the sign; therefore, by chance alone, among the y_1 patients with the sign according to observer B, observer A would find the sign in (w_1/N) times y_1 or (w_1y_1/N) patients (i.e., this is the *number* of patients in which both observers agree the sign is present, by chance alone). Similarly, both observers would agree the sign is absent by chance alone in (w_2y_2/N) patients. Therefore, the expected chance agreement (P_E) is their sum, divided by N:

$$P_E = \frac{(w_1y_1 + w_2y_2)}{N^2}$$

This equation shows that agreement by chance alone (P_E) approaches 100% as both w_1 and y_1 approach 0 or N (i.e., both clinicians agree that a finding is rare or that it is very common).

The κ-statistic is the increment in observed agreement beyond that expected by chance $(P_O–P_E)$, divided by the maximal increment that could have been observed had the observed agreement been perfect $(1–P_E)$:

$$\kappa = \frac{(P_O - P_E)}{(1 - P_E)}$$

For example, Fig. 5.1 depicts the observations of two observers in a study of 100 patients with dyspnea. Both agree the third heart sound is present in 5 patients and absent in 75 patients; therefore, simple agreement is (5 + 75)/100 or 0.80. By chance alone, they would have agreed about the sound being present in (10 × 20)/100 patients (i.e., 2 patients) and absent in (90 × 80)/100 patients (i.e., 72 patients); therefore, chance agreement is (2 + 72)/100 patients or 0.74. The κ-statistic for this finding becomes (0.80–0.74)/(1–0.74) = (0.06)/(0.26) = 0.23.

References may be accessed online at *Elsevier eBooks for Practicing Clinicians.*

PART 3

General Appearance
of the Patient

Mental Status Examination

I. Introduction

Dementia is a clinical syndrome characterized by deteriorating cognition, behavior, and autonomy. Dementia affects 9% to 13% of adults older than 65 years living in the community.[1] Before diagnosing dementia, clinicians must exclude delirium (i.e., acute confusion; see the section on diagnosis of delirium).

Of the many simple and rapid bedside tests developed to diagnose dementia, the most extensively investigated ones are the clock-drawing test, Mini-Cog test, and Mini-Mental Status Examination (MMSE).

II. Clock-Drawing Test

The clock-drawing test was originally developed in the early 1900s to evaluate soldiers who had suffered head wounds to the occipital or parietal lobes, injuries that often led to difficulty composing images with the appropriate number of parts of correct size and orientation (i.e., constructional apraxia).[2] To depict a clock, patients must be able to follow directions, comprehend language, visualize the proper orientation of an object, and execute normal movements, all tasks that may be disturbed in dementia.

A. TECHNIQUE AND SCORING

There are 20 or more different methods for performing and scoring the clock-drawing test, some with intricate grading systems that defeat the test's simplicity.[3,4] In a simple and well-investigated method,[5] the clinician gives the patient a piece of paper with a preprinted circle 4 inches in diameter and states to the patient "draw a clock." If the patient has any questions, the clinician only repeats the same instructions and gives no other guidance. The patient may take as long as he or she wants to complete the task. Fig. 6.1 describes how to score the drawing.

Normal patterns:

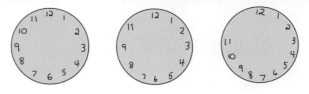

Abnormal patterns:

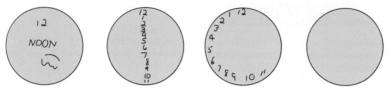

Fig. 6.1   The clock-drawing test (Wolf-Klein method). The clock-drawing is normal if the patient has included most of the 12 numbers in the correct clockwise orientation. The patient does not need to draw the hands of the clock, and abnormal spacing of the numbers, however inappropriate, is still regarded normal as long as the numbers are in correct order and near the rim. Normal clock-drawing patterns, from left to right, are "normal," "missing one number," and "inappropriate spacing." Abnormal clock-drawing patterns, from left to right, are "irrelevant figures," "unusual arrangement" (i.e., vertical orientation of numbers), "counterclockwise rotation," and "absence of numbers." Adapted with permission from Wolf-Klein GP, Silverstone FA, Levy AP, Brod MS, Breuer J. Screening for Alzheimer's disease by clock drawing. *J Am Geriatr Soc.* 1989;37:730–734.

B. CLINICAL SIGNIFICANCE

In patients without other known causes of constructional apraxia (e.g., parietal lobe lesion), a positive clock-drawing test increases the probability of dementia (likelihood ratio [LR] = 4, EBM Box 6.1). A normal clock-drawing test is a less useful result, being elicited from many patients with dementia as defined by other measures. In contrast to the MMSE, the clock-drawing test is unaffected by the patient's level of education.[6]

III. Mini-Cog Test

A. TECHNIQUE AND SCORING

The Mini-Cog test combines a clock-drawing test with tests of recall to provide a brief screening tool suitable for primary care patients, even those who do not speak English as their native language.[12] To perform the test, the clinician asks the patient to register three unrelated words (e.g., *banana, sunrise,* and *chair*) and then asks him or her to draw a clock, stating "Draw a large circle, fill in the numbers on a clock face, and set the hands at 8:20." The patient is allowed 3 minutes to draw the clock, and instructions may be repeated if necessary. After drawing the clock (or after 3 minutes have elapsed), the patient is asked to recall the three words. The Mini-Cog is scored by assigning 1 point for each word recalled (score, 0 to 3) and 2 points for a "normal" clock, which should have the correct orientation and spacing of numbers and hands. An "abnormal" clock receives 0 points, thus creating possible score range of 0 to 5.[44]

EBM BOX 6.1	Dementia and Delirium*

Finding (Reference)[†]	Sensitivity (%)	Specificity (%)	Likelihood Ratio[‡] if Finding Is Present	Likelihood Ratio[‡] if Finding Is Absent
Dementia				
Abnormal clock drawing test[5–11]	36–75	72–98	4.0	0.5
Mini-Cog score 2 or less[12–17]	75–99	59–93	4.5	0.1
Mini-Mental Status Examination: traditional threshold				
23 or less[13,17–32]	47–100	71–99	7.8	0.2
Mini-Mental Status Examination: 3 levels[20,22–24,29]				
20 or less	29–69	93–99	14.4	...
21–25	26–57	...	2.1	...
26 or more	4–14	14–31	0.1	...
Delirium				
Positive test using "confusion assessment method"[33–43]	46–98	83–99	11.5	0.2

*Diagnostic standard: for *dementia*, dementia by NINCDS-ADRDA criteria,[5,6] DMS criteria,[8–19,21,22,24,26,27,29,31,32] CAMDEX instrument,[20] AGECAT,[25,28] or neurologist opinion;[23,30] for *delirium*, the DMS criteria.[33–43]

[†]Definition of findings: for *abnormal clock drawing test*, see Fig. 6.1; for *Mini-Cog test* and *confusion assessment method*, see text.

[‡]Likelihood ratio (LR) if finding present = positive LR; LR if finding absent = negative LR.

NS, Not significant.

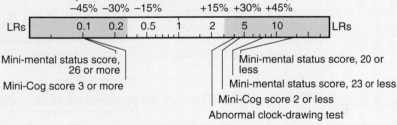

DEMENTIA
Probability

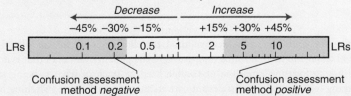

DELIRIUM
Probability

B. CLINICAL SIGNIFICANCE

As displayed in EBM Box 6.1, a Mini-Cog score of 2 or less increases the probability of dementia (LR = 4.5). A score of 3 or more decreases probability of dementia (LR = 0.1).

IV. Mini-Mental Status Examination (MMSE)

A. INTRODUCTION

The MMSE was introduced by Folstein in 1975 as an 11-part bedside test requiring only 5 to 10 minutes to administer, a much briefer time compared to the 1 to 2 hours required by more formal tests of dementia.[45] The 30-point test combines questions addressing the patient's orientation, registration, recall, and language. Historically the MMSE has been widely distributed, but now its use is copyrighted and the test may be administered free of charge only from memory, by consultation of the original paper, or by using forms sold by the copyright owner.[46]

B. CLINICAL SIGNIFICANCE

EBM Box 6.1 illustrates that, assuming there is no evidence of delirium (see section on diagnosis of delirium), a MMSE score of 23 or less increases the probability of dementia (LR = 7.8) whereas a score 24 to 30 decreases it (LR = 0.2). Nonetheless, because false-positive results become a concern when applying this threshold to large populations with a low incidence of dementia (such as elderly persons living independently), some experts prefer interpreting the MMSE score in 3 ranges (see EBM Box 6.1): a score of 20 or less rules-in dementia (LR = 14.4); one of 26 or more rules-out dementia (LR = 0.1); and scores 21 to 25 are regarded as less conclusive (LR = 2.1), thus prompting further investigation.

The MMSE score may be used to follow patients over time, but only changes of 4 points or more reliably indicate a change of cognition.[47] The level of the patient's education also affects the MMSE score, regardless of the presence of dementia,[19,48] and some have suggested adjusting the threshold for a positive test downward slightly in more poorly educated persons.[19]

V. Diagnosis of Delirium (Confusion Assessment Method)

Delirium is an acute and reversible confusional state that affects up to 50% of elderly patients hospitalized with acute medical illnesses.[49] Of the several screening tools available to diagnose delirium, one simple and well-investigated one is the confusion assessment method.[33]

A. SCORING

When administering the confusion assessment method, the clinician looks for the following four clinical features: (1) change in mental status (compared to the patient's baseline) that is *acute* and *fluctuating*; (2) difficulty focusing attention or trouble keeping track of what is being said; (3) disorganized thinking (e.g., rambling or irrelevant conversation, unpredictable switching between subjects, illogical flow of ideas), and (4) altered level of consciousness (e.g., lethargic, stuporous, or hyperalert).

A positive test requires both features (1) and (2) *and* either (3) or (4).

B. CLINICAL SIGNIFICANCE

As illustrated in EBM Box 6.1, a positive test argues strongly *for* delirium (LR = 11.5) and a negative test argues *against* delirium (LR = 0.2). This test has been adapted with similar accuracy to mechanically ventilated patients who cannot talk[50] and to patients in emergency departments.[51] In any patient with delirium, positive bedside tests for *dementia* are inaccurate because of a high false-positive rate.

References may be accessed online at *Elsevier eBooks for Practicing Clinicians.*

Stance and Gait

- Observation of the patient's gait helps diagnose important neurologic and musculoskeletal problems and allows clinicians to predict the patient's risk of falls.
- Gait abnormalities may be symmetric or asymmetric. Pain, immobile joints, and muscle weakness cause *asymmetric* gaits. Rigidity, proprioceptive disorders, cerebellar diseases, and problems with central control all cause *symmetric* gaits. Spasticity may cause asymmetric gait abnormalities (i.e., hemiplegia) or symmetric ones (i.e., paraplegia).
- Simple observation may result in prompt diagnosis. Examples include the *lateral lurch* of hip disease, the *backward lean* of gluteus maximus weakness, the *Trendelenburg gait* of gluteus medius weakness (often after hip replacement), the *steppage gait* and *foot slap* of foot drop, the *leg circumduction* of hemiplegia, and the *shuffling steps with narrow base and flexed posture* of Parkinson disease.
- Gait abnormalities are prominent in Lewy body dementia and vascular dementia but are uncommon in Alzheimer dementia until late in its course.
- The timed-up-and-go test, stops-talking-when-walking test, and observation of the patient's ability to stand with feet together for 10 seconds all accurately assess the elderly patient's risk of falls.

I. Introduction

Observation of gait not only uncovers important neurologic and musculoskeletal problems (e.g., Parkinson disease, hemiparesis, spinal stenosis, hip disease), but it also provides clues to the patient's emotions, overall function, and even prognosis. For example, the speed of an elderly person's gait accurately predicts falls, future disability, and risk of institutionalization.[1–4] In patients with congestive heart failure, gait speed predicts cardiac index, future hospitalization, and mortality as well as the ejection fraction and better than the treadmill test.[5,6] Even depressed patients have a characteristic gait, marked by an abnormally short stride and weak lift-off of the heel.[7]

The phases of the normal gait are depicted in Fig. 7.1.

II. Etiology of Gait Disorders

Among patients presenting to neurologists, the most common causes of gait disorder are stroke and Parkinson disease, followed by frontal gait disorder, myelopathy (e.g., cervical spondylosis, B$_{12}$ deficiency), peripheral neuropathy, and cerebellar disease.[8,9] Among patients presenting to general clinicians, most gait abnormalities are caused by arthritis, followed by orthostatic hypotension, stroke, Parkinson disease, and intermittent claudication.[10]

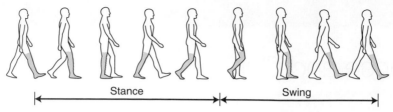

| ◄─────────── Stance ───────────► | ◄─────────── Swing ───────────► |

Fig. 7.1   Normal gait. This figure illustrates the phases of normal gait, focusing on the right leg (*shaded*). Normal gait consists of the *stance phase* (the period during which the leg bears weight) and *swing phase* (the period during which the leg advances and does not bear weight). The stance and swing make up the *stride*, which is the interval from the time one heel strikes the ground to when it again strikes the ground. During the normal stance phase, it is the *extensor* muscles that contract—the gluteus maximus in early stance, the quadriceps in mid stance, and the plantar flexors (soleus and gastrocnemius) in terminal stance pushing off the heel. The healthy swing, in contrast, requires contraction of the *flexor* muscles, all of which are activated early in the swing phase—hip flexors (iliopsoas muscles), knee flexors (hamstring muscles), and ankle flexors (tibialis anterior and toe extensor muscles).[11,12] Figure adapted with permission from The Pathokinesiology service and the physical therapy department of the Rancho Los Amigos Medical Center. *Observational Gait Analysis*. 4th ed. Downey, CA: Los Amigos Research and Educatio Institute, Inc.; 2001.

III. Types of Gait Disorders and Their Significance

Disorders of gait reflect one of four possible problems: pain, immobile joints, muscle weakness, or abnormal limb control. Abnormal limb control, in turn, may result from spasticity, rigidity, diminished proprioception, cerebellar disease, or problems with cerebral control.

When analyzing a patient's gait, the most important initial question is whether the gait is symmetric or asymmetric. Pain, immobile joints, and muscle weakness are usually unilateral and thus cause *asymmetric* abnormalities of gait. Rigidity, proprioceptive disorders, cerebellar diseases, and problems with central control all cause *symmetric* abnormalities of the gait. Spasticity may cause *asymmetric* gait abnormalities (hemiplegia) or *symmetric* ones (paraplegia).

A. PAINFUL GAIT (ANTALGIC GAIT)

If bearing weight on a limb is painful, patients adopt an antalgic gait to minimize the pain. (*Antalgic* is from the Greek *an* and *algesis*, meaning "against pain.") All antalgic gaits are characterized by a short contralateral step, along with other characteristic features.

1. Short Contralateral Step

After bearing weight on the affected leg, patients with pain quickly step onto the sound leg. The short contralateral step produces an uneven cadence, one identical to that produced by a rock in one shoe.

2. Other Characteristic Features

Depending on whether the pain is located in the foot, knee, or hip, each antalgic gait is distinctive, allowing diagnosis from a distance.

a. Foot Pain

In patients with foot pain, the foot contacts the ground abnormally. For example, patients may bear weight during stance on their heel only, forefoot only, or along the lateral edge of the foot.

b. Knee Pain

Patients with knee pain display a stiff knee that does not extend or flex fully during stride.[13]

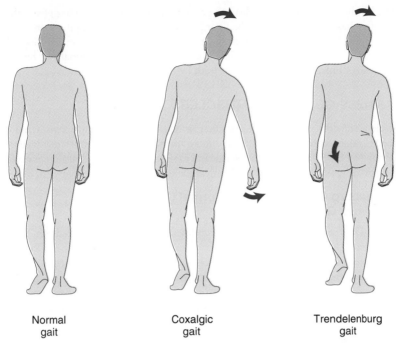

| Normal
gait | Coxalgic
gait | Trendelenburg
gait |

Fig. 7.2   Comparison of coxalgic and Trendelenburg gaits. In both abnormal gaits (*middle and right figures*), the trunk may lean over the abnormal leg during stance (*top arrow*), but in patients with hip pain (coxalgic gait, *middle figure*), the trunk lean and accompanying ipsilateral arm movement (*bottom arrow*) is more dramatic (the so-called "lateral lurch") and the opposite pelvis does not fall excessively. In the Trendelenburg gait (from ineffective or weak hip abductors, *right figure*), the opposite pelvis falls excessively (*bottom arrow*), and the conspicuous but opposing swings of the upper body and pelvis create the impression of a hinge between the sacral and lumbar spine. In these figures, the patient is bearing weight on the affected side, i.e., *right* hip pain (coxalgic gait) and ineffective *right* hip abductors (Trendelenburg gait).

c. Hip Pain (Coxalgic Gait)

Patients with hip pain limit the amount of hip extension during late stance (when the normal hip extends 20 degrees). Even so, the most characteristic feature of the coxalgic gait is the so-called **lateral lurch**: When bearing weight on the painful limb, there is an excessive asymmetric lateral shift of the patient's upper body toward the weight-bearing side, causing the trunk to lean and ipsilateral arm to abduct (Fig. 7.2).[14,15]

Lateral lurch reduces the pain of patients with hip disease because it minimizes the need to activate the ipsilateral hip abductor muscles. These muscles normally support the upper body during swing of the other leg, but when activated can easily put 400 pounds of pressure on the femoral head, an intolerable force if there is hip disease. By leaning over the painful limb during stance, patients effectively balance their center of gravity over the painful limb and thus avoid activation of the hip abductors.

B. IMMOBILE JOINTS

Most clinicians do not consider immobile joints as a cause of abnormal gait, but the condition is well known to physiatrists. A common example is plantar flexion contracture, a complication that may occur after prolonged periods of plaster immobilization or confinement to bed. Affected patients may place their weight on the forefoot during initial stance (instead of the heel) or, during mid-stance, lift their heel too early or lean their trunk forward. During swing phase, the abnormally flexed foot has difficulty clearing the floor, leading the patient to drag the foot or develop an unusual movement to clear it, such as contralateral trunk lean or contralateral vaulting.[11,12]

The clinician can easily identify immobile joints as the cause of abnormal gait by testing the range of motion of hips, knees, and ankles of both legs.

C. WEAKNESS OF SPECIFIC MUSCLES

Three muscle groups, when weak, cause specific gait abnormalities: (1) hip extensor and abductor muscles (i.e., gluteus maximus and medius/minimus muscles), (2) knee extensors (quadriceps muscle), and (3) foot and toe dorsiflexors (tibialis anterior and toe extensor muscles). The gluteus maximus and quadriceps gaits were frequently observed historically as complications of poliomyelitis or diphtheria.

1. Trendelenburg Gait and Sign (Abnormal Gluteus Medius And Minimus Gait)

a. Definition Of Trendelenburg Gait (Or Trendelenburg's Symptom; Friedrich Trendelenburg, 1844 to 1924)

The Trendelenburg gait occurs when the gluteus medius and minimus do not function properly. These two muscles abduct the hip, an action that supports the opposite pelvis and prevents it from dropping excessively during the normal single-limb stance. During walking, a slight dip of the opposite pelvis is normal during stance phase on one limb. An excessive drop of the opposite pelvis indicates an abnormal Trendelenburg gait. When the abnormality is bilateral, the pelvis waddles like that of a duck.

Like patients with the coxalgic gait (see previous section on hip pain/coxalgic gait), patients with Trendelenburg gait may lean their trunk over the abnormal leg during stance, but the lean lacks the dramatic lurch seen in coxalgic gait, and the opposing sways of the ipsilateral shoulder and opposite pelvis make it appear as if patients with Trendelenburg gait have a hinge between their sacral and lumbar spine (Fig. 7.2).[15,16]

b. Etiology of Trendelenburg Gait

Causes include (1) neuromuscular weakness of the hip abductors and (2) hip disease. Although poliomyelitis and progressive muscular atrophy were important causes historically, this gait now occurs as a complication of hip arthroplasty using a lateral approach, which risks damage to the superior gluteal nerve or gluteus medius muscle.[17] Another common cause is congenital dislocation of the hip and coxa vara (i.e., "bent hip," a deformity in which the angle between femoral neck and body is significantly decreased). In both congenital hip dislocation and coxa vara, the abnormal upward displacement of the greater trochanter shortens the fibers of the gluteus medius, rendering them more horizontal than vertical and thus abolishing their role as abductors.

c. Trendelenburg Sign

In 1895, before use of roentgenography, Friedrich Trendelenburg was the first to show that the waddling gait of patients with congenital dislocation of the hip was due to weak abductor function, not the upward movement of the femur during stance (which was what his contemporaries believed). He successfully argued this by inventing a simple test, now known as Trendelenburg sign. In this test, the patient is asked to stand on one leg with the other hip flexed to 90 degrees (the clinician may help the patient balance by supporting the ipsilateral arm to align the ipsilateral shoulder over the hip being tested).[18] In patients with normal abductor strength, the contralateral buttock rises, but if the abductor muscles are weak, the contralateral buttock falls. (The buttock falls until the ipsilateral femur and pelvis come into contact.) It is important to remember that the side being tested is the one bearing the weight. Some deformities of the leg, such as severe genu varum, may cause a false-positive result.[19]

d. Clinical Significance

In one study of patients clinical diagnosed with "trochanteric bursitis" (i.e., lateral hip pain and maximal tenderness over the greater trochanter),[20] the finding of *both* a positive Trendelenburg sign and gait on the symptomatic side accurately detected the MRI finding of a tear in the gluteus medius tendon (sensitivity = 73%, specificity = 77%, positive likelihood ratio [LR] = 3.2, negative LR not significant). This sign was superior to directly testing gluteus medius strength (by resisting the patient's active hip abduction or internal rotation, LRs not significant). The results of this study suggest that some patients with "trochanteric bursitis" actually have tendonitis or tears of gluteus medius tendon, a discovery analogous to the historic realization that many patients with "subacromial bursitis" (in the shoulder) actually have disorders of the rotator cuff tendons.

In patients with a foot drop, the presence of ipsilateral hip abductor weakness argues that the foot drop is from lumbosacral radiculopathy and not peroneal nerve palsy (see Chapter 64). In one study of patients with foot drop from various causes, ipsilateral hip abductor weakness was a compelling sign of lumbosacral radiculopathy (positive LR = 24; see Chapter 64).[21] Although hip abductor weakness in this study was identified by manual resistance testing, the abnormality is often first suspected by observing a Trendelenburg gait.

2. Gluteus Maximus Gait

If the hip extensors are weak, the patient develops a characteristic abnormal backward trunk lean during early stance, which places the patient's center of gravity behind the hip joint line and removes the need for the gluteus maximus muscle to contract (Fig. 7.3).

3. Weak Quadriceps Gait

If the knee extensors are weak, two different abnormalities of gait may appear. Some patients develop a characteristic hyperextension of the knee during stance (Fig. 7.3). At first this seems paradoxical because the normal action of the quadriceps is knee extension, which should therefore be weak in these patients. However, the main role of the quadriceps during gait is to support the flexed knee during stance, and patients with weak quadriceps avoid bearing weight on a flexed knee by hyperextending the joint (i.e., genu recurvatum). They can fully extend the knee because their hip flexes strongly during swing and then decelerates abruptly, which whips the tibia forward.[9] Alternatively, other patients with weak quadriceps may place their hand just above the knee to support the weak leg and prevent the knee from buckling during stance (Fig. 7.3). Most patients with weak quadriceps muscles have great difficulty walking on uneven ground.

4. Foot Drop (Weak Tibialis Anterior and Toe Extensor Muscles)

There are two characteristic features: (1) "foot slap," which is the uncontrolled slap of the forefoot immediately after the heel makes contact, thus producing (in patients with *unilateral* foot drop) a characteristic cadence of two sounds alternating with a single sound (i.e., stance of abnormal foot alternating with that of normal foot): "dada…da….dada….da"; and (2) "steppage gait," which occurs during the forward swinging phase of the affected foot, when the patient flexes the hip and knee excessively in order to clear the foot from the ground (thus creating the appearance of the abnormal foot "stepping over" an invisible object (Fig. 7.3).[8]

D. SPASTICITY

Spasticity is a feature of weakness of the upper motor neuron type (see Chapter 61). Characteristic gaits are the hemiplegic gait and diplegic (paraplegic) gait.

1. Hemiplegic Gait

This gait is the result of poor control of the flexor muscles during swing phase and spasticity of the extensor muscles acting to lengthen the affected leg (compared to the healthy side). The ankle

Weak gluteus maximus gait

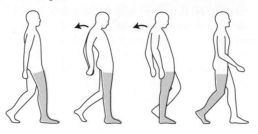

Weak quadriceps gait

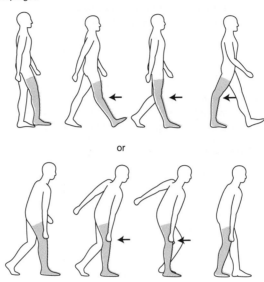

or

Footdrop gait

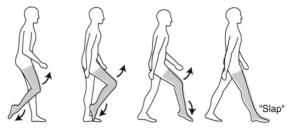

"Slap"

Fig. 7.3　Characteristic gaits of weak muscles. In each figure, the *shading* indicates the limb with the weak muscle and the *black arrows* indicate the diagnostic movements. Because both the gluteus maximus and quadriceps muscles are *extensor* muscles, abnormalities of these muscles produce characteristic findings during the *stance* phase. Because the foot dorsiflexors (i.e., the weak muscles causing foot drop) are *flexor* muscles, abnormalities produce characteristic findings during the *swing* phase. In the weak gluteus maximus gait (*top row*), there is an abnormal backward lean during stance. In the weak quadriceps gait (*middle rows*), patients may hyperextend their knee during stance (i.e., genu recurvatum, *second row*) or place their ipsilateral arm on the leg to prevent the knee from buckling (*third* row). In the foot drop gait (*bottom row*), the actual foot weakness is conspicuous (*bottom arrows*), and there is excessive flexion of the hip and knee during the swing phase (*upper arrow*) and a slapping sound of the foot when it strikes the ground.

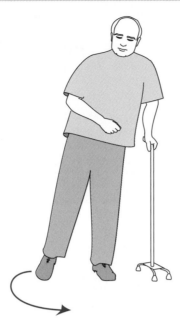

Fig. 7.4   Hemiplegic gait. In a patient with right hemiparesis, the paretic arm is flexed and paretic leg is hyperextended. In order to clear the extended right leg from the floor, the patient leans over the healthy left leg and slowly advances the stiffened, paralyzed right leg with a circumducting movement (*arrow*).

is abnormally flexed downward and inward (equinovarus deformity), and initial contact during stance is abnormal, along the lateral edge of the foot or forefoot. The knee is stiff, hyperextends during stance, and does not flex normally during swing. The contralateral step often advances just to meet the position of the paralyzed limb, instead of advancing normally beyond it.

Because the paralyzed leg is hyperextended, and therefore longer than the sound leg, the patient may drag the toe of the affected leg during swing or adopt abnormal movements to clear that limb during the swing phase. These movements include contralateral trunk lean, which raises the ipsilateral pelvis to clear the paralyzed leg, and circumduction, an abnormal movement in which the toe traces a semicircle on the floor, first moving outward and then inward as it advances, instead of the normal straightforward movement (Fig. 7.4).

According to classic teachings, the clinician should suspect mild hemiplegia if a patient swings his or her arms asymmetrically while walking, although this finding appears in 11% to 70% of normal persons[22,23] and the sign did not accurately detect focal cerebral disease in one study (sensitivity 22%, specificity 89%, positive and negative LRs not significant).[22]

2. Diplegic Gait

Diplegic gait affects patients with spinal cord disease (e.g., spinal cord trauma, cervical spondylosis, B_{12} deficiency). The combinations of spasticity and abnormal proprioception cause a characteristic slow, laborious, and stiff-legged gait. In some spastic diplegias of childhood, adductor spasm causes the feet to cross in front of each other (scissors gait).

E. RIGIDITY

Chapter 61 describes the characteristic features of rigidity and distinguishes it from spasticity. The most common gait abnormality due to rigidity is the parkinsonian gait.

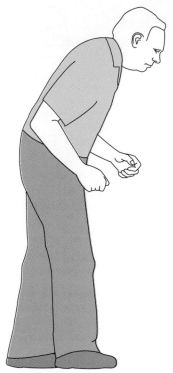

Fig. 7.5   **Parkinsonian gait.** The characteristic features are flexed posture (trunk, neck, and arms), diminished arm swing, narrow-based gait, and shuffling steps.

1. The Parkinsonian Gait (Fig. 7.5)

The characteristic features are (1) flexed posture of the arms, hips, trunk, and neck; (2) rigidity of movement (en bloc turning, difficulty initiating gait); (3) steps that are flat-footed, small, shuffling, with a narrow base; (4) diminished arm swing (normal arm excursion, measured at the wrist, averages 16 inches; the average value for patients with Parkinson disease is 5 inches); (5) involuntary hastening of gait (festination); and (6) poor postural control (retropulsion).

2. Differential diagnosis

Patients with spinal stenosis superficially resemble those with Parkinson disease in that they have a flexed stance (simian stance), which reduces the tension on the lumbosacral nerves.[24] Patients with spinal stenosis, however, complain of pain and otherwise have a normal gait.

The distinguishing features of the frontal gait disorder, which also may superficially resemble the parkinsonian gait, are discussed later in the section on Frontal Gait Disorder.

3. Clinical Significance

Patients presenting with parkinsonism (i.e., bradykinesia in combination with rigidity, resting tremor, or both) have either Parkinson disease (a disorder from pathologic depigmentation of the substantia nigra that responds to levodopa) or a group of mimicking disorders called Parkinson-plus syndromes (disorders with distinct pathologic findings that respond less well to levodopa; e.g., progressive supranuclear palsy and multiple system atrophy, see Chapter 66).

The gait of patients with Parkinson disease has a narrower base than the gait of patients with the Parkinson-plus syndromes, suggesting that Parkinson-plus patients may have greater instability during tandem gait. In clinical studies of patients *with parkinsonism*, the ability to successfully walk 10 tandem steps without errors thus increases probability of Parkinson disease (LR = 4.6, EBM Box 7.1); inability to complete 10 tandem steps, in contrast, increases probability of a Parkinson-plus syndrome (LR = 4.9) (see Chapter 66).

F. ATAXIA

The characteristic features of the ataxic gait are its wide base and the irregular, uneven, and sometimes staggering steps (the normal base, measured when one limb swings past the other at mid-stance, is 2 to 4 inches). There are two types of ataxia, sensory ataxia and cerebellar ataxia.

EBM BOX 7.1   **Gait Abnormalities, in Patients with Parkinsonism or Dementia***

Finding (Reference)[†]	Sensitivity (%)	Specificity (%)	Likelihood Ratio[‡] if Finding Is Present	Absent
Detecting Parkinson disease, in patients with parkinsonism				
Able to perform 10 perfect tandem steps[25-27]	67–92	77–91	4.6	0.2
Detecting type of dementia[§]				
Any gait or balance disorder (moderate or worse), detecting Alzheimer dementia [28]	16	25	0.2	3.4
Parkinsonian gait, detecting Lewy body dementia or Parkinson disease with dementia[28]	78	91	8.8	0.2
Frontal gait, detecting vascular dementia[28]	56	91	6.1	0.5

*Diagnostic standard: for *Parkinson-plus disorder*, the conventional diagnostic criteria for multiple system atrophy, progressive supranuclear palsy, Lewy body dementia, corticobasal degeneration, or vascular dementia[25-27]; for *Alzheimer dementia*, conventional diagnostic criteria.
[†]Definition of findings: for *unable to perform tandem gait*, the patient was instructed to take 10 consecutive tandem steps along a straight line without walking aids and support, with eyes open. One or more observed side steps indicates a positive test.[25]
[‡]Likelihood ratio (LR) if finding present = positive LR; LR if finding absent = negative LR.
[§]All patients have dementia.

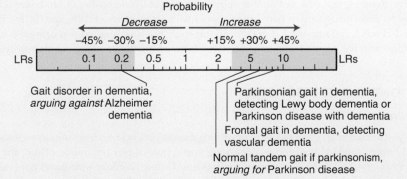

GAIT IN PARKINSONISM OR DEMENTIA
Probability

Decrease   *Increase*

−45% −30% −15%   +15% +30% +45%

LRs   0.1   0.2   0.5   1   2   5   10   LRs

Gait disorder in dementia, *arguing against* Alzheimer dementia

Parkinsonian gait in dementia, detecting Lewy body dementia or Parkinson disease with dementia

Frontal gait in dementia, detecting vascular dementia

Normal tandem gait if parkinsonism, *arguing for* Parkinson disease

1. Sensory Ataxia

Sensory ataxia affects patients with significant proprioceptive loss (see Chapter 62). Characteristically, the patient looks down and walks as if throwing his feet, which tend to slap on the ground. Smooth, familiar routes cause less trouble than uneven, rough ones.

2. Cerebellar Ataxia

Affected patients place their feet too far apart or too close together irregularly, and they sway, stagger, and reel in all directions as if intoxicated by alcohol. In contrast to sensory ataxia, patients with cerebellar ataxia have other cerebellar signs, including dysmetria, hypotonia, intention tremor, dysarthria, and nystagmus (see Chapter 65).

3. Romberg Sign

a. Introduction

In his famous textbook, written between 1840 and 1846, Moritz Romberg described the sign now bearing his name as a finding in patients with severe sensory ataxia from syphilitic damage to the dorsal columns of the spinal cord (tabes dorsalis). According to Romberg, when a patient with tabes dorsalis stands and closes his eyes, "he immediately begin to move from side to side, and the oscillations soon attain such a pitch that unless supported, he falls to the ground."[29] Most authors claim that Romberg sign is negative in patients with cerebellar ataxia, although Romberg did not make this claim (cerebellar disease was not defined during his time; Duchenne and Babinski later added this diagnostic point).[30]

b. Definition of a Positive Romberg Sign

One problem with Romberg sign is that various authors define the positive test differently: some state that it is the increased swaying that occurs when the eyes close, while others require the patient to be on the verge of falling down.[29] Increased swaying alone seems inadequate, because most normal persons sway more when they close their eyes, as do patients with vestibular, cerebellar, and Parkinson disease.[31]

The best definition of a positive Romberg sign is inability to stand for 60 seconds with feet together and eyes closed. In one study, every healthy person and over half of the patients with cerebellar ataxia could maintain this position for 60 seconds, whereas half of the patients with sensory ataxia lasted only 10 seconds before beginning to topple over.[32]

A related sign, the sharpened Romberg sign,[33] in which patients must stand with one foot in front of the other with eyes closed, has little proven diagnostic value. Many normal persons, especially elderly ones, are unable to stand like this for very long.[32]

c. Romberg Test and Back Pain

In one study of 93 patients with chronic back pain (mean duration of 37 months), the finding of a positive Romberg test detected lumbar spinal stenosis (i.e., compression of lumbosacral nerve roots by an abnormally narrow bony spinal canal) with a sensitivity of 39%, specificity of 91%, positive LR = 4.3, and negative LR of 0.7.[34] In this study, the Romberg test was defined as inability to stand with feet together and eyes closed for 10 seconds without taking compensatory steps.

G. FRONTAL GAIT DISORDER

1. Definition

Frontal gait disorder is an imprecise term describing a combination of findings seen in patients with cerebral tumors, subdural hematomas, dementing illness, normal pressure hydrocephalus, and multiple lacunar infarcts.[35,36] The characteristic findings are (1) slow, shuffling, wide-based gait (*marche a petis pas*); (2) hesitation in starting to walk (ignition failure); (3) difficulty picking feet off the floor (magnetic foot response); and (4) poor postural control. Motor function of the legs is sometimes much better when these patients are seated or lying, suggesting an element of gait apraxia.

Some of these findings resemble parkinsonism, but the distinguishing features of the frontal gait disorder are its wide base, normal arm swing, absence of other parkinsonian features, more upright posture, and higher incidence of dementia and urinary incontinence.

2. Clinical Significance

In studies of elderly patients undergoing computed tomography (CT) of the head because of neurologic symptoms, the finding of a frontal gait disorder correlates strongly with the CT finding of ventricular enlargement.[9,37,38] Only a minority of these patients, however, meet the criteria for normal pressure hydrocephalus, suggesting that the findings of ventricular enlargement and gait disturbance are general ones occurring in many different forebrain disorders.[9,37]

Analysis of gait assists diagnosis of patients with dementia. The presence of a gait disturbance makes Alzheimer disease less likely (especially if the gait disturbance appears early during the patient's course; LR = 0.2, EBM Box 7.1); a parkinsonian gait in patients with dementia increases the probability of Lewy body dementia or Parkinson disease with dementia (LR = 8.8), and a frontal gait increases probability of vascular dementia (LR = 6.1).

IV. Evaluation of Gait Disorders

The methods of evaluating gait range from very simple tests that require minutes to complete (e.g., assessing the fall risk in elderly patients) to comprehensive observational gait analysis, which physiatrists use to break down complicated gait abnormalities into smaller components to direct treatment.[12] Most clinicians adopt an intermediate approach and ask the patient first to walk back and forth several strides at a time, and then again on the toes, heels, and using tandem steps, all maneuvers that may bring out weak muscles or difficulties with balance.

Testing gait is essential, whatever the method, because patients often appear normal during conventional tests of motor, sensory, musculoskeletal, and visual function, yet, when asked to stand and walk, demonstrate abnormal balance and gait.[39]

A. OBSERVATIONAL GAIT ANALYSIS[11,12]

Using this method, the clinician focuses on one limb at a time as the patient walks, first observing the ankle, then the knee, hip, pelvis, and trunk. At each joint, the clinician considers each of the four fundamental ingredients of abnormal gait: pain, immobile joints, muscle weakness, and abnormal limb control.

As an example, the differential diagnosis of "abnormal ipsilateral trunk lean during stance" includes ipsilateral hip pain, ipsilateral short limb (>1.5 inches shorter), or intentional attempts to clear the contralateral limb during swing (e.g., drop foot or extended limb). Or, "dragging of the foot or toe during swing" may occur because of weak ipsilateral ankle dorsiflexor muscles, ipsilateral plantar flexion contractures, inadequate ipsilateral hip or knee flexion, or impaired proprioception. An excellent manual of observational gait analysis by the Rancho Los Amigos Medical Center has been published.[14]

B. PREDICTING FALLS

Thirty percent of persons over the age of 65 living in the community fall each year.[4] Of the many brief tests designed to identify patients at higher risk for falls, the best studied are "stops walking when talking" and "timed up-and-go" tests. In studies of these tests, the history of a prior fall during the previous year predicts another fall in the next 6 to 12 months, with a sensitivity of 20% to 62%, specificity of 71% to 93%, and positive LR of = 2.4.[4,40,41]

1. The Findings

a. Stops Walking When Talking

The premise behind this test is that elderly patients at risk for falls have difficulty completing separate tasks simultaneously. To perform the test, the patient is accompanied while walking and then observed what happens when the examiner initiates conversation. If the patient stops walking when talking, the test is positive.

b. Timed Up-and-Go Test[3]

The clinician measures the time it takes the patient to rise from a standard chair, walk to a line on the floor 3 meters away, turn, return, and sit down again. They are instructed to walk at normal speed and are allowed one trial before timing. The timing starts when the patient's back comes off the chair and ends when their buttocks touch the seat of the chair.

2. Clinical Significance

According to the LRs presented in EBM Box 7.2, the most compelling findings increasing a patient's risk of falls are failure to stand with feet together and eyes open for 10 seconds

---

EBM BOX 7.2	**Predicting Falls[a]**				
				Likelihood Ratio[‡] if Finding Is	
Finding (Reference)[†]		**Sensitivity (%)**	**Specificity (%)**	**Present**	**Absent**
Neurologic Examination					
Palmomental reflex present[4]		31	89	2.8	0.8
Failure to stand with feet together and eyes open for 10 seconds [40]		4	99	**4.5**	NS
Failure to tandem walk (>2 errors) [40]		53	70	1.7	0.7
Special Tests					
Stops walking when talking[2,42–44]		14–53	70–97	**3.0**	NS
Timed-up-and-go test[41]					
	<15 sec	4	67	**0.1**	...
	15–35 sec	60	...	NS	...
	≥35 sec	36	86	2.6	...

*Diagnostic standard: for *falls*, ≥1 fall during 6 month follow-up[2,41–44] or 12 month follow-up.[4,40,42]
†Definition of findings: for *palmomental reflex*, see Chapter 63; for all other tests, see text.
‡Likelihood ratio (LR) if finding present = positive LR; LR if finding absent = negative LR.
NS, not significant.

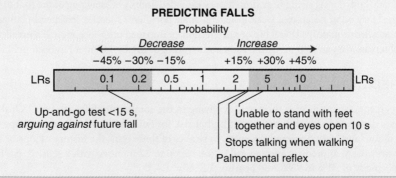

PREDICTING FALLS

Probability

(LR = 4.5), a positive "stops walking when talking" test (LR = 3), a positive palmomental reflex (LR = 2.8, see Chapter 63), and a "timed-up-and-go" test of 35 seconds or more (LR = 2.6). A timed-up-and-go test result of less than 15 seconds identifies patients at low risk of falls (LR = 0.1). The cutoff points used for the timed-up-and-go test vary greatly and likely depend on methodology and specific population studied[45]; the LRs in EBM Box 7.2 are derived from study of frail nursing home residents.

In patients with parkinsonism, a timed-up-and-go test result >16 seconds increases probability of a Parkinson-*plus* disorder (LR = 5.6) and *decreases* probability of Parkinson disease (LR = 0.2).[27] This finding is consistent with the observation that patients with Parkinson-plus disorders have more difficulty with gait and balance than those with Parkinson disease, especially early on in the course of their disease (see Parkinsonian gait above).

V. Canes

Physical examination of gait is incomplete without considering the length of the patient's cane and which arm the patient uses to hold the cane.

A. LENGTH OF CANE

Twenty-three percent to 42% of the time, the patient's cane is too long or too short by 5 cm or more.[46,47] An appropriately fitted cane should extend the distance from the distal wrist crease to the ground when the patients wear everyday shoes and dangle their arms at their sides.[48]

B. CONTRALATERAL VERSUS IPSILATERAL USE OF CANE

In patients with hip and knee arthritis, patients are conventionally taught to hold the cane in the contralateral hand, although compelling evidence for contralateral cane use exists only for patients with hip arthritis.[49,50] By placing just 20, 33, or 38 pounds of pressure on a cane contralateral to a diseased hip when standing on that hip, the patient can *reduce* the pressure on the diseased femoral head by 165, 272, or 319 pounds, respectively.[49]

References may be accessed online at *Elsevier eBooks for Practicing Clinicians*.

Jaundice

I. Introduction

Jaundice is an abnormal yellowish discoloration of the skin and mucous membranes caused by accumulation of bile pigment. There are three forms: (1) hemolytic jaundice (due to increased bilirubin production from excessive breakdown of red cells), (2) hepatocellular jaundice (due to disease of the liver parenchyma, e.g., alcoholic liver disease, drug-induced liver disease, viral hepatitis, or metastatic carcinoma), and (3) obstructive jaundice (due to mechanical obstruction of the biliary ducts outside the liver, e.g., choledocholithiasis or pancreatic carcinoma). In most published series of jaundiced patients, hemolysis is uncommon, and the usual task of the clinician at the bedside is to distinguish hepatocellular disease from obstructed biliary ducts.[1,2]

II. The Findings

A. JAUNDICE

Jaundice is usually first noted in the eyes, but the traditional term for this finding (scleral icterus) is actually a misnomer because pathologic studies reveal most of the pigment to be deposited in the conjunctiva, not the avascular sclera.[3] As jaundice progresses and the serum bilirubin increases, the face, mucous membranes, and eventually the entire skin acquire a yellow or orange hue.

Prominent yellowish subconjunctival fat may be mistaken for conjunctival jaundice, but fat is usually limited to the conjunctival folds and, unlike jaundice, spares the area near the cornea. Patients with carotenemia (from excess carrot or multivitamin ingestion) also develop a yellowish discoloration of the skin, especially the palms, soles, and nasolabial fold, but in contrast to jaundice the conjunctiva are spared.[4]

B. ASSOCIATED FINDINGS

According to classic teachings, several findings distinguish hepatocellular disease from obstructed biliary ducts.

1. Hepatocellular Jaundice

Characteristic findings are spider telangiectasia, palmar erythema, gynecomastia, dilated abdominal wall veins, splenomegaly, asterixis, and fetor hepaticus.

a. Spider Telangiectasia (Spider Angiomas)

Spider telangiectasia are dilated cutaneous blood vessels with three components: (1) a central arteriole (the "body" of the spider) that can be seen to pulsate when compressed slightly with a glass slide; (2) multiple radiating "legs"; and (3) surrounding erythema, which may encompass the entire lesion or only its central portion.[5] After blanching, the returning blood fills the central arteriole first before traveling to the peripheral tips of each leg. Spiders are most numerous on the face and neck, followed by the shoulders, thorax, arms, and hands. They are rare on the palms, scalp, and below the umbilicus.[5] This peculiar distribution may reflect the neurohormonal properties of the microcirculation, because it is similar to the distribution of where blushing is most intense.[5]

Acquired vascular spiders are associated with three clinical conditions: liver disease, pregnancy, and malnutrition.[6] In patients with liver disease, the spiders advance and regress with disease severity,[7] and their appearance correlates somewhat with an abnormally increased ratio of serum estradiol to testosterone levels.[8] In pregnant women, spiders typically appear between the second and fifth months and usually disappear within days after delivery.[6] Vascular spiders also have been described in normal persons, but these lesions, in contrast to those of liver disease, are always small in number (average, three) and size.[5]

Vascular spiders were first described by the English physician Erasmus Wilson in 1867.[5]

b. Palmar Erythema

Palmar erythema is a symmetric reddening of the surfaces of the palms, most pronounced over the hypothenar and thenar eminences.[6] Palmar erythema occurs in the same clinical conditions as vascular spiders, and the two lesions tend to come and go together.[6]

c. Gynecomastia and Diminished Body Hair

Many patients with liver disease have gynecomastia (defined as a palpable, discrete button of firm subareolar breast tissue 2 or more cm in diameter) and diminished pubic and body hair, both findings attributed to increased circulating estrogen-to-testosterone levels.

d. Dilated Abdominal Veins

In some patients with cirrhosis, elevated portal venous pressures lead to the development of collateral vessels from the portal venous to systemic venous systems. One group of such vessels surrounds the umbilicus, decompressing the left portal vein via paraumbilical vessels into abdominal wall veins.[9] Sometimes these abdominal wall veins become so conspicuous they resemble a cluster of serpents, thus explaining their common label *caput medusae*.[10] Collateral vessels may generate a continuous humming murmur heard during auscultation between the xiphoid and umbilicus.[11]

Collateral abdominal vessels also may appear in patients with the superior vena cava syndrome (if the obstruction also involves the azygous system)[12] or inferior vena cava syndrome.[13] In these disorders, however, the vessels tend to appear on the lateral abdominal wall. A traditional test to distinguish inferior vena cava obstruction from portal hypertension is to strip abdominal wall veins below the umbilicus and see which way blood is flowing. (In portal-systemic collaterals, blood should flow away from the umbilicus towards the patient's feet, whereas in inferior vena cava collaterals, flow is reversed and toward the head.) Even so, this test is unreliable because most dilated abdominal vessels lack competent valves, and the clinician can "demonstrate" blood to flow in either direction in most patients with both conditions.

e. Palpable Spleen

One of the principal causes of splenomegaly is portal hypertension from severe hepatocellular disease.[14] Therefore, a traditional teaching is that the finding of splenomegaly in a jaundiced patient increases the probability of hepatocellular disease.

f. Asterixis

Originally described by Adams and Foley in 1949,[15,16] asterixis is one of the earliest findings of hepatic encephalopathy and is thus a finding typical of hepatocellular jaundice. To elicit the sign, the patient holds both arms outstretched with fingers spread apart. After a short latent period, both fingers and hands commence to "flap," with abrupt movements occurring at irregular intervals of a fraction of a second to seconds (thus earning the name *liver flap*). The fundamental problem in asterixis is the inability to maintain a fixed posture (the word *asterixis* comes from the Greek *sterigma*, meaning "to support"), and consequently asterixis can also be demonstrated by having the patient elevate the leg and dorsiflex the foot, close the eyelids forcibly, or protrude the tongue.[15] Because some voluntary contraction of the muscles is necessary to elicit asterixis, the sign disappears once coma ensues (although some comatose patients exhibit the finding during the grasp reflex; see Chapter 63).[15]

Electromyography reveals that asterixis represents the abrupt disappearance of electrical activity in the muscle (i.e., negative myoclonus).[17] Asterixis is not specific to liver disease but also appears in encephalopathy from other causes, such as hypercapnia or uremia.[18] Unilateral asterixis indicates structural disease in the contralateral brain.[19,20]

g. Fetor Hepaticus

Fetor hepaticus is the characteristic breath of patients with severe hepatic parenchymal disease, an odor likened to a mixture of rotten eggs and garlic. Gas chromatography reveals that the principal compound causing the odor is dimethylsulphide.[21] Fetor hepaticus correlates best with severe portal-systemic shunting, not encephalopathy per se, because even alert patients with severe portal-systemic shunting may have the characteristic breath.[22]

2. Obstructive Jaundice: Palpable Gallbladder (Courvoisier Sign)

The presence of a smooth, nontender, distended gallbladder in a patient with jaundice is a traditional sign of obstructive jaundice. Courvoisier sign refers to the association of the palpable gallbladder and extrahepatic obstruction, a sign discussed fully in Chapter 51.

III. Clinical Significance

A. DETECTION OF JAUNDICE

Although many textbooks claim jaundice becomes evident once the serum bilirubin exceeds 2.5 to 3 mg/dL, clinical studies reveal that only 70% to 80% of observers detect jaundice at this threshold.[23,24] The sensitivity of examination increases to 83% when bilirubin exceeds 10 mg/dL and 96% when it exceeds 15 mg/dL.

B. HEPATOCELLULAR VERSUS OBSTRUCTIVE JAUNDICE

Studies show that clinicians accurately distinguish hepatocellular from obstructive jaundice more than 80% of the time by just using bedside and basic laboratory findings (i.e., before

EBM BOX 8.1	Diagnosing Hepatocellular Disease in Patients with Jaundice*			
Finding (Reference)[†]	Sensitivity (%)	Specificity (%)	Likelihood Ratio[‡] if Finding Is	
			Present	Absent
General appearance				
Weight loss[25,27]	10–49	21–97	NS	NS
Skin				
Spider angiomas[25,27]	35–47	88–97	**4.7**	0.6
Palmar erythema[25]	49	95	**9.8**	0.5
Dilated abdominal veins[25]	42	98	**17.5**	0.6
Abdomen				
Ascites[25]	44	90	**4.4**	0.6
Palpable spleen[25,27]	29–47	83–90	2.9	0.7
Palpable gallbladder[25]	0[†]	69	**0.04**	1.4
Palpable liver[25,27]	71–83	15–17	NS	NS
Liver tenderness[25,27]	37–38	70–78	NS	NS

*Diagnostic standard: for *nonobstructive (vs. obstructive) jaundice*, needle biopsy of liver, surgical exploration, or autopsy.

[†]None of the 41 patients with medical jaundice in this study had a palpable gallbladder; for calculation of the likelihood ratios (LRs), 0.5 was added to all cells of the 2 × 2 table.

[‡]LR if finding present = positive LR; LR if finding absent = negative LR. *NS*, not significant.

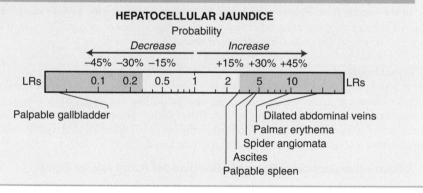

HEPATOCELLULAR JAUNDICE

clinical imaging).[25,26] In EBM Box 8.1, *disease* is arbitrarily defined as hepatocellular disease: therefore, likelihood ratios (LRs) with large positive values *increase* the probability of hepatocellular disease, whereas those with values close to zero decrease it and thus *increase* probability for obstructive disease.

These studies show that in patients presenting with jaundice, the physical signs of portal hypertension (dilated abdominal veins, LR = 17.5; ascites, LR = 4.4; and palpable spleen, LR = 2.9), palmar erythema (LR = 9.8), and spider angiomas (LR = 4.7) all increase probability of hepatocellular jaundice. The only finding arguing strongly *against* hepatocellular jaundice is the palpable gallbladder (LR = 0.04; in other words, the finding of a palpable gallbladder argues *for* obstructed bile ducts with an LR of 26, the inverse of 0.04).

Weight loss does not discriminate well between hepatocellular and obstructive etiologies. Other unhelpful signs are liver tenderness and a palpable liver. The palpable liver remains unhelpful even when defined as a liver edge extending more than four to five fingerbreaths below the right costal margin.[25]

| EBM BOX 8.2 | **Diagnosing Cirrhosis in Patients with Chronic Liver Disease*** |

Finding (Reference)†	Sensitivity (%)	Specificity (%)	Likelihood Ratio‡ if Finding Is Present	Absent
Skin				
Spider angiomas[28-39]	33–84	48–98	4.2	0.5
Palmar erythema[29,31,32,34,37,39]	12–70	49–98	3.7	0.6
Gynecomastia[29,37]	18–58	92–97	7.0	NS
Reduction of body or pubic hair[29,37]	24–51	94–97	8.8	NS
Jaundice[29,33,35,37,40]	16–44	83–99	3.8	0.8
Dilated abdominal wall veins[29,34,37]	9–51	79–100	9.5	NS
Abdomen				
Hepatomegaly[29,32-36,38,41]	31–96	20–96	2.3	0.6
Palpable liver in epigastrium[35,38]	50–86	68–88	2.7	0.3
Liver edge firm to palpation[32,41,42]	71–78	71–90	3.3	0.4
Splenomegaly[28,30-36,38,40,41]	5–85	35–100	2.5	0.8
Ascites[28,29,31,33-35,40]	14–52	82–99	6.6	0.8
Other				
Peripheral edema[29,33,34]	24–56	87–92	3.0	0.7
Encephalopathy[28,29,31]	9–29	98–99	8.8	NS

*Diagnostic standard: for *cirrhosis*, needle biopsy of liver.
†Definition of findings: for *hepatomegaly* and *splenomegaly*, examining clinician's impression using palpation, percussion, or both; *encephalopathy*, disordered consciousness and asterixis.[15]
‡Likelihood ratio (LR) if finding present = positive LR; LR if finding absent = negative LR.

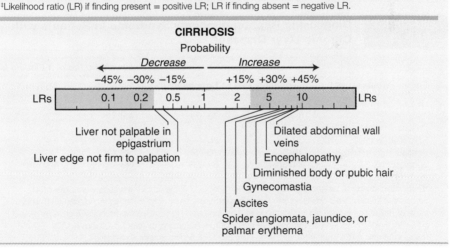

C. DIAGNOSIS OF CIRRHOSIS

The diagnosis of cirrhosis in patients with liver disease has important prognostic and therapeutic implications. EBM Box 8.2 displays the diagnostic accuracy of physical findings in detecting cirrhosis, determined from hundreds of patients presenting with diverse chronic liver diseases. According to this EBM Box, the findings increasing the probability of cirrhosis the most are dilated abdominal wall veins (LR = 9.5) encephalopathy (irrational behavior, disordered consciousness, or asterixis; LR = 8.8), reduced body or pubic hair (LR = 8.8), gynecomastia (LR = 7), ascites (LR = 6.6), spider angiomas (LR = 4.2), jaundice (LR = 3.8), palmar erythema (LR = 3.7), a liver edge that is firm to palpation (LR = 3.3), and peripheral edema (LR = 3). Other helpful findings (though less compelling ones) are a palpable liver in the epigastrium (LR = 2.7), and splenomegaly (LR = 2.5). The only findings decreasing the probability of cirrhosis in these patients are *absence* of a palpable liver in the epigastrium (LR = 0.3) and *absence* of a firm liver edge (LR = 0.4).

D. DETECTING LARGE GASTROESOPHAGEAL VARICES IN PATIENTS WITH CIRRHOSIS

In studies of more than 750 patients with cirrhosis who have not had prior gastrointestinal bleeding, no physical finding reliably predicts which patients have significant gastroesophageal varices (as detected by endoscopy). For all findings—caput medusae, spider angiomas, jaundice, hepatomegaly, splenomegaly, or hepatic encephalopathy—the LRs are 1.5 or less or not significant.[43-47]

E. DETECTING HEPATOPULMONARY SYNDROME

Hepatopulmonary syndrome is a serious complication of cirrhosis causing intrapulmonary vascular shunting and significant hypoxemia. In 12 studies of more than 1000 patients with cirrhosis, most of them awaiting liver transplantation, the findings of cyanosis (LR = 4.4) and finger clubbing (LR = 4.3) increased probability of hepatopulmonary syndrome (EBM Box 8.3). In these patients, the symptom of dyspnea also increases probability (LR = 3.3), whereas the symptom of platypnea greatly increases probability of hepatopulmonary syndrome (LR = 10.6).[55] (Platypnea

EBM BOX 8.3	Diagnosing Hepatopulmonary Syndrome in Patients with Chronic Liver Disease*			
			Likelihood Ratio[†] if Finding Is	
Finding (Reference)	Sensitivity (%)	Specificity (%)	Present	Absent
Clubbing[48-56]	12–91	64–96	4.3	0.6
Cyanosis[48,49,53,55-58]	8–87	75–99	4.4	0.7
Palmar erythema[48,55,59]	31–80	54–78	1.7	NS
Spider angioma[48-53,55,56,59]	39–97	26–87	2.1	0.4
Ascites[50-52,54,55,57]	49–94	20–57	NS	NS
Jaundice[55,57]	24–38	64–77	NS	NS

*Diagnostic standard: for *hepatopulmonary syndrome*, all 3 of the following criteria were present: (1) cirrhosis, (2) contrast echocardiography revealing intrapulmonary right-to-left shunting, and (3) hypoxemia, variably defined as arterial pO_2 < 70 mm Hg[56,59] or < 80 mm Hg[48,52], alveolar-arterial pO_2 gradient (AapO$_2$) ≥15 mm Hg[51,53-55,57,58]; or >20 mm Hg,[49] or *either* pO_2 < 70 mm Hg or AapO$_2$ >20 mm Hg.[50]
[†]Likelihood ratio (LR) if finding present = positive LR; LR if finding absent = negative LR.
NS, Not significant.

HEPATOPULMONARY SYNDROME
Probability

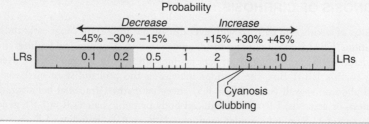

EBM BOX 8.4 — Diagnosing Pulmonary Hypertension in Patients with Cirrhosis*

Finding[60]	Sensitivity (%)	Specificity (%)	Likelihood Ratio[†] if Finding Is	
			Present	Absent
Vital signs				
Blood pressure ≥ 140/90	63	91	7.3	NS
Oxygen saturation < 92%	25	89	NS	NS
Heart examination				
Elevated neck veins	13	94	NS	NS
Right ventricular heave	38	96	8.8	NS
Loud P2	38	98	17.6	NS
Other				
Ascites, edema, or both	75	36	NS	NS

*Diagnostic standard: for *pulmonary hypertension*, measured mean pulmonary artery pressure ≥ 25 mm Hg.
†Likelihood ratio (LR) if finding present = positive LR; LR if finding absent = negative LR.
NS, Not significant.

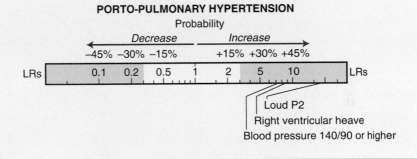

is the paradoxical increase of dyspnea when the patient moves from a supine to upright position, see Chapter 19). A Child C classification (compared to class A or B*) increased probability of hepatopulmonary syndrome only a small amount (LR = 2.2).[52,53,55]

F. DETECTING PORTOPULMONARY HYPERTENSION

Some patients with end-stage liver disease develop pulmonary hypertension, a significant complication because it greatly increases the surgical risk of liver transplantation. In one study of 80 consecutive liver transplant candidates, three physical findings accurately detected pulmonary hypertension (mean pulmonary artery pressure of 25 mm Hg or higher): a loud P2 (pulmonary component of the second heart sound, EBM Box 8.4; LR = 17.6), right ventricular heave (LR = 8.8), and systemic hypertension (blood pressure 140/90 or higher, LR = 7.3).[60] At first glance, the association between systemic and pulmonary hypertension may be unexpected, but most patients with end-stage liver disease

---

*The Child score (or Child-Pugh score) predicts the prognosis of patients with chronic liver disease by addressing five clinical variables (bilirubin, albumin, prothrombin times, ascites, and hepatic encephalopathy) and scoring each 1 to 3 based on levels of abnormality. The combined score distinguishes Child classes A (best prognosis), B, and C (worst prognosis).

actually have a normal or low blood pressure from systemic vasodilation, suggesting that the association between pulmonary and systemic hypertension represents a generalized abnormality of vascular tone.

The presence of oxygen desaturation, elevated neck veins, ascites, or edema does not affect the probability of pulmonary hypertension in these patients (EBM Box 8.4).

References may be accessed online at *Elsevier eBooks for Practicing Clinicians.*

Cyanosis

I. Definitions

Cyanosis is an abnormal bluish discoloration of the skin and mucous membranes, caused by blue-colored blood circulating in the superficial capillaries and venules. The blue color usually represents excessive amounts of deoxygenated hemoglobin, although in some patients it results from increased amounts of methemoglobin or sulfhemoglobin. Cyanosis may be central or peripheral. In central cyanosis the blood leaving the heart is colored blue; in peripheral cyanosis, the blood leaving the heart is red but becomes blue by time it reaches the fingers and toes. Pseudocyanosis, in contrast, refers to a permanent bluish discoloration caused by deposition of blue pigments in the skin.

Cyanosis was first described in 1761 by Morgagni, who attributed it to pulmonary stenosis.[1] In 1869, Claude Bernard described the qualitative difference in blood gases between blue venous and red arterial blood. The first person to quantify the amount of deoxygenated hemoglobin necessary to produce the blue color was Lundsgaard in 1919.[1]

II. Pathogenesis

A. THE BLUE COLOR

Blood becomes blue when an absolute amount of blue pigment (usually deoxyhemoglobin) accumulates, probably because only then is the blue color deep enough to be seen through the opaque epidermis.[1-4] Once this minimal amount of deoxyhemoglobin accumulates and cyanosis appears, the amount of additional red blood (or oxyhemoglobin) matters little to the overall skin color.

The color of the skin depends on the color of blood flowing through the dermal capillaries and subpapillary venous plexus, not the arteries and veins that lie too deep to contribute to skin color.[1,5] There has been much confusion over the absolute concentration of deoxyhemoglobin required for cyanosis, primarily because some investigators have mistakenly equated the arterial levels of deoxyhemoglobin, which are easy to measure, with the capillary levels thereof, which impart the blue color but must exceed the measured arterial levels. In patients with central cyanosis, the *average* amount of *arterial* deoxyhemoglobin is 3.48 ± 0.55 g/dL (or 5.35 g/dL in the capillaries and small venules). The *minimal* amount of *arterial* deoxyhemoglobin causing cyanosis is 2.38 g/dL (or 4.25 g/dL in the capillaries and small venules).[*,4]

Because cyanosis depends on the absolute quantity of deoxyhemoglobin, not the relative amount, the appearance of cyanosis also depends on the patient's total hemoglobin concentration (i.e., 5 g/dL of capillary deoxyhemoglobin represents a higher percent of oxygen desaturation for an anemic patient, who has less total hemoglobin, than it does for a polycythemic patient). Table 9.1 displays this relationship: polycythemic patients (haemoglobin = 20 g/dL) may appear cyanotic with only mild hypoxemia (i.e, oxygen saturation [SaO_2] = 88% or pO_2 = 56 mm Hg), yet anemic patients (haemoglobin = 8 g/dL) do not develop the finding until the hypoxemia is severe (i.e., SaO_2 = 70% or pO_2 = 36 mm Hg). These figures are calculated as follows: for the polycythemic patient (haemoglobin = 20 g/dL), 2.38 g/dL of arterial deoxyhemoglobin indicates that there is 20 − 2.38 or 17.62 g/dL of arterial oxyhemoglobin. The oxygen saturation, therefore, is (17.62)/(20) = 0.88, or 88%. For the anemic patient, the calculation is (8 − 2.38)/8 = 0.7, or 70% saturation.

B. PERIPHERAL CYANOSIS

In peripheral cyanosis, the blood leaving the heart is red; however, because of increased extraction of oxygen by the peripheral tissues, enough deoxyhemoglobin accumulates to render it blue in the subepidermal blood vessels of the feet and hands. The clinician can easily demonstrate peripheral cyanosis by wrapping a rubber band around his or her own finger and watching the distal digit turn blue as oxygen continues to be extracted from the stagnant blood.

TABLE 9.1 ■ Cyanosis and Hemoglobin Concentration.

| Hemoglobin concentration (g/dL) | Cyanosis appears at:* | |
	Oxygen saturation (%) below:	Arterial pO_2 (mm Hg) below:
6	60	31
8	70	36
10	76	40
12	80	45
14	83	47
16	85	50
18	87	54
20	88	56

*These figures assume that central cyanosis begins to appear when 2.38 g/dL deoxygenated hemoglobin accumulates in the arterial blood (see text for calculations). The corresponding pO_2 was obtained from standard hemoglobin dissociation curves for oxygen.

[*]Capillary deoxyhemoglobin is 1.87 g/dL more than arterial levels, based on three assumptions: (1) the difference in oxygen content between the arteries and veins is 5 mL of oxygen/dL blood; (2) the amount of deoxyhemoglobin in the capillaries is midway between that of the arteries and vein; and (3) 1.34 mL of oxygen binds to 1 g of saturated hemoglobin. Therefore, $5/(2 \times 1.34) = 1.87$.

III. The Finding

Cyanosis is best appreciated in areas where the overlying epidermis is thin and subepidermal vessels are abundant, such as the lips, nose, cheeks, ears, hands, feet, and the mucous membranes of the oral cavity.[1,6] Cyanosis is detected more easily with fluorescent lighting than with incandescent lighting or daylight.[4]

A. CENTRAL CYANOSIS

Patients with central cyanosis have blue discoloration of the lips, tongue, and sublingual tissues, as well as the hands and feet. The correlation between severity of oxygen desaturation and the depth of the cyanotic color is best appreciated by examining the patient's lips and buccal mucosa.[7,8] Some patients with longstanding central cyanosis have associated clubbing (see Chapter 28).

When central cyanosis is suspected yet administration of oxygen fails to diminish the blue color, the clinician should consider methemoglobinemia or sulfhemoglobinemia. The color of patients with methemoglobinemia often has a characteristic brownish hue (so-called **chocolate cyanosis**).[9]

Because cyanosis depends on blue blood being present in the underlying blood vessels, maneuvers that express blood out of the vessels (e.g., pressure on the skin) make the blue color temporarily disappear.

B. PERIPHERAL CYANOSIS

Peripheral cyanosis causes blue hands and feet, although the mucous membranes of the mouth are pink. Warming the patient's limb skin often diminishes peripheral cyanosis because blood flow to the involved area improves, whereas the color of central cyanosis is unchanged or deepens after warming of the skin.

C. PSEUDOCYANOSIS

In patients with pseudocyanosis, the mucous membranes of the mouth are pink, and pressure on the skin fails to blanch the abnormal color.[6]

D. CYANOSIS AND OXIMETRY

Cyanosis affects co-oximetry (i.e., blood gas analysis in the laboratory) differently from how it affects pulse oximetry (i.e., equipment used at the bedside; see Chapter 20). Because co-oximetry can distinguish deoxyhemoglobin from other abnormal hemoglobins, it indicates hypoxemia only in patients with central cyanosis (i.e., it samples *arterial* blood and therefore indicates normal oxygen levels in peripheral cyanosis). Pulse oximetry, in contrast, detects the *color* of the pulsatile waveform in the digit. Although it also indicates hypoxemia in patients with central cyanosis, pulse oximetry may falsely indicate arterial hypoxemia in patients with peripheral cyanosis or with abnormal hemoglobin (see Chapter 20). Both co-oximetry and pulse oximetry indicate normal oxygen levels in pseudocyanosis.

IV. Clinical Significance

A. CENTRAL CYANOSIS

Any disorder causing hypoxemia may generate sufficient deoxyhemoglobin in the blood leaving the heart to produce central cyanosis. The typical etiologies are pulmonary edema, pneumonia, and intracardiac right-to-left shunts. The finding of central cyanosis increases the probability of

| EBM BOX 9.1 | Central Cyanosis, Detecting Arterial Deoxyhemoglobin ≥2.38 g/dL* |

Finding (Reference)	Sensitivity (%)	Specificity (%)	Likelihood Ratio[†] if Finding Is Present	Likelihood Ratio[†] if Finding Is Absent
Central cyanosis[2,4]	79–95	72–95	7.4	0.2

*Corresponding to O_2 saturation of 80% and pO_2 of 45 mm Hg if hemoglobin concentration is 12 g/dL (see Table 9.1).
[†]Likelihood ratio (LR) if finding present = positive LR; LR if finding absent = negative LR.

CYANOSIS
Probability

Decrease ←   → Increase
−45% −30% −15%   +15% +30% +45%

LRs | 0.1 0.2 0.5   1   2   5   10 | LRs

Absence of cyanosis, *arguing against* arterial deoxyhemoglobin >2.38 g/dL

Presence of cyanosis, detecting arterial deoxyhemoglobin >2.38 g/dL

hypoxemia greatly (likelihood ratio [LR] = 7.4, see EBM Box 9.1). In these studies, hypoxemia is defined as arterial deoxyhemoglobin level ≥2.38 g/dL, corresponding to SaO_2 ≤80% and pO_2 ≤45 mm Hg in patients with normal amounts of hemoglobin (see Table 9.1). The absence of central cyanosis decreases the likelihood of such severe hypoxemia (LR = 0.2, EBM Box 9.1).

In patients with chronic liver disease, the finding of cyanosis increases the probability of hepatopulmonary syndrome (LR = 4.4; see Chapter 8).

B. PERIPHERAL CYANOSIS

In clinical practice, the common causes of peripheral cyanosis are low cardiac output, arterial disease or obstruction (e.g., Raynaud disease), and venous disease.

C. PSEUDOCYANOSIS

Pseudocyanosis may occur after exposure to metals (*argyria* from topical silver compounds; *chrysiasis* of gold therapy) or drugs (amiodarone, minocycline, chloroquine, or phenothiazines).[10,11]

References may be accessed online at *Elsevier eBooks for Practicing Clinicians.*

Anemia

I. Introduction

Anemia refers to an abnormally low number of circulating red cells, caused by blood loss, hemolysis, or underproduction of cells by the bone marrow. In patients with acute blood loss, the abnormal vital signs of hypovolemia are the most prominent physical findings (see Chapter 17), but in chronic anemia (the subject of this chapter) physical findings reflect instead changes in color of the skin and conjunctiva.

II. The Findings

Chronic anemia causes the skin and conjunctiva to appear abnormally pale because of reduced amounts of red-colored oxyhemoglobin that circulate in the dermal and subconjunctival capillaries and venules.[1] Nonetheless, pallor does not always indicate anemia, because skin color also depends on the diameter of these minute vessels, the amount of circulating deoxyhemoglobin, and the patient's natural skin pigments.[1] Vasoconstriction from cold exposure or sympathetic stimulation also may cause pallor, and the pallor of anemia may be obscured by the red color of vasodilation (inflammation or permanent vascular injury from ischemia, cold, or radiation), the blue color of cyanosis (see Chapter 9), or the brown pigments of dark-skinned persons. Theoretically, examination of the conjunctiva, nailbeds, and palms avoids the effects of the patient's natural skin pigments.

Most clinicians assess for pallor subjectively, by comparing the patient's skin color with their own color or their recollection of normal skin color. One definition of pallor, however, is more objective: **conjunctival rim pallor** is present if examination of the lower lid's conjunctiva reveals the color of the anterior rim to have the same pale fleshy color of the deeper posterior aspect of the palpebral conjunctiva (see Fig. 10.1).[2] In persons without anemia, the normal bright red color of the anterior rim contrasts markedly with the fleshy color of the posterior portion.

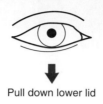

Pull down lower lid

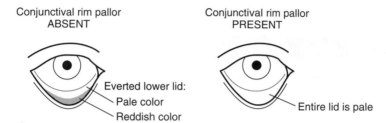

Conjunctival rim pallor
ABSENT

Conjunctival rim pallor
PRESENT

Everted lower lid:
Pale color
Reddish color

Entire lid is pale

Fig. 10.1   Conjunctival rim pallor. After gently pulling down the patient's lower lid (*top*), the clinician observes the lid's inner surface, comparing the color of the lid margin (its rim) with that of the conjunctival surface nearer the globe. In patients without anemia (*bottom left*), there are two zones of color: a reddish color at the rim (due to its prominent vascular supply) and a contrasting paler color nearer the globe (from prominent lymphoid tissue.) In patients with anemia (*bottom right*), the entire inner surface of the lower lid has a pale color (i.e., conjunctival rim pallor.)

III. Clinical Significance

EBM Box 10.1 presents the diagnostic accuracy of physical signs for chronic anemia as applied to hundreds of patients. These studies excluded patients with acute bleeding or those who had recently received transfusions. As much as possible, the color of skin and conjunctiva was determined using natural lighting.

According to EBM Box 10.1, the finding of conjunctival rim pallor (likelihood ratio [LR] = 16.7), increases the probability of anemia the most, followed by palmar crease pallor (LR = 7.9), palmar pallor (LR = 5.6), conjunctival pallor (i.e., not specifically conjunctival rim pallor, LR = 4.7), nailbed pallor (LR = 4.3), facial pallor (light-skinned persons only, LR = 3.8), and tongue pallor (LR = 3.7). Importantly, no physical sign convincingly *decreases* the probability of anemia (i.e., no LR <0.4).

EBM BOX 10.1	Anemia*			
			Likelihood Ratio‡ if Finding Is	
Finding (Reference)†	**Sensitivity (%)**	**Specificity (%)**	**Present**	**Absent**
Pallor at any site [3-9]	22–77	66–92	3.8	0.5
Facial pallor [4]	46	88	3.8	0.6
Nailbed pallor[4,5,8]	41–60	66–93	4.3	0.5
Palmar pallor[4,5]	58–64	74–96	5.6	0.4
Palmar crease pallor[4]	8	99	7.9	NS
Conjunctival pallor[4,5,10,11]	31–62	82–97	4.7	0.6

Continued

| EBM BOX 10.1 | Anemia*—Con'td | | | | |

Finding (Reference)[†]	Sensitivity (%)	Specificity (%)	Likelihood Ratio[‡] if Finding Is Present	Absent
Tongue pallor[12]	48	87	**3.7**	0.6
Conjunctival rim pallor[2]				
Pallor present	10	99	**16.7**	...
Pallor borderline	36	...	2.3	...
Pallor absent	53	16	0.6	...

*Diagnostic standard: for *anemia*, hematocrit less than 35%,[4] hemoglobin (Hb) less than 7 g/dL,[9] Hb less than 9 g/dl,[12] Hb less than 10,[6] Hb less than 11 g/dl,[2,5,7,10,11] or Hb less than 11 g/dl in women and less than 13 g/dl in men.[3,8]

[†]Definition of findings: for *pallor at any site*, examination of skin, nailbeds, and conjunctiva[3-5,8]; for *facial pallor*, the study excluded black patients; for *palmar crease pallor*, examination after gentle extension of the patient's fingers; for *conjunctival rim pallor*, see Fig. 10.1.

[‡]Likelihood ratio (LR) if finding present = positive LR; LR if finding absent = negative LR.

NS, Not significant.

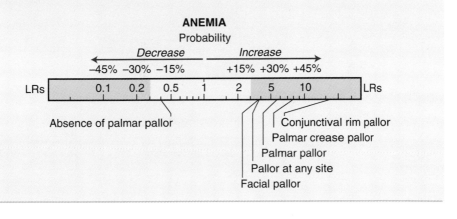

References may be accessed online at *Elsevier eBooks for Practicing Clinicians.*

Hypovolemia

I. Introduction

The term *hypovolemia* refers collectively to two distinct disorders: (1) **volume depletion**, which describes the loss of sodium from the extracellular space (i.e., intravascular and interstitial fluid) that occurs during gastrointestinal hemorrhage, vomiting, diarrhea, and diuresis; and (2) **dehydration**, which refers to the loss of intracellular water (and total body water) that ultimately causes cellular desiccation and elevates the plasma sodium concentration and osmolality.[1] Chapter 17 discusses the accuracy of abnormal vital signs in patients with volume depletion; this chapter discusses assorted additional findings.

II. The Findings and Their Pathogenesis

Many of the traditional signs of hypovolemia—dry mucous membranes, sunken eyes, shriveled skin, poor skin turgor, and confusion—were originally described in patients with cholera near vascular collapse.[2] Presumably, cellular dehydration, interstitial space dehydration, and poor perfusion contribute to these signs.

Poor skin turgor refers to the slow return of skin to its normal position after being pinched between the examiner's thumb and forefinger.[3,4] In one study, persistence of skin tenting 3 or more seconds after 3 seconds of pinching was defined as abnormal.[5] The protein elastin is responsible for the recoil of skin, and *in vitro* experiments show that its recoil time increases forty-fold after loss of as little as 3.4% of its wet weight.[3] Elastin also deteriorates with age, however, suggesting that the specificity of poor skin turgor diminishes as patients age.

III. Clinical Significance

EBM Box 11.1 presents clinical studies comparing traditional signs to laboratory tests of hypovolemia (i.e., increased serum urea-to-creatinine, serum osmolarity, or serum sodium levels). These studies enrolled mostly elderly patients presenting to emergency departments with vomiting, decreased oral intake, or diarrhea. Few if any were as desperately hypovolemic as patients with classic cholera.

EBM BOX 11.1	Hypovolemia*				

Finding (Reference)[†]	Sensitivity (%)	Specificity (%)	Likelihood Ratio[‡] if Finding Is	
			Present	Absent
Skin, eyes, and mucous membranes				
Dry axilla[6-8]	40–57	82–93	**3.8**	0.5
Dry mucous membranes of mouth and nose[5,8,9]	49–85	58–88	2.8	0.4
Dry tongue[8,9]	59–73	73–85	**3.6**	0.4
Longitudinal furrows on tongue[9]	85	58	NS	**0.3**
Sunken eyes[7,9]	33–62	82–93	**3.7**	0.6
Abnormal skin turgor (subclavicular area)[5]	73	79	**3.5**	**0.3**
Neurologic findings				
Confusion[5,9]	49–57	73–99	NS	0.5
Weakness[9]	43	82	NS	NS
Speech unclear or rambling[9]	56	82	NS	0.5

*Diagnostic standard: for *hypovolemia*, serum urea nitrogen-creatinine ratio >25, osmolarity >295-300 mOsm/L, or serum sodium >145-150 mEq/L.
[†]Definition of findings: for *abnormal skin turgor*, see text.
[‡]Likelihood ratio (LR) if finding present = positive LR; LR if finding absent = negative LR.
NS, Not significant.

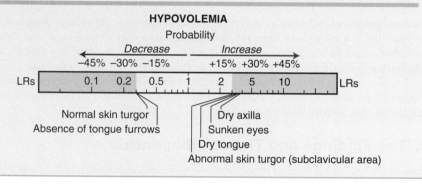

These studies indicate that the presence of dry axilla (likelihood ratio [LR] = 3.8, EBM Box 11.1), sunken eyes (LR = 3.7), dry tongue (LR = 3.6), abnormal skin turgor (tested in the subclavicular area, LR = 3.5), and dry mucous membranes (LR = 2.8) *increase* the probability of hypovolemia. Testing skin turgor over the thighs, sternum, or subclavicular area was more accurate than testing skin over the forearms.[5] The *absence* of tongue furrows and presence of normal skin turgor *decrease* the probability of hypovolemia (LR = 0.3 for both findings). The presence or absence of confusion, weakness, or abnormal speech had little diagnostic value in these studies.

Although poor capillary refill time has been advanced as a reliable sign of hypovolemia, it lacked diagnostic value in one study[9] (see Chapters 54 and 70).

References may be accessed online at *Elsevier eBooks for Practicing Clinicians*.

Protein-Energy Malnutrition and Weight Loss

PROTEIN-ENERGY MALNUTRITION

I. Introduction

The most common cause of malnutrition worldwide is inadequate food supply, although in industrialized countries malnutrition usually reflects increased nutrient loss (e.g., malabsorption, diarrhea, nephrotic syndrome), increased nutrient requirements (e.g., fever, cancer, infection, or surgery), or both. Among patients admitted to surgical services in industrialized nations, 9% to 27% have signs of severe malnutrition.[1,2]

II. The Findings

In children of developing nations, there are two distinct syndromes of protein-energy malnutrition: **marasmus** (profound weight loss, muscle wasting, and fat wasting) and **kwashiorkor** (abdominal distention, edema, and hypopigmented hair). In industrialized countries, however, most malnourished patients have less dramatic findings and present instead with combinations of low body weight, atrophy of muscle and subcutaneous fat, weakness, and various laboratory abnormalities (e.g., low albumin or other serum proteins).

A. ARM MUSCLE CIRCUMFERENCE

Arm muscle circumference is a decades-old anthropometric measurement of the amount of muscle in the arm, which theoretically reflects the total amount of muscle or protein in the body. The clinician measures the upper arm circumference (C_a, using a flexible tape measure) and the triceps skinfold thickness (h, using calipers) and estimates arm muscle circumference (AMC) with the following formula:

$$AMC = C_a - \pi h$$

Age- and sex-standardized values of the normal AMC have been published.[3] The technique for forearm muscle circumference is similar.

B. GRIP STRENGTH

Based on the hypothesis that malnutrition influences the outcome of surgical patients and that muscle weakness is an important sign of malnutrition, Klidjian in 1980 investigated 102 surgical patients and demonstrated that hand grip strength accurately predicts postoperative complications.[4] In his method the patient squeezes a simple handheld spring dynamometer three times, resting 10 seconds between each attempt, and the clinician records the highest value obtained (patients with arthritis, stroke, or other obvious causes of weakness are excluded).

Age- and sex-standardized values of normal grip strength have been published.[5] Clinical studies of grip strength usually test the nondominant arm, but this may be unnecessary because studies show both arms are similar.[5]

Historically, clinicians measured grip strength by rolling up an adult aneroid blood pressure cuff (making a cylinder of about 2 inches in diameter with rubber bands on each end), inflating the cuff to 20 mm Hg, and then asking the patient to squeeze the cuff. The subsequent sphygmomanometer reading (in mm Hg) is a measure of grip strength; formulas for converting these readings to dynamometer readings (in kilograms or pounds) have been published.[6]

III. Clinical Significance

EBM Box 12.1 addresses the accuracy of physical examination in predicting significant postoperative complications among patients undergoing major surgery. In these studies, complications are significant if they prolong hospital stay, threaten the patient's life, or cause death (e.g., sepsis, wound infections, myocardial infarction, or stroke).

In these studies, the findings of reduced arm or forearm muscle circumference (likelihood ratio [LRs] = 2.5 to 3.2), reduced grip strength (LR = 2.6), and low body weight (LR = 2) all modestly increase the probability of postoperative complications. Normal grip strength *decreases* the probability of complications (LR = 0.4). Interestingly, the presence of recent weight loss has little diagnostic value in predicting complications, possibly because this finding not only identifies patients with weight loss from malnutrition (which should increase complications) but also overweight patients who voluntarily lose weight before surgery (which should decrease complications).

WEIGHT LOSS

I. Introduction

Involuntary weight loss reflects either diuresis, decreased caloric intake, or the increased caloric requirements of malabsorption, glucosuria, or a hypermetabolic state. In series of patients

---

*This formula assumes that the arm is a cylinder of only skin and muscle (i.e., it disregards the humerus). To derive this formula: (1) $AMC = \pi d_1$ (d_1=diameter of muscle component of the arm); (2) $d_1 = d_2 - h$ (d_2=diameter of arm; h=skinfold thickness, which, since the skin is pinched, actually includes a *double* layer of skin and subcutaneous tissue); (3) Therefore $AMC = \pi d_1 = \pi(d_2 - h) = \pi d_2 - \pi h = C_a - \pi h$. If the clinician desires to directly enter the skinfold thickness in mm (as it is measured), 0.314 is substituted for π in the formula (i.e., AMC and C_a are measured in centimeters).

EBM BOX 12.1   Protein-Energy Malnutrition and Major Surgical Complications*

Finding (Reference)[†]	Sensitivity (%)	Specificity (%)	Likelihood Ratio[‡] if Finding Is Present	Absent
Body weight				
Weight loss >10%[4,7–10]	15–75	47–88	1.4	NS
Low body weight[4,8,9,11]	11–35	83–97	2.0	NS
Anthropometry				
Upper arm muscle circumference <85% predicted[4,8,9]	26–38	83–91	2.5	0.8
Forearm muscle circumference <85% predicted[4,8,9]	14–42	85–97	**3.2**	0.8
Muscle strength				
Reduced grip strength[4,5,8,9,12–16]	33–90	46–93	2.6	0.4

*Diagnostic standard: in each of these studies, *disease* is defined as a major postoperative complication, including those prolonging hospital stay, threatening the patient's life, or causing death.
†Definition of findings (all findings from preoperative physical examination): for *weight loss >10%*, (recalled usual weight – measured weight)/(recalled usual weight) >10%; for *low body weight*, weight-for-height less than normal lower limit,[11] <90% of predicted,[4] or <85% of predicted;[8,9,14,15] for *predicted arm muscle circumference*, published standardized values;[3] for *forearm muscle circumference <85%*, <20 cm in men and <16/3 cm in women;[4,9] and for *reduced grip strength*, specific thresholds differ but all correspond closely to published age- and sex-standardized abnormal values based upon reference 5.
‡Likelihood ratio (LR) if finding present = positive LR; LR if finding absent = negative LR.
NS, Not significant.

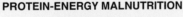

PROTEIN-ENERGY MALNUTRITION

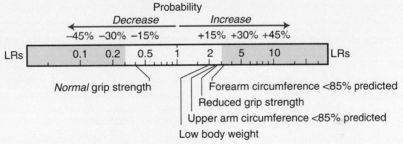

presenting with involuntary weight loss (exceeding 5% of their usual weight), organic disease is diagnosed in 65% of patients (most commonly cancer and gastrointestinal disorders, although virtually any chronic disease may cause weight loss) and psychiatric disorders are diagnosed in 10% of patients (depression, anorexia nervosa, schizophrenia). In 25% of patients, the cause remains unknown despite at least 1 year of follow-up.[17–21]

II. Clinical Significance

Weight loss is rarely due to occult disease, and most diagnoses are made during the initial evaluation, including the patient interview, physical examination, and basic laboratory testing.[17,18,20,21]

In patients with involuntary weight loss, the presence of alcoholism (LR = 4.5) and cigarette smoking (LR = 2.2) increase the probability that an organic cause will be discovered during 6 months follow-up, whereas prior psychiatric disease (LR = 0.2) and a *normal* initial physical examination (LR = 0.4) decrease the probability of discovering organic disease.[22] Also, the patient's perceptions of the weight loss—whether he or she significantly underestimates or overestimates it—helps predict the final diagnosis. The patient is asked to estimate his or her weight before the illness (W) and the amount of weight lost (E). The observed weight loss (O) is the former weight (W) minus the current measured weight. Significant *underestimation* of weight loss, defined as (O − E) greater than 0.5 kg, predicts an *organic* cause of weight loss with a sensitivity of 40%, specificity of 92%, positive LR of 5.4, and negative LR of 0.6.[23] Significant *overestimation* of weight loss, defined as (E − O) greater than 0.5 kg, predicts a *nonorganic* cause of weight loss with a sensitivity of 70%, specificity of 81%, positive LR of 3.6, and negative LR of 0.4.[23]

References may be accessed online at *Elsevier eBooks for Practicing Clinicians.*

CHAPTER 13

Obesity

KEY TEACHING POINTS

- Obesity increases the risk of diabetes, cardiovascular disease, and overall mortality.
- The best measures of obesity are body mass index (BMI) and waist circumference. Thresholds predicting increased mortality are BMI > 25 kg/m² and waist circumference >102 cm (>40 inches) in men and >88 cm (>35 inches) in women.
- Abdominal obesity (elevated waist-to-hip ratio [WHR]) indicates a worse prognosis that gluteal-femoral obesity (reduced WHR).

I. Introduction

Obesity increases the risk of coronary artery disease, diabetes, hypertension, osteoarthritis, cholelithiasis, certain cancers, and overall mortality.[1] Clinicians have recognized the hazards of obesity for thousands of years (according to one Hippocratic aphorism, "Sudden death is more common in those who are naturally fat than in the lean").[2] Two-thirds of U.S. adults are overweight or obese.[3]

II. The Findings and Their Significance

Several different anthropometric parameters have been used to identify those patients at greatest risk for the medical complications of obesity. The most important ones are body-mass index (BMI), skinfold thickness, waist-to-hip ratio (WHR), waist circumference, and abdominal sagittal diameter.

A. BODY MASS INDEX (BMI)

1. The Finding

BMI (or the Quetelet index) is the patient's weight in kilograms divided by the square of his height in meters (kg/m²). If pounds and inches are used, the quotient should be multiplied by 703.5 to convert the units to kg/m². An individual is overweight if the BMI exceeds 25 kg/m², and obese if the BMI exceeds 30 kg/m².[3]

BMI was derived by a 17th century Belgian mathematician and astronomer, Lambert-Adolphe-Jacques Quetelet, who discovered that this ratio best expressed the natural relationship between weight and height.[4]

2. Clinical Significance

BMI is an easy and reliable measurement that correlates well with precise measures of total body fat (r = 0.70 to 0.96), much better that other formulas of weight (W) and height (H) (e.g., W/H, W/H^3, $W/H^{0.3}$).[5,6] BMI also correlates significantly with a patient's cholesterol level, blood pressure, incidence of coronary events, and overall mortality.[7,8]

The arbitrary cutoff of $25 \, \text{kg/m}^2$ was chosen in part because it reflects the level at which there is a significant increase in mortality. Many studies of BMI and mortality revealed a J-shaped relationship (i.e., both lean and overweight patients have increased mortality), but the increased risk of lean individuals is likely explained by cigarette use, short duration of follow-up, and illness-related weight loss.[7,8]

B. SKINFOLD THICKNESS

Another measure of obesity is *total skinfold thickness*, which is estimated by adding together the skinfold thickness (measured with calipers) of multiple sites (mid-biceps, mid-triceps, subscapular, and supra-iliac area). These sums are then converted by formulae into estimates of total body fat, which correlate well with more traditional measures (r = 0.7 to 0.8).[5] Measurements of skinfold thickness are rarely used today, in part because of their complexity, but mostly because relatively few studies show the parameter is clinically significant.

C. WAIST-TO-HIP RATIO

1. The Finding

WHR is the circumference of the waist divided by that of the hips. It is based on the premise that the most important characteristic of obesity is its distribution, not its quantity. *Abdominal obesity* (also called android, upper body, or apple-shaped obesity; Fig. 13.1) has a much worse prognosis than *gluteal-femoral obesity* (also called gynoid, lower body, or pear-shaped obesity).

Most authorities measure the waist circumference at the midpoint between the lower costal margin and the iliac crest and the hip circumference at the widest part of the gluteal region. Adverse health outcomes increase significantly when the WHR exceeds 1 in men and 0.85 in women, values that are close to the top quintiles in epidemiologic studies.[9]

The French diabetologist Jean Vague is usually credited with making the observation in the 1940s that abdominal obesity, more common in men, is associated with worse health outcomes than obesity over the hips and thighs, more common in women (even so, American life insurance companies made the same observation in the late 1800s).[10] Vague's original *index of masculine differentiation*, a complicated index based on skinfolds and limb circumferences,[11] is no longer used, having been replaced in the 1980s by the much simpler WHR.

2. Clinical Significance

Even after controlling for the effects of BMI, WHR correlates significantly with blood pressure, cholesterol level, incidence of diabetes mellitus, stroke, coronary events, and overall mortality.[12-14]

3. Pathogenesis

The main contributor to abdominal obesity is visceral fat (i.e., omental, mesenteric, and retroperitoneal fat), not subcutaneous fat. Visceral fat is metabolically active, constantly releasing free fatty acids into the portal circulation, which probably contributes to hyperlipidemia, atherogenesis, and hyperinsulinemia.[15] Gluteal-femoral fat, on the other hand, is metabolically inactive except during pregnancy and the postpartum period, which has led some to suggest that the role of lower body

Abdominal obesity

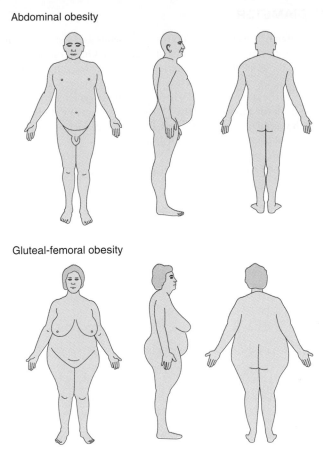

Gluteal-femoral obesity

Fig. 13.1 Comparison of abdominal and gluteal-femoral obesity. Abdominal obesity is depicted in the *top row*; gluteal-femoral obesity in the *bottom row*. The drawings in this figure are adapted from photographs published by Jean Vague,[11] who is credited with first associating adverse health outcomes with abdominal obesity.

fat is to help guarantee the survival of the species, by providing a constant source of energy to the lactating female even when external nutrients are unavailable.

D. WAIST CIRCUMFERENCE

Waist circumference is simply the numerator of the WHR calculation. It has the advantages of being simpler to measure and of avoiding attention to the hips, which, because they encompass bone and skeletal muscle as well as fat, should have no biologically plausible relationship to diabetes, hypertension, and atherosclerosis. Recommended cutoffs for increased health risk are a waist circumference >102 cm (>40 inches) for men and >88 cm (>35 inches) for women.[16]

Waist circumference is strongly associated with risk of death, independent of BMI.[13,17] Waist circumference is also a criterion for the **metabolic syndrome** (defined as the presence of three or more of the following five variables: large waist circumference, hypertension, elevated triglycerides, reduced high-density lipoprotein cholesterol, and elevated fasting glucose).[18]

E. SAGITTAL DIAMETER

Because waist circumference encompasses both subcutaneous and visceral fat, investigators have looked for better anthropometric measures of just visceral fat. One proposed measure is the sagittal diameter, which is the total anterior-posterior distance between the anterior abdominal wall of the *supine* patient and the surface of the examining table. Theoretically, visceral fat maintains the abdominal depth in the supine patient, whereas subcutaneous fat allows the abdominal depth to partially collapse from the force of gravity.[19] Even so, there are few studies of this measure and most correlate it with variables of uncertain clinical significance such as cardiovascular risk factors or the amount of visceral fat visualized on body imaging.[15]

References may be accessed online at *Elsevier eBooks for Practicing Clinicians*.

Cushing Syndrome

I. Introduction

Cushing syndrome refers to those clinical findings induced by excess circulating glucocorticoids, such as hypertension, central obesity, weakness, hirsutism (in women), depression, skin striae, and bruises. The most common cause is exogenous administration of corticosteroid hormones.[1] Endogenous Cushing syndrome results from pituitary tumors producing adrenocorticotropic hormone (ACTH) (i.e., Cushing disease, 60% to 70% of all endogenous cases), ectopic production of ACTH (usually by small cell carcinoma of the lung or carcinoid tumors of the lung or mediastinum, 5% to 10% of cases), adrenal adenomas (10% to 20% of cases), or adrenal carcinoma (5% to 7% of cases).[1,2] Cushing disease and the ectopic ACTH syndrome are referred to as **ACTH-dependent disease**, because the elevated cortisol levels are accompanied by inappropriately increased ACTH levels. Adrenal tumors are **ACTH-independent disease**.

The bedside findings of Cushing syndrome were originally described by Harvey Cushing in 1932.[3] Corticosteroid hormones were first used as therapeutic agents to treat patients with rheumatoid arthritis in 1949; within 2 years, clear descriptions of exogenous Cushing syndrome appeared.[4]

II. The Findings and Their Pathogenesis

Table 14.1 presents the physical signs of more than 1500 patients with Cushing syndrome.

A. BODY HABITUS

Patient with Cushing syndrome develop **central obesity** (also known as **truncal obesity** or **centripetal obesity**), a term describing accumulation of fat centrally on the neck, chest, and abdomen, which contrasts conspicuously with the muscle atrophy affecting the extremities. There are three definitions of central obesity: (1) obesity sparing the extremities (a subjective definition and also the most common one);[5,6] (2) the **central obesity index**, a complicated ratio of the sum of 3 truncal circumferences (neck, chest, and abdomen) divided by the sum of 6 limb circumferences (bilateral arms, thighs, and lower legs), in which a value greater than 1 is abnormal;[7] (3) obesity as defined by an abnormal waist-to-hip circumference ratio (i.e., >1 in men and >0.85 in women; see Chapter 13).[8] The abnormal waist-to-hip circumference is not recommended because there are many false positives (i.e., for Cushing syndrome).

Other characteristic features of the Cushing body habitus are accumulation of fat in the bitemporal region (**moon facies**),[9] between the scapulae and behind the neck (**buffalo hump** or **dorsal cervical fat pad**), in the supraclavicular region (producing a "collar" around the base of the neck),[8] and in front of the sternum (**dewlap,** named after its resemblance to the hanging fold of skin at the base of the bovine neck, see Fig. 14.1).[10] Morbid obesity is rare in Cushing syndrome.[11]

TABLE 14.1 ■ Cushing Syndrome – Frequency of Individual Findings*

Physical Finding[†]	Frequency (%)[‡]
Vital signs	
Hypertension	64–88
Body habitus	
Moon facies	67–92
Central obesity	44–97
Buffalo hump	34–75
Skin findings	
Thin skin	27
Plethora	28–94
Hirsutism, women	48–81
Ecchymoses	23–75
Red or purple striae	46–68
Acne	21–52
Extremity findings	
Proximal muscle weakness	39–68
Edema	15–66
Other	
Significant depression	12–40

*Information is based on 1522 patients from references.[5,31,34,35,40-44] Each study enrolled >50 patients with disease.
[†]*Diagnostic standard*: for *Cushing syndrome*, elevated daily cortisol or corticosteroid metabolites, or both, with loss of circadian rhythm and with abnormal dexamethasone suppression tests.
[‡]Results are overall mean frequency or, if statistically heterogenous, the range of values.

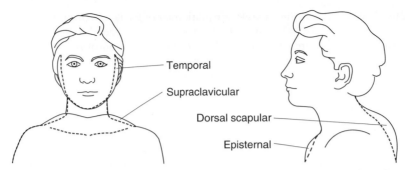

Fig. 14.1   Distribution of adipose tissue in Cushing syndrome. Rounding of cheeks and prominent bitemporal fat produces the characteristic moon facies. Fat also may accumulate bilaterally above the clavicles (supraclavicular collar), in front of the sternum (episternal area, or dewlap), and over the back of the neck (dorsal cervical fat pad, or buffalo hump). .In these drawings, the *dotted line* depicts normal contours of patients without Cushing syndrome

The truncal obesity of Cushing syndrome reflects increased intraabdominal visceral fat, not subcutaneous fat,[12] probably from glucocorticoid-induced reduction in lipolytic activity and activation of lipoprotein lipase, which allows tissues to accumulate triglyceride.

B. HYPERTENSION

Hypertension is present in three of four patients with Cushing syndrome. The pathogenesis of hypertension in Cushing syndrome is complex and incompletely understood. Proposed mechanisms include changes in the renin-angiotensin system, mineralocorticoid activity, sympathetic system reactivity, and vasoactive substances.[13,14]

C. SKIN FINDINGS

The characteristic skin findings are thin skin, striae, plethora, hirsutism (in women), acne, and ecchymoses.

Significant thinning of the skin probably arises from corticosteroid-induced inhibition of epidermal cell division and dermal collagen synthesis.[8,14] To measure skin thickness, many experts recommend using calipers (either skinfold calipers or electrocardiograph calipers) on the back of the patient's hand, an area lacking significant subcutaneous fat and thus representing just epidermis and dermis.[15,16] In women of reproductive age, this skinfold should be thicker than 1.8 mm.[15] Precise cutoffs have not been established for men, whose skin is normally thicker than women's, or for elderly patients, whose skin is normally thinner than younger patients.[16]

The striae in patients presenting with Cushing syndrome are wide (>1 cm) and colored deep red or purple, in contrast to the thinner, paler pink or white striae that occur normally during rapid weight gain from other causes.[5,17,18] Striae are usually found on the lower abdomen, but may occur on the buttocks, hips, lower back, upper thighs and arms. In one of Cushing original patients, wide striae extended from the lower abdomen to the axillae.[3] Pathologically, striae are dermal scars, with collagen fibers all aligned in the direction of stress, covered by an abnormally thin epidermis.[19] The pathogenesis of striae is not understood, but they may result from rupture of the weakened connective tissue of the skin, under tension from central obesity, which leaves a thin translucent window to the red and purple colored dermal blood vessels. Striae are more common in younger patients with Cushing syndrome than older patients.[17,20]

Plethora is an abnormal diffuse purple or reddish color of the face.[5] Hirsutism and acne occur because of increased adrenal androgens.[8,17] Ecchymoses probably appear because the blood vessels, lacking connective tissue support and protection, are more easily traumatized.

The severity of striae, acne, and hirsutism correlate poorly with cortisol levels, indicating that other factors—temporal, biochemical, or genetic—play a role in these physical signs.[17]

D. PROXIMAL WEAKNESS

Painless proximal weakness of the legs is common and prominent in Cushing syndrome, especially in elderly patients.[20] Because the weakness is a true myopathy, patients lack fasciculations, sensory changes, or reflex abnormalities. Chapter 61 discusses how to assess proximal muscle strength.

E. DEPRESSION

Patients with Cushing syndrome may have crying episodes, insomnia, impaired concentration, difficulty with memory, and suicide attempts.[21,22] The severity of depression correlates with the cortisol level,[21] and unless the depression antedates the endocrine symptoms by years, it usually improves dramatically after treatment.[22]

F. PSEUDO-CUSHING SYNDROME

Several disorders, including chronic alcoholism, depression, and HIV infection, may mimic the physical or biochemical findings of Cushing syndrome. Patients with chronic alcoholism may develop the physical findings or the biochemical abnormalities associated with Cushing syndrome, or both, most likely due to the overproduction of ACTH by the hypothalamic-pituitary axis, an abnormality that resolves after several weeks of abstinence.[23,24] Depressed patients may have the biochemical abnormalities of Cushing syndrome, but they usually lack the physical findings.[25] Patients with HIV infection, particularly if they are receiving protease inhibitors, may develop some of the physical findings (especially the buffalo hump and truncal obesity) but rarely the biochemical abnormalities.[26–29*]

III. Clinical Significance

A. DIAGNOSTIC ACCURACY OF FINDINGS

EBM Box 14.1 presents the diagnostic accuracy of individual physical signs for Cushing syndrome, as applied to over 650 patients with suspected disease. The findings that significantly *increase* the probability of Cushing syndrome are thin skinfold (likelihood ratio [LR] = 115.6), ecchymoses (LR = 4.5), proximal muscle weakness (LR = 3.8), central obesity (LR = 3), and plethora (LR = 2.7). (The astronomical LR for thin skinfold thickness [LR = 115.6] derives from young women presenting with hirsutism and menstrual irregularity and thus applies only to similar patients.) The findings that *decrease* the probability of Cushing syndrome are generalized obesity (LR = 0.1), absence of moon facies (LR = 0.1), absence of central obesity (LR = 0.2), and normal skinfold thickness (LR = 0.2).

---

*The term "pseudo-Cushing syndrome" is usually applied to patients with *both* clinical *and* biochemical evidence of hypercortisolism. Therefore, the term does not usually include HIV-infected patients with buffalo humps or truncal obesity, because these patients usually lack biochemical abnormalities.

EBM BOX 14.1	Cushing Syndrome*			

Finding (Reference)[†]	Sensitivity (%)	Specificity (%)	Likelihood Ratio[‡] if Finding Is	
			Present	Absent
Vital signs				
Hypertension[5,6]	25–38	83–94	2.3	0.8
Body habitus				
Moon faciesf[6]	98	41	1.6	**0.1**
Dorsal cervical fat pad[45]	50	78	2.3	0.6
Central obesity[5-7]	72–90	62–97	**3.0**	**0.2**
Generalized obesity[5]	4	38	**0.1**	2.5
BMI >30 kg/m[2 30,45]	31–85	4–26	NS	**3.1**
Skin findings				
Thin skinfold[15]	78	99	**115.6**	**0.2**
Plethora[5]	83	69	2.7	**0.3**
Hirsutism, in women[5,6,30,45]	31–76	48–79	1.4	NS
Ecchymoses[5,6,30]	38–71	69–94	**4.5**	0.6
Red or blue striae[5,6,30,45]	15–52	61–93	1.7	NS
Acne[5,30]	25–52	61–76	NS	NS
Extremity findings				
Muscle weakness[5,6,30,45]	28–63	69–98	**3.8**	NS
Edema[5,6]	38–57	56–83	1.8	0.7

*Diagnostic standard: for *Cushing syndrome*, elevated daily cortisol or corticosteroid metabolites, or both, with loss of circadian rhythm and with abnormal dexamethasone suppression.
[†]Definition of findings: for *hypertension*, diastolic blood pressure >105 mm Hg; for *central obesity*, central obesity index exceeds 1 or subjective appearance of central obesity sparing the extremities;[5,6,7] for *thin skinfold*, skinfold thickness on back of hand <1.8 mm (women of reproductive age only).[15]
[‡]Likelihood ratio (LR) if finding present = positive LR; LR if finding absent = negative LR.
NS, Not significant.

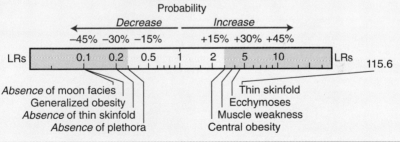

In these same studies, one of the more powerful predictors of Cushing syndrome is osteoporosis (sensitivity of 32% to 63%, specificity of 90% to 97%, positive LR = 8.6, and negative LR = 0.5).[5,6,30] Osteoporosis was identified radiographically in these studies, but it is often apparent at the bedside from vertebral fractures, kyphosis, and loss of height. Presumably, these bedside findings also accurately identify Cushing syndrome.

B. ETIOLOGY OF CUSHING SYNDROME AND BEDSIDE FINDINGS

Patients who take exogenous corticosteroids have the same frequency of central obesity, moon facies, and bruising as patients with endogenous Cushing, but a significantly lower incidence of hypertension, hirsutism, acne, striae, and buffalo humps.[31]

Patients with the ectopic ACTH syndrome from small cell carcinoma are more often male, have Cushing syndrome of rapid onset (over months instead of years), and present with prominent weight loss, myopathy, hyperpigmentation, and edema.[25,32,33] The irregular hepatomegaly of metastatic disease may suggest this diagnosis.[32] In studies of patients with ACTH-dependent Cushing syndrome, two findings significantly increase the probability of ectopic ACTH syndrome: weight loss (positive LR = 20) and symptom duration less than 18 months (positive LR = 15). Male sex increases the probability of ectopic ACTH syndrome a smaller amount (LR = 2.9).[32,34-36]

Hirsutism and acne may occur in any woman with endogenous Cushing syndrome, but the presence of virilization (i.e., male pattern baldness, deep voice, male musculature, clitoromegaly) argues strongly for adrenocortical carcinoma.[37-39]

References may be accessed online at *Elsevier eBooks for Practicing Clinicians*.

Vital Signs

Pulse Rate and Contour

PULSE RATE

I. Introduction

Taking the patient's pulse is one of the oldest physical examination techniques, practiced as long ago as 3500 BC by ancient Egyptian physicians, who believed a weakening pulse indicated advancing disease.[1] The pulse was one of Galen's (ca. 129–200 AD) favorite subjects, occupying several treatises that directed clinicians to observe the pulse's speed, force, and duration.[2,3] The first accurate observations of heart rate in disease were by John Foyer (1649–1734), who published his clinical observations in 1707 based on his invention, the pulse-watch.[3] The first clinicians to establish the significance of bradycardia were Adams and Stokes, who, between 1827 and 1846, pointed out that not all seizures and fainting represented disease of the brain but instead could occur because of the slow pulse of heart block.[1]

II. Technique

Most clinicians determine the pulse rate by palpating the radial pulse or, less often, by listening to the heart tones with the stethoscope (i.e., apical rate). Counting the pulse for 30 seconds and doubling the result is more accurate than 15 seconds of observation.[4] In patients with fast heart rates, especially if the patient has atrial fibrillation, counting the apical rate is more accurate than counting the radial pulse, and 60 seconds of observation is more accurate than shorter periods.[5]

A difference between the radial pulse rate and apical rate (the apical rate always being greater if there is a difference) is called the **pulse deficit**. A pulse deficit has traditionally been associated with atrial fibrillation, although it is a common finding with extrasystoles and all fast heart rates and by itself has little diagnostic significance.[6,7]

III. The Finding

Many textbooks state that the normal sinus rate ranges from 60 beats/min to 100 beats/min, but evidence indicates that the heart rate of 95% of healthy persons instead ranges from 50 beats/min to 95 beats/min.[8] **Bradycardia** is a pulse rate less than 50 beats/min; **tachycardia** is a rate greater than 100 beats/min.

IV. Clinical Significance

An important role of any vital sign is to provide the clinician an early indication that trouble is afoot for the patient. EBM Box 15.1 shows that the finding of tachycardia serves this role well. In a wide variety of clinical disorders, including septic shock, pneumonia, myocardial infarction, upper gastrointestinal hemorrhage, gallstone pancreatitis, and pontine hemorrhage, the finding of tachycardia (variably defined as rate >85 beats/min to >125 beats/min) predicts both increased complications and worse survival (likelihood ratios [LRs] = 1.5 to 25.4). In patients with myocardial infarction, the increased risk of adverse outcome is a continuum, being greater for patients with higher heart rates and persisting whether or not the patient has a low ejection fraction, takes beta-blocker medications, or receives thrombolytic therapy.[13,24–27] Tachycardia continues to predict increased mortality when detected during the first year after myocardial infarction.[28] In patients with septic shock, the relationship between tachycardia and mortality is independent of whether the patient receives vasopressor medications,[11] and in patients with pontine hemorrhage, tachycardia is a better predictor of mortality than other neurologic findings such as extensor posturing or the absence of withdrawal to pain.[20] The *absence* of tachycardia, on the other hand, decreases the probability of hospital mortality in patients with trauma, septic shock, and pontine hemorrhage (LRs = 0.1 to 0.3; see EBM Box 15.1) and argues *against* the presence of active bleeding during endoscopy for upper gastrointestinal hemorrhage (LR = 0.3).

Bradycardia is also an ominous finding in acute disorders. In patients with severe trauma, a pulse rate of 50 or less predicts mortality with a sensitivity of 17%, specificity of 99%, and positive LR of 20.7.[29] In acutely ill patients presenting to emergency departments for a variety of reasons, a pulse rate of 40 or less predicts hospital mortality with sensitivity of 9%, specificity of 100%, and positive LR of 39.1.[30]

Heart rates less than 50 beats/min or greater than 120 beats/min may also indicate heart rhythms other than sinus rhythm (e.g., complete heart block, atrial flutter), a subject discussed fully in Chapter 16.

ABNORMALITIES OF PULSE CONTOUR

I. Pulsus Alternans

A. THE FINDING

Pulsus alternans describes a regular pulse that has alternating strong and weak beats (Fig. 15.1). The pulse must be absolutely regular to diagnose pulsus alternans and distinguish it from the bigeminal pulse, which also has beats of alternating strength although that rhythm is irregular (see

EBM BOX 15.1	Tachycardia, Predicting Patient Outcome			
			Likelihood Ratio* if Finding Is	
Finding (Reference)	Sensitivity (%)	Specificity (%)	Present	Absent
Heart rate >85 beats/min				
Predicting postoperative complications, if lung cancer surgery[9]	71	81	**3.8**	0.4
Heart rate >90 beats/min				
Predicting hospital mortality, if trauma and hypotension[10]	94	38	1.5	**0.2**
Heart rate >95 beats/min				
Predicting hospital mortality, if septic shock[11]	97	53	2.0	**0.1**
Heart rate >100/min				
Predicting hospital mortality, if myocardial infarction[12–16]	6–40	88–98	**3.0**	0.9
Predicting active bleeding on urgent endoscopy, if UGI hemorrhage[17]	71	86	**4.9**	0.3
Predicting postoperative complications, if hernia surgery[18]	54	90	**5.6**	0.5
Predicting complications, if gallstone pancreatitis[19]	86	87	**6.8**	NS
Heart rate >110 beats/min				
Predicting hospital mortality, if pontine hemorrhage[20]	70	97	**25.4**	0.3
Heart rate >125 beats/min				
Predicting hospital mortality, if pneumonia[21–23]	6–33	86–98	2.6	NS

*Likelihood ratio (LR) if finding present = positive LR; LR if finding absent = negative LR.
NS, Not significant; *UGI*, upper gastrointestinal.

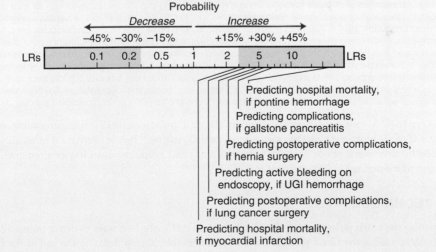

TACHYCARDIA
Probability
Decrease   Increase
−45% −30% −15%   +15% +30% +45%

LRs   0.1   0.2   0.5   1   2   5   10   LRs

Predicting hospital mortality, if pontine hemorrhage

Predicting complications, if gallstone pancreatitis

Predicting postoperative complications, if hernia surgery

Predicting active bleeding on endoscopy, if UGI hemorrhage

Predicting postoperative complications, if lung cancer surgery

Predicting hospital mortality, if myocardial infarction

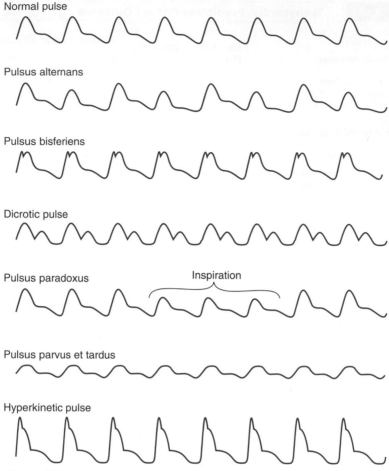

Fig. 15.1   Abnormalities of pulse contour. The normal pulse tracing (*top row*) is displayed with six tracings of abnormal pulse contours (*bottom rows*). **Pulsus alternans** (*second row*) is a *regular* pulse that has alternating strong and weak beats. Both **pulsus bisferiens** (*third row*) and the **dicrotic pulse** (*fourth row*) have two beats per cardiac cycle: in pulsus bisferiens both beats are systolic, whereas in the dicrotic pulse one is systolic and the other diastolic. **Pulsus paradoxus** (*fifth row*) is a pulse whose systolic blood pressure decreases more than 10 to 12 mm Hg during inspiration. **Pulsus parvus et tardus** (*sixth row*) is a pulse that has a small volume and rises slowly. The **hyperkinetic pulse** (*last row*) is a pulse with unusually abrupt and strong force; it may have a normal diastolic blood pressure (e.g., severe mitral insufficiency) or low diastolic blood pressure (e.g., severe aortic regurgitation). These tracings are facsimiles of actual pulse tracings made over 100 years ago. See text for pathogenesis and clinical significance.

Chapter 16).[31] In rare cases of pulsus alternans, the weak pulse is so small it is imperceptible, with only half of the beats reaching the radial artery (total alternans).[32] Pulsus alternans is often accompanied by alternation of the intensity of heart sounds and murmurs (auscultatory alternans).[31,33] Traube first described pulsus alternans in 1872.[34]

B. TECHNIQUE

Palpating the radial pulse or using the blood pressure cuff is the best ways to detect pulsus alternans. When using the blood pressure cuff, the clinician should stop deflating the cuff at the first appearance of Korotkoff sounds and hold the cuff pressure for several beats just below systolic blood pressure. In patients with pulsus alternans, only the Korotkoff sounds belonging to the strong beats are heard. Further deflation of the cuff allows cuff pressure to fall below the systolic pressure of the weaker beats, causing the cadence of Korotkoff sounds to suddenly double. The usual difference in systolic pressure between the strong and weak beats is only 15 to 20 mm Hg.[32]

Pulsus alternans often is most prominent in the several beats immediately after a pause in the heart rhythm. Typically, the pause is caused by a premature beat or the abrupt termination of a paroxysmal tachycardia.[35]

C. CLINICAL SIGNIFICANCE

In patients with normal heart rates, the finding of pulsus alternans indicates severe left ventricular dysfunction, caused by ischemic or valvular heart disease, long-standing hypertension, or idiopathic cardiomyopathy.[36–38] In one series of patients presenting for cardiac catheterization, investigators specifically looked for pulsus alternans after premature beats or 10 seconds of pacemaker-induced atrial tachycardia: those with pulsus alternans had worse ejection fractions and higher left ventricular filling pressures than those without the finding.[35]

In patients with rapid heart rates, pulsus alternans has less significance because even patients with normal hearts sometimes develop the finding during paroxysmal tachycardia.[39] Moreover, pulsus alternans rarely may reflect an intermittent left bundle branch block that alternates with ventricular beats having normal conduction.[40]

D. PATHOGENESIS

There has been considerable debate regarding whether the primary cause of pulsus alternans is alternation of intrinsic contractility of the heart (contractility argument) or alternation of filling of the ventricles (hemodynamic argument).

One version of the hemodynamic argument is particularly compelling.[34,41] In patients with a *regular* pulse, the sum of the length of systole and the length of the subsequent diastole must be constant. If systole lengthens for any reason, the subsequent diastole must be shorter; if systole shortens for any reason, the subsequent diastole must be longer. In patients with left ventricular dysfunction, a sudden increase in ventricular filling (such as that induced by a postextrasystolic pause) causes the subsequent systole to produce a strong beat, although it takes longer than normal for the weakened heart to eject this blood (i.e., thus lengthening systole). By prolonging systole, the strong beat thus shortens the next diastole, which reduces filling of the heart and causes the next beat to be weaker. The weaker beat is ejected more quickly, shortening systole and causing the next diastole to be longer, thus perpetuating the alternating pulse.

Nonetheless, the hemodynamic argument does not explain how pulsus alternans ever gets started when there is no pause in the rhythm from an extrasystole or termination of a tachycardia. Most experts now believe that alternation of intrinsic contractility is the fundamental problem in pulsus alternans, because alternation can even be demonstrated in vitro in isolated muscles at constant length and resting tension.[37,38] Once alternans begins, however, the hemodynamic effects probably contribute to the alternating amplitude of the pulse.

II. Pulsus Bisferiens
A. THE FINDING

Pulsus bisferiens (Latin *bis*, meaning "twice" and Latin *ferire*, meaning "to beat") has two beats per cardiac cycle, both of which occur in systole (the first beat is called the percussion wave; the second, the tidal wave, see Fig. 15.1).[31] Descriptions of pulsus bisferiens appear in the writings of Galen.[42]

B. TECHNIQUE

Pulsus bisferiens is detected by palpating the brachial or carotid pulse with moderate compression of the vessel, or by using the blood pressure cuff.[43] When using the blood pressure cuff, the clinician hears a quick double tapping sound instead of the typical single sound (the clinician can mimic the double sound by saying "pa-da…pa-da" as fast as possible).[44]

C. CLINICAL SIGNIFICANCE

Pulsus bisferiens is a finding in patients with moderate-to-severe aortic regurgitation.[42,44,45] Pulsus bisferiens also occurs in patients with combined aortic stenosis and regurgitation, though the principal lesion is usually the regurgitation and the stenosis is mild.[42,45,46] There are exceptional cases of the finding in severe aortic stenosis.[43]

Pulsus bisferiens is sometimes described in patients with hypertrophic cardiomyopathy,[47] although almost always as a finding seen on direct intraarterial pressure tracings, not as one palpated at the bedside.[48,49]

D. PATHOGENESIS

The bisferiens pulse probably results from rapid ejection of blood into a flexible aorta. Because of the Venturi effect, the rapidly moving bloodstream temporarily draws the walls of the aorta together, reducing flow momentarily and producing a notch with two systolic peaks in the waveform (in hypertrophic cardiomyopathy, the Venturi effect draws the anterior leaflet of the mitral valve and the interventricular septum together.).[43,50] Although this hypothesis was proposed over 50 years ago, direct evidence supporting it is difficult to find.

III. Pulsus Paradoxus

A. THE FINDING

Pulsus paradoxus is an exaggerated decrease of systolic blood pressure during inspiration (see Fig. 15.1).[31,51] Although the usual definition is an inspiratory decrease in systolic blood pressure exceeding 10 mm Hg, a better threshold may be 12 mm Hg, which is the upper 95% confidence interval for inspiratory decline in normal persons (i.e., the average inspiratory decrease in systolic pressure of normal persons is 6 ± 3 mm Hg).[52] In patients with pulsus paradoxus, the systolic blood pressure and pulse pressure fall dramatically during inspiration, though the diastolic blood pressure changes little.[51,52]

In 1873, Kussmaul first described pulsus paradoxus in three patients with pericardial disease.[53,54] Kussmaul called the finding "paradoxical" because the pulse of his patients disappeared during inspiration even though the apical beat persisted throughout the respiratory cycle. The term is unfortunate, because the finding is nothing more than an exaggeration of normal physiologic change.

B. TECHNIQUE

When checking for pulsus paradoxus, the clinician should have the patient breathe quietly and regularly, because even normal persons can induce a pulsus paradoxus with vigorous respirations. Pulsus paradoxus is detected by palpating the pulse or using the blood pressure cuff, although only paradoxical pulses exceeding 15 to 20 mm Hg are palpable.[55,56] For this reason, most clinicians use the blood pressure cuff, which has the added advantage of quantifying the finding (Fig. 15.2).

Pulsus paradoxus also has been noted in pulse oximetry tracings as respiratory movement of the tracing's baseline.[57] The amplitude of this oscillation correlates with the severity of pulsus

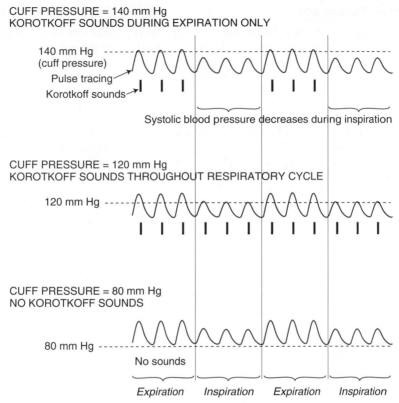

CUFF PRESSURE = 140 mm Hg
KOROTKOFF SOUNDS DURING EXPIRATION ONLY

140 mm Hg
(cuff pressure)
Pulse tracing
Korotkoff sounds

Systolic blood pressure decreases during inspiration

CUFF PRESSURE = 120 mm Hg
KOROTKOFF SOUNDS THROUGHOUT RESPIRATORY CYCLE

120 mm Hg

CUFF PRESSURE = 80 mm Hg
NO KOROTKOFF SOUNDS

80 mm Hg

No sounds

Expiration   Inspiration   Expiration   Inspiration

Fig. 15.2 Technique for measuring pulsus paradoxus. The figure simultaneously depicts the pressure in the blood pressure cuff (*dashed horizontal line*), the patient's pulse tracing (*solid line*), and Korotkoff sounds (*solid vertical bars* under pulse tracing) during two breaths (expiration and inspiration are separated by *vertical lines*). The pulse tracing shows the decrease in systolic pressure during inspiration, which is characteristic of pulsus paradoxus. To detect and measure the paradoxical pulse, the clinician begins by checking the blood pressure in the usual way but slowly deflates the cuff to precisely identify the *cuff pressure* at three points: First, the moment Korotkoff sounds first appear (*top tracing*). In patients with pulsus paradoxus, cuff pressure will fall below the systolic pressure of just the expiratory beats, and the Korotkoff sounds will repeatedly come and go during quiet respiration, disappearing with inspiration and reappearing with expiration. Second, the moment when Korotkoff sounds persist throughout the respiratory cycle (*middle tracing*). At this point cuff pressure has fallen below systolic blood pressure of all beats. Third, the moment when Korotkoff sounds disappear (i.e., the diastolic pressure, *bottom tracing*). In this patient, only expiratory Korotkoff sounds are heard between cuff pressures of 140 mm Hg and 120 mm Hg, but Korotkoff sounds are heard throughout the respiratory cycle between pressures of 120 mm Hg and 80 mm Hg. The patient's blood pressure is therefore "140/80 mm Hg with a paradox of 20 mm Hg" (i.e., 20 = 140 − 120).

paradoxus.[57] When using the blood pressure cuff to quantify pulsus paradoxus, clinicians may actually look at the visual display of the pulse oximeter placed on the patient's finger (distal to the cuff) instead of listening to the Korotkoff sounds.[58]

C. CLINICAL SIGNIFICANCE

Pulsus paradoxus is a common finding in two conditions, cardiac tamponade and acute asthma.

1. Cardiac Tamponade

Pulsus paradoxus of more than 10 mm Hg occurs in 98% of patients with cardiac tamponade (i.e., a pericardial effusion under high pressure compressing the heart and compromising cardiac output; see Chapter 47). Because it is one of three key findings of tamponade—the others being elevated neck veins (sensitivity = 100%) and tachycardia (sensitivity = 81% to 100%)— the clinician should consider tamponade and check for pulsus paradoxus in any patient suspected of having pericardial disease, such as those with elevated neck veins, unexplained dyspnea, pericardial rub, or known pericardial effusion.[56]

In patients with pericardial effusions, the finding of pulsus paradoxus of more than 12 mm Hg discriminates patients with tamponade from those without tamponade with a sensitivity of 98%, specificity of 83%, positive LR of 5.9, and negative LR of 0.03*.[52]

In another study of 74 patients with suspected tamponade,[59] clinicians printed out the patients' pulse oximetry tracings and measured the vertical amplitude (nadir-to-peak) of the tallest and shortest waveforms. After calculating the "oximetry paradoxus" ratio (tallest amplitude divided by shortest amplitude), these clinicians showed that a value less than 1.2 (i.e., minimal respiratory variation of the waveforms) argued compellingly *against* tamponade, as defined by subsequent echocardiography and right heart catheterization (LR = 0.05).[59]

2. Cardiac Tamponade without Pulsus Paradoxus

In only 2% of patients with tamponade, pulsus paradoxus is absent. These patients usually have one of five disorders: (1) atrial septal defect, (2) severe left ventricular dysfunction (especially those with uremic pericarditis),[60] (3) regional tamponade (tamponade affecting only one or two heart chambers, a complication of cardiac surgery),[61] (4) severe hypotension,[62-64] or (5) aortic regurgitation. Knowing that aortic regurgitation may eliminate pulsus paradoxus is especially significant, because patients with proximal (type A) aortic dissection and hemopericardium usually lack the paradoxical pulse despite significant tamponade, and the unaware clinician may exclude the possibility of tamponade to the harm of the patient.

The section on pathogenesis explains why pulsus paradoxus is absent in these clinical disorders.

3. Asthma

EBM Box 15.2 shows that, in patients with acute asthma, pulsus paradoxus exceeding 20 mm Hg almost certainly indicates severe bronchospasm (LR = 8.2). Nonetheless, pulsus paradoxus has limited clinical utility in patients with acute asthma, for two reasons. First, up to half of patients with severe bronchospasm lack a pulsus paradoxus greater than 10 mm Hg (EBM Box 15.2). The sensitivity is low because in asthma pulsus paradoxus depends on both respiratory rate and effort, even when the degree of airway obstruction remains constant.[66,68] Second, the best measure of bronchospasm (and the criterion standard in EBM Box 15.2) is peak expiratory flow rate. In a busy emergency department with an anxious and dyspneic patient, it is much more convenient to measure peak flow rates using handheld flow meters than trying to interpret the coming and going of Korotkoff sounds.

In patients being mechanically ventilated, the amount of pulsus paradoxus, as reflected in the changing baseline of the pulse oximeter tracing, correlates with the degree of the patient's auto-PEEP (a measure of expiratory obstruction in ventilated patients).[57]

---

*Tamponade was defined in this study as improvement in cardiac output of 20% or more following pericardiocentesis. See Chapter 47.

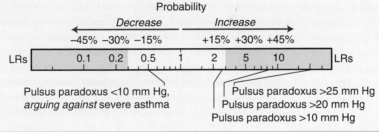

EBM BOX 15.2   **Pulsus Paradoxus Predicting Severe Asthma***

Finding (Reference)	Sensitivity (%)	Specificity (%)	Likelihood Ratio† if Finding Is	
			Present	Absent
Pulsus paradoxus >10 mm Hg[55,65-67]	52–68	69–92	2.7	0.5
Pulsus paradoxus >20 mm Hg[55,65,66]	19–39	91–100	**8.2**	0.8
Pulsus paradoxus >25 mm Hg[67]	16	99	**22.6**	0.8

*Diagnostic standard: for *severe asthma*, a FEV₁/forced vital capacity <50%,[55] FEV1 < 1.0 L,[65] peak flow < 200 L/min,[67] and peak flow < 30% predicted.[66] All patients in these studies had acute asthma.
†Likelihood ratio (LR) if finding present = positive LR; LR if finding absent = negative LR.
FEV_1, Forced expiratory volume in 1 second; *FVC*, forced vital capacity.

SEVERE ASTHMA
Probability

```
          Decrease              Increase
      ←—————————————         —————————————→
    -45%  -30%  -15%        +15%  +30%  +45%

LRs [    0.1    0.2    0.5    1    2    5    10    ] LRs
```

Pulsus paradoxus <10 mm Hg,   Pulsus paradoxus >25 mm Hg
arguing against severe asthma   Pulsus paradoxus >20 mm Hg
    Pulsus paradoxus >10 mm Hg

4. Pulsus Paradoxus in Other Conditions

Pulsus paradoxus has been described in constrictive pericarditis, right ventricular infarction, pulmonary embolism, tension left hydrothorax, and severe pectus excavatum,[51,69,70] although in each of these disorders it is an uncommon finding (see Chapter 47).

5. Reversed Pulsus Paradoxus[71]

Reversed pulsus paradoxus is a systolic blood pressure that falls more than 10 mm Hg *during expiration*. It has been described in three clinical disorders: (1) hypertrophic cardiomyopathy, (2) isorhythmic dissociation (i.e., inspiration accelerates the sinus rate, which temporarily positions the P waves before the QRS complex, thus coordinating the atrial and ventricular contractions and raising blood pressure; expiration slows the sinus rate, removes atrioventricular coordination, and lowers blood pressure), and (3) intermittent inspiratory positive-pressure breathing in the presence of left ventricular failure (this is a variation of the Valsalva square wave response in heart failure. See Chapter 48).

D. PATHOGENESIS

1. Cardiac Tamponade

Tamponade develops when the pressure of fluid inside the pericardial space exceeds the diastolic filling pressure of the heart chambers. Once this occurs, the diastolic pressure in the heart chambers, reflected in the neck veins, becomes a measurement of the force acting to compress the heart. The four chambers, now smaller in size, begin to compete for space, and an increase in the size of one comes at the expense of the size of another. Inspiration increases filling to the right side of the heart and shifts the interventricular septum to the left and posteriorly, thus obliterating the left ventricular chamber and causing the cardiac output to decrease. During expiration, filling of the right side of the heart is less, which increases left ventricular size, and both cardiac output and blood pressure increase.[51,61,72–75]

This explains why pulsus paradoxus is absent in regional tamponade and tamponade associated with atrial septal defect, severe left ventricular dysfunction, and aortic insufficiency (see the section on cardiac tamponade without pulsus paradoxus). Inspiratory movement of the interventricular septum is prevented when the right ventricle does not fill more during inspiration (atrial septal defect, see Chapter 40), when the left ventricular pressures are very high (severe left ventricular dysfunction), or when the left ventricle fills from some source other than the left atrium (aortic insufficiency). Regional tamponade, by definition, compresses only one or two chambers, enough to impair cardiac output but too confined to cause the heart chambers to compete for space.

2. Asthma

The mechanism of pulsus paradoxus in asthma is complex and not fully understood. Difficulty breathing causes wide swings of intrapleural pressure, which then are transmitted directly to the aorta, contributing to the paradoxical pulse. This is not a complete explanation, however, because the amount of pulsus paradoxus in asthma often exceeds the pressure shifts of these respiratory excursions.[68] Furthermore, the pulse pressure also declines during inspiration of some asthma patients, which would not happen if transmission of pressures were the only cause. Other proposed mechanisms are an inspiratory reduction in pulmonary venous return to the left heart[51,68,76,77] and the compressive action of the hyperinflated chest, which, like tamponade, may reduce the size of the heart chambers and cause them to compete for space.[66,78]

IV. Pulsus Parvus Et Tardus

A. THE FINDING AND TECHNIQUE

Pulsus parvus et tardus describes a carotid pulse with a small volume (pulsus parvus) that rises slowly and has a delayed systolic peak (pulsus tardus, see Fig. 15.1).[31] It is routinely detected by palpation.

B. CLINICAL SIGNIFICANCE

Pulsus parvus et tardus is a finding of aortic stenosis. Of its two components, pulsus tardus is the better discriminator, detecting severe aortic stenosis with a sensitivity of 31% to 91%, specificity of 68% to 93%, positive LR of 3.5, and negative LR of 0.4 (see Chapter 44).

C. PATHOGENESIS

Pulsus tardus depends on both the severity of obstruction to flow and the compliance of the vessel distal to the obstruction. The pulse waveform rises rapidly in stiff vessels, but slowly in more compliant vessels that act like low-pass filters and remove the high frequency components of the waveform.[79] That the delay in the pulse reflects the severity of obstruction is a principle also used by Doppler sonography to gauge the severity of renal artery stenosis.[79]

V. Dicrotic Pulse

A. THE FINDING AND TECHNIQUE

The **dicrotic pulse** has two beats per cardiac cycle, but unlike pulsus bisferiens one peak is systolic and the other is diastolic (Fig. 15.1).[31] It is usually detected by palpation of the carotid artery.[80]

The second wave of the dicrotic pulse is identical in timing to the small dicrotic wave of normal persons, obvious on arterial pressure tracings but never palpable. The dicrotic wave is felt to represent rebound of blood against the closed aortic valve.

B. CLINICAL SIGNIFICANCE

The dicrotic pulse occurs in younger patients with severe myocardial dysfunction, low stroke volumes, and high systemic resistance.[80,81] In patients who have had valvular replacement surgery, the finding of a persistent dicrotic pulse is associated with a poor prognosis.[81]

C. PATHOGENESIS

A dicrotic pulse relies on the simultaneous presence of two conditions: (1) low stroke volume, which significantly reduces the height of the pulse's initial systolic wave, thus increasing the chances that the dicrotic wave will be palpable[82]; and (2) a resilient arterial system, which amplifies the rebound of the pulse waveform during diastole. The importance of a resilient arterial system may explain why the dicrotic pulse usually occurs in young patients with cardiomyopathy, who have more compliant vessels than older patients.[80,81]

The importance of a low stroke volume to the dicrotic pulse is illustrated by the observation that the dicrotic pulse sometimes disappears with beats that have larger stroke volumes, such as the beat after a premature beat, the stronger beats of pulsus alternans, and the expiratory beats of pulsus paradoxus.[80,82] Vasodilators often cause the dicrotic pulse to disappear, perhaps because of better forward flow and a greater stroke volume.[80]

VI. Hyperkinetic Pulse

A. THE FINDING

The hyperkinetic pulse strikes the examiner's fingers with unusually abrupt and strong force (see Fig. 15.1). Hyperkinetic pulses may have either a normal pulse pressure (e.g., severe mitral regurgitation, hypertrophic obstructive cardiomyopathy) or increased pulse pressure (e.g., aortic insufficiency and other disorders with abnormal aortic runoff).[31] In both severe mitral regurgitation and hypertrophic obstructive cardiomyopathy, the blood is ejected rapidly from the left ventricle but the integrity of the aortic valve preserves a normal arterial diastolic and pulse pressure.[83] In aortic regurgitation, the rapid ejection of blood is accompanied by an incompetent aortic valve, which causes a very low diastolic pressure in the aortic root, thus increasing the pulse pressure and causing the Corrigan or water-hammer pulse characteristic of this disorder (see Chapter 45).

B. CLINICAL SIGNIFICANCE

Chapter 45 discusses the significance of the water hammer pulse and large pulse pressure of aortic regurgitation.

In patients with mitral stenosis, the pulse is characteristically normal or diminished. If the clinician instead finds a hyperkinetic pulse in these patients, the probability is high that additional

| EBM BOX 15.3 | Pulses and Hypovolemic Shock[86*] |

Finding (Reference)	Sensitivity (%)	Specificity (%)	Likelihood Ratio[†] if Finding Is	
			Present	Absent
Detecting systolic blood pressure ≥60 mm Hg				
Carotid pulse present	95	22	NS	NS
Femoral pulse present	95	67	2.9	**0.1**
Radial pulse present	52	89	NS	0.5

*Diagnostic standard: for *systolic blood pressure* ≥ 60 mm Hg, invasive arterial blood pressure measurements.
[†]Likelihood ratio (LR) if finding present = positive LR; LR if finding absent = negative LR.
NS, Not significant.

SYSTOLIC BLOOD PRESSURE ≥60 mm Hg (IF HYPOVOLEMIC SHOCK)
Probability

Decrease   Increase

−45% −30% −15%   +15% +30% +45%

LRs   0.1   0.2   0.5   1   2   5   10   LRs

Femoral pulse *absent*   Femoral pulse *present*
Radial pulse *absent*

valvular disease is present, such as significant mitral regurgitation (sensitivity 71%, specificity 95%, positive LR = 14.2, negative LR = 0.3, see Chapter 46).[84,85]

VII. Pulses and Hypovolemic Shock

In patients with hypovolemic shock, the peripheral pulses provide a rough guide to the patient's systolic blood pressure.[86] As blood pressure progressively diminishes, the radial pulse generally disappears first, then the femoral pulse, and finally the carotid pulse. In one study of 20 patients with hypovolemic shock, summarized in EBM Box 15.3, the femoral pulse had the greatest diagnostic accuracy in determining severity of shock: the presence of a palpable femoral pulse increased probability of a systolic blood pressure greater than 60 mm Hg (LR = 2.9), whereas its absence decreased the probability of a blood pressure this high (LR = 0.1).

References may be accessed online at *Elsevier eBooks for Practicing Clinicians.*

Abnormalities of Pulse Rhythm

I. Introduction

In the late 19th and early 20th centuries, before the introduction of electrocardiography, clinicians could examine the patient's arterial pulse, heart tones, and jugular venous waveforms and, from these observations alone, diagnose atrial and ventricular premature contractions, atrial flutter, atrial fibrillation, complete heart block, Mobitz 1 and 2 atrioventricular block, and sinoatrial block.[1-3] In fact, clinicians were familiar enough with the bedside findings of these arrhythmias that early textbooks of electrocardiography included tracings of the arterial and venous pulse to help explain the electrocardiogram (ECG; see Fig. 16.1).[4]

The bedside diagnosis of arrhythmias today is probably little more than an intellectual endeavor, because all significant arrhythmias require electrocardiography for confirmation and monitoring. Nonetheless, bedside diagnosis of arrhythmias is still possible, using principles discovered 100 years ago by Mackenzie, Wenckebach, and Lewis. These principles, based on extensive investigation and many polygraph recordings of the arterial and venous pulse,[1-4] allow diagnosis of simple arrhythmias when the electrocardiograph is not immediately available.

Normal sinus rhythm

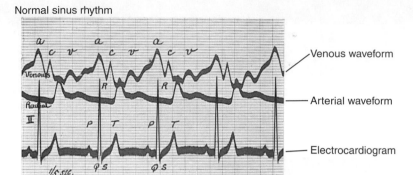

Venous waveform

Arterial waveform

Electrocardiogram

Complete heart block

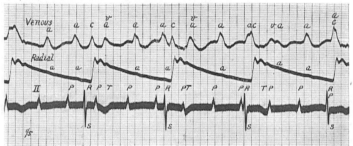

Atrial fibrillation

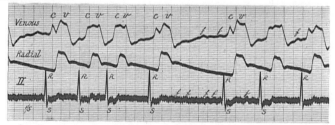

Fig. 16.1 Simultaneous venous, arterial, and electrocardiographic curves. To help clinicians understand the P, QRS, and T waves of the newly introduced electrocardiogram, early textbooks displayed simultaneous venous and arterial waveforms with the electrocardiogram. These examples, reproduced from Sir Thomas Lewis's 1925 *Mechanism and graphic registration of the heart beat*,[4] depict normal sinus rhythm (*top*), complete heart block (*middle*), and atrial fibrillation (*bottom*). See the text.

II. Technique

The first step in diagnosing arrhythmias is to determine the basic rhythm of the patient's radial pulse. Most arrhythmias can be classified into one of five basic abnormalities: (1) the pause, (2) regular bradycardia, (3) regular tachycardia, (4) irregular rhythm that varies with respiration, and (5) irregularly irregular (or chaotic) rhythm (see Fig. 16.2).

The radial pulse may not correspond to the ventricular pulse (or apical pulse), as determined by auscultation of the heart tones or palpation of the cardiac impulse, because some ventricular

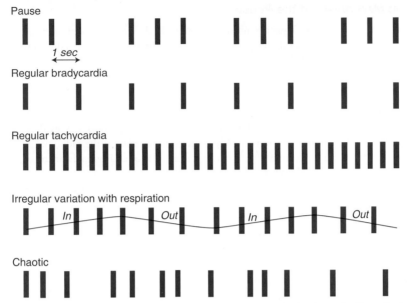

Fig. 16.2   Basic abnormalities of pulse rhythm. (1) The pause, (2) regular bradycardia, (3) regular tachycardia, (4) irregular rhythm that varies with respiration ("in" depicts inspiration and "out" depicts expiration), and (5) irregularly irregular (or "chaotic") rhythm. See the text.

contractions are too weak to propel blood to the radial artery. Although the clinician must compare the radial pulse with the ventricular pulse to diagnose arrhythmias, the difference in *rate* between the two by itself indicates no particular diagnosis.

After the basic rhythm of the radial pulse is identified, analysis of the jugular venous waveforms, heart tones, and response of the heart rhythm to vagal maneuvers may further distinguish the various causes.

III. The Findings and Their Clinical Significance

A. THE PAUSE

The pause has two important causes, premature contractions (common) and heart block (uncommon).

1. Terminology

When the radial pulse consists of the regular repetition of two beats followed by a pause, the term **bigeminal pulse** or **bigeminal rhythm** is used. When there are three radial pulse beats between each pause, the appropriate term is **trigeminal pulse** or **trigeminal rhythm**. The finding of several beats between each pause is usually called **group beating**, and even longer periods of regular rhythm interrupted by the rare pause is sometimes referred to as **pulse intermissions**. The basic mechanism for all of these rhythm disturbances is the same, only the frequency of premature beats or heart block differs among them.

Because the cadence of these rhythms becomes predictable after short periods of observation, the term *regularly irregular* is sometimes used. This term, however, inaccurately conveys to others what actually is going on and is best discarded.

2. Basic Mechanism of the Pause

The pause has three basic mechanisms, illustrated in Fig. 16.3. The two most important questions that distinguish these mechanisms are the following: (1) Is there a premature radial pulse immediately preceding the pause? (2) Do additional ventricular beats (identified by listening to the heart tones or palpating the apical pulse) occur during the pause?

a. Premature Beat

Patients with premature contractions (the first two examples in Fig. 16.3) have evidence of a premature ventricular beat during or immediately preceding the pause in the radial pulse. This early beat is always evident in the form of a palpable apical impulse or additional heart tones, although it may not be felt in the radial artery.

Some premature contractions are strong enough to open the aortic valve (first example in Fig. 16.3). If so, the clinician will feel a quick beat in the radial pulse just preceding the pause,

Premature beat opens aortic valve:

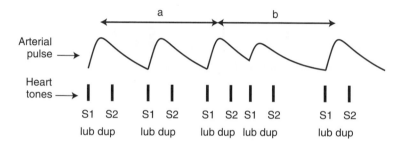

Premature beat fails to open aortic valve:

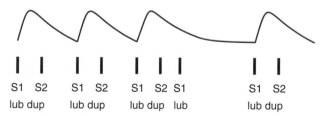

Heart block:

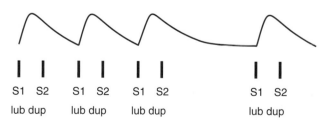

Fig. 16.3 **Mechanism of the pause.** The radial pulse tracing and heart tones are presented, illustrating the three mechanisms for the pause: (1) premature contraction that opens the aortic valve, (2) premature contraction that fails to open the aortic valve, and (3) heart block. Onomatopoeia of the heart tones appears below each tracing ("lub" is the first heart sound, "dup" is the second heart sound). See the text.

although the quick beat is usually not as strong as a normal sinus beat. When listening to the heart tones, the clinician will hear both the first and second heart sounds of the early beat, which produces the following characteristic cadence:

lub dup   *lub dup*   *lub dup lub dup*   *lub dup*

(In this and the following two examples, *lub* is the first heart sound and *dup* is the second sound; each rhythm begins with three normal beats, i.e., three *lub dups*.)

If the premature contraction is too weak to open the aortic valve (second example in Fig. 16.3), the clinician palpating the pulse will not detect the quick beat but will only feel the pause. Listening to the heart, he or she will hear only the first sound of the premature beat (S_2 is absent because the aortic valve never opens):

lub dup   *lub dup*   *lub dup lub*   *lub dup*

b. Heart Block

Patients with heart block (third example in Fig. 16.3), whether sinoatrial or atrioventricular, lack a palpable apical impulse or extra heart tones during the pause. The cadence of heart tones contrasts with those of the premature beat:

lub dup   *lub dup*   *lub dup*   *lub dup*

3. Bigeminal and Trigeminal Rhythms, and Grouped Beating

Based upon the mechanisms previously discussed, there are three causes of the bigeminal pulse rhythm: (1) alternating normal and premature contractions; (2) premature contractions occurring every third beat, although the premature contraction is too weak to open the aortic valve; and (3) 3:2 heart block (atrioventricular or sinoatrial). In causes 2 and 3, both beats of the couplet are strong, but cause 2 has evidence of a ventricular contraction during the pause whereas cause 3 does not.

The same analysis is used for trigeminal rhythms and grouped beating (i.e., in trigeminal rhythms, possible causes are premature contractions after every two or three normal beats or 4:3 heart block).

4. Atrial vs. Ventricular Premature Contractions

Two helpful bedside findings distinguish atrial premature contractions from ventricular ones:

a. Compensatory Pause

Beats that originate in the ventricle usually do not upset the underlying sinus rhythm, causing the beat immediately following the pause to fall exactly when the clinician anticipates it. Tapping the foot during the normal regular rhythm helps determine this. In Fig. 16.3, the distance "b" equals "a," meaning there is a "complete compensatory pause."

Beats that originate in the atria, in contrast, often reset the sinus node, causing the next beat to appear earlier than expected. In Fig. 16.3, "b" would be less than "a," and the clinician tapping the foot would find that the basic meter of rhythm changes.

This rule is more helpful when the pause is not compensatory (i.e., b < a, indicating the beat is atrial), because many atrial premature contractions also seem to have a complete compensatory pause at the bedside.

b. Cannon A Waves

The appearance of a sudden prominent venous wave in the neck (cannon A wave) *during the pause* indicates that the premature beat was ventricular (see also Chapter 36). This occurs because the right atrium, still beating under the direction of the uninterrupted sinus impulses, contracts after the ventricular premature contraction has closed the tricuspid valve. Rarely, extremely premature ectopic atrial beats may also produce cannon A waves, but these waves precede the first heart sound of the premature contraction, whereas cannon A waves from ventricular premature contractions always follow the first heart sound of the premature beat.

B. REGULAR BRADYCARDIA

Regular bradycardia is a heart rate of less than 50 beats/min. There are three causes of regular bradycardia that are recognizable at the bedside: sinus bradycardia, complete heart block, and halved pulse.

1. Sinus Bradycardia

This arrhythmia resembles the normal rhythm in every way except for the abnormally slow rate: the venous waveforms in the neck are normal, the intensity of the first heart sound is the same with each beat, and there is no evidence of ventricular contractions between radial pulsations (as determined by palpation of apical impulse or auscultation of the heart tones).

2. Complete Heart Block

In complete heart block, the atria and ventricles beat independently of each other (i.e., atrioventricular dissociation). Sometimes the atrial and ventricular contractions are contiguous, and sometimes they are far apart. Atrioventricular dissociation causes two important bedside findings: changing intensity of the first heart sound and intermittent cannon A waves in the venous pulse.

a. Changing Intensity of the First Heart Sound

In complete heart block, the first heart sound of most beats is faint. Intermittently, however, the atrium contracts just before the ventricle contraction, which results in a first heart sound of booming intensity (named **bruit de canon** because of its explosive quality; see Chapter 40 for the pathophysiology of S_1 intensity).[5]

The finding of a changing first heart sound is only significant when the pulse is regular, because in irregular rhythms its intensity naturally varies with the length of the previous diastole (i.e., long diastoles intensify the first heart sound of the next beat; short diastoles diminish it). If the ventricular pulse is regular, however, a changing intensity of the first heart sound (or intermittent "booming" of the first heart sound) indicates only one diagnosis, atrioventricular dissociation.

b. Intermittent Appearance of Cannon A Waves in the Venous Pulse

In complete heart block, when an atrial contraction falls intermittently just after a ventricular contraction, the right atrium will contract against a closed tricuspid valve, causing an abrupt systolic outward wave in the jugular venous pulse (i.e., cannon A wave; see also Chapter 36).

In many different arrhythmias, cannon A waves appear with *every* arterial pulse. If cannon A waves appear *intermittently*, however, in a patient whose ventricular pulse is *regular*, the only possible diagnosis is atrioventricular dissociation.

c. Other Evidence of Atrioventricular Dissociation

Other uncommon signs of atrioventricular dissociation are regular small A waves in the venous pulse; regular muffled fourth heart sounds at the apex; or, in patients with mitral stenosis, regular short murmurs from the atrium pushing blood across the stenotic valve. All of these findings represent regular atrial contractions that continue during the long ventricular diastoles.

A rare sign of complete heart block is an intermittently audible summation gallop (or third heart sound; see Chapter 41).[6]

3. Halved Pulse

Halved pulse refers to the finding of twice as many ventricular beats as radial pulse beats. This is almost always due to premature contractions that appear every other beat but are too weak to open the aortic valve and reach the radial pulse. Rarely, pulsus alternans may be the cause (**total alternans**),[7] although in these patients the heart tones at the apex are regular, whereas in premature contractions they are bigeminal.

C. REGULAR TACHYCARDIA

The regular tachycardias that *sometimes* are recognizable at the bedside include sinus tachycardia, atrial flutter, paroxysmal supraventricular tachycardia, and ventricular tachycardia. The bedside observations that distinguish these arrhythmias are response to vagal maneuvers, signs of atrioventricular dissociation, and abnormalities of the neck veins. Even so, bedside examination is diagnostic in only the minority of patients with rapid rates, and the careful clinician always relies on electrocardiography for diagnosis.

1. Vagal Maneuvers

The usual maneuvers are the Valsalva maneuver and carotid artery massage.

a. Technique

Both maneuvers are performed when the patient is supine. To perform the Valsalva maneuver, the clinician asks the patient to bear down and strain against a closed glottis as if "having a bowel movement." Patients who have difficulty following this instruction sometimes respond better when asked to put the tip of their own thumb in their mouth and pretend it is a balloon to blow up. In patients with supraventricular tachycardia, 15 seconds of straining is as effective as 30 seconds.[8] The Valsalva maneuver increases vagal tone and has its maximal effect on tachycardias *after* the release of the Valsalva, not while the patient is straining.[8]

In carotid artery massage, the clinician finds the bifurcation of one carotid artery, located at the point of maximal carotid pulsation just below the angle of the jaw,[9] and massages or presses on it for 5 seconds.[8,10,11]

The Valsalva maneuver is preferred for two reasons: (1) It tends to be more efficacious, terminating supraventricular tachycardia 20% to 50% of the time, compared with only a 10% efficacy using carotid massage,[8,12] and (2) in elderly patients with carotid artery disease, carotid artery massage may rarely cause a stroke.[13,14]

b. Response of Regular Tachycardias to Vagal Maneuvers[10]

Transient slowing of the pulse during a vagal maneuver indicates sinus tachycardia. **Abrupt termination** of the tachycardia indicates paroxysmal supraventricular tachycardia (this occurs with both nodal re-entry tachycardias and reciprocating tachycardias from accessory pathways). **Abrupt halving** of the rate may occur in atrial flutter. **No response** is unhelpful, being characteristic of ventricular tachycardia[15] but also occurring with every other regular tachycardia.[8,12]

2. Atrioventricular Dissociation

Any finding of atrioventricular dissociation in patients with regular tachycardia indicates the rhythm is ventricular tachycardia. These findings include the *intermittent* appearance of cannon A waves in the neck veins*, changing intensity of the first heart sound, and changing systolic blood pressure (usually detected with the blood pressure cuff).[16,17] In one study of patients with ventricular tachycardia, in which atrioventricular association or dissociation was determined by pacing (EBM Box 16.1), the finding of a changing S_1 increased probability of atrioventricular dissociation (likelihood ratio [LR] = 24.4) and the *absence* of intermittent cannon A waves decreased probability of atrioventricular dissociation (LR = 0.1).

Even so, these LRs are misleading because some patients with ventricular tachycardia lack atrioventricular dissociation and instead have 1:1 retrograde conduction or atrial fibrillation.[15] Given the serious consequences of misdiagnosing the regular tachycardia rhythm, an ECG should always be obtained.

3. Flutter Waves in the Venous Pulse

In elderly patients with a ventricular pulse of 130 to 160 beats/min, the clinician should suspect atrial flutter with 2:1 conduction. In addition to performing vagal maneuvers, the clinician may see rapid, small undulations (with a rate about 300/min) in the venous pulse, which are called flutter waves (or f waves) and correspond to the wave of the same name on the ECG.[19]

4. Sensation of Pounding in the Neck

A common cause of regular tachycardia is atrioventricular nodal reentrant tachycardias. In patients with this arrhythmia, the retrograde P wave of every beat coincides with the QRS complex, resulting in simultaneous cannon A venous pulsations and carotid arterial pulsations in the neck of affected patients, thus creating conspicuous pounding neck palpitations. Other causes of regular tachycardias are less likely to create neck palpitations because the atrial and ventricular contractions occur at slightly different times (in patients with reciprocating tachycardias from accessory pathways, for example, the atrial contraction occurs after the ventricular contraction).

In studies of patients referred to electrophysiology specialists because of intermittent rapid palpitations, the symptom of *rapid, regular* pounding in the neck during the palpitations distinguished atrioventricular nodal reentrant tachycardia from other causes of tachycardia with a sensitivity of 20% to 92%, specificity of 83% to 100%, positive LR of 7.7, and negative LR of 0.6.[20–23]

D. IRREGULAR RHYTHM THAT VARIES WITH RESPIRATION

This rhythm is sinus arrhythmia, an especially common and prominent arrhythmia of younger patients. The pulse characteristically quickens during inspiration and slows during exhalation (see Fig. 16.2).[24] The slowing during expiration is sometimes so conspicuous it mimics the finding of a pause.

E. IRREGULARLY IRREGULAR RHYTHM (CHAOTIC RHYTHM)

This term describes a cadence of ventricular and radial beats that is completely irregular and unpredictable. The diagnosis is usually atrial fibrillation. In studies of over 2000 patients, the finding of an *irregular* radial pulse increases the probability of atrial fibrillation (LR = 6.4, EBM Box 16.2), whereas the absence of this finding (i.e., the pulse is *regular*) decreases probability of atrial fibrillation (LR = 0.1). In one of these studies, using just 20 seconds of observation, the finding of a **chaotic pulse** markedly increased probability of atrial fibrillation (LR = 24.1).

---

*A video demonstrating the intermittent cannon A waves of ventricular tachycardia appears in the reference by Ali.[16]

| EBM BOX 16.1 | **Atrioventricular Dissociation and Ventricular Tachycardia**[*] | | | |

Finding (Reference)[†]	Sensitivity (%)	Specificity (%)	Likelihood Ratio[‡] if Finding Is Present	Likelihood Ratio[‡] if Finding Is Absent
Varying arterial pulse[18]	63	70	NS	NS
Intermittent cannon A waves, neck veins[18]	96	75	3.8	0.1
Changing intensity S_1[18]	58	98	24.4	0.4

[*]Diagnostic standard: for *atrioventricular dissociation*, ventricular-paced rhythm at a rate independent of the atrial rate.
[†]Definition of findings: for *varying arterial pulse*, varying amplitude of radial or carotid pulse by palpation.
[‡]Likelihood ratio (LR) if finding present = positive LR; LR if finding absent = negative LR.
NS, Not significant.

ATRIOVENTRICULAR DISSOCIATION (IF TACHYCARDIA)

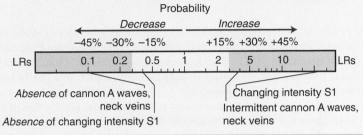

Absence of cannon A waves, neck veins
Absence of changing intensity S1

Changing intensity S1
Intermittent cannon A waves, neck veins

| EBM BOX 16.2 | **Atrial Fibrillation**[*] |

Finding (Reference)[†]	Sensitivity (%)	Specificity (%)	Likelihood Ratio[‡] if Finding Is Present	Likelihood Ratio[‡] if Finding Is Absent
Pulse *not* regular[25–30]	80–98	70–97	6.4	0.1
Chaotic pulse[27]	54	98	24.1	0.5

[*]Diagnostic standard: for *atrial fibrillation*, electrocardiography.
[†]Definition of findings: for *chaotic pulse*, "frequent or continuous irregularity" during 20 second examination of the radial pulse.
[‡]Likelihood ratio (LR) if finding present = positive LR; LR if finding absent = negative LR.

ATRIAL FIBRILLATION

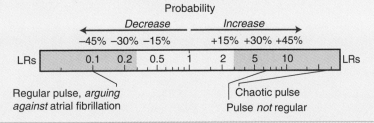

Regular pulse, *arguing against* atrial fibrillation

Chaotic pulse
Pulse *not* regular

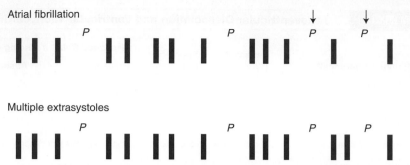

Fig. 16.4 The chaotic rhythm. The irregularly irregular or chaotic rhythm may represent atrial fibrillation (*top*) or sinus rhythm with multiple extrasystoles (*bottom*). "P" marks conspicuous pauses that appear in the cadence of *apical* heart tones. (Each bar depicts one cardiac cycle, or one *lub dup*.) In this example, the cadence of the two arrhythmias is identical until the end of the tracing: in atrial fibrillation, two pauses occur in a row (*arrows*), thus distinguishing it from the pauses of multiple extrasystoles that are flanked by quick beats or beats of normal cadence. See the text.

Frequent multifocal premature contractions may sometimes seem chaotic at the bedside, but two findings distinguish this rhythm from atrial fibrillation: **(1) Venous pulse**. In atrial fibrillation, the venous pulse is simple and consists of only one wave per cardiac cycle (i.e., there is no A wave and the x' descent is diminished, revealing a solitary y descent; see Chapter 36). In frequent premature contractions, in contrast, the venous pulse is complex and consists of intermittent cannon A waves superimposed on two venous movements per cardiac cycle. **(2) Rhythm of ventricular pulse** (Fig. 16.4). In atrial fibrillation, the interval between ventricular beats is random, and it is quite common to have one pause followed by an even longer pause. In frequent premature contractions, this is impossible because the pause must be followed by another quick beat or the normal sinus interval. This difference in rhythm, which again focuses on the ventricular rhythm at the apex, not the radial pulse, is quite conspicuous once the clinician is aware of it.

References may be accessed online at *Elsevier eBooks for Practicing Clinicians*.

Blood Pressure

- There are two methods of blood pressure measurement, the traditional auscultatory method (using the stethoscope to detect Korotkoff sounds) and the oscillometric method (automated machines). Only the auscultatory method detects pulsus paradoxus, pulsus alternans, and pulsus bisferiens. The oscillometric method, in contrast, reduces observer biases and avoids the error of the auscultatory gap.
- Hypotension is an ominous finding in hospitalized patients, predicting increased mortality and adverse outcomes.
- A difference of more than 20 mm Hg in the systolic blood pressure of the arms is abnormal, suggesting either subclavian steal syndrome (in patients with symptoms of vertebrobasilar ischemia) or aortic dissection (in patients with acute chest pain).
- In patients with known cardiomyopathy, a *narrow* pulse pressure (i.e., proportional pulse pressure less than 0.25) increases probability of low cardiac output. In patients with the murmur of aortic regurgitation, a wide pulse pressure (80 mm Hg or more) increases probability of moderate-to-severe regurgitation.
- When measuring postural vital signs (i.e., comparing supine and standing positions), hypovolemia is likely if there is *either* a pulse increment of 30/min or more *or* the patient cannot stand because of dizziness.

I. Introduction

Systolic blood pressure is the maximal pressure within the artery during ventricular systole, **diastolic blood pressure** is the lowest pressure in the vessel just before the next systole, and **pulse pressure** is the difference between the systolic and diastolic values. Pulse pressure may be normal, abnormally small (narrow), or abnormally large (wide; see the section on abnormal pulse pressure). The mean arterial pressure can be estimated by $(S + 2D)/3$, where S is systolic blood pressure and D is diastolic blood pressure.[1]

The first person to measure blood pressure was Stephen Hales, an English clergyman of creative genius, who in 1708 directly connected the left crural artery of a horse to a 9-foot tall glass manometer using brass tubes and a trachea of goose.[2,3] Vierordt of Germany introduced the indirect method of measuring blood pressure in 1855, based on the principle that blood pressure is equal to the amount of external pressure necessary to obliterate the distal pulse. Indirect measurements required cumbersome mechanical devices and were not widely accepted until 1896, when the Italian Riva-Rocci invented the blood pressure cuff.[2,3]

Blood pressure was the last of the four traditional vital signs to be routinely monitored in hospitalized patients. In 1901, after Harvey Cushing first brought the blood pressure cuff to America and encouraged its use in neurosurgical patients, most clinicians resisted using it because they believed palpation of pulse revealed much more information, including its "fullness," "tension," "rate," "rhythm," "size," "force," and "duration."[4,5] Two events were responsible for clinicians eventually accepting the blood pressure cuff: (1) Korotkoff described his sounds in 1905, which allowed clinicians to easily measure systolic and diastolic blood pressure using a stethoscope, and: (2) Janeway published his book *Clinical Study of Blood Pressure* in 1907, which proved that monitoring blood pressure was clinically useful. Janeway showed, for example, that the first sign of intestinal perforation or hemorrhage in patients with typhoid fever was progressive hypotension.[6] By the time of the First World War, blood pressure was routinely recorded by most clinicians along with the patient's pulse rate, respiratory rate, and temperature.[5,7,8]

II. Technique

A. AUSCULTATORY VERSUS OSCILLOMETRIC METHODS

There are two methods of measuring blood pressure: The **auscultatory method** (the traditional method) uses a stethoscope to detect Korotkoff sounds in the brachial artery as a blood pressure cuff is slowly manually deflated. Aneroid manometers have largely replaced the original standard for this method, the mercury sphygmomanometer, because of mercury's environmental risks and bans on its use.[9] The **oscillometric method** analyzes pressure oscillations within the cuff itself and uses proprietary computer programs to calculate the blood pressure and display the result digitally.[9]

The auscultatory method has the advantage of being able to detect abnormalities of pulse contour, such as pulsus paradoxus, pulsus alternans, and pulsus bisferiens, all abnormalities missed using the oscillometric method (see Chapter 15). The oscillometric method, in contrast, has the advantages of convenience, reduced observer bias, and elimination of the auscultatory gap. (See subsequent sections on terminal digit preference and auscultatory gap.)

B. RECOMMENDED TECHNIQUE[9,10]

Published recommendations for measuring blood pressure are based on the consensus opinion of expert committees who have reviewed all available scientific evidence. These recommendations, however, are designed to avoid misdiagnosis of hypertension and may not be as relevant to clinicians using the blood pressure cuff to diagnose other abnormalities, such as hypotension or abnormalities of pulse contour. (See Chapter 15 and the section on clinical significance later in this chapter.)

The important elements of the correct technique are as follows: (1) The patient should sit in a chair with his or her back supported and should rest for at least 5 minutes before the blood pressure is measured. (2) The patient's arm should be at the level of the heart. (3) The length of the blood pressure cuff's bladder should encircle at least 80% of the arm's circumference. (4) The clinician should inflate the cuff to a pressure 20 to 30 mm Hg above the systolic pressure, as first identified by palpation of the distal pulse (i.e., the pulse disappears when cuff pressure exceeds systolic pressure). (5) The pressure in the cuff should be released at a rate of 2 mm Hg per second. (6) The clinician should obtain at least two readings separated by at least 30 seconds and average them; if these differ by more than 5 mm Hg, additional readings are necessary. (7) The readings should be rounded off to the nearest 2 mm Hg.

In some clinical scenarios, described in the section "Findings and Their Clinical Significance," additional measurements are necessary, including those of the legs or opposite arm, or measurements taken with the patient in different positions.

C. KOROTKOFF SOUNDS (AUSCULTATORY METHOD)

1. Definition of Systolic and Diastolic Blood Pressure

As the cuff is slowly deflated from a point above systolic pressure, the first appearance of sound (Korotkoff phase 1) indicates systolic blood pressure.* Clinicians have debated for decades whether the muffling of sound (Korotkoff phase 4) or disappearance of sound (Korotkoff phase 5) better indicates diastolic blood pressure, although now all experts favor using phase 5 for the following reasons: (1) In most studies phase 5 sounds correlate better with intraarterial measurements of diastolic blood pressure[14,15]; (2) many persons lack phase 4 sounds[14,16]; (3) interobserver agreement is better for phase 5 sounds than phase 4 sounds[14,16]; and, most importantly, (4) long-term observational and treatment studies correlating hypertension and cardiovascular risk events used phase 5 sounds for definition of diastolic blood pressure.

2. Pathogenesis

Korotkoff sounds are produced underneath the *distal* half of the blood pressure cuff.[17] The sounds appear when cuff pressures are between systolic and diastolic blood pressure, because the underlying artery is collapsing completely and then reopening with each heartbeat. The artery collapses because cuff pressure exceeds diastolic pressure; it opens again with each beat because cuff pressure is less than systolic pressure. The sound represents the sudden deceleration of the rapidly opening arterial walls, which causes a snapping or tapping sound just like the sail of a boat snaps when it suddenly tenses after tacking in the wind or a handkerchief snaps when its ends are suddenly drawn taut.[17-21] Once cuff pressure falls below the diastolic blood pressure, the sound disappears because the vessel wall no longer collapses but instead gently ebbs and expands with each beat, being held open by diastolic pressure.

The genesis of the Korotkoff sounds, therefore, is similar to the genesis of other snapping or tapping sounds produced by the sudden deceleration of other biologic membranes, such as the normal first and second heart sounds or the femoral pistol shot sounds of aortic regurgitation (see Chapters 40 and 45).

D. MEASUREMENT USING PALPATION

Even before the discovery of Korotkoff sounds, clinicians used the blood pressure cuff to measure both systolic and diastolic blood pressure.[6] Systolic blood pressure was simply the amount of cuff pressure necessary to obliterate the pulse. Clinicians still use this technique to measure the blood pressure of hypotensive patients (a setting when Korotkoff sounds are often too faint to hear) or to determine whether the patient has an auscultatory gap. (See the subsequent section on the auscultatory gap.)

To identify diastolic pressure, clinicians can use one of two methods. In the first method, the clinician applies light pressure to palpate the brachial artery just below the blood pressure cuff. As the cuff is deflated, the first appearance of a pulse indicates systolic blood pressure. As the cuff pressure decreases and approaches diastolic pressure, the pulsatile forces distending the artery distal to the cuff progressively grow, eventually causing a sudden shock to strike the clinician's fingers as the artery abruptly opens and then completely collapses with each beat. (This abrupt tapping sensation is similar to the **water-hammer pulse** of aortic regurgitation.).[18] At the moment the cuff

---

*There are five Korotkoff phases, numbered in order as they appear during deflation of the cuff. The initial tapping sound at systolic blood pressure is phase 1; a swishing murmur is phase 2; the reappearance of a softer tapping sound is phase 3; the disappearance of the tapping and appearance of a much softer murmur ("muffling") is phase 4; and the disappearance of all sound is phase 5.[2] Korotkoff described only four of these sounds (phases 1, 2, 3, and 5). Ettinger added the muffling point (phase 4) in 1907.[7,11,12] All five phases are audible with electronic stethoscopes in 40% of adults.[13]

pressure falls below diastolic blood pressure, the shocking sensations disappear, being replaced by a much gentler pulse, because the underlying artery no longer collapses completely between beats. The cuff pressure at this *lower limit of maximal pulsation* indicates the diastolic blood pressure.[6]

A second method requires a rigid and tightly applied cuff, so that the arterial pulsations under the cuff are actually transmitted to the manometer. As the cuff pressure decreases, the indicator needle of an aneroid manometer starts to bob with increasing amplitude, until the bobbing suddenly disappears at the moment cuff pressure falls below diastolic pressure.[6] Many patients with tightly applied cuffs experience similar pounding sensations in their arms near the diastolic pressure, which abruptly disappear the moment cuff pressure falls below diastolic blood pressure.

Measurements of systolic and diastolic blood pressure by palpation differ from readings by auscultation by only 6 to 8 mm Hg or less.[22,23]

E. POSTURAL VITAL SIGNS[24]

When obtaining postural vital signs (i.e., comparison of measurements when the patient is supine with those when the patient is upright), clinicians should wait 2 minutes before measuring the supine vital signs and 1 minute after standing before measuring the upright vital signs. These recommendations are based on the following observations: (1) shorter periods of supine rest significantly reduce the sensitivity of postural vital signs for detecting blood loss, and (2) after normal persons stand, the pulse rate stabilizes after 45 to 60 seconds and the blood pressure stabilizes after 1 to 2 minutes. Counting the heart rate first, beginning at 1 minute, allows more time for the blood pressure to stabilize.

Supine vital signs should always be compared with standing vital signs, because sitting instead of standing significantly reduces the clinician's ability to detect postural changes after blood loss.[25,26]

F. COMMON ERRORS

Biologic variation of blood pressure is common, and many studies show that blood pressure measurements vary with physical activity, smoking, caffeine ingestion, emotional state, ambient temperatures, and different seasons.[27-29] In addition, the blood pressure measurement may be inaccurate because of inappropriate technique, improper equipment, or other biases related to the observer.[12,28]

1. Wrong Cuff Size

In 1901, Von Recklinghausen discovered that Riva-Rocci's original blood pressure cuff, whose bladder was about the size of a bicycle tire, was too narrow and often overestimated the true blood pressure, especially in larger arms.[7,30,31] Subsequent investigations have shown that both the bladder width and length affect the measurement, although if the bladder encircles at least 80% of the arm's circumference, the effect of width is minimized.[15,30,32] The bladder of the standard cuff measures 12 × 23 cm and thus is appropriate only for arm circumferences up to 28 cm, which includes just 60% to 70% of the adult population.[30]

Cuffs that are too short overestimate blood pressure because they transmit cuff pressure inefficiently to the underlying soft tissues. Much higher cuff pressures are then necessary to cause collapse of the artery, leading the clinician to misdiagnose hypertension when it is not present.[32] This error is greater the farther the *center* of the bladder is positioned from the brachial artery.[15]

The significance of the opposite error—underestimation of true blood pressure by using a cuff that is too large—is controversial, although most studies show that such an error is small. Table 17.1 presents the mean errors resulting from using cuffs too small or too large.[33] These data are based on measurements of blood pressure in the same individual with three cuffs of different sizes, assuming that the most accurate measurement is the one made with the smallest cuff encircling 80% of the arm. The greatest errors, according to these data, occur from using too small of a cuff; the risk of underestimating true pressure with too large a cuff is relatively minor.

TABLE 17.1 ■ **Blood Pressure Cuff Size and Error in Measurement***

Cuff Bladder Size (cm)	Arm Circumference		
	28 cm or less	**29 to 42 cm**	**43 cm or more**
Regular (12 × 23 cm)	Accurate	Overestimates SBP by 4–8 mm Hg DBP by 3–6 mm Hg	Overestimates SBP by 16–17 mm Hg DBP by 10–11 mm Hg
Large (15 × 33 cm)	Underestimates SBP by 2–3 mm Hg DBP by 1–2 mm Hg	Accurate	Overestimates SBP by 5–7 mm Hg DBP by 2–4 mm Hg
Thigh (18 × 36 cm)	Underestimates SBP by 5–7 mm Hg DBP by 1–3 mm Hg	Underestimates SBP by 5–7 mm Hg DBP by 2–4 mm Hg	Accurate

Overestimation means that hypertension may be diagnosed in someone with normal blood pressure; *underestimation* means that the blood pressure reading may be normal in someone who actually has high blood pressure. See text for further discussion.
Data from Maxwell MH, Waks AU, Schroth PC, Karam M, Dornfeld LP. Error in blood-pressure measurement due to incorrect cuff size in obese patients. *Lancet*. 1982;2:33–35.
DBP, Diastolic blood pressure reading; *SBP,* systolic blood pressure reading.

2. Auscultatory Gap

Up to 20% of elderly patients with hypertension have an **auscultatory gap,** which means that the phase 1 Korotkoff sounds normally appear at systolic pressure but then disappear for varying lengths of time before they reappear above the diastolic pressure.[34] This auscultatory gap is important because inflation of the cuff just to the initial disappearance of sounds (i.e., auscultatory gap) significantly underestimates the true systolic blood pressure. Because the distal pulse persists during the auscultatory gap, however, clinicians can avoid this mistake by palpating the systolic pressure before using the stethoscope.

The cause of the auscultatory gap remains a mystery. Patients with auscultatory gaps have twice as much arterial atherosclerotic plaque as those without a gap, suggesting perhaps that the gap is somehow related to arterial stiffness.[34] Venous congestion also seems to promote auscultatory gaps, because slow cuff inflation (which increases venous congestion) may produce an auscultatory gap and elevation of the arm before inflating the cuff may make the gap disappear.[31]

The auscultatory gap was discovered by Krylov in 1906, one year after Korotkoff's discovery.[11] In part, the discovery of the auscultatory gap was responsible for the initial reluctance of clinicians to adopt Korotkoff's method of indirect blood pressure measurement.[7]

3. Inappropriate Level of the Arm

The recommended position of the patient's elbow is the "level of the heart," which is usually regarded to be the fourth intercostal space at the sternum. If the seated patient's arm is instead 6 to 7 cm higher (e.g., level of the sternomanubrial junction), both the systolic and diastolic readings will be about 5 mm Hg lower. If the arm is 7 to 8 cm lower (e.g., level of the xiphisternal junction), the pressures will be about 6 mm Hg higher.[35]

These errors are largely explained by the hydrostatic effect. When the arm is at the lower position, for example, the measured pressure is the sum of the blood pressure in the artery plus the weight of a column of blood 8 cm high: 8 cm blood = $(8 \div 13.6) \times 1.06 = 0.6$ cm or 6 mm Hg (13.6 = density of mercury; 1.06 = density of blood).[10,35,36]

4. Terminal Digit Preference (Auscultatory Method)[27,28]

Clinicians often tend to round off blood pressure readings to the nearest 0, 5, or other preferred number, a bias called **terminal digit preference**. Clinical studies minimize this and other observer biases by using oscillometric devices or a random zero sphygmomanometer (an instrument that blinds the clinician to the true reading).[29,37]

G. OTHER VARIABLES

For years clinicians believed that pressing too firmly with the stethoscope artificially decreased diastolic blood pressure readings, but recent studies show this is not true.[38] Whether the bell or diaphragm of the stethoscope are used[39,40] or whether the stethoscope is placed under the cuff or just outside the cuff[38] does not significantly affect the measurement. Raising the patient's arm overhead for 30 seconds before returning it to the normal position and inflating the cuff will intensify Korotkoff sounds without significantly changing the pressure reading.[41]

III. The Findings and Their Clinical Significance

A. HYPERTENSION

1. Essential Hypertension

Essential hypertension is defined as three or more blood pressure readings taken over three visits separated by weeks whose average exceeds 130/80 (i.e., systolic blood pressure of 130 mm Hg and diastolic blood pressure of 80mm Hg)[†]. Detecting essential hypertension is the reason blood pressure should be measured in every person, even when asymptomatic, because the disorder is common and treatable and because treatment reduces cardiovascular morbidity and overall mortality.[42]

2. Pseudohypertension and Osler Sign

Pseudohypertension describes the finding of elevated indirect measurements in persons who have normal intraarterial pressure. The traditional explanation for pseudohypertension is that the artery under the cuff is so stiff and calcified it remains open long after the cuff pressure exceeds systolic blood pressure, continuing to produce Korotkoff sounds.

The diagnosis of pseudohypertension requires direct cannulation of the patient's artery, which is of course inappropriate and impractical during daily routine. A single study from 1985 proposed that a simple physical finding, **Osler sign**, accurately identifies patients with pseudohypertension.[43] This sign is positive if the patient's radial or brachial artery distal to the cuff remains palpable after inflation of the cuff above systolic blood pressure.

Osler sign, however, has limited clinical value. It occurs commonly in elderly individuals, whether or not they have hypertension (11% over the age of 75 years and 44% over 85 years have a positive Osler sign).[44] Other investigators have shown that almost all patients with Osler sign do not have pseudohypertension but instead have direct measurements that exceed the indirect ones.[45,46]

Although pseudohypertension remains an important problem in blood pressure measurements of the legs, especially in diabetic patients with intermittent claudication (see Chapter 54), undue emphasis on pseudohypertension in the brachial artery misses the point that all clinical studies

---

[†]The precise definition of hypertension has changed in recent years based on analysis of new evidence addressing cardiovascular morbidity and benefits of antihypertension treatment.

demonstrating the benefits of treating essential hypertension used the blood pressure cuff and indirect measurements, not intra-arterial ones.

B. HYPOTENSION

In patients with acute illness, hypotension is ominous. It predicts death in patients hospitalized in the intensive care unit (likelihood ratio [LR] = 3.1, EBM Box 17.1); with acute illness in the emergency department (LR = 15.3); or hospitalized with bacteremia (LR = 4.9), pneumonia (LR = 5.3), or myocardial infarction (LR = 15.5). Presumably, it predicts mortality in many other acute disorders as well. The APACHE scoring system, which predicts the risk of hospital mortality among patients in the intensive care unit, assigns greater risk to severe hypotension than to any other vital sign or laboratory variable.[47]

Hypotension also predicts adverse outcomes besides death. In patients with myocardial infarction, a systolic blood pressure of less than 80 mm Hg predicts an increased incidence of congestive heart failure, ventricular arrhythmias, and complete heart block.[48] In patients presenting with syncope, an initial systolic blood pressure of less than 90 mm Hg increases the probability of adverse events in the next 7 days (sensitivity 8% to 18%, specificity 95% to 99%, positive LR 4.2).[49–53] Finally, in hospitalized patients with a wide variety of problems, low blood pressure readings increase greatly the risk of serious adverse outcomes in the next 24 hours (systolic BP ≤90 mm Hg, LR = 4.7; ≤85 mm Hg, LR = 9; ≤80 mm Hg, LR = 16.7; see EBM Box 17.1)[‡].

C. DIFFERENCES IN PRESSURE BETWEEN THE ARMS

The average difference in systolic blood pressure between the two arms is 6 to 10 mm Hg.[54,55] Differences of 20 mm Hg or more are uncommon and detect obstructed flow in the subclavian artery (i.e., >50–60% obstruction) of the arm with the lower pressure (sensitivity 70% to 90%, specificity 99%, positive LR = 89.1, and negative LR = 0.2).[56,57] This is a significant finding in two clinical settings:

1. Subclavian Steal Syndrome

The finding of one weak radial pulse in a patient with symptoms of vertebral-basilar ischemia (episodic vertigo, visual complaints, hemiparesis, ataxia, or diplopia) suggests the **subclavian steal syndrome**. In this syndrome, stenosis or occlusion of one subclavian artery proximal to the origin of the vertebral artery reduces the pressure distal to the obstruction, which causes the flow in the vertebral artery to reverse directions: instead of traveling normally up the vertebral artery to perfuse the brain, blood flow courses downward to perfuse the arm (i.e., the arm *steals* blood from the posterior cerebral circulation).[58,§] Ninety-four percent of patients with subclavian steal have an interarm systolic blood pressure difference of 20 mm Hg or more (the mean difference between arms is 45 mm Hg in affected patients).[60] Most patients have an ipsilateral radial pulse that is diminished or absent and a systolic bruit over the ipsilateral subclavian artery.[60] The left side is affected in 70% and the right side in 30%.[60]

[‡]Two out of three of these adverse outcomes were unexpected transfer to intensive care unit care. Although this suggests circular reasoning (i.e., hypotension was likely a principal reason for transfer), the remaining one of the three adverse events was *unexpected cardiac arrest* or unexpected death on the general medicine ward.

[§]An excellent online video of vertebral retrograde flow in a patient with subclavian stenosis is available in the supplementary material of Aithal and Ulrich.[59]

EBM BOX 17.1	Hypotension and Prognosis*

Finding (reference)	Sensitivity (%)	Specificity (%)	Likelihood Ratio[†] if Finding Is	
			Present	Absent
Predicting hospital mortality				
Systolic blood pressure <90 mm Hg				
Patients in intensive care unit[97,98]	21–78	67–95	**3.1**	NS
Patients with bacteremia[99,100]	13–71	85–98	**4.9**	NS
Patients with pneumonia[101–105]	11–47	87–99	**5.3**	0.7
Patients with acute illness in the emergency department[106]	12	99	**15.3**	0.9
Systolic blood pressure ≤80 mm Hg				
Patients with acute myocardial infarction[48]	32	98	**15.5**	0.7
Predicting adverse outcome in hospitalized patients[107]				
Systolic blood pressure ≤90 mm Hg	34	93	**4.7**	0.7
Systolic blood pressure ≤85 mm Hg	25	97	**9.0**	0.8
Systolic blood pressure ≤80 mm Hg	21	99	**16.7**	0.8

*Diagnostic standard: for *adverse outcome*, unexpected cardiac arrest, unplanned intensive care unit (ICU) admission, or unexpected death.
[†]Likelihood ratio (LR) if finding present = positive LR; LR if finding absent = negative LR.
NS, Not significant.

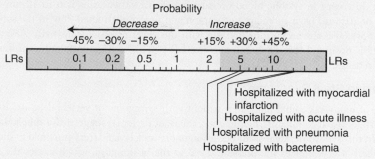

HYPOTENSION, PREDICTING MORTALITY

Hospitalized with myocardial infarction
Hospitalized with acute illness
Hospitalized with pneumonia
Hospitalized with bacteremia

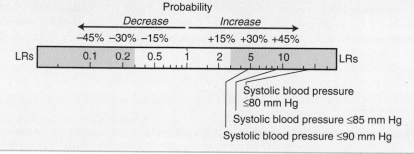

HYPOTENSION, PREDICTING ADVERSE OUTCOME

Systolic blood pressure ≤80 mm Hg
Systolic blood pressure ≤85 mm Hg
Systolic blood pressure ≤90 mm Hg

EBM BOX 17.2	**Aortic Dissection***				

Finding (Reference)†	Sensitivity (%)	Specificity (%)	Likelihood Ratio‡ if Finding Is	
			Present	Absent
Individual findings				
Pulse deficit[61,62,66,108-110]	13–49	79–100	**4.3**	0.8
Aortic regurgitation murmur[61-63,66,108,109]	5–49	45–100	1.6	NS
Focal neurologic signs[62,108,109]	13–20	93–100	**13.8**	0.9
Systolic blood pressure <90 mm Hg[108,109]	9–22	96–99	**5.6**	NS
Combined findings[62]				
0 predictors	4	47	**0.1**	...
1 predictor	20	...	0.5	...
2 predictors	49	...	5.3	...
3 predictors	27	100	65.8	...

*Diagnostic standard: for *aortic dissection*, transesophageal echocardiography,[61,63] aortography,[66] or any of a variety of tests (i.e., computed tomography, magnetic resonance imaging, transesophageal echocardiography, or digital angiography).[62,108-110]

†Definition of findings: for *pulse deficit*, absent extremity or carotid pulse[61,66] or 20 mm Hg difference in blood pressure in the arms, absent extremity or carotid pulse, or both[62,108,109]; for *combined findings*, see text.

‡Likelihood ratio (LR) if finding present = positive LR; LR if finding absent = negative LR.
NS, Not significant.

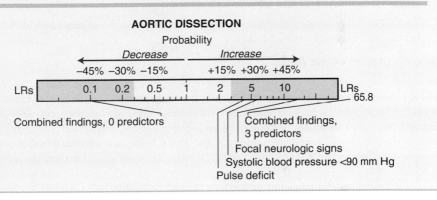

AORTIC DISSECTION

2. Aortic Dissection

The finding of a difference in blood pressure between the two arms in a patient with acute chest pain suggests aortic dissection. EBM Box 17.2 presents the accuracy of physical examination in over 3600 patients presenting to emergency departments with acute chest or upper back pain suspicious for aortic dissection. In these studies, the presence of focal neurologic signs (LR = 13.8), systolic blood pressure <90 mm Hg (LR = 5.6), or a pulse deficit (i.e., absent extremity or carotid pulse; interarm systolic difference >20 mm Hg; LR = 4.3) increased probability of aortic dissection. Mediastinal or aortic widening on chest radiography also increased the probability of dissection, although only modestly (LR = 2); the *absence* of mediastinal widening *decreased* probability (LR = 0.3).[61-63]

In these studies, the murmur of aortic regurgitation was diagnostically unhelpful, possibly because of the highly selected nature of enrolled patients: overall, enrolled patients represented only 0.3% of patients with chest or back pain evaluated in these centers[62]; one-quarter had the murmur of aortic regurgitation, and one-half had the diagnosis of dissection eventually confirmed.

Von Kodolitsch and others[62] have identified three independent predictors of aortic dissection in patients with acute chest pain: (1) pain that is tearing or ripping, (2) pulse deficits, blood pressure differentials (>20 mm Hg), or both, and (3) mediastinal or aortic widening on chest radiography. The absence of all three predictors *decreases* probability of dissection (LR = 0.1; see EBM Box 17.2); two predictors increases probability of dissection (LR = 5.3), and the presence of all three predictors is pathognomonic for dissection (LR = 65.8).

Rare patients with aortic dissection present with the physical findings of pulsatile sternoclavicular joints[64] or unilateral femoral pistol shot sounds (see Chapter 45).[65]

In patients with established aortic dissection, three findings increase the probability that the dissection involves the proximal aorta (i.e., it is a type A dissection, not a type B dissection): systolic blood pressure less than 100 mm Hg (LR = 5), murmur of aortic regurgitation (LR = 5), and a pulse deficit (LR = 1.9).[61,64,66–69] In patients with acute type A dissection, pulse deficits are associated with increased hospital mortality.[70]

D. DIFFERENCES IN PRESSURE BETWEEN ARMS AND LEGS

This finding is valuable in two clinical settings:

1. Chronic Ischemia of the Lower Extremities

Chapter 54 describes calculation of the ankle-arm index, which is the principal bedside tool used in patients with intermittent claudication.

2. Coarctation of the Aorta

In young patients with hypertension, the finding of an unobtainable blood pressure in the legs or a blood pressure that is much lower in the legs than arms suggests the diagnosis of coarctation of the aorta.[71,72] These patients also have hypertension of the arms (96% have a blood pressure >140/90), femoral pulses that are absent or diminished and delayed (100%), augmented carotid pulsations, various murmurs (usually a systolic murmur at the sternal border and a continuous murmur posteriorly over the upper spine), and visible collateral arteries (usually around the scapula, intercostal spaces, or axilla).[71,72]

During simultaneous palpation of the femoral and radial arteries of healthy persons, it is impossible to tell which comes first. In patients with coarctation, however, the femoral pulse is delayed, due both to delay in arrival at the legs and to more rapid than normal conduction of the wave to the arms.[73]

In one study of 1206 children with unexplained heart murmurs, clinicians correctly diagnosed coarctation of the aorta in 18 of 22 affected patients (in this study, the overall accuracy for detecting coarctation by bedside examination—presumably using arm-to-leg blood pressure or pulse discrepancies—was sensitivity of 82%, specificity of 100%, positive LR = 242, and negative LR = 0.2).[74]

E. ABNORMAL PULSE CONTOUR

The three abnormalities of pulse contour—pulsus paradoxus, pulsus alternans, and pulsus bisferiens—are easily detectable with the blood pressure cuff using the auscultatory method (see Chapter 15).

F. ABNORMAL PULSE PRESSURE

1. Abnormally Small Pulse Pressure

Since the pulse pressure depends on stroke volume, clinicians have tried for decades to use it as a way to quantify cardiac output. This relationship has been validated in one setting, patients with known left ventricular dysfunction: In these patients, the finding of a proportional pulse pressure less than 0.25 (proportional pulse pressure = pulse pressure divided by systolic pressure) detects a cardiac index less than 2.2 L/min/m^2 with a sensitivity of 70% to 91%, specificity of 83% to 93%, positive LR = 6.9, and negative LR = 0.2.[75,76]

In contrast to conventional teachings, many patients with significant aortic stenosis have a normal pulse pressure (see Chapter 44).[77] Chapter 70 discusses using changes in pulse pressure after passive leg elevation as a sign of volume responsiveness in critically ill patients.

2. Abnormally Large Pulse Pressure

In patients with the murmur of aortic insufficiency, a pulse pressure of 80 mm Hg or more increases probability that the regurgitation is moderate or severe, with a sensitivity of 57%, specificity of 95%, and positive LR = 10.9.[78]

G. ORTHOSTATIC HYPOTENSION

When a person stands, 350 to 600 mL of blood shifts to the lower body. Normally, the blood pressure remains relatively stable during this shift because of compensatory increases in cardiac output, heart rate, and systemic vascular resistance, and transfer of blood from the pulmonary circulation to the systemic side.[24] Orthostatic hypotension, usually defined as a fall in systolic blood pressure of 20 mm Hg or more when the patient stands from the supine position, may occur if (1) compensatory mechanisms fail (i.e., autonomic insufficiency) or (2) the patient has lost excessive amounts of fluid from the vascular space (e.g., acute blood loss).

1. Postural Vital Signs in Healthy Persons

As normovolemic persons stand up from the supine position, the pulse increases on average by 10.9 beats/min, systolic blood pressure decreases by 3.5 mm Hg, and diastolic blood pressure increases by 5.2 mm Hg.[24] Postural hypotension, defined as a decrement in systolic blood pressure of 20 mm Hg or more, occurs in 10% of normovolemic individuals younger than 65 years and in 11% to 30% older than 65 years.[24] As persons age, the postural pulse increment diminishes (r = −0.50, p < 0.02); this phenomenon and the observation that older persons have more postural hypotension suggests that autonomic reflexes decline as persons age.

2. Vital Signs and Hypovolemia

Table 17.2 presents the vital signs from normal persons before and after phlebotomy of 450 to 630 mL (moderate blood loss) or 630 to 1150 mL (large blood loss)¶. Chapter 11 reviews the other physical findings of hypovolemia.

a. Postural Change in Pulse

Table 17.2 shows that the most valuable observation is *either* a postural pulse increment of 30/min or more *or* the inability of the patient to stand long enough for vital signs because of severe dizziness. Virtually all persons have one or both of these findings after large amounts of blood loss

---

¶Calculating LRs for these data is inappropriate, because *acute blood loss* has endless gradations of severity, many of which are important to the clinician. For example, the LR of physical signs for moderate blood loss are of little use to the clinician who, when taking care of the patient with melena, regards blood loss of 400 mL (*disease-negative* according to the LR) to be as significant as a loss of 500 mL (*disease-positive*). Table 17.2 instead just illustrates the general trends of vital signs with increasing amounts of blood loss.

TABLE 17.2 ■ Vital Signs and Acute Blood Loss*

Physical Finding (Ref)[†]	Moderate Blood Loss, Sensitivity (%)	Large Blood Loss, Sensitivity (%)	Specificity (%)
Postural pulse increment ≥30/min or severe postural dizziness[25,81,90,91]	7–57	98	99
Postural hypotension (≥20 mm Hg decrease in SBP)[81,90]	9	…	90–98
Supine tachycardia (pulse >100/min)[26,91-94]	1	10	99
Supine hypotension (SBP <95 mm Hg)[26,92,93,95,96]	13	31	98

Data from McGee S, Abernethy WB, Simel DL. Is this patient hypovolemic? *JAMA.* 1999;281:1022–1029.
*Data obtained from 568 normal persons, mostly young and healthy, after "moderate" blood loss (phlebotomy of 450–630 mL) or "large" blood loss (phlebotomy of 630–1150 mL). "Specificity" from same patients when euvolemic, before blood loss. Results are overall mean frequency or, if statistically heterogenous, the range of values.
[†]*Definition of finding*: for *postural*, the difference between supine and standing measurements; for *postural hypotension* (≥20 mm Hg decrease in SBP), the finding applies only to patients able to stand without severe dizziness.
SBP, Systolic blood pressure.

(sensitivity = 98%), but only 1 of 5 persons develop either of them after moderate blood loss (sensitivity ranges from 7% to 57%, Table 17.2).[24] These findings are durable after hemorrhage, lasting at least 12 to 72 hours if intravenous fluids are withheld.[26,79,80]

b. Postural Change in Blood Pressure

After excluding those patients unable to stand for vital signs (which includes almost all patients after large amounts of blood loss), the finding of postural hypotension (a postural decrement in systolic blood pressure of 20 mm Hg or more) has no proven value, being found just as often in patients before blood loss as after it. For example, in persons younger than 65 years, postural hypotension is found in 8% before moderate blood loss and 9% after blood loss. For those 65 years or older, postural hypotension is detected in 11% to 30% before blood loss and about 25% after blood loss.[24,81]

Obviously, because severe dizziness with standing is a valuable finding, but postural hypotension of 20 mm Hg is inaccurate, there must be an intermediate level of postural fall (e.g., 30 mm Hg, 40 mm Hg, or another value), not yet identified, that better discriminates between patients with and without blood loss.

c. Supine Pulse and Supine Blood Pressure

In patients with suspected blood loss, both supine tachycardia and supine hypotension are specific indicators of significant blood loss, although both findings are infrequent. After moderate blood loss, 1% have tachycardia in the supine position and only 13% have supine hypotension; after large blood loss, only 10% have tachycardia and 31% have hypotension.

Sinus bradycardia, in contrast, is a common arrhythmia after blood loss and frequently precedes the drop in blood pressure that causes patients to faint.[24]

H. BLOOD PRESSURE AND IMPAIRED CONSCIOUSNESS

Patients with impaired consciousness may have either a structural intracranial lesion (e.g., stroke or brain tumors) or metabolic encephalopathy (e.g., hepatic encephalopathy, diabetic coma, drug intoxication, or sepsis). Patients with structural lesions tend to have higher blood pressures (from reflex responses to increases in intracranial pressure—the Cushing reflex—or from the etiologic association of hypertension and stroke) than patients with metabolic encephalopathy (whose severe comorbidities often are associated with lower blood pressure). In two studies of consecutive

EBM BOX 17.3	Systolic Blood Pressure and Impaired Consciousness			
Finding (Reference)	Sensitivity (%)	Specificity (%)	Likelihood Ratio* if Finding Is	
			Present	Absent
Detecting structural brain lesion				
Systolic blood pressure ≥160 mm Hg[111,112]	37–58	93–94	**7.3**	0.6

*Likelihood ratio (LR) if finding present = positive LR; LR if finding absent = negative LR.

STRUCTURAL BRAIN LESION (IF COMA)

Probability

Decrease ← → Increase

−45% −30% −15%   +15% +30% +45%

LRs 0.1 0.2 0.5 1 2 5 10 LRs

Systolic blood pressure ≥160mm Hg

patients with impaired consciousness (i.e., Glasgow Coma Scale less than 15) but no history of head trauma, a systolic blood pressure of 160 mm Hg or more significantly increased the probability of a structural lesion (LR = 7.3, EBM Box 17.3).

I. CAPILLARY FRAGILITY TEST (RUMPEL-LEEDE TEST)

Traditionally, the blood pressure cuff was used to test capillary fragility, although measurements of blood pressure were not part of the test. Capillary fragility tests were designed to detect abnormally weakened capillary walls in the skin that would burst more easily when distended, resulting in appearance of high numbers of petechiae. The diseases associated with capillary fragility were legion, ranging from coagulopathies, vitamin deficiencies (e.g., scurvy), infectious diseases (e.g., scarlet fever), endocrine disorders (e.g., hyperthyroidism), to dermatologic disorders (e.g., Osler-Weber-Rendu syndrome).[82]

Both negative and positive pressure methods were used. The negative pressure technique applied suction to a defined area of the skin, a technique whose undoing was the eventual demonstration that the number of resulting petechiae depended on not only the age of patient, but also on the time of day, season, and psychic influences.[83] Positive pressure methods, introduced at the turn of the century by Drs. Rumpel and Leede, consisted of raising the venous pressure by a tourniquet or blood pressure cuff around the arm and counting petechiae that subsequently developed in a defined area distally. This test was eventually standardized,[83] but interest fell after the introduction of better diagnostic tests for coagulation and the other associated disorders. More recently, increased capillary fragility was believed to represent a sign of diabetic retinopathy,[84] but this was soon disproven.[85]

Nonetheless, a variation of this Rumpel-Leede test (called the **tourniquet test**#) remains important in the developing world as a diagnostic test for dengue fever and its complications. In patients with undifferentiated fever presenting to clinicians working in tropical settings, a positive tourniquet test detected confirmed dengue infection with a sensitivity of 34% to 68%, specificity of 84% to 99%, and positive LR = 6.8.[86–89]

References may be accessed online at *Elsevier eBooks for Practicing Clinicians.*

#In the standard method of the tourniquet test, the clinician inflates the blood pressure cuff midway between the systolic and diastolic blood pressures for 5 minutes and then counts the number of petechiae that form in a 2.5 cm² area just distal to the antecubital fossa. The positive test is 20 petechiae or more.

Temperature

I. Introduction

Fever is a fundamental sign of almost all infectious diseases and many noninfectious disorders. Clinicians began to monitor the temperature of febrile patients in the 1850s and 1860s, after Traube introduced the thermometer to hospital wards and Wunderlich published an analysis based on observation of an estimated 20,000 subjects that convinced clinicians of the value of graphing temperature over time.[1-3] These temperature charts, the first vital sign to be routinely recorded in hospitalized patients, were originally named **Wunderlich curves**.[4]

II. Technique

A. SITE OF MEASUREMENT

Thermometers are used to measure the temperature of the patient's oral cavity, rectum, axilla, tympanic membrane, or forehead (i.e., temporal artery). Because of potential toxicity from mercury exposure, the time-honored mercury thermometer has been replaced by electronic thermometers with thermistors (oral, rectal, and axillary measurements) and infrared thermometers (tympanic or forehead measurements). These instruments provide more rapid results than does the traditional mercury thermometer.

Normal body temperature varies widely, depending in part on the site measured. Rectal readings are on average 0.4° to 0.6°C higher than oral ones, which are 0.1° to 0.2°C higher than axillary readings.[5-9] Temporal (forehead) measurements typically fall between rectal and oral readings.[7,10,11] Tympanic readings are the most variable, some studies showing them to be systematically higher than rectal readings[9,12] and others showing them to be systematically lower than oral readings.[13,14]

Even so, these studies, which are designed to detect *systematic differences* between instruments, do not reflect the variability observed in individual patients. For example, comparisons of sequential rectal and oral readings measured in large numbers of patients reveal the *rectal-minus-oral difference* to be 0.6 ± 0.5°C.[9,12] This indicates that *on average* rectal readings are 0.6°C greater than the oral readings (i.e., the *systematic difference*), but it also indicates that the rectal reading of a particular patient may vary from as much as 0.4°C *lower* than the oral reading to 1.6°C *higher* than the oral reading.* Similar variability is observed when any of the 5 sites are compared to each other in the same patient (e.g., oral vs temporal, axillary vs rectal, etc.).

A better question is how well different instruments detect infection. In one study of elderly patients presenting to an emergency department, three different techniques—rectal, temporal, and tympanic measurements—had similar diagnostic accuracy for infection (likelihood ratios [LRs] 4.2 to 8.5; see EBM Box 18.1), although each instrument had a different definition of fever (rectal T >37.8°C; forehead T >37.9°C; tympanic T >37.5°C).[10]

B. VARIABLES AFFECTING THE TEMPERATURE MEASUREMENT

1. Eating and Smoking[5,15-17]

The *oral* temperature measurement increases about 0.3°C after sustained chewing and stays elevated for up to 20 minutes, probably because of increased blood flow to the muscles of mastication. Drinking hot liquids also increases oral readings about 0.6° to 0.9°C, for up to 15 to 25 minutes, and smoking a cigarette increases oral readings about 0.2°C for 30 minutes. Drinking ice water causes the oral reading to fall 0.2° to 1.2°C, a reduction lasting about 10 to 15 minutes.

EBM BOX 18.1	**Temperature Measurement at Different Sites, Detecting Infection[10,*]**			
Finding (Reference)	**Sensitivity (%)**	**Specificity (%)**	**Likelihood Ratio[†] if Finding Is**	
			Present	**Absent**
Rectal temperature >37.8°C	44	93	**6.1**	0.6
Forehead temperature >37.9°C	38	91	**4.2**	0.7
Tympanic temperature >37.5°C	34	96	**8.5**	0.7

*Diagnostic standard: for *infection*, consensus diagnosis from chart review.
[†]Likelihood ratio (LR) if finding present = positive LR; LR if finding absent = negative LR.

---

*This is calculated as follows: the 95% confidence interval (CI) equals 2 × standard deviation (i.e., 2 × 0.5°C = 1°C). A rectal-minus-oral difference of 0.6 ± 0.5°C, therefore, indicates the variation ranges from –0.4 (i.e., 0.6 – 1.0; rectal is 0.4°C lower than oral) to +1.6 (i.e., 0.6 + 1.0; rectal is 1.6°C higher than oral).

2. Tachypnea

Tachypnea reduces the *oral* temperature reading about 0.5°C for every 10 breaths/min increase in the respiratory rate.[18,19] This phenomenon probably explains why marathon runners, at the end of their race, often have a large discrepancy between normal oral temperatures and high rectal temperatures.[20]

In contrast, administration of oxygen by nasal canula does not affect oral temperature.[21]

3. Cerumen

Cerumen lowers *tympanic* temperature readings by obstructing radiation of heat from the tympanic membrane.[5]

4. Hemiparesis

In patients with hemiparesis, *axillary* temperature readings are about 0.5°C lower on the weak side compared with the healthy side. The discrepancy between the two sides correlates poorly with the severity of the patient's weakness, suggesting that it is not due to difficulty holding the thermometer under the arm, but instead to other factors, such as differences in cutaneous blood flow between the two sides.[22]

5. Mucositis

Oral mucositis, a complication of chemotherapy, increases oral readings on average by 0.7°C,[23] even without fever. This increase in temperature likely reflects inflammatory vasodilation of the oral membranes.

III. The Finding

A. NORMAL TEMPERATURE AND FEVER

In healthy persons, the mean oral temperature is 36.5°C (97.7°F), a value slightly lower than Wunderlich's original estimate of 37°C (98.6°F), which in turn had been established using foot-long axillary thermometers that may have been calibrated higher than the thermometers used today.[1] The temperature is usually lowest at 6 AM and highest at 4 PM to 6 PM (a variation called *diurnal variation*).[24] One investigator has defined fever as the 99th percentile of maximum temperatures in healthy persons, or an *oral* temperature greater than 37.7°C (99.9°F).[24] Most studies show that a temperature >37.8°C with any instrument is abnormal (and, therefore, indicative of fever).[6]

B. FEVER PATTERNS

In the early days of clinical thermometry, clinicians observed that prolonged fevers could be categorized into one of four fever patterns—sustained, intermittent, remittent, and relapsing (Fig. 18.1).[3,25–27] **(1) Sustained fever**. In this pattern the fever varies little from day to day (the modern definition is variation ≤0.3°C [≤0.5°F] each day); **(2) Intermittent fever**. In this pattern the temperature returns to normal between exacerbations. If the exacerbations occur daily, the fever is *quotidian*; if they occur every 48 hours, it is *tertian* (i.e., they appear again on the third day); and if they occur every 72 hours, it is *quartan* (i.e., they appear again on the fourth day). **(3) Remittent**. Remittent fevers vary at least 0.3°C (0.5°F) each day but do not return to normal. **Hectic fevers** are intermittent or remittent fevers with wide swings in temperature, usually greater than 1.4°C (2.5°F) each day. **(4) Relapsing fevers**. These fevers are characterized by periods of fever lasting days interspersed by equally long afebrile periods.

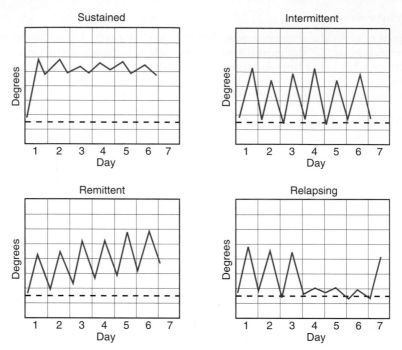

Fig. 18.1 Fever patterns. The four basic fever patterns are sustained, intermittent, remittent, and relapsing fever. The *dashed line* in each chart depicts normal temperature. See text for definitions and clinical significance.

Each of these patterns was associated with prototypic diseases: sustained fever was associated with lobar pneumonia (lasting 7 days until it disappeared abruptly by *crisis* or gradually by *lysis*); intermittent fever with malarial infection; remittent fever with typhoid fever (causing several days of ascending remittent fever, whose curve resemble climbing steps, before becoming sustained); hectic fever with chronic tuberculosis or pyogenic abscesses; and relapsing fever with relapse of a previous infection (e.g., typhoid fever). Other causes of relapsing fever are the Pel-Ebstein fever of Hodgkin disease,[28] rat-bite fever (*Spirillum minus* or *Streptobacillus moniliformis*),[29] and *Borrelia* infections.[30]

Despite these etiologic associations, early clinicians recognized that the diagnostic significance of fever patterns was limited.[31] Instead, they used these labels more often to communicate a specific observation at the bedside rather than imply a specific diagnosis, much like we use the words "systolic murmur" or "lung crackle" today.

C. ASSOCIATED FINDINGS

1. Focal Findings

Over 80% of patients with bacterial infections have specific focal signs or symptoms that point the clinician to the correct diagnosis.[32] There are countless focal signs associated with febrile illness (e.g., the tender swelling of an abscess or the diastolic murmur of endocarditis), which are reviewed in detail in infectious diseases textbooks. One potentially misleading focal sign, however, is jaundice. Although fever and jaundice are often due to hepatitis or cholangitis, jaundice is also a nonspecific complication of bacterial infection distant to the liver, occurring in 1% of all bacteremias.[33,34] This *reactive hepatopathy of bacteremia* was recognized over a century ago by Osler, who wrote that jaundice appeared in pneumococcal pneumonia with curious irregularity in different outbreaks.[31]

2. Relative Bradycardia

Relative bradycardia, a traditional sign of intracellular bacterial infections (e.g., typhoid fever), refers to a pulse rate that is inappropriately slow for the patient's temperature. On average, the expected heart rate increases 10 beats/min for each 1°C increment in body temperature.[35] One rigorous definition of relative bradycardia is a pulse rate that is lower than the 95% confidence limit for the patient's temperature, which can be estimated by multiplying the patient temperature in degrees Celsius times 10 and then subtracting 323.[35] For example, if the patient's temperature is 39°C, relative bradycardia would refer to pulse rates below 67/min (i.e., 390–323).[†]

3. Anhidrosis

Classically, patients with heat stroke have "bone-dry skin," but most modern studies show that anhidrosis appears very late in the course of heat stroke and has a sensitivity of only 3% to 60%.[36-38] In contrast, 91% of patients with heat stroke have significant pyrexia (exceeding 40°C), and 100% have abnormal mental status.

4. Muscle Rigidity

Muscle rigidity suggests the diagnosis of neuroleptic malignant syndrome (a febrile complication from dopamine antagonists) or serotonin syndrome (from proserotonergic drugs).[39,40]

IV. Clinical Significance

A. DETECTION OF FEVER

Two findings increase probability of fever: the patient's subjective report of fever (LR = 5.3) and the clinician's perception that the patient's skin is abnormally warm (LR = 2.8, EBM Box 18.2). When either of these findings is absent, the probability of fever decreases (LR = 0.2 to 0.3).

B. PREDICTORS OF BACTEREMIA IN FEBRILE PATIENTS

In patients hospitalized with fever, 8% to 37% will have documented bacteremia,[46-54] a finding associated with an increased hospital mortality.[55] Of all the bedside findings that help diagnose bacteremia, the most important are the patient's underlying disorders, in particular the presence of renal failure (LR = 4.6, EBM Box 18.3), hospitalization for trauma (LR = 3), and poor functional status (i.e., bedridden or requiring attendance, LR = 3.6).[‡] Two studies even showed that the amount of food consumed by a febrile hospitalized patient was predictive of bacteremia: low food consumption (i.e., less than half of the meal served just before the blood culture) increased probability of bacteremia slightly (LR = 1.9), whereas high food consumption (more than 80% consumed) decreased it (LR = 0.2).[66,68] A few physical findings also modestly increase the probability of bacteremia: presence of an indwelling urinary catheter (LR = 2.7), presence of a central venous catheter (LR = 2.4), and hypotension (LR = 2.3). Age under 50 years decreases probability of bacteremia (LR = 0.3).

In 12 studies of almost 8000 patients with fever, the presence of **chills** modestly increased probability of bacteremia (sensitivity 24% to 95%; specificity 45% to 90%; positive LR = 2, negative LR = 0.7).[48,50,51,53,54,58-61,64,69,70] If chills are instead prospectively defined as **shaking chills** (i.e., the patient feels so cold that his or her body involuntarily shakes even under thick clothing or blanket), the

---

[†]This formula combines separate formulas for women (<11 × T° C − 359) and men (<10.2 × T° C − 333) provided in reference.[35]

[‡]For comparison, the LRs of these findings are superior to those for traditional laboratory signs of bacteremia, such as leucocytosis and bandemia. In detecting bacteremia, a WBC >15,000 has a LR of only 1.6,[32,47,54,58,67] whereas a band count >1,500 has an LR of 2.6.[32,47,50]

EBM BOX 18.2	Detection of Fever*				
Finding (reference)	Sensitivity (%)	Specificity (%)	Likelihood Ratio† if Finding Is	
			Present	Absent
Patient's report of fever[41–43]	80–90	55–95	5.3	0.2
Patient's forehead abnormally warm[42,44,45]	67–85	72–74	2.8	0.3

*Diagnostic standard: for *fever*, measured axillary temperature >37.5°C,[42,45] oral temperature >38°C,[41,43] or rectal temperature >38.1°C.[44]
†Likelihood ratio (LR) if finding present = positive LR; LR if finding absent = negative LR.

DETECTION OF FEVER
Probability

finding of shaking chills accurately detects bacteremia (sensitivity 24% to 90%, specificity 74% to 95%, positive LR = 4.1).[60,68,71] The presence of **toxic appearance** fails to discriminate serious infection from trivial illness.[32,72]

C. EXTREME PYREXIA AND HYPOTHERMIA

Extreme pyrexia (i.e., temperature exceeding 41.1°C [106°F]) has diagnostic significance because the cause is usually gram negative bacteremia or problems with temperature regulation (heat stroke, intracranial hemorrhage, severe burns).[38]

In a wide variety of disorders, the finding of a very high or low temperature indicates a worse prognosis.[73,74] For example, temperatures >39°C are associated with an increased risk of death in patients with pontine hemorrhage (LR = 23.7, EBM Box 18.4). Very low temperatures are associated with an increased risk of death in patients hospitalized with congestive heart failure (LR = 5.3), pneumonia (LR = 3.5), and bacterial sepsis (LR = 3.6).

D. FEVER PATTERNS

Most fevers today, whether infectious or noninfectious in origin, are intermittent or remittent and lack any other characteristic feature.[83,84] Antibiotic medications have changed many traditional fever patterns. For example, the fever of lobar pneumonia, which in the preantibiotic era was sustained and lasted 7 days, now lasts only 2 to 3 days.[85,86] The double quotidian fever pattern (i.e., 2 daily fever spikes), a feature of gonococcal endocarditis present in 50% of cases during the preantibiotic era, is consistently absent in reported cases from the modern era.[87] The characteristic tertian or quartan intermittent fever of malaria infection also is uncommon today, because most patients are treated before the characteristic synchronization of the malaria cycle.[88]

EBM BOX 18.3 — Detection of Bacteremia in Febrile Patients*

Finding (Reference)[†]	Sensitivity (%)	Specificity (%)	Likelihood Ratio[‡] if Finding Is Present	Absent
Risk factors				
Age 50 years or more[32,47]	89–95	32–33	1.4	**0.3**
Renal failure[48]	19–28	95	**4.6**	0.8
Hospitalization for trauma[46,56]	12–63	79–98	**3.0**	NS
Intravenous drug use[51,57]	2–7	98–99	NS	NS
Previous stroke[48,58]	13–17	85–94	NS	NS
Diabetes mellitus[32,47,48,50,54,57–62]	17–38	70–90	1.4	0.9
Poor functional performance[48]	48–61	83–87	**3.6**	0.6
Rapidly fatal disease (<1 mo)[51,53]	2–30	88–99	2.7	NS
Physical examination				
Indwelling lines and catheters				
Indwelling urinary catheter present[47,48,50,54,57,58,63]	3–38	83–99	2.7	NS
Central intravenous line present[46,57,63–65]	8–24	90–97	2.4	0.9
Vital signs				
Temperature ≥38.5°C[50,65]	62–87	27–53	1.2	0.7
Tachycardia[46,54,58,60,65,66]	53–73	40–57	1.2	0.8
Respiratory rate >20/minute[54,58,60]	37–76	28–74	NS	NS
Hypotension[50,51,54,58,60–62,65]	7–38	82–99	2.3	0.9
Other findings				
Acute abdomen[51,53,58,64]	2–22	89–100	1.9	NS
Confusion or depressed sensorium[46,50,54,58,59,61,64]	5–52	68–96	1.5	NS

*Diagnostic standard: for *bacteremia*, true bacteremia (not contamination), as determined by number of positive cultures, organism type, and results of other cultures.

†Definition of findings: for *renal failure*, serum creatinine >2 mg/dL, for *rapidly fatal disease*, >50% probability of fatality within 1 month (e.g., relapsed leukemia without treatment, hepatorenal syndrome); for *poor functional status*, see text; for *tachycardia*, pulse rate >90 beats/min[46,66] or >100 beats/min (all other studies); for *hypotension*, systolic blood pressure <100 mm Hg,[54] "shock,"[50] or <90 mm Hg (all other studies).

‡Likelihood ratio (LR) if finding present = positive LR; LR if finding absent = negative LR.

NS, Not significant.

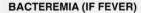

BACTEREMIA (IF FEVER)

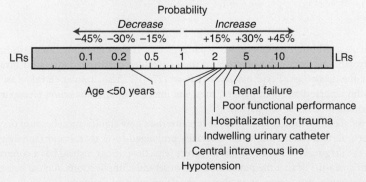

| EBM BOX 18.4 | **Extremes of Temperature and Prognosis** |

Finding (Reference)*	Sensitivity (%)	Specificity (%)	Likelihood Ratio[†] if Finding Is Present	Absent
Temperature >39°C				
Predicting hospital mortality in patients with pontine hemorrhage[75]	66	97	**23.7**	0.4
Hypothermia*				
Predicting hospital mortality in patients with congestive heart failure[76,77]	20–29	95–96	**5.3**	NS
Predicting hospital mortality in patients with pneumonia[78,79]	14–43	93	**3.5**	NS
Predicting hospital mortality in patients with sepsis[80–82]	7–15	96–98	**3.6**	NS

*Definition of findings: for *hypothermia*, temperature <35.2°C,[76] ≤35.5°C,[77] <36°C,[81,82] <36.1°C,[79] <36.5°C,[80] or <37.0°C.[78]
[†]Likelihood ratio (LR) if finding present = positive LR; LR if finding absent = negative LR.
NS, Not significant.

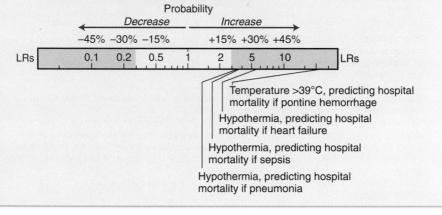

Nonetheless, although traditional fever patterns may be less common, they still have significance. In tropical countries, the presence of the **stepladder remittent pattern** of fever is highly specific for the diagnosis of typhoid fever (LR = 177.4).[89] Also, among travelers with malarial infection who reported a tertian pattern, most are infected with *Plasmodium vivax* (traditionally the most common cause of this pattern).[90]

Moreover, the antibiotic era has given fever patterns a new significance, because once antibiotics have been started, the finding of an unusually prolonged fever is an important sign indicating either that the diagnosis of infection was incorrect (e.g., the patient instead has a connective tissue disorder or neoplasm) or that the patient has one of several complications, such as resistant organisms, superinfection, drug fever, or an abscess requiring surgical drainage.

E. RELATIVE BRADYCARDIA

Clinical studies demonstrate that some infections, such as intracellular bacterial infections (e.g., typhoid fever and Legionnaire disease) and arboviral infections (e.g., sand-fly fever and dengue fever), do produce less tachycardia than other infections, but few patients with these infections actually have a relative bradycardia as defined earlier in the Findings section. Furthermore, most studies supporting the value of relative bradycardia fail to define the finding.

Nonetheless, in one study of 100 febrile patients admitted to a Singapore hospital, a pulse rate of 90/min or less increased probability of dengue infection (LR = 3.3) and a pulse rate of 80/min or less increased probability even more (LR = 5.3).[91] Another study of febrile patients returning from the tropics showed that the finding of relative bradycardia changed probability of enteric fever very little (LR = 1.7).[92, §]

F. FEVER OF UNKNOWN ORIGIN (FUO)

Fever of unknown origin is defined as a febrile illness lasting at least 3 weeks without an explanation after at least 1 week of investigation. Most etiologies of FUO are noninfectious, particularly malignancies and noninfectious inflammatory disorders. In 3 studies of almost 300 patients with FUO, two physical findings modestly increased the probability that a bone marrow examination would be diagnostic (usually of a hematologic malignancy): splenomegaly (sensitivity 35% to 53%; specificity 82% to 89%, LR = 2.9) and peripheral lymphadenopathy (sensitivity 21% to 30%; specificity 83% to 90%; LR = 1.9).[93–95]

References may be accessed online at *Elsevier eBooks for Practicing Clinicians.*

---

§This study applied a more liberal definition of relative bradycardia: for temperature of 101° F, pulse < 110/min; 102° F, <120/min; 103° F, <120/min; 104° F, <130/min; and 105° F, < 140/min.

CHAPTER 19

Respiratory Rate and Abnormal Breathing Patterns

KEY TEACHING POINTS

- Respirations should be observed for at least 60 seconds, not only to increase the detection of tachypnea but also to uncover unusual breathing patterns, such as Cheyne-Stokes breathing.
- Tachypnea is a valuable diagnostic and prognostic sign in a varisssety of conditions. In patients with altered mental status, bradypnea (≤12 breaths/min) increases probability of opiate intoxication.
- In hospitalized patients, Cheyne-Stokes breathing is an accurate sign of left ventricular dysfunction, especially in patients aged ≤80 years. It is present in one out of three patients with reduced ejection fraction.
- Abnormal respiratory abdominal movements—abdominal paradox and asynchronous breathing—are best observed when the patient is supine. These signs indicate respiratory muscle weakness, either diaphragm paralysis (abdominal paradox) or a patient who is tiring from the distress of bronchospasm (asynchronous breathing).
- Orthopnea, trepopnea, platypnea, and bendopnea each describe tachypnea that appears abruptly in particular patient positions. Each has specific diagnostic significance.

RESPIRATORY RATE

I. Introduction

The respiratory rate (i.e., number of breaths per minute) is one of the four traditional vital signs, the others being heart rate, blood pressure, and temperature. One of the first clinicians to recommend routine measurement of the respiratory rate was Stokes in 1825,[1] although routine charting of this vital sign was infrequent until the late 19th century.[2,3]

II. Technique

The respiratory rate is usually measured while the clinician is holding the patient's wrist and ostensibly counting the pulse, primarily because the respiratory rate may change if attention is drawn to it. This practice seems reasonable, because the respiratory rate is the only vital sign under voluntary control.

As routinely recorded in the patient's hospital record, the respiratory rate is often inaccurate.[4,5] In studies of patients whose actual respiratory rates ranged from 10 to more than 30 breaths/min, the recorded rates clustered around 16 to 22 breaths/min 75% to 98% of the time.[5-8] These errors usually reflect too short a period of observation (i.e., the clinician counting the number of breaths in 15 seconds and multiplying the result times 4); in one study, 15 seconds of observation detected only 23% of tachypneic patients, whereas 60 seconds of observation detected every tachypneic patient.[6] Consequently, respirations should be observed for at least 60 seconds, not only to increase accuracy of the measured rate[7] but also to allow detection of unusual breathing patterns, such as Cheyne-Stokes respirations (see later).

III. Finding

A. THE NORMAL RESPIRATORY RATE

The normal respiratory rate averages 20 breaths/min (range 16 to 25 breaths/min), based on careful measurement in persons without fever, heart disease, or lung disease.[9,10] This estimate is identical to that made over 150 years ago by Lambert Quetelet, who was the first to compile and analyze vital and social statistics.[11] Quetelet's 1835 monumental treatise also provided our current formula for body mass index, known as the Quetelet index (see Chapter 13). For unclear reasons, many textbooks, citing no data, mistakenly record the normal rate as 12 to 18 breaths/min.[9]

B. TACHYPNEA

Definitions of tachypnea vary, but the most commonly applied definition, based on the normal range and clinical studies, is respirations of 25 breaths/min or more.

C. BRADYPNEA

Bradypnea is variably defined as respiratory rates less than 8 to 12 breaths/min. In patients receiving epidural opiate analgesia, respiratory rates less than 8 to 10/min are the best definition of respiratory depression, a finding heralding respiratory failure.[12] In patients with altered mental status who are evaluated by medics, a respiratory rate of 12 breaths/min or less best identifies those intoxicated with opiates. (See the section on clinical significance.)[13]

IV. Clinical Significance

A. TACHYPNEA

The finding of tachypnea has both diagnostic and prognostic value. As a diagnostic sign, tachypnea argues modestly for the diagnosis of pneumonia in outpatients with cough and fever (likelihood ratio [LR] = 2.7, see EBM Box 19.1). Tachypnea also increases probability of pneumonia in hospitalized patients, the abnormal sign sometimes appearing as early as 1 to 2 days before the diagnosis is apparent by other means.[10,33] In patients with pneumatosis intestinalis (i.e., small cysts of gas in the bowel wall on radiologic images), tachypnea increases the probability that the surgeon will find bowel ischemia or obstruction at laparotomy (LR = 5.9).*

---

*In these patients, tachypnea was more accurate than other computed tomography findings, such as portal venous gas (LR = 3.2), dilated loops of bowel (LR = 1.3), or pneumoperitoneum (LR = NS). In this study about half of patients with pneumatosis intestinalis had bowel ischemia or obstruction; the other half had more benign etiologies.

EBM BOX 19.1	Tachypnea*

Finding (Reference) (breaths/min)	Sensitivity (%)	Specificity (%)	Likelihood Ratio† if Finding Is Present	Likelihood Ratio† if Finding Is Absent
Rate >20 Detecting operative finding of intestinal ischemia or obstruction, in patients with pneumatosis intestinalis[14,15]	27–29	93–98	**5.9**	0.8
Rate >24 Predicting failure of weaning from the ventilator, in intubated patients[16]	94	68	2.9	NS
Rate >26-27 Predicting cardiopulmonary arrest, in medical inpatients[17,18]	25–54	82–96	**4.3**	0.7
Rate >28 Detecting pneumonia, in patients with cough and fever[19–22]	7–36	80–99	2.7	0.9
Rate >30 Predicting hospital mortality, in patients with pneumonia[23–32]	9–85	63–99	2.4	0.9

*Diagnostic standard: for *failure of weaning*, progressive hypoxemia or respiratory acidosis; for *pneumonia*, infiltrate on chest radiograph.
†Likelihood ratio (LR) if finding present = positive LR; LR if finding absent = negative LR.
NS, Not significant.

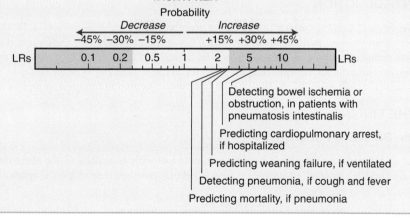

TACHYPNEA
Probability
Decrease | Increase
−45% −30% −15% | +15% +30% +45%
LRs 0.1 0.2 0.5 1 2 5 10 LRs

Detecting bowel ischemia or obstruction, in patients with pneumatosis intestinalis
Predicting cardiopulmonary arrest, if hospitalized
Predicting weaning failure, if ventilated
Detecting pneumonia, if cough and fever
Predicting mortality, if pneumonia

One characteristic of a vital sign is that it accurately predicts the patient's prognosis, and EBM Box 19.1 shows that tachypnea predicts subsequent cardiopulmonary arrest in hospitalized patients (LR = 4.3), better than does tachycardia or abnormal blood pressure.[17,18] During trials of weaning from a ventilator, tachypnea is a significant though modest predictor of weaning failure (LR = 2.9).[16,34] In patients hospitalized with pneumonia, severe tachypnea (i.e., rate >30 breaths/min) predicts subsequent hospital death (LR = 2.4).

B. TACHYPNEA AND OXYGEN SATURATION

The respiratory rate correlates poorly with the patient's level of oxygen desaturation (r = 0.16).[35] Although this initially seems surprising (i.e., the lower the oxygen level, the more rapid a patient should breathe), this actually is expected because some hypoxemic patients, by breathing rapidly, are able to restore a more normal oxygen level (i.e., hyperventilation increases arterial oxygen levels) and because other patients are hypoxemic simply because they have a primary hypoventilatory disorder. Consequently, the respiratory rate and oxygen saturation are both valuable to the clinician, each providing information independent of the other.

C. BRADYPNEA

In a study of patients seen by medics for altered mental status, the finding of a respiratory rate of 12 breaths/min or less predicted a positive response to naloxone, thus confirming the clinical impression of opiate intoxication (sensitivity of 80%, specificity of 95%, positive LR = 15.5, and negative LR = 0.2).[13]

ABNORMAL BREATHING PATTERNS

I. Cheyne-Stokes Breathing (Periodic Breathing)

A. INTRODUCTION

Cheyne-Stokes breathing consists of alternating periods of apnea and hyperpnea (Fig. 19.1). Some authors equate the term **periodic breathing** with Cheyne-Stokes breathing,[36,37] while others reserve the term periodic breathing for oscillations of tidal volume that lack intervening periods of apnea.[38]

Cheyne-Stokes breathing was described by John Cheyne in 1818 and William Stokes in 1854.[39]

B. THE FINDING

1. The Breathing Pattern

At the end of each apneic period, breathing commences with excursions of the chest that initially are small but gradually increase for several breaths and then diminish until apnea returns.

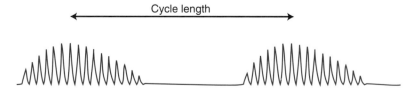

Fig. 19.1 Cheyne-Stokes respiration. There are alternating cycles of hyperpnea and apnea. During the hyperpnea phase only the tidal volume oscillates; the respiratory frequency is constant.

The respiratory rate is constant during the hyperpnea phase and does not gradually increase and then decrease as often surmised.[40] Cheyne-Stokes breathing often first appears when the patient lies down, probably because this position reduces the patient's functional residual capacity, thus diminishing the lung's ability to buffer changes in carbon dioxide.[37,41] (See the section on pathogenesis later.)

The time between two consecutive peaks of hyperpnea is called the **cycle length** or **period**. Each cycle length is divided into a hyperpnea phase (lasting about 30 seconds on average in patients with congestive heart failure) and an apnea phase (lasting about 25 seconds on average).[42,43]

2. Associated Bedside Observations

Several additional findings appear in patients with Cheyne-Stokes breathing. During the hyperpnea phase, the patient is alert and sometimes agitated, with dilated pupils, hyperactive muscle stretch reflexes, and increased muscle tone. During the apnea phase, the patient appears motionless and asleep with constricted pupils, hypoactive reflexes, and reduced muscle tone.[44,45] The agitation of the hyperpnea phase can easily startle a patient out of sleep, a symptom that clinicians can mistake for the paroxysmal nocturnal dyspnea of heart failure caused by transient pulmonary edema.[46,47]

C. CLINICAL SIGNIFICANCE

1. Associated Conditions

Cheyne-Stokes breathing affects 30% of patients with stable congestive heart failure.[38,43] The breathing pattern also appears in many neurologic disorders, including hemorrhage, infarction, tumors, meningitis, and head trauma involving the brainstem or higher levels of the central nervous system.[44,48] Normal persons often develop Cheyne-Stokes breathing during sleep[36] or at high altitudes.[44]

In patients hospitalized on an inpatient medicine service, the finding of Cheyne-Stokes respirations increases the probability left ventricular systolic dysfunction (i.e., ejection fraction less than 40%; LR = 5.4, EBM Box 19.2). The finding is more accurate in patients under the age of 80 years (LR = 8.1) than in patients over the age of 80 years (LR = 2.7), suggesting that alternative explanations of Cheyne-Stokes breathing (e.g., central nervous system injury) are more important in older patients.[43]

2. Prognostic Importance

Although Dr. Stokes originally believed that Cheyne-Stokes respirations implied a poor prognosis in patients with heart failure, modern studies demonstrate contradictory results, some showing that the finding implies worse survival,[49] while others showing no independent association with increased mortality.[43,50]

D. PATHOGENESIS

The fundamental problem causing Cheyne-Stokes breathing is enhanced sensitivity to carbon dioxide. The circulatory delay between the lungs and systemic arteries, caused by poor cardiac output, also contributes to the waxing and waning of breaths. Cerebral blood flow increases during hyperpnea and decreases during apnea, perhaps explaining the fluctuations of mental status.[42,51]

1. Enhanced Sensitivity to Carbon Dioxide

Whether because of congestive heart failure or neurologic disease, patients with Cheyne-Stokes breathing have 2 to 3 times the normal sensitivity to carbon dioxide.[48,52] This causes patients to hyperventilate excessively, eventually driving the carbon dioxide level so low that central apnea

EBM BOX 19.2	**Cheyne-Stokes Breathing, Detecting Reduced Ejection Fraction[43,*]**

Finding (reference)	Sensitivity (%)	Specificity (%)	Likelihood Ratio[†] if Finding Is Present	Absent
All adults	33	94	**5.4**	0.7
Patients aged ≤80 years	32	96	**8.1**	0.7
Patients aged >80 years	42	84	2.7	NS

*Diagnostic standard: for *reduced ejection fraction*, <40% by transthoracic echocardiography.
[†]Likelihood ratio (LR) if finding present = positive LR; LR if finding absent = negative LR.
NS, Not significant.

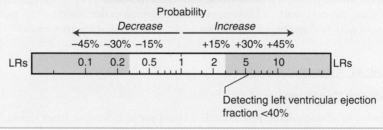

CHEYNE-STOKES BREATHING

results. After they stop breathing, carbon dioxide levels again rise, eliciting another hyperventilatory response and thus perpetuating the alternating cycles of apnea and hyperpnea.

Mountain climbers develop Cheyne-Stokes breathing because hypoxia induces hypersensitivity to carbon dioxide. In contrast, their native Sherpa guides, who are acclimated to hypoxia, lack an exaggerated ventilatory response and do not develop Cheyne-Stokes breathing.[44]

2. Circulatory Delay between Lungs and Arteries

Ventilation is normally controlled by the medullary respiratory center, which monitors arterial carbon dioxide levels and directs the lungs to ventilate more if carbon dioxide levels are too high and less if levels are too low. The medulla signals the lungs almost immediately, the message traveling via the nervous system. The feedback to the medulla, however, is much slower because it requires circulation of blood from lungs back to systemic arteries.

In Cheyne-Stokes breathing, the carbon dioxide levels in the alveoli and those of the systemic arteries are precisely out of sync. During peak hyperpnea, carbon dioxide levels in the alveoli are very low, yet the medulla is just beginning to sample blood containing high carbon dioxide levels from the previous apnea phase and thus still directs the lungs to continue breathing deeply.[44] The delay in feedback to the medulla contributes to the gradual waxing and waning of tidal volume.

The length of circulatory delay also governs the cycle length of Cheyne-Stokes breathing, the two correlating closely (r = 0.8 between cycle length and circulation time from lung to arteries, p <0.05).[42,51] The cycle length is about 2 times the circulation time, just as would be expected from the observation that carbon dioxide levels in the lungs and arteries are precisely out of sync. Nonetheless, one study showed poor correlation between cycle length and ejection fraction, indicating either that ejection fraction is a poor measure of circulation time or that variables other than cardiac performance govern cycle length.

II. Kussmaul Respiration

Kussmaul respirations are rapid and deep and appear in patients with metabolic acidosis.[53] The unusually deep respirations are distinctive, because other causes of tachypnea, such as heart and lung disease, reduce vital capacity and thus cause rapid, *shallow* respirations.

In children with severe malaria, the finding of Kussmaul respirations detects severe metabolic acidosis with a sensitivity of 19% to 91%, specificity of 81% to 97%, and positive LR = 5.3.[54–56]

III. Grunting Respirations

A. DEFINITION

Grunting respirations are short, explosive sounds of low-to-medium pitch produced by vocal cord closure during expiration. The actual sound is the rush of air that occurs when the glottis opens and suddenly allows air to escape. Grunting respirations are more common in children,[57] although the finding also has been described in adults as a sign of respiratory muscle fatigue[58] and, in the preantibiotic era, as a cardinal sign of lobar pneumonia, usually appearing after 4 to 6 days of illness.[3,59]

B. PATHOGENESIS

Grunting respirations slow down expiration and allow more time for maximal gas exchange.[58] In animal experiments, artificial mimicking of grunting respirations causes the pO_2 to increase by 10% and the pCO_2 to fall by 11%, whether or not the animal has pneumonia.[60] Grunting respirations also produce positive pressure exhalation that may reduce exudation of fluid into the alveoli, based on an old observation that administration of morphine to patients with pneumonia often reduced grunting respirations but was sometimes immediately followed by fatal pulmonary edema.[59]

IV. Abnormal Abdominal Movements

A. NORMAL ABDOMINAL MOVEMENTS

In the absence of massive gaseous distention, the abdominal viscera are noncompressible and act like hydraulic coupling fluid that directly transmits movements of the diaphragm to the anterior abdominal wall.[61] Abdominal respiratory movements, therefore, indicate indirectly how the diaphragm is moving. During normal respiration, the chest and abdomen move synchronously: both out during inspiration and both in during expiration (Fig. 19.2). The chest wall moves more when the person is upright, and the abdomen moves more when the person is supine.[62,63]

B. ABNORMAL ABDOMINAL MOVEMENTS

Two abnormal abdominal movements are signs of chronic airflow obstruction or respiratory muscle weakness: **asynchronous breathing** and **paradoxical abdominal movements**.

1. Asynchronous Breathing

a. Findings
Asynchronous breathing is an abnormal *expiratory* movement that sometimes develops in patients with chronic airflow obstruction. In these patients, the normal smooth inward abdominal movement during expiration is replaced by an abrupt inward and then outward movement (see Fig. 19.2).[64,65]

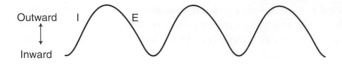

Chest wall movements:

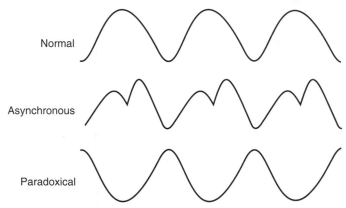

Outward I

Inward E

Abdominal wall movements:

Normal

Asynchronous

Paradoxical

Fig. 19.2 **Respiratory abdominal movements.** Chest movements are depicted in the first row. "I" denotes inspiration and "E," expiration. *Upward sloping lines* on the drawing indicate outward body wall movements; *downward sloping lines,* inward movements. In normal persons, the abdominal and chest wall movements are completely in sync. In asynchronous breathing, only expiratory abdominal movements are abnormal. In paradoxical abdominal movements, both inspiratory and expiratory abdominal movements are abnormal. See text.

b. Clinical Significance

In patients with chronic airflow obstruction, asynchronous breathing correlates with lower forced expiratory volumes and a much poorer prognosis.[65] Among patients with chronic airflow obstruction who develop acute respiratory symptoms, the presence of an asynchronous breathing pattern predicts subsequent hospital death or the need for artificial ventilation with a sensitivity of 64%, specificity of 80%, and positive LR of 3.2 (negative LR not significant).[64]

c. Pathogenesis

The outward abdominal movement during expiration probably reflects the strong action of chest wall accessory muscles during expiration, which push the flattened diaphragm temporarily downward, and thus the abdomen abruptly outward.[62,64]

2. Paradoxical Abdominal Movements

a. Finding

Paradoxical abdominal movements are completely out of sync with those of the chest wall. During inspiration the abdomen moves in as the chest wall moves out; during expiration, the abdomen moves out as chest moves in.[61,66–68]

b. Clinical Significance

Paradoxical abdominal movements are a sign of bilateral diaphragm weakness. Most of these patients also complain of severe orthopnea. In one study of patients with dyspnea and neuromuscular disease, the finding of paradoxical abdominal movements detected diaphragm weakness with a sensitivity of 95%, specificity of 70%, and positive LR = 3.2 (in this study, the definition of paradoxical movements was any inspiratory inward abdominal movement, and the definition of diaphragm weakness was a maximal transdiaphragmatic pressure ≤30 cm H_2O; the normal sniff transdiaphragmatic pressure is >98 cm H_2O).[66]

c. Pathogenesis
If the diaphragm is totally paralyzed, the inspiratory outward movement of the chest wall will draw the diaphragm upward, and thus the abdomen inward. The weight of the abdominal viscera probably also plays a role, because paradoxical movements are most obvious in affected patients who are positioned supine and are often absent when the patient is upright.[66]

A mimic of paradoxic abdominal movements is seen in patients with tetraplegia. In these patients, respiratory motion relies entirely on the diaphragm: as it descends during inspiration, pushing the abdominal wall out, the paralyzed chest wall may be drawn inward. The chest and abdomen are completely out of sync in these patients, but in contrast to the paradoxical abdominal movements of diaphragm weakness, the abdominal wall of tetraplegic patients moves *outward* during inspiration, not *inward*.

V. Orthopnea, Trepopnea, Platypnea, and Bendopnea

These terms describe tachypnea (and dyspnea) that appears abruptly in particular positions: when the patient is supine (**orthopnea**), lying on one side (**trepopnea**), upright (**platypnea**), or bending over (**bendopnea**). These findings are often first diagnosed during observation of the patient's respirations at the bedside.

A. ORTHOPNEA

1. Finding

Orthopnea describes dyspnea that appears when the patient lies down but is relieved when the patient sits up (from the Greek words *ortho* meaning straight or vertical, and *pnea* meaning to breathe).

2. Clinical Significance

Orthopnea occurs in a variety of disorders, including massive ascites, bilateral diaphragm paralysis, pleural effusion, morbid obesity, and severe pneumonia, although its most important clinical association is congestive heart failure.[66,67,69] In one study of patients with known chronic obstructive pulmonary disease, the finding of orthopnea distinguished between those patients with abnormally low ejection fraction (less than 50%) and those with normal ejection fraction with a sensitivity of 97%, specificity of 64%, positive LR = 2.7, and negative LR = 0.04.[70] This suggests that, in patients with lung disease, the *presence* of orthopnea has limited value (i.e., occurs in both lung and heart disease), but the *absence* of orthopnea is more compelling, *decreasing* the probability of associated left ventricular dysfunction (LR = 0.04).

3. Pathogenesis

In patients with orthopnea, lung compliance and vital capacity decrease significantly after moving from the upright to supine position. This explains in part why dyspnea worsens in the supine position and why orthopnea is a finding common to so many different clinical conditions.[69,71,72] Nonetheless, orthopnea cannot be entirely caused by postural changes in lung mechanics, for several reasons. First, orthopnea is uncommon in other disorders with similar reductions of vital capacity and compliance (e.g., interstitial fibrosis). Second, in patients with congestive heart failure, orthopnea correlates poorly with the pulmonary artery wedge pressure, which should have some relation to interstitial edema and pulmonary mechanics.[73] Finally, elevation of the head alone brings prompt relief to some orthopneic patients. It was once believed that elevation of the head relieved dyspnea because it reduced intracranial venous pressure and thus improved cerebral perfusion, although this hypothesis has been experimentally disproved.[69]

B. TREPOPNEA

1. Finding

Trepopnea[†] (from Greek *trepo* meaning twist or turn) describes dyspnea that is worse in one lateral decubitus position and relieved in the other.

2. Clinical Significance

There are three principal causes of trepopnea.

a. Unilateral Parenchymal Lung Disease[76,77]

Affected patients usually prefer to position their healthy lung down, which improves oxygenation because blood preferentially flows to the lower lung.

b. Congestive Heart Failure from Dilated Cardiomyopathy[74,75,78]

Patients usually prefer to have their right side down. Whether this is due to positional changes in lung mechanics (e.g., left lung atelectasis from cardiomegaly), right ventricular preload, or airway compression is unclear. The preference for the right side down in heart failure may contribute to the right-sided predilection of pleural effusions in these patients.[79]

c. Mediastinal or Endobronchial Tumor

Tumors may compress the airways or central blood vessels in one position but not the other.[80–82] A clue to this diagnosis is a localized wheeze that appears in the position causing symptoms.[80]

d. Other Causes

Rare reports of trepopnea include a patient with position-dependent right-to-left intracardiac shunting[83] and a patient with unilateral diaphragmatic paralysis.[84] The patient with hemidiaphragm paralysis (on the right side) had left-sided trepopnea, possibly because this position increased the weight of abdominal viscera against the only functioning half of the diaphragm.[84]

C. PLATYPNEA

1. Finding

Platypnea (from the Greek *platus*, meaning "flat") is the opposite of orthopnea: patients experience worse dyspnea when upright (sitting or standing) and relief after lying down (a related term, *orthodeoxia*, describes a similar deterioration of oxygen saturation in the upright position). This rare syndrome was first described in 1949, and the term *platypnea* was first coined in 1969.[85,86]

[†]In 1937, Drs. Wood and Wolferth first described trepopnea in patients with congestive heart failure.[74] In searching for a name for the finding, a patent lawyer suggested to them *rolling relief*, which they translated into *rotopnea*, until a Dr. Kern pointed out that roto was a Latin root and the pure Greek term *trepopnea* would be better.[75]

2. Clinical Significance

Platypnea occurs in patients with right-to-left shunting of blood through intracardiac or intra-pulmonary shunts.[87]

a. Right-to-Left Shunting of Blood through a Patent Foramen Ovale or Atrial Septal Defect

These patients often first develop the finding after undergoing pneumonectomy or developing a pulmonary embolus or pericardial effusion, which for unclear reasons promotes right-to-left shunting in the upright position.[88–93]

b. Right-To-Left Shunting of Blood through Intrapulmonary Shunts

Right-to-left shunting of blood through intrapulmonary shunts located in the bases of the lungs occurs in the hepatopulmonary syndrome, a complication of chronic liver disease (see Chapter 8)[94] and hereditary hemorrhagic telangiectasia.[95] In these patients, the upright position causes more blood to flow to the bases, thus aggravating the right-to-left shunting of blood and the patient's hypoxemia. In one series of 110 patients with chronic liver disease, the symptom of platypnea detected hepatopulmonary syndrome with a sensitivity of 66%, specificity of 94%, positive LR = 10.6, and negative LR = 0.4 (see Chapter 8).[96]

D. BENDOPNEA

1. Finding

Bendopnea describes shortness of breath that develops when a seated patient bends over. Chapter 48 describes a specific bedside test for bendopnea.

2. Clinical Significance

In patients with heart failure, a positive bendopnea test increases probability that the patient's pulmonary capillary wedge pressure is 22 mm Hg or more (LR = 3.2).[97] The pathogenesis and clinical significance of this finding are fully discussed in Chapter 48.

References may be accessed online at *Elsevier eBooks for Practicing Clinicians*.

Pulse Oximetry

I. Introduction

Pulse oximetry measures the arterial oxygen saturation rapidly and conveniently. It is regarded the fifth vital sign,[1,2] although some clinicians argue that pulse oximetry is a diagnostic test, not a physical sign, because it requires special equipment. Measurement of oxygen saturation, however, is no different from the other vital signs whose measurement requires a thermometer, sphygmomanometer, or stopwatch.

Takuo Aoyagi of Japan discovered the basic principle of pulse oximetry—pulsatile transmission of light through tissue depends on the patient's arterial saturation—in the mid-1970s.[3] The first pulse oximeters were successfully marketed in the 1980s.[4]

II. The Finding

Measurements are obtained by using a self-adhesive or clip-type probe attached to the patient's finger, nose, forehead, or earlobe.[5] The oximeter makes several hundred measurements each second and then displays an average value based on the previous 3 to 6 seconds, a value that is updated about every second.[6] Although the digital display of pulse oximeters creates a sense of precision, studies show that, between oxygen saturation levels of 70% and 100%, pulse oximeters are only accurate within 5% (i.e., ±2 standard deviations) of measurements made by in vitro arterial blood gas analysis using co-oximetry.[4,7,8]

The most common causes of inadequate oximeter signals are poor perfusion (due to cold or hypotension) and motion artifact. The clinician can sometimes correct these problems and thus improve the signal by warming or rubbing the patient's hand, repositioning the probe, or resting the patient's hand on a soft surface.[6] If inadequate signals persist, the clinician should try obtaining measurements with the clip probe attached to the lobule or pinna of the patient's ear.

In patients with hemiparesis, the results of pulse oximetry on the right and left sides of the body are the same.[9]

III. Clinical Significance

A. ADVANTAGES OF PULSE OXIMETRY

As a sign of low oxygen levels, pulse oximetry is superior to the physical sign of cyanosis, because of oximetry is more sensitive and because readings do not depend on the patient's hemoglobin level (see Chapter 9). Consequently, pulse oximetry has become indispensable in the monitoring of patients in emergency departments, recovery and operating rooms, pulmonary clinics, and intensive care units, where measurements often reveal unsuspected oxygen desaturation, leading to changes in diagnosis and treatment. Oxygen therapy prolongs survival of some hypoxemic patients, such as patients chronically hypoxemic from lung disease.[10,11] Presumably, oxygen therapy benefits patients with acute hypoxemia as well.

In hospitalized patients, an O_2 saturation of less than 90% predicts hospital mortality (likelihood ratio [LR] = 4.5, EBM Box 20.1). As a diagnostic sign, an O_2 saturation of less than 96% increases probability of hepatopulmonary syndrome in patients with chronic liver disease

---

EBM BOX 20.1	Oxygen Saturation by Pulse Oximetry*			
			Likelihood Ratio[†] if Finding Is	
Finding (reference)	**Sensitivity (%)**	**Specificity (%)**	**Present**	**Absent**
Predicting hospital mortality in hospitalized patients				
Oxygen saturation <90%[12,13]	21–39	87–97	**4.5**	0.8
Detecting hepatopulmonary syndrome in patients with chronic liver disease				
Oxygen <96%[14,15]	28–39	91–94	**4.3**	0.7
Detecting pneumonia in outpatients with cough and fever				
Oxygen <95%[16-19]	32–52	80–99	**3.0**	0.7

*Diagnostic standard: for *hepatopulmonary syndrome*, triad of cirrhosis, intrapulmonary shunting by contrast echocardiography, and arterial alveolar to arterial oxygen gradient >20 mm Hg; for *pneumonia*, chest radiography.
[†]Likelihood ratio (LR) if finding present = positive LR; LR if finding absent = negative LR.

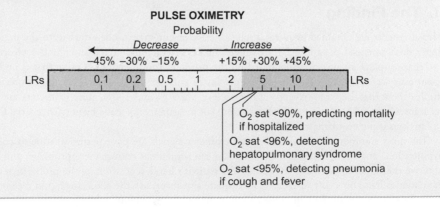

PULSE OXIMETRY
Probability

(LR = 4.3), and an O_2 saturation of less than 95% increases probability of pneumonia in patients with cough and fever (LR = 3). The use of pulse oximetry and its waveform to diagnose pulsus paradoxus, peripheral vascular disease, and aspiration in patients with stroke are discussed in Chapters 15, 54, and 60.

B. LIMITATIONS OF PULSE OXIMETRY[4,5,7,20]

Because pulse oximetry readings indicate only the degree of oxygen saturation of hemoglobin, they fail to detect problems of poor oxygen delivery (e.g., anemia, poor cardiac output), hyperoxia, and hypercapnia. Other limitations of pulse oximetry measurements are discussed below.

1. Dyshemoglobinemias

The pulse oximeter interprets carboxyhemoglobin to be oxyhemoglobin and therefore seriously underestimates the degree of oxygen desaturation in patients with carbon monoxide poisoning. In patients with methemoglobinemia, the pulse oximetry readings decrease initially but eventually plateau at around 85%, despite true oxyhemoglobin levels that continue to decrease to much lower levels.

2. Dyes

Methylene blue causes a spurious decrease in oxygen saturation readings. Darker colors of nail polish reduce oxygen saturation readings, although the error is small when using modern oximeters.[21,22] Even so, clinicians should remove all pigments from the patient's fingers before pulse oximetry (a procedure that may reveal additional nail findings). Hyperbilirubinemia and jaundice do not affect oximeter accuracy.

3. Low Perfusion Pressure

In patients with hypotension or peripheral vascular disease, the arterial pulse may be so weak that the pulse oximeter is unable to pick up the arterial signal, thus making measurements difficult or impossible.

4. Exaggerated Venous Pulsations

In patients with right-sided heart failure or tricuspid regurgitation, the oximeter may mistake the venous waveform for the arterial one, leading to spuriously low oxygen saturation readings.

5. Ambient Light

Excessive ambient light has long been felt to affect oximeter readings, although one study comparing various types of lamps (fluorescent, incandescent, infrared heat, quartz-halogen, and bilirubin lamps) failed to show any clinically significant effect on oximeter readings.[23]

References may be accessed online at *Elsevier eBooks for Practicing Clinicians*.

Head and Neck

Head and Neck

The Pupils

NORMAL PUPILS

I. Introduction

The integrity of the pupil depends on the iris, cranial nerves II and III, and the sympathetic nerves innervating the eye.

II. Size

The size of the normal pupil decreases as persons grow older (r = −0.75, p <0.001): At 10 years of age the mean diameter is 7 mm, at 30 years it is 6 mm, and at 80 years it is 4 mm.[1,2] Throughout human history, large pupils have been associated with youth, beauty, and vigor, explaining why the plant yielding the pupillary dilator atropine was named *belladonna*, which literally means "beautiful lady."

III. Hippus

Under steady illumination the normal pupil is in continual motion, repeatedly dilating and contracting small amounts. This restless undulation, called **hippus** or **pupillary unrest**, is more prominent in younger patients and during exposure to bright light. Clinicians of the 19th century associated hippus with diverse disorders, ranging from myasthenia gravis to brain tumors, but hippus is now known to be a normal phenomenon.[3] The oscillations of the right and left pupil are synchronous, a finding suggesting hippus is under central control.

IV. Simple Anisocoria

Simple anisocoria, a normal finding, is defined as a difference in pupil diameter of 0.4 mm or more that cannot be attributed to any of the pathologic pupils discussed later, intraocular drugs, ocular injury, or ocular inflammation.[2] Simple anisocoria affects up to 38% of healthy persons (only half of whom have anisocoria at any given moment) and is a constant finding in 3% of persons. As simple anisocoria waxes and wanes over time, it is the usually same eye that displays the larger pupil.[2]

The difference in pupil size in simple anisocoria rarely exceeds 1 mm.[2] Other features distinguishing it from pathologic anisocoria are described later, in the section on abnormal pupils.

V. Normal Light Reflex

A. ANATOMY

Fig. 21.1 illustrates the nerves responsible for the normal light reflex. Because both pupillary constrictor muscles normally receive identical signals from the midbrain, they constrict the same amount, which may be small or large depending on the *summation* of light intensity coming into *both* eyes. For example, both pupils dilate the same amount in darkness, constrict an identical small amount when a dim light is held in front of one eye, and constrict an identical larger amount when a bright light is held in front of one eye.

With a light held in front of one eye, ipsilateral pupillary constriction is called **direct reaction** to light and contralateral constriction is called **consensual reaction**.

B. CLINICAL SIGNIFICANCE

The anatomy of the normal light reflex has two important clinical implications:

1. Anisocoria Is Absent in Disorders of the Optic Nerve or Retina (i.e., Afferent Connections)

Because the signal in both outgoing third nerves is identical in these disorders, representing the summation of light intensity from both eyes, the pupils are the same size. Unilateral afferent disease is similar to the experiment of holding a bright light in front of one eye (i.e., the opposite eye thus mimicking one with an afferent defect): despite the asymmetry of light signals in the two optic nerves, both pupils have identical diameter.

2. Anisocoria Indicates Asymmetric Disease of the Iris, Cranial Nerve III, or Sympathetic Nerves (Efferent Connections and Iris)

Asymmetric disease of the efferent connections guarantees that the signals arriving at the pupil are different and, therefore, that the pupil size will be different.

VI. Near Synkinesis Reaction

The near synkinesis reaction occurs when a person focuses on a near object. The reaction has three parts: (1) constriction of the pupils (pupilloconstrictor muscle), (2) convergence of eyes (medial rectus muscles), and (3) accommodation of the lenses (ciliary body).

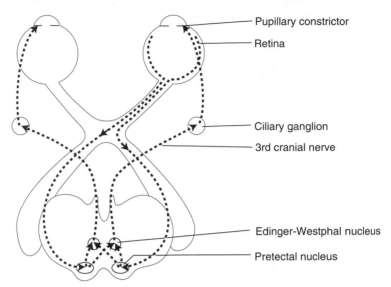

Pupillary constrictor

Retina

Ciliary ganglion

3rd cranial nerve

Edinger-Westphal nucleus

Pretectal nucleus

Fig. 21.1 **Anatomy of the pupillary light reflex.** The *dotted lines* show how nerve impulses from the retina and optic nerve on one side (right eye in this example), contribute to the nerve impulses of both third nerves, via the crossing of the nerve impulses from the nasal retina in the optic chiasm and the abundant interconnections between both pretectal nuclei and both Edinger-Westphal nuclei. Unless there is asymmetric disease of the efferent pathway (i.e., third nerve, ciliary ganglion and postganglionic fibers, iris), the pupils are thus symmetric.

ABNORMAL PUPILS

I. Relative Afferent Pupillary Defect (Marcus Gunn Pupil)

A. INTRODUCTION

The relative afferent pupillary defect is the most common abnormal pupillary finding, more common than all other pupillary defects combined.[4]

Although the relative afferent pupillary defect was described by R. Marcus Gunn in 1904, it is clear from his report that the sign was generally known to clinicians of his time. Kestenbaum named the finding in 1946 after Marcus Gunn,[4] and in 1959, Levatin introduced the swinging flashlight test, which is how most clinicians now elicit the finding.[5]

B. THE FINDING

Because the pupils are equal in patients with disorders of the retina and optic nerves (see the section on normal pupils, earlier, and Fig. 21.1), the **swinging flashlight test** is necessary to uncover disorders of the afferent half of the light reflex. This test compares the amount of pupilloconstriction produced by illuminating one eye with that produced by illuminating the other.

To perform the test, the clinician swings the flashlight back and forth from eye to eye, holding it over each pupil 1 to 3 seconds before immediately shifting it to the other (see Fig. 21.2). Both pupils constrict strongly when the light is shining into the normal eye, but, as the light swings over to illuminate the abnormal eye, both pupils dilate (dilation occurs because the pupils respond as if the light were much dimmer, producing *less* bilateral constriction—or net dilation—compared to when the light is shining in the normal eye).[4,6] As long as the clinician swings the light back and

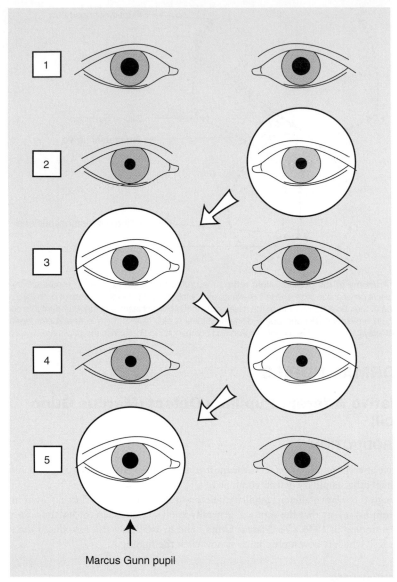

Marcus Gunn pupil

Fig. 21.2 **The relative afferent pupillary defect (Marcus Gunn pupil).** The figure depicts a patient with an abnormal *right* optic nerve. Under normal room light illumination (row 1), the pupils are symmetric. During the swinging flashlight test, the pupils constrict when the patient's normal left eye is illuminated (rows 2 and 4) but dilate when the abnormal right eye is illuminated (rows 3 and 5). Although both pupils constrict or dilate simultaneously, the clinician is usually focused on just the illuminated pupil. The pupil that dilates during the swinging flashlight test has the relative afferent pupillary defect and is labeled the Marcus Gunn pupil. See the text.

forth, the reaction persists—pupils constrict when illuminating the normal eye and dilate when illuminating the abnormal eye. Because clinicians usually focus on the illuminated pupil, the one that dilates is labeled as having a **relative afferent pupillary defect** or the **Marcus Gunn pupil.***

---

*An excellent video of the Marcus Gunn pupil appears in reference 7.

There has been some debate whether eyes with afferent defects also display abnormal pupillary release (i.e., **pupillary release** is the small amount of pupillary dilatation immediately following initial constriction during steady illumination).[8] Nonetheless, two studies demonstrated that only the swinging flashlight test reliably uncovers the afferent defect.[9,10]

Light reflecting off the cornea may sometimes obscure the movements of the pupils. To overcome this, the clinician should angle the light by holding the light source slightly below the horizontal axis.

Interpreting the swinging flashlight test has three caveats:[6]

1. **Correct interpretation of the test ignores hippus**, which otherwise can make interpretation difficult.

2. **The clinician should avoid the tendency to linger with the flashlight on the eye suspected to have disease**. Uneven swinging of the light may temporarily bleach the retina being illuminated more, thus eventually producing a relative pupillary defect and erroneously confirming the initial suspicion. To avoid this and ensure equal illumination of both retinas, the clinician should silently count: "one, two, switch, one two, switch," and so on.

3. **Only one working iris is required to interpret this pupillary sign**. If the patient has only one pupil that reacts to light (see the section on anisocoria), the test is performed the same way, although the clinician focuses only on the normal iris to interpret the results.

C. CLINICAL SIGNIFICANCE

A relative afferent defect implies ipsilateral optic nerve disease or severe retinal disease.

1. Optic Nerve Disease

Patients with optic nerve disease (e.g., optic neuritis, ischemic optic neuropathy, glaucomatous optic nerve damage) have the most prominent relative afferent pupillary defects. If the disease is asymmetric, the sensitivity of the finding is 92% to 98%, much higher than that for other tests of afferent function, including visual acuity, pupil cycle times, and visual evoked potentials.[11,12] Even compared to optical coherence tomography, the Marcus Gunn pupil is accurate, detecting the asymmetric thickness of the retinal nerve fiber layer in patients with glaucoma (sensitivity of 92%, specificity of 78%, positive likelihood ratio [LR] = 4.2, negative LR = 0.1)[13] and multiple sclerosis (sensitivity of 50%, specificity of 86%, positive LR = 3.6).[14] In patients with glaucoma, a Marcus Gunn pupil increases probability there will be significant cup-to-disc ratio asymmetry on fundoscopy (sensitivity of 75%, specificity of 84%, and positive LR = 4.8).[15]

Even so, the Marcus Gunn pupil depends on *asymmetric* optic nerve function (hence the word *relative* in its label); consequently, if patients with suspected unilateral disease lack the afferent pupillary finding, bilateral optic nerve disease is eventually found in 65%.[12]

2. Retinal Disease

Severe retinal disease may cause a relative afferent pupillary defect, although the retinal disease must be markedly asymmetric to produce the finding and, once the finding appears, it is subtle compared with that seen in optic nerve disease.[16]

3. Cataracts do not Cause the Relative Afferent Pupillary Defect[17]

Although this seems surprising, it is because the retina, if healthy, compensates over minutes for any diminished brightness, just as it does after a person walks into a dark movie theater. In fact, during the time of Galen, the classical Roman physician, clinicians tested the pupillary light reaction of patients with cataracts to determine whether vision could be restored after couching (couching was an ancient treatment for cataracts that used a needle to displace the cataract posteriorly; a preserved light reaction indicated that the retina and optic nerve behind the cataract were intact).[18]

4. Unilateral Visual Loss and the Marcus Gunn Pupil

Unilateral visual loss could result from refractive errors (e.g., near-sightedness, far-sightedness, astigmatism), optic nerve disorders (ischemic optic neuropathy, optic neuritis), extensive retinal disease (retinal detachment, central retinal vein or artery occlusion), macular disease (e.g., macular degeneration), or abnormalities of the optic media (e.g., cataracts, vitreous hemorrhage). Clinicians can easily identify visual loss from refractive errors by having the patient look through a pinhole aperture, which will focus light and improve acuity for those with refractive errors but not those with other ocular diseases (e.g., of the optic nerve, retina, macula, or media).

In one study of patients with unilateral visual loss not made better with a pinhole aperture (i.e., not due to refractive errors), the presence of the Marcus Gunn pupil greatly *increased* probability of optic nerve or retinal disease (sensitivity of 71%, specificity of 96%, positive LR = 16.8) and *decreased* probability of disorders of the macula or optic media (LR = 0.1).[19]

II. Argyll Robertson Pupils

A. THE FINDING[20,21]

Argyll Robertson pupils have four characteristic findings: (1) bilateral involvement, (2) small pupils that fail to dilate fully in dim light, (3) no light reaction, and (4) brisk constriction to near vision and brisk redilation to far vision.[†]

Originally described by Douglas Moray Cooper Lamb Argyll Robertson in 1868, this finding had great significance a century ago because it settled a long-standing debate whether general paresis and tabes dorsalis were the same disease. The pupillary abnormality was found in a high proportion of patients with both diseases and was limited to these diseases, arguing for a common syphilitic origin of both. The introduction of Wasserman's serologic test for syphilis in 1906 confirmed that the two diseases had the same cause.

B. CLINICAL SIGNIFICANCE

1. Associated Disorders

In addition to neurosyphilis, there are rare, scattered reports of Argyll Robertson pupils in patients with various other disorders, including diabetes mellitus, neurosarcoidosis, and Lyme disease (see also the section on diabetic pupil).[20] The responsible lesion is probably located in the dorsal midbrain, where damage would interrupt the light reflex fibers but spare the more ventrally located fibers innervating the Edinger-Westphal nuclei that control the near reaction[23,24]

2. Differential Diagnosis of Light-Near Dissociation

Argyll Robertson pupils display light-near dissociation, that is, they fail to react to light but constrict during near vision. Other causes of light-near dissociation include the following:
a. **Adie Tonic Pupil** (see later)
b. **Optic Nerve or Severe Retinal Disease**
   Either of these disorders may eliminate the light reaction when light is directed into the abnormal eye, although the pupils still constrict with the near synkinesis. In contrast to other causes of light-near dissociation, however, optic nerve and retinal disease severely impair vision.

[†]An excellent video of the Argyll Robertson pupil in a patient with tabes dorsalis appears in reference 22.

c. **Dorsal Midbrain Syndrome (Parinaud syndrome, Sylvian Aqueduct Syndrome, Pretectal Syndrome).**[25,26] Characteristic findings of the dorsal midbrain syndrome are light-near dissociation, vertical gaze palsy, lid retraction, and convergence-retraction nystagmus (a rhythmic inward movement of both eyes from co-contraction of the extra-ocular muscles, usually elicited during convergence on upward gaze; many neuro-ophthalmologists use a optokinetic drum rotating downward to elicit the finding). Common causes of the dorsal midbrain syndrome are pinealoma in younger patients and multiple sclerosis and basilar artery strokes in older patients.

d. **Aberrant Regeneration of the Third Nerve.** After damage to the third nerve (from trauma, aneurysms, or tumors, but *not* ischemia), regenerating fibers originally destined for the medial rectus muscle may instead re-innervate the pupillary constrictor, thus causing pupillary constriction during convergence but the absence of reaction to light. Unlike Argyll Robertson pupils, however, this finding is unilateral, and most patients also have anisocoria, ptosis, and diplopia.[27]

3. Near-Light Dissociation

The phenomenon opposite to light-near dissociation, **near-light dissociation**, describes pupils that react to light but not during near synkinesis. Near-light dissociation was historically associated with von Economo encephalitis lethargica, although experts now believe it indicates that the patient is not trying hard enough to focus on the near object.[20] For this reason, many neuro-ophthalmologists save time during their examination and skip testing the near response unless the patient demonstrates the absence of pupillary light reaction.

III. Oval Pupil

There are three causes of the oval pupil.

A. EVOLVING THIRD NERVE PALSY FROM BRAIN HERNIATION

These patients are invariably comatose from cerebral catastrophes causing elevated intracranial pressure.[28–30] As the pupil enlarges, it may appear oval for a short time before it becomes fully round, dilated, and fixed.

B. ADIE TONIC PUPIL (SEE LATER)

The Adie tonic pupil may sometimes appear oval from segmental iris palsy.[31] These patients are alert and, if complaining of anything, describe blurring of vision in the involved eye (from paralysis of accommodation).

C. PREVIOUS SURGERY OR TRAUMA TO THE IRIS

IV. Anisocoria

A. DEFINITION

Anisocoria is defined as a difference of 0.4 mm or more in the diameter of the pupils. It represents either a problem with the pupillary constrictor muscle (parasympathetic denervation, iris disorder, pharmacologic pupil) or the pupillary dilator muscle (sympathetic denervation, simple anisocoria).

B. TECHNIQUE

Figs. 21.3 and 21.4 summarize the initial approach to anisocoria. The most important initial questions follow:

1. **Is anisocoria old or new?** Examination of a driver's license photograph or other facial photograph, magnified with the direct ophthalmoscope (using the +10 lens), may reveal a preexisting pupillary inequality.[32]
2. **Do both pupils constrict normally during the light reflex?** If there is a poor light reaction in the eye with the larger pupil, the pupillary constrictor of that eye is abnormal. If there is a good light reaction in both eyes, the pupillary dilator of the eye with the smaller pupil is abnormal.
3. **Is anisocoria worse in bright light or dim light/darkness?** If anisocoria is worse in light than in darkness, the pupillary constrictor of the eye with the larger pupil is abnormal. If anisocoria is worse in darkness than in light, the pupillary dilator of the eye with the smaller pupil is abnormal (see Fig. 21.4).[33,‡]

C. ABNORMAL PUPILLARY CONSTRICTOR MUSCLE

If an abnormal pupillary constrictor muscle is present, the *fixed, dilated pupil* is due to parasympathetic defect, iris disorder, or pharmacologic blockade. The most important questions in these patients are (1) is there a full third nerve palsy or are the findings confined to the pupillary constrictor? (Fig. 21.5) and (2) is there altered mental status or other neurologic findings?

1. Full Third Nerve Palsy: Associated Ptosis and Paralysis of Ocular Movements

Because the third cranial nerve controls the levator palpebrae (which lifts the eyelid) and four of six eye muscles (medial, inferior, and superior rectus muscles and inferior oblique muscle), a full third nerve palsy causes a dilated pupil, ptosis, and ophthalmoplegia with the eye deviated outward and downward (see Fig. 21.5, *top row*). In patients with anisocoria, this has the following two important causes:

a. Ipsilateral Brain Herniation (Hutchinson Pupil)[34,35]

These patients are in the midst of a neurologic catastrophe from an expanding unilateral cerebral mass that causes coma, damage to the ipsilateral third nerve (dilated pupil, ptosis, and ophthalmoplegia), and eventually damage to the contralateral cerebral peduncle (which may lead to the false localizing sign of hemiplegia on the *same* side of the lesion). Although the involvement of the extraocular muscles may be difficult to recognize, most patients have narrowing of the ipsilateral palpebral fissure and an eye that (if not dysconjugate) moves poorly during the vestibulo-ocular reflex (doll's-eye maneuver or response to calorics).

Examination of the pupils is essential in patients with acute neurologic catastrophes: (1) In patients with **head trauma** and acute **subdural hematomas,** about 40% have anisocoria, and the dilated pupil is *ipsilateral* to the expanding mass about 90% of the time, just as Hutchison suggested (hence the eponym "Hutchinson pupil").[36–39] In addition, the presence of anisocoria or absent light reaction in patients with subdural hematomas predicts a worse outcome after craniotomy (sensitivity of 63% to 69%, specificity of 70% to 88%, positive LR = 3.4; worse outcome is defined as dependence on others, persistent vegetative state, or death)[40,41]; (2) In patients with **coma** (i.e., Glasgow Coma Scale ≤7),[42] anisocoria of more than 1 mm increases the probability of

---

‡To determine the amount of anisocoria in darkness, neuro-ophthalmologists often take flash photographs of patients in darkness. Because there is a delay of approximately 1.5 seconds between the flash of light and subsequent pupillary constriction, a photograph that is synchronous with the initial flash will actually reflect pupil size in darkness (this delay explains why modern cameras reduce "red eye" by flashing repeatedly before the photograph is taken).[4]

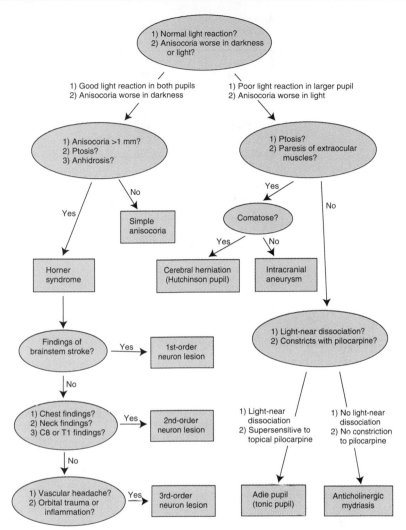

Fig. 21.3 Summary of approach to anisocoria. The first two questions (Is there a normal light reaction? and Is anisocoria worse in darkness or light?) (see also Fig. 21.4) distinguish problems with the pupillary dilator muscle (i.e., Horner syndrome, simple anisocoria; *left side* of figure) from problems with the pupillary constrictor muscle (i.e., third cranial nerve, iris; *right side* of Fig. 21.3). Two other tests distinguish Horner syndrome from simple anisocoria: the cocaine or apraclonidine eyedrop tests (see text) and pupillary dilator lag (i.e., the pupil dilates slowly in darkness, as documented by photographs; see the text). Data from Czarnecki JSC, Pilley SFJ, Thompson HS. The analysis of anisocoria: the use of photography in the clinical evaluation of unequal pupils. *Can J Ophthalmol* 1979;14(4):297–302; Thompson HS, Pilley SFJ. Unequal pupils. A flow chart for sorting out the anisocorias. *Surv Ophthalmol*. 1976;21(1):45–48.

an intracranial structural disorder (e.g., expanding hemispheric or posterior fossa mass; LR = 9, EBM Box 21.1), whereas preservation of light reactions in both pupils decreases the probability of a structural disorder (LR = 0.2) and thus makes metabolic encephalopathy more likely (e.g., drug overdose, hypoglycemia, sepsis, uremia, or another metabolic disorder); and (3) In patients with **stroke**, anisocoria and full third nerve palsy increases the probability of intracranial hemorrhage (LR = 3.2, EBM Box 21.1), thus decreasing the probability of ischemic cerebral infarction.

Anisocoria worse in *light;*
pupillary constrictor abnormal

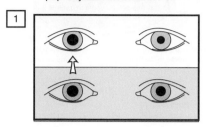

Anisocoria worse in *darkness;*
pupillary dilator abnormal

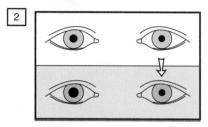

Fig. 21.4   Comparing anisocoria in light and darkness. Patient 1 (*top*) has more prominent anisocoria in light than darkness, indicating that the pupillary *constrictor* of the *larger* pupil is abnormal (i.e., it fails to constrict in light, *arrow*). Patient 2 has more prominent anisocoria in darkness than light, indicating that the pupillary *dilator* of the *smaller* pupil is abnormal (i.e., it fails to dilate in darkness, *arrow*). The diagnosis in patient 1 (abnormal pupillary constrictor) could be a third nerve palsy, tonic pupil, pharmacologic mydriasis, or a disorder of the iris (*right side* of Fig. 21.3). The diagnosis in patient 2 (abnormal pupillary dilator, *left side* of Fig. 21.3) could be Horner syndrome or simple anisocoria. In patient 2, both pupils will react to light, whereas the larger pupil of patient 1 does not react well to light.

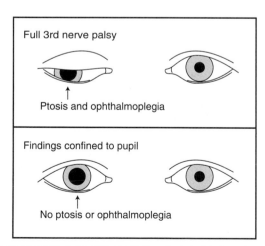

Fig. 21.5   Types of abnormal pupillary constrictor. Both patients in this figure have a paralyzed right pupillary constrictor (i.e., a dilated pupil that fails to react well to light; see Fig. 21.4). The patient in the *top row* also has ptosis and ophthalmoplegia (i.e., eyes not aligned), indicating a full third nerve palsy: possible diagnoses are transtentorial herniation (if comatose) or intracranial aneurysm (if mentally alert). The patient in the *bottom row* lacks ptosis and ophthalmoplegia, indicating that the findings are confined to the pupil itself: possible diagnoses are the tonic pupil, pharmacologic mydriasis, or a disorder of the iris. See the text.

EBM BOX 21.1	Pupils and Anisocoria*				
				Likelihood Ratio‡ if Finding Is	
Finding (Reference)†		**Sensitivity (%)**	**Specificity (%)**	**Present**	**Absent**
Patients with coma[42]					
Anisocoria >1 mm, detecting intracranial structural lesion		39	96	**9.0**	0.6
Absent light reflex in at least one eye, detecting intracranial structural lesion		83	77	**3.6**	0.2
Patients with stroke					
Anisocoria and full third nerve palsy, detecting intracranial hemorrhage[43]		34	90	**3.2**	0.7
Horner syndrome, detecting posterior circulation disease[44]		4	100	**72.0**	NS
Patients with third nerve palsy[45-47]					
Anisocoria or abnormal light reaction, detecting intracranial aneurysm		80–93	62–75	2.4	0.2
Patients with unilaterally red eye					
Anisocoria with *smaller* pupil in red eye, detecting serious eye disease[48]		19	97	**6.5**	0.8
Anisocoria with *larger* pupil in red eye, detecting acute angle closure glaucoma[49]		90	98	**57.6**	NS

*Diagnostic standard: for *structural lesion*, supratentorial and subtentorial lesions with gross anatomical abnormality, including cerebrovascular disease, intracranial hematoma, tumor, and contusion; for *intracranial hemorrhage*, computed tomography; for *posterior circulation stroke* (vs. anterior circulation), MRI; for *intracranial aneurysm*, contrast arteriography or rupture[47] or CT/MRI angiography;[45,46] for *serious eye disease*, corneal foreign body or abrasion, keratitis, or uveitis; for *acute angle closure glaucoma*, examination by ophthalmologist.

†Definition of finding: for *anisocoria with smaller pupil in red eye*, difference in pupil size is 1 mm or more; for *anisocoria with larger pupil in red eye*, all patients had 3 additional findings (according to the authors' algorithm): (1) no eyelashes touching the eyeball, (2) normal eyelid closure strength, and (3) no staining of cornea with fluorescein.

‡Likelihood ratio (LR) if finding present = positive LR; LR if finding absent = negative LR.

CT, Computed tomography; *MRI*, magnetic resonance imaging.

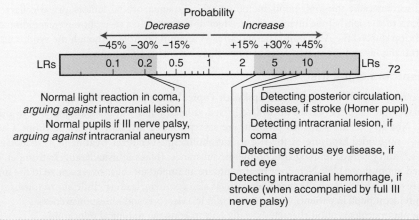

ANISOCORIA

Probability

Decrease   *Increase*

−45% −30% −15%   +15% +30% +45%

LRs   0.1   0.2   0.5   1   2   5   10   LRs 72

Normal light reaction in coma,
arguing against intracranial lesion
Normal pupils if III nerve palsy,
arguing against intracranial aneurysm

Detecting posterior circulation,
disease, if stroke (Horner pupil)
Detecting intracranial lesion, if
coma
Detecting serious eye disease, if
red eye
Detecting intracranial hemorrhage, if
stroke (when accompanied by full III
nerve palsy)

b. Posterior Communicating Artery Aneurysm

The most common of all intracranial aneurysms, posterior communicating artery aneurysm presents with ipsilateral third nerve palsy (thus dilating the pupil) up to 60% of the time.[50] It is essential to recognize this disorder promptly because of the risk of subsequent, devastating subarachnoid hemorrhage. Importantly, the abnormal pupil is almost always accompanied by at least some degree of ptosis and ophthalmoplegia (i.e., features of a full third nerve palsy, see Fig. 21.5); isolated anisocoria is rare.

In alert patients with new-onset third nerve palsy (i.e., at least some degree of ptosis and ophthalmoplegia), the presence of a normal pupil decreases the probability of an intracranial aneurysm or other compressive lesion (LR = 0.2, EBM Box 21.1; see also pupil-sparing rules in Chapter 59), although almost all patients with this finding should now undergo noninvasive neurovascular imaging to exclude intracranial aneurysms.[51]

2. The Tonic Pupil

a. The Finding

The tonic pupil has five important features (Fig. 21.6): (1) unilateral dilation of a pupil, (2) poor or absent response to light, (3) extensive, slow (over seconds), and long-lasting constriction during near vision (this is why the pupil is called "tonic"; i.e, it is analogous to myotonia), (4) disturbances of accommodation (which causes the main concern for many patients, i.e., inability of the involved eye to focus), and (5) supersensitivity of pupillary constriction to pilocarpine.[31,52,53]

Although both the Argyll Robertson pupil and the tonic pupil display light-near dissociation, they are easily distinguished by the characteristics in Table 21.1.

b. Pathogenesis

The tonic pupil occurs because of injury to the ciliary ganglion and postganglionic fibers (see Fig. 21.1) and subsequent misdirection of nerve fibers as they regenerate from the ciliary ganglion to the eye. In the normal eye, the ciliary ganglion sends 30 times the number of nerve fibers to the ciliary body (the muscle that focuses the lens during the near synkinesis) as to the iris (i.e., the pupillary constrictor).[54] Once these fibers are disrupted, odds are thus 30 to 1 that the iris will receive regenerating fibers originally intended for the ciliary body instead of those participating in the light reaction. The pupil of these patients thus fails to respond to light, although during near vision, which normally activates the ciliary body, the misdirected fibers to the iris cause the pupil to constrict (i.e., light-near dissociation).

c. Clinical Significance

Because the ciliary ganglion and postganglionic fibers are contiguous to the eyeball, a variety of local disorders cause the tonic pupil, including orbital trauma, orbital tumors, or varicella-zoster infections of the ophthalmic division of the trigeminal nerve. Most cases, however, are idiopathic, a condition dubbed the **Adie pupil** (named after William John Adie, although the syndrome was more thoroughly and accurately described by others before his 1931 paper).[52]

3. Disorders of the Iris

a. Pharmacologic Blockade of the Pupil with Topical Anticholinergic Drugs

Pharmacologic blockade causes an isolated fixed, dilated pupil without paralysis of eye movements. Not all patients with this problem are surreptitiously instilling mydriatic drops. Causes include unintended exposure of the eye to anticholinergic nebulizer treatments,[55] scopolamine patches,[56] and plants containing anticholinergic substances (blue nightshade, angel's trumpet, jimsonweed, moonflower).[57,58] Nebulizer treatments are an important cause to recognize in the intensive care unit, where metabolic encephalopathy is also common, leading clinicians to misdiagnose the Hutchison pupil in patients with pharmacologic anisocoria and unresponsiveness.

The pharmacologic pupil characteristically fails to constrict to topical pilocarpine.

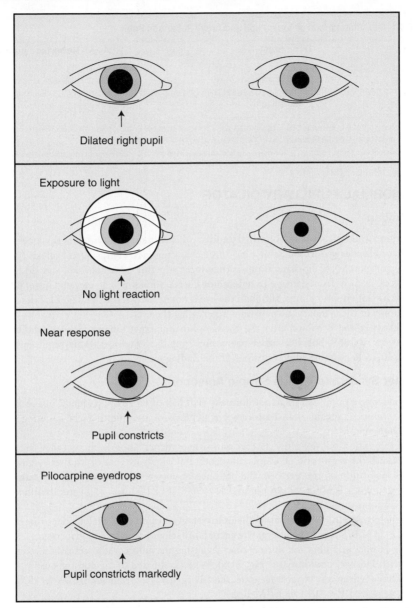

Fig. 21.6 **Tonic pupil (Adie pupil).** The patient in this figure has a *right* tonic pupil. At baseline, there is anisocoria with the right pupil larger than the left (*first row*). The dilated pupil fails to react to light (*second row*) but constricts slowly (i.e., tonic contraction) when the patient focuses on a near object (*third row*). After instillation of dilute pilocarpine eyedrops (*fourth row*), the pupil constricts markedly.

4. The Poorly Reactive Pupil—Response to Pilocarpine

In difficult diagnostic problems, especially when pharmacologic blockade is a consideration, the pupil's response to topical pilocarpine solution is helpful. Pilocarpine constricts the Adie pupil and the dilated pupil from parasympathetic denervation (Hutchinson pupil or intracranial aneurysm) but not the dilated pupil from pharmacologic blockade.[59]

TABLE 21.1 ■ Comparison of Tonic Pupil and Argyll Robertson Pupil

Finding	Tonic pupil	Argyll Robertson pupils
Pupil size	Large	Small
Laterality	Mostly unilateral	Mostly bilateral
Reaction to near vision	Extremely slow and prolonged with slow redilation	Normal with brisk redilation

From Loewenstein O, Loewenfeld IR. Pupillotonic pseudotabes (syndrome of Markus-Weill and Reys-Holmes-Adie): a critical review of the literature. *Surv Ophthalmol.* 1967;10:129–185.

D. ABNORMAL PUPILLARY DILATOR

1. Definition

The most important cause of an abnormal pupillary dilator muscle is sympathetic denervation of the pupil, or **Horner syndrome**, which has three characteristics: (1) ipsilateral miosis (paralyzed pupillodilator muscle), (2) ipsilateral ptosis (paralyzed superior tarsal muscle), and (3) ipsilateral anhidrosis of the face (from damage to sudomotor fibers). Sometimes, an elevated lower lid creates the appearance of enophthalmos, although the eye is not actually retracted. Fig. 21.7 describes the neuroanatomy of the sympathetic pathways innervating the eye.

Horner syndrome is named after the Swiss ophthalmologist Johann Horner, who described the syndrome in 1869, but, like other eponymous pupillary findings (Adie pupil and Marcus Gunn pupil), earlier published descriptions of the finding exist.[60]

2. Horner Syndrome Versus Simple Anisocoria

When evaluating a pupil that dilates abnormally (left half of Fig. 21.3; patient 2 in Fig. 21.4), the finding of anisocoria greater than 1 mm, associated ptosis, or asymmetric facial sweating indicates Horner syndrome.

In difficult cases, the definitive test of sympathetic denervation is the cocaine test (cocaine drops diminish the anisocoria of simple anisocoria but aggravate that of Horner syndrome; Fig. 21.8).[61] In one study of 169 persons, the presence of post-cocaine anisocoria of 1 mm or more was pathognomonic for Horner syndrome (LR = 96.8, see EBM Box 21.2) and its absence made Horner syndrome unlikely (LR = 0.1).

Nonetheless, cocaine eyedrops are difficult to obtain and store, and they render urine drug tests positive for up to 48 hours.[70] An alternative agent is apraclonidine, a topical glaucoma eyedrop that dilates the Horner pupil but not normal ones,[71] causing the anisocoria to actually reverse sides in patients with Horner syndrome (see Fig. 21.8). When compared to the cocaine eyedrop test, the apraclonidine eyedrop test is quite accurate: sensitivity of 95%, specificity of 90% to 95%, positive LR = 14, negative LR = 0.1 (see EBM Box 21.2).

Because the apraclonidine response relies on sympathetic denervation supersensitivity, the test may be falsely negative early after onset of Horner syndrome before supersensitivity has had time to develop. Nonetheless, one patient with Horner syndrome from a lateral medullary infarct developed a positive apraclonidine test just 36 hours after symptom onset.[72]

3. Clinical Significance of Horner Syndrome

a. Etiology

Which etiologies of Horner syndrome a clinician is likely to see depends on the clinician's specialty. On a neurologic service, 70% of patients with Horner syndrome have lesions in the first-order neuron, usually strokes in the brainstem (see Table 62.2 in Chapter 62).[73] On a medical

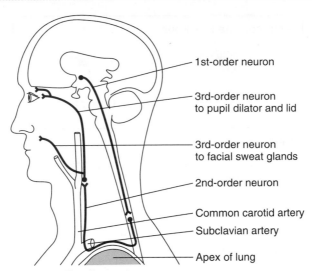

1st-order neuron

3rd-order neuron
to pupil dilator and lid

3rd-order neuron
to facial sweat glands

2nd-order neuron

Common carotid artery

Subclavian artery

Apex of lung

Fig. 21.7   Anatomy of the sympathetic pathways to the eye. The sympathetic innervation of the eye consists of three neurons connected in series: first-order neurons, second-order neurons, and third-order neurons. The first-order neurons (central neurons) extend from the posterior hypothalamus to the C8 to T2 level of the spinal cord. The second-order neurons (preganglionic neurons) leave the spinal cord and travel over the lung apex, around the subclavian artery, and along the carotid artery to the superior cervical ganglion. The third-order neurons (postganglionic neurons) diverge and take two paths: those to the pupil and lid muscles travel along the internal carotid artery through the cavernous sinus to reach the orbit; those to the facial sweat glands travel with the external carotid artery to the face. Lesions in any of these neurons cause Horner syndrome and distinct associated physical signs (see Fig. 21.3 and text).

service, 70% of afflicted patients have lesions in the second-order neuron, usually from tumors (e.g., lung and thyroid) or trauma (e.g., to the neck, chest, spinal nerves, subclavian or carotid arteries).[74] Causes of third order neuron lesions are vascular headache, carotid artery dissection, skull fracture, and cavernous sinus syndrome.

b. Localizing the Lesion

(1) Associated Findings. Helpful features include the following: (1) findings of deficits in the ipsilateral brainstem (e.g., lateral medullary syndrome), pointing to a first-order neuron lesion (see Table 62.2 in Chapter 62); in patients hospitalized with stroke, the finding of Horner syndrome is a compelling argument for a posterior (vertebrobasilar) circulation stroke (*not* anterior circulation stroke; LR = 72, EBM Box 21.1; see also Chapter 61); (2) abnormal chest or neck findings, a supraclavicular mass, or motor, reflex, or sensory findings of the ipsilateral C8 to T1 spinal roots, all pointing to the second-order neuron lesion; and (3) orbital trauma, orbital inflammation, migraine or neck pain, pointing to a third-order neuron lesion. An acute *painful* Horner syndrome suggests dissection of the carotid artery.[75]

(2) Facial Sweating. The sudomotor sympathetic fibers to the face diverge from the sympathetic pathway at the bifurcation of the carotid artery and therefore do not accompany the sympathetic nerves to the pupil and lid. Theoretically, therefore, Horner syndrome from a third-order neuron lesions would preserve facial sweating, whereas Horner syndrome from a first- and second-order neurons would cause asymmetric facial sweating. Nonetheless, in one study this finding lacked diagnostic value (LR not significant; see EBM Box 21.2).

(3) Distinguishing Third Nerve Lesions from First and Second Nerve Lesions: The Eyedrop Tests. When the cause of Horner syndrome remains unexplained despite careful bedside

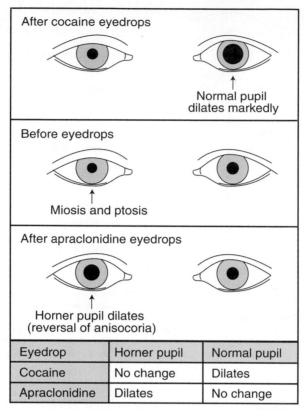

Fig. 21.8   Confirmation of Horner syndrome: the cocaine and apraclonidine eyedrop tests. This patient has a right Horner syndrome with right miosis and ptosis (*middle row*). Forty-five minutes after installation of cocaine drops into each eye (*top row*), the Horner pupil fails to dilate but the normal pupil dilates, markedly aggravating the anisocoria and confirming the diagnosis of Horner syndrome. Forty-five minutes after installation of apraclonidine drops into each eye (performed on a different day than the cocaine test, *bottom row*), the right Horner pupil dilates but there is no response in the normal pupil, thus reversing the anisocoria and also confirming the diagnosis of Horner syndrome. Cocaine eyedrops block the reuptake of norepinephrine at the myoneural junction of the iris dilator, causing the pupil to dilate unless norepinephrine is absent because of sympathetic denervation. Apraclonidine eyedrops have no effect on normal pupils, but after sympathetic denervation from Horner syndrome the affected pupil is supersensitive to their effect. Apraclonidine may also cause elevation of the lid in Horner syndrome (*bottom row*), although only the response of the pupil is used when interpreting the test.

examination, most clinicians now routinely order magnetic resonance imaging to investigate the entire sympathetic pathway to the eye. Before the advent of modern neuroimaging, however, eyedrop tests were used to distinguish first/second nerve lesions from third nerve lesions. The classic eyedrop test was the **Paredrine test** (i.e., topical hydroxyamphetamine). Dilation of the Horner miotic pupil after topical Paredrine indicates a first- or second-order neuron lesion (LR = 9.2, EBM Box 21.2). Nonetheless, Paredrine is now difficult to obtain, and some investigators have recommended substituting dilute phenylephrine eyedrops (in this test, the *absence of dilation* of the Horner miotic pupil after topical phenylephrine indicates a first-/second-order neuron lesion; LR = 4.2, EBM Box 21.2).

EBM BOX 21.2	Horner Syndrome, Eyedrop Tests*			
			Likelihood Ratio[†] if Finding Is	
Finding (Reference)	Sensitivity (%)	Specificity (%)	Present	Absent
Detecting Horner syndrome				
Anisocoria ≥1 mm after topical cocaine[62,63]	95	99	**96.8**	0.1
Reversal of anisocoria after topical apraclonidine[64,65]	95	90–95	**14.0**	0.1
Diagnosing first- or second-order nerve lesion in Horner syndrome				
Small pupil dilates with topical hydroxyamphetamine (Paredrine)[66,67]	83–92	79–96	**9.2**	0.2
Small pupil fails to dilate with dilute phenylephrine[68]	88	79	**4.2**	NS
Asymmetric facial sweating[69]	53	78	NS	0.6

*Diagnostic standard: for *Horner syndrome* (cocaine drop testing), combined clinical follow-up and dilation lag of pupil during infrared video recording;[62,63] for *Horner syndrome* (apraclonidine drop testing), cocaine drop testing;[64,65] for *localization of Horner syndrome*, clinical evaluation,[66,67] clinical evaluation plus Paredrine testing,[69] or magnetic resonance imaging.[68]

[†]Likelihood ratio (LR) if finding present = positive LR; LR if finding absent = negative LR.
NS, Not significant.

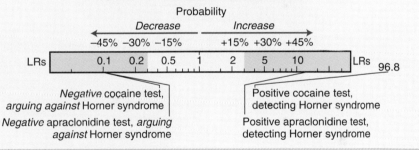

HORNER SYNDROME: EYEDROP TESTS

Probability

Decrease | Increase

−45% −30% −15% | +15% +30% +45%

LRs 0.1 0.2 0.5 1 2 5 10 LRs 96.8

Negative cocaine test, arguing against Horner syndrome

Negative apraclonidine test, arguing against Horner syndrome

Positive cocaine test, detecting Horner syndrome

Positive apraclonidine test, detecting Horner syndrome

E. INTRAOCULAR INFLAMMATION

As part of the eye's response to intraocular inflammation, the ipsilateral pupil often constricts. In one study of 317 patients with the unilaterally red eye, anisocoria of 1 mm or more (with the *smaller* pupil in the red eye) significantly increased the probability of serious eye disease (i.e., corneal foreign body, corneal abrasion, keratitis, or uveitis, LR = 6.5, EBM Box 21.1) and thus decreased the probability of more benign problems (i.e., subconjunctival hemorrhage, conjunctivitis, or episcleritis; see Chapter 23).

Rarely, the pupil of the inflamed eye is larger than that of the contralateral pupil (relative *mydriasis*), a finding indicating acute angle-closure glaucoma. The mydriasis results from ischemia and infarction of the iris tissue itself (i.e., the pupillary constrictor muscle). In one study of patients with a unilaterally red eye, the finding of anisocoria (with the *larger* pupil in the red eye) was diagnostic for acute angle closure glaucoma (LR = 57.6, EBM Box 21.2).[§]

V. Diabetes and the Pupil

The pupils of patients with long-standing diabetes show signs of sympathetic denervation (small size and poor dilation in darkness), parasympathetic denervation (sluggish light reaction), and decreased amplitude of hippus.[76] Even so, denervation alone does not explain all of the diabetic pupillary abnormalities, because the pupils of many diabetic patients respond poorly to dilating and constricting eyedrops, a finding suggesting additional problems in the iris itself (i.e., denervated pupils are classically supersensitive to eyedrops).[77] Some reviews state that diabetes causes the Argyll Robertson pupil, but the data for this are meager and what exists suggests that the finding is very rare.[20]

VI. Pinpoint Pupils and Altered Mental Status

In one study of patients with altered mental status, the finding of pinpoint pupils predicted a positive response to naloxone (LR = 8.5), thus confirming the diagnosis of opiate intoxication.[78] The absence of pinpoint pupils argued strongly against opiate intoxication (LR = 0.1).

References may be accessed online at *Elsevier eBooks for Practicing Clinicians*.

---

[*]All patients in this study had 3 additional findings (according to the author's algorithm): (1) no eyelashes touching the eyeball, (2) normal eyelid closure strength, and (3) no staining of cornea with fluorescein.[49] These findings exclude trichiasis, facial palsy, and corneal disorders, respectively, as the cause of the red eye, though none of these disorders would cause mydriasis.

Diabetic Retinopathy

I. Introduction

Diabetic retinopathy is the leading cause of blindness in adults aged 20 to 74 years.[1] Whether a patient develops retinopathy depends on the type and duration of diabetes: those with type 1 diabetes have a 0% risk of proliferative retinopathy at 5 years after diagnosis, 4% at 10 years and 50% at 20 years, whereas those with type 2 diabetes, especially if taking insulin, the risk is 3% to 4% at the time of diagnosis, 10% at 10 years and 20% at 15 years.[2] Once retinopathy develops, however, the best predictor of progression to sight-threatening retinopathy is the extent of retinopathy during the baseline examination: the higher the grade of retinopathy during the initial examination, the greater the risk of progression (Table 22.1). In type 1 diabetics, pregnancy increases the risk of progression 2.3-fold.[2]

In large cross-sectional surveys of diabetic patients seen by general practitioners, sight-threatening retinopathy (i.e., proliferative retinopathy and more severe forms of nonproliferative retinopathy) is found in 5% to 15% of patients.[6–10]

II. The Findings

The findings of diabetic retinopathy are divided into nonproliferative changes, which occur *within* the retina, and proliferative changes, which are located on the inner surface of the retina or in the vitreous.[11] The terms *background retinopathy* and *preproliferative retinopathy* are outdated and no longer recommended, having been replaced by the grades of retinopathy shown in Table 22.1. Diabetic retinopathy progresses in an orderly fashion through these grades.

A. NONPROLIFERATIVE CHANGES (FIG. 22.1)[3]

The earliest changes to appear in diabetic retinopathy are **microaneurysms**, which are distinct red, round spots less than one-twelfth the diameter of an average optic disc, or 125 μm in its

TABLE 22.1 ■ Progression to High-Risk Proliferative Diabetic Retinopathy*

Grade of Baseline Retinopathy	Principal Clinical Findings	Cumulative Risk (%) of High-Risk Proliferative Retinopathy at:	
		1 year	5 years
Nonproliferative retinopathy			
Mild	Microaneurysms	1	16
	Dot and blot hemorrhages		
	Soft exudates		
Moderate	Extensive microaneurysms and hemorrhages	3–8	27–39
	IRMA		
	Venous beading		
Severe	Same as moderate[†]	15	56
Very severe	Same as moderate[†]	45	71
Proliferative retinopathy[‡]			
	Neovascularization	22–46	64–75
	Preretinal/vitreous hemorrhages		
	Fibrovascular proliferation		

*High-risk proliferative retinopathy is NVD >0.25 of disc area, NVD <0.25 of disc area *and* vitreous or preretinal hemorrhage, OR NVE >0.5 disc area *and* vitreous or preretinal hemorrhage. These figures assume that the patient is untreated.

[†]Moderate, severe, and very severe nonproliferative retinopathy share the same fundoscopic findings, although they differ in severity (based on standardized photographs) and the number of retinal quadrants involved.[3–5]

[‡]Percentages are for patients whose baseline evaluation reveals proliferative retinopathy with less than high-risk characteristics.

IRMA, Intraretinal microvascular abnormalities; *NVD*, neovascularization within one disc diameter of the optic disc; *NVE*, neovascularization elsewhere, i.e., beyond one disc diameter of the optic disc; see the text.

longest dimension (the average optic disc is about 1500 μm in diameter; 125 μm is approximately the width of an average major vein at the disc margin). **Dot hemorrhages** are larger red dots with sharp borders; red spots with indistinct borders are **blot hemorrhages**. Both dot and blot hemorrhages are located in the inner retinal layers. **Hard exudates** (deposition of lipids in the inner retina) are small, white or yellowish-white deposits with sharp margins that often have a waxy or glistening appearance. **Soft exudates** (or **cotton wool exudates**) are ischemic swellings of the superficial nerve fiber layer, which appear as white, round, or oval patches with ill-defined, feathery edges. As retinal ischemia progresses, two other abnormalities appear: venous beading (veins resembling a string of beads) and intraretinal microvascular abnormalities (IRMA), which are extra tortuous vessels *within* the retina that may be either new vessels or dilated preexisting capillaries.

B. PROLIFERATIVE RETINOPATHY

Proliferative retinopathy is new vessel formation (i.e., neovascularization) on the inner surface of the retina or vitreous, which threatens vision by increasing the risk of retinal detachment or vitreous hemorrhage. These new vessels often resemble a small wagon wheel, with individual vessels radiating like spokes to a circumferential vessel forming the rim.[12] New vessel formation is subdivided into neovascularization of the disc (within one disc diameter of the optic disc, abbreviated [NVD]) and neovascularization elsewhere (NVE). Of the two, NVD has a much worse visual prognosis.[5]

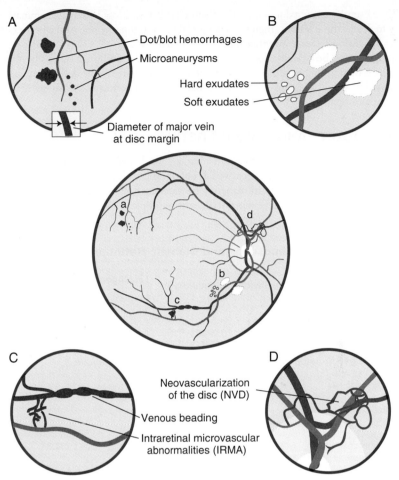

Fig. 22.1 Types of diabetic retinopathy. The center figure depicting the fundus of a patient with diabetic retinopathy is surrounded by four enlarged views, each labeled with a letter (A to D) corresponding to specific locations on the center figure. (A) Microaneurysms and dot/blot hemorrhages. The diameter of microaneurysms is less than the width of a major vein at the disc margin (reproduced in square inset). (B) Hard and soft exudates. (C) Venous beading and intraretinal microvascular abnormalities (IRMA). (D) Neovascularization, which may be located within one disc diameter of the optic disc (NVD) or elsewhere (NVE). Although both IRMA and neovascularization represent the formation of new blood vessels, IRMA is confined to the layers of the retina, whereas neovascularization is on the inner surface of the retina or vitreous (see the text).

C. MACULAR EDEMA

Macular edema, which may accompany any stage of nonproliferative or proliferative retinopathy, is very difficult to visualize using the direct ophthalmoscope, although important clues are rings of hard exudates (often surrounding the edematous area) and diminished visual acuity.[11]

III. Clinical Significance

In patients with high-risk proliferative retinopathy or those with clinically significant macular edema, laser photocoagulation or intravitreal injections of anti–vascular endothelial growth factor (anti-VEGF) significantly reduces the risk of subsequent visual loss.[1] Retinal examination is the only way to detect these lesions, thereby making diabetic retinopathy one of the best examples of a disorder benefiting from an attentive physical examination.

The findings that best predict subsequent proliferative retinopathy are venous beading, intra-retinal microvascular abnormalities, and the extent of microaneurysms and hemorrhages. Soft exudates are less predictive, and the extent of hard exudates correlates poorly with subsequent proliferative retinopathy.[5]

A. VISUAL ACUITY AND DIABETIC RETINOPATHY

Diminished visual acuity per se is a poor screening test for diabetic retinopathy (EBM Box 22.1: positive likelihood ratio [LR] = 1.5, negative LR not significant [NS]). Indeed, the most common causes of diminished visual acuity in diabetics are cataracts (49% of diabetics with diminished acuity) and macular degeneration (29%), not diabetic retinopathy (15%).[14]

EBM BOX 22.1	Ophthalmoscopy and Diabetic Retinopathy*			
			Likelihood Ratio‡ if Finding Is	
Finding (Reference)†	**Sensitivity (%)**	**Specificity (%)**	**Present**	**Absent**
Detecting any diabetic retinopathy				
Visual acuity 20/40 or worse[13,14]	21–28	82–86	1.5	NS
Detecting sight-threatening retinopathy, using the following technique				
Direct ophthalmoscopy, nondilated pupils[15]	50	92	**6.2**	0.5
Direct ophthalmoscopy, dilated pupils, general providers[8,9,16–18]	53–69	91–96	**9.4**	0.4
Direct ophthalmoscopy, dilated pupils, specialists[6–10]	48–82	90–100	**25.5**	0.3

*Diagnostic standard: for *sight-threatening retinopathy*, retinal photographs through dilated pupils or slit-lamp biomicroscopy reveal proliferative retinopathy, macular edema, or both.
†Definition of findings: for *sight-threatening retinopathy*, proliferative retinopathy, macular edema, or both.
‡Likelihood ratio (LR) if finding present = positive LR; LR if finding absent = negative LR.
NS, Not significant.

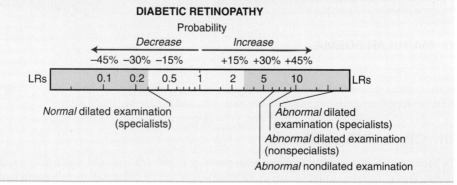

DIABETIC RETINOPATHY
Probability

TABLE 22.2 ■ Recommended Ophthalmologic Examination Schedule for Patients With Diabetes Mellitus

Time of Onset of Diabetes	Recommended First Examination	Minimal Routine Follow-Up
Less than 30 years of age*	Within 5 years after diagnosis of diabetes	Yearly†
30 years of age or older*	At time of diagnosis of diabetes	Yearly†
Pregnancy in preexisting diabetes	Prior to conception and during first trimester	Physician discretion pending results of first trimester examination

*Less than 30 years and greater than 30 years are operational definitions of type 1 and type 2 diabetes used in the Wisconsin Epidemiologic Study of Diabetic Retinopathy.
†In some patients with normal eye examinations, eye specialists may advise less frequent examinations (every 2 to 3 years).[1]

B. DIAGNOSTIC ACCURACY OF OPHTHALMOSCOPY

EBM Box 22.1 displays the accuracy of various methods in detecting sight-threatening retinopathy (i.e., proliferative changes and macular edema), using multiview dilated pupil retinal photographs or slit-lamp biomicroscopy as the diagnostic standard. Not surprisingly, specialists using direct ophthalmoscopy perform better than general clinicians, and dilated examinations are superior to nondilated ones (LRs 6.2 to 25.5; EBM Box 22.1). In comparison, many diabetic centers now routinely screen their patients for retinopathy using nonmydriatic photography, a test with excellent diagnostic accuracy (positive LR = 24.5, negative LR = 0.1).[19*]

Macular edema is rarely detected by general providers using direct ophthalmoscopy (sensitivity is close to 0%).[20] Because many patients with macular edema have normal visual acuity (i.e., the sensitivity of "visual acuity worse than 20/30" for macular edema is only 38%),[20] clinicians who screen for macular edema using just visual acuity are missing many patients who would benefit from treatment.

C. SCREENING RECOMMENDATIONS

Diabetic retinopathy is common, treatable, and detectable using simple tools. Consequently, it is the prototype of a disease that would benefit from organized screening. Table 22.2 reviews the screening schedule recommended by the American Diabetes Association.[1] Given the stakes of missing serious retinopathy and the suboptimal performance of general clinicians using direct ophthalmoscopy, only clinicians with training and experience—in most cases, optometrists and ophthalmologists—should screen patients. Any patient with macular edema, more than moderate nonproliferative retinopathy, or proliferative retinopathy should be seen by eye care providers with experience in the management of diabetic retinopathy.

References may be accessed online at *Elsevier eBooks for Practicing Clinicians*.

---

*The LRs of 24.5 and 0.1 (from reference 19) refer to >2 field nonmydriatic photographs in detecting "any diabetic retinopathy" compared to retinal photographs through dilated pupils or slit-lamp biomicroscopy.

The Red Eye

I. Introduction

The term **red eye** refers to several acute inflammatory disorders of the eye, all of which produce prominent ocular erythema. For clinicians evaluating patients with the red eye, the most important decision is to distinguish serious disorders (e.g., iritis, keratitis, corneal abrasion, scleritis, or acute glaucoma) from more benign disorders of the conjunctiva (e.g., conjunctivitis, episcleritis, or subconjunctival hemorrhage). All patients with serious disorders require urgent referral to an eye specialist. In patients with suspected conjunctivitis, distinguishing bacterial conjunctivitis from nonbacterial (viral, allergic) conjunctivitis is important because only bacterial conjunctivitis benefits from administration of topical antimicrobial eye drops.[1] This chapter therefore focuses on those bedside findings that assist clinicians with identifying serious disease and on those distinguishing bacterial from nonbacterial conjunctivitis.

Descriptions of the red eye are as old as ophthalmologic records, figuring prominently in descriptions from ancient Egypt and classical Greece and Rome.[2] Many patients in these ancient descriptions likely suffered from trachoma or other contagious diseases of the eye.[3] The French ophthalmologist Charles Saint Yves (1667–1736) is credited with the first clear description of iritis, including its characteristic redness, photophobia, pain, and decreased pupillary diameter.[2]

II. The Findings

A. DISTINGUISHING SERIOUS FROM BENIGN DISEASE

The traditional signs of serious causes of the red eye are significant eye pain, visual blurring, photophobia, and abnormalities of the pupil.

1. Visual Acuity

Benign causes of the red eye do not affect visual acuity, except for the temporary effects of purulent exudate in bacterial conjunctivitis, a blurriness that resolves when secretions are wiped away. In

contrast, corneal disease and iritis may cause significant blurriness of vision, either from opacifi-
cation of the cornea (corneal infiltrates) or from inflammatory exudate and cells in the anterior
chamber (iritis).

2. Pupillary Abnormalities

In benign disease, the pupils are normal. Serious causes of the red eye, however, may produce
anisocoria (i.e., unequal pupils, see Chapter 21). Usually, the smaller pupil is in the inflamed eye
(i.e., relative *miosis*), either from inflammatory congestion of the iris itself, associated ciliary muscle spasm, or both. Rarely the pupil of the inflamed eye is larger than that of the contralateral
pupil (relative *mydriasis*), a finding of acute angle-closure glaucoma, which produces ischemia and
infarction of the iris tissue itself (i.e., the pupillary constrictor muscle).

3. Pupil Constriction Tests

In serious eye disorders, pupillary constriction may be painful, which explains why many affected
patients experience *photophobia* (i.e., pain during exposure to light). Painful pupillary constriction
is the basis for three different pupillary constriction tests. These tests differ in how the pupillary
constriction is produced, but in all tests the positive response is pain in the *affected* red eye.

a. Direct Photophobia Test
The clinician shines a penlight into the affected eye. (See the section on the normal light reflex in
Chapter 21.)

b. Indirect (Consensual) Photophobia Test
The clinician shines a penlight into the *contralateral* (i.e., uninflamed) eye. (See the section on the
normal light reflex in Chapter 21.)

c. Finger-to-Nose Convergence Test
The patient focuses on his or her outstretched finger and slowly moves the finger toward his or her
nose. (See the section on the near synkinesis reaction in Chapter 21.)

B. DISTINGUISHING BACTERIAL CONJUNCTIVITIS
FROM NONBACTERIAL CAUSES

According to traditional teachings, bacterial conjunctivitis is more likely if disease onset is during
the winter months or if there is a purulent exudate,[4] which may cause stickiness of the eyelids in
the morning. Viral conjunctivitis is traditionally thought to be more likely if there is watery discharge, conjunctival follicles, or preauricular adenopathy. Allergic conjunctivitis is suggested by a
stringy mucoid discharge and itchiness of the eyes.

1. Normal Conjunctival Anatomy
The normal anatomy of the conjunctiva appears in Fig. 23.1.

2. Papillary Conjunctivitis vs. Follicular Conjunctivitis

In conjunctivitis, combinations of hyperemia (vasodilation), edema, and hemorrhage produce a
red color, which is most prominent on the undersurface of the lids and the more peripheral portions of the globe (see Fig. 23.2). Some patients develop small projections on the conjunctival surface of the upper and lower lids (the *palpebral* or *tarsal* conjunctiva). These elevations are classified
as *papillae* or *follicles* (i.e., papillary conjunctivitis or follicular conjunctivitis, see Fig. 23.2). Papillae
characteristically appear in bacterial or allergic conjunctivitis. Follicles suggest viral or chlamydial
conjunctivitis and are often associated with preauricular adenopathy.

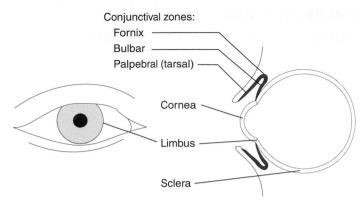

Conjunctival zones:
Fornix
Bulbar
Palpebral (tarsal)

Cornea

Limbus

Sclera

Fig. 23.1 Normal conjunctival anatomy. The figure compares the frontal view of the normal eye (*left*) to its corresponding sagittal section (*right*). The normal conjunctiva (*heavy blue line, right*) is a continuous translucent membrane that lines the undersurface of both eyelids (**tarsal or palpebral conjunctiva**), reflects backwards (at the *fornix*), and then covers the anterior globe (**bulbar conjunctiva**). The conjunctiva ends at the **limbus**, the peripheral border of the cornea where it joins the **sclera**.

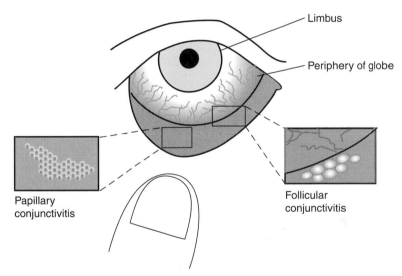

Limbus

Periphery of globe

Papillary
conjunctivitis

Follicular
conjunctivitis

Fig. 23.2 Conjunctivitis: papillary vs follicular. The erythema of conjunctivitis (*shaded dark grey*) is most intense on the inside surface of the eyelids (tarsal conjunctiva) and peripherally on the globe (near the fornices), while the erythema is less intense centrally near the limbus. In more severe conjunctivitis, the entire conjunctival surface (both tarsal and bulbar) is red. This pattern of erythema contrasts with iritis, which causes more intense erythema centrally around the limbus, a finding called *circumlimbal flush* or *ciliary flush*. In patients with conjunctivitis, the clinician should inspect the everted upper or lower lids, noting whether the inner membrane has its normal smooth surface or instead has small projections, which are characterized as either *papillae* or *follicles*. In this example, the clinician has used his thumb to gently evert the lower lid for inspection. Papillae (*left bottom*) are contiguous red vascular bumps; the center of each papilla contains a blood vessel. They are red on the surface and pale at the base. Papillae are often so tiny that the conjunctiva acquires a velvety appearance and only magnification reveals their true nature. Other times, papillae may become large and produce a cobblestone appearance. Follicles (*right bottom*) are discrete 1 to 2 mm diameter white bumps consisting of aggregates of lymphoid tissue; the center of each is avascular. They are pale on the surface and red at the base. See text for the significance of these findings.

III. Clinical Significance

A. DISTINGUISHING SERIOUS FROM BENIGN DISEASE

In 5 studies of 957 consecutive patients with red eye, all 3 pupillary constriction tests increased probability of serious disease: indirect photophobia test (likelihood ratio [LR] = 28.8; EBM Box 23.1), finger-to-nose convergence test (LR = 21.4), and direct photophobia test (LR = 8.3). The *absence* of pain in the affected eye during the finger-to-nose convergence test *decreases* probability of serious disease (LR = 0.3). In these studies, most patients with serious disease had anterior uveitis (iritis) or corneal disorders (herpes simplex infection, corneal abrasion, and miscellaneous causes of keratitis). The presence of anisocoria is also helpful: anisocoria with the *smaller* pupil in the affected red eye (*relative miosis*) increased probability of serious disease (LR = 6.5), and anisocoria with the *larger* pupil in the affected red eye (*relative mydriasis*) was diagnostic of acute glaucoma (LR = 57.6).

EBM BOX 23.1 | **The Red Eye, Diagnosing Serious Eye Disease***

Finding (Reference)[†]	Sensitivity (%)	Specificity (%)	Likelihood Ratio[‡] if Finding Is Present	Absent
Detecting serious eye disease				
Direct photophobia[5-7]	54–77	80–98	**8.3**	0.4
Indirect photophobia[5]	44	98	**28.8**	0.6
Finger-to-nose convergence test[8]	74	97	**21.4**	**0.3**
Anisocoria with smaller pupil in red eye (difference >1 mm)[9]	19	97	**6.5**	0.8
Detecting acute angle closure glaucoma				
Anisocoria with larger pupil in red eye[10]	90[§]	98	**57.6**	NS

*Diagnostic standard: for *serious eye disease*, slit-lamp biomicroscopy revealing iritis, keratitis, corneal abrasion, scleritis, or acute narrow angle glaucoma.
[†]Definition of findings: for *pupillary constriction tests* (direct photophobia, indirect photophobia, finger-to-nose convergence test), see text.
[‡]Likelihood ratio (LR) if finding present = positive LR; LR if finding absent = negative LR.
[§]All of the patients with acute glaucoma in this study had a mydriatic pupil (i.e., sensitivity = 100%); for calculations of the LRs, 0.5 was added to all cells of the 2 × 2 table.

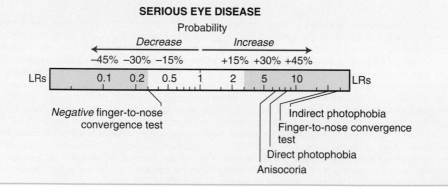

SERIOUS EYE DISEASE
Probability

EBM BOX 23.2	Conjunctivitis, Diagnosing Bacterial Etiology*			
			Likelihood Ratio‡ if Finding Is	
Finding (Reference)†	Sensitivity (%)	Specificity (%)	Present	Absent
Redness of conjunctiva				
Peripheral only[12,13]	30	59	NS	NS
Red eye observed at 20 feet[14]	94	36	1.5	0.2
Redness completely obscures tarsal vessels[14]	33	93	4.6	NS
Discharge[14,15]				
None	12–28	41–56	0.4	…
Watery	6–12	…	NS	…
Mucous	6–44	…	NS	…
Purulent	32–50	85–94	3.9	…
Follicular conjunctivitis[15]	50	48	NS	NS
Papillary conjunctivitis[15]	24	95	NS	NS
Preauricular adenopathy[14,15]	6–16	70–88	NS	NS

*Diagnostic standard: for *bacterial conjunctivitis*, recovery of a known pathogen from conjunctival secretions (i.e., *Streptococcus pneumonia, Hemophilus influenzae, Moraxella catarrhalis,* or *Staphylococcus aureus*).
†Definition of findings: for *follicular* and *papillary conjunctivitis*, see Fig. 23.2.
‡Likelihood ratio (LR) if finding present = positive LR; LR if finding absent = negative LR.
NS, Not significant.

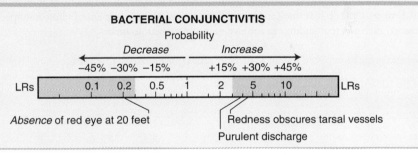

BACTERIAL CONJUNCTIVITIS
Probability

In general, the sensitivity of other classic findings is poor: 23% to 56% of patients with serious pathology lack photophobia, and 81% lack anisocoria. Also, even though abnormal visual acuity is a clue to serious eye disease, up to half of patients with proven iritis have a visual acuity of 20/60 or better.[11] The clinician should never use the finding of *normal* visual acuity as an argument *against* serious eye disease.

B. DISTINGUISHING BACTERIAL CONJUNCTIVITIS FROM NONBACTERIAL CAUSES

1. Individual Findings

In the 3 studies enrolling 281 consecutive patients with conjunctivitis summarized in EBM Box 23.2, investigators excluded patients with previous eye trauma, eye surgery, chemical injury, visual blurring, contact lenses, conspicuous iritis (circumlimbal flush), or obvious deep orbital pathology. In these studies, the presence or absence of matting of the eyes was the most helpful historical item: matting of both eyes in the morning increased probability of bacterial conjunctivi-tis (LR = 2.6), and absence of matting in both eyes decreased it (LR = 0.3).[12,13]

Two physical findings increased probability of bacterial conjunctivitis: complete redness of the conjunctiva obscuring the tarsal vessels (LR = 4.6, EBM Box 23.2) and observed purulent discharge (LR = 3.9). Absence of red eye when observed at 20 feet decreased probability of a bacterial cause (LR = 0.2). The symptoms of itching or burning and the findings of preau-ricular adenopathy, conjunctival follicles, or conjunctival papillae were diagnostic unhelpful (LRs not significant).[12,13,15] Finally, even though the physical sign of purulent secretions was accurate, the patient's report of "purulent" secretions was diagnostically unhelpful (LR not significant).

2. Combined Findings

One study of 700 patients[16] demonstrated that eye specialists using combinations of bedside find-ings could accurately diagnose the cause of conjunctivitis. The diagnostic standard in this study was cytology and cultures of conjunctival secretions: bacterial conjunctivitis was defined by posi-tive bacterial culture and neutrophils; viral conjunctivitis by positive viral inclusions, mononuclear cells and negative bacterial cultures; and allergic conjunctivitis by conjunctival eosinophils. The clinicians based the diagnosis of bacterial conjunctivitis on the findings of mucopurulent drainage and absence of follicles and adenopathy: this combination of findings accurately detected a bacte-rial cause (positive LR = 5.3; negative LR = 0.2). Combinations of scanty watery discharge, fol-licles, and preauricular adenopathy accurately diagnosed a viral cause (positive LR = 3.5; negative LR = 0.4). Finally, combinations of *allergic chemosis* (a pale swollen conjunctiva with a jelly-like appearance) and stringy mucoid discharge indicated an allergic cause (positive LR = 16.4, nega-tive LR = 0.01). Still, it is unclear from the study how these experienced clinicians specifically combined each of these findings to achieve such spectacular accuracy.

References may be accessed online at *Elsevier eBooks for Practicing Clinicians.*

Hearing

I. Introduction

Hearing loss, which affects approximately 50% of all individuals over the age of 65, is associated with difficulty communicating and higher rates of depression, frailty, and falls.[1] Clinicians using casual assessment in the office overlook significant hearing loss about half the time.[2] The causes of hearing loss are either **neurosensory** (i.e., damage to the auditory nerve or cochlear hair cells) or **conductive** (i.e., damage to the parts of the ear that conduct sound from air to the cochlea). Most neurosensory hearing loss is due to presbycusis (the degenerative hearing loss of aging). Less common causes are Meniere disease and acoustic neuroma. The most common causes of conductive loss are impacted cerumen, otitis media, perforated eardrum, and otosclerosis.[1]

II. Technique
A. WHISPERED VOICE TEST

Many tests of hearing are available to general clinicians, some more formal (hand-held audiometer) than others (listening to a whispered voice or to a watch, finger rub, or tuning fork). One validated test not requiring special tools is the whispered voice test. In this test, the clinician whispers a combination of three letters or numbers (e.g., 5, B, 6) while standing at arm's length (i.e., approximately 2 feet) behind the patient and then asks the patient to repeat the sequence. If the patient answers correctly, hearing is considered normal and testing is stopped. If the patient misidentifies any of the three items, the clinician repeats different triplets of numbers or letters 1 or 2 more times. If 50% or more of the items in the two or three triplets are incorrect, the test is abnormal.

The clinician stands behind the patient to prevent lip-reading. Only one ear is tested at a time, the other being masked by the examiner's finger, which occludes the external auditory canal and makes continuous circular rubbing motions (occlusion without rubbing is insufficient masking). The clinician should quietly exhale before whispering to produce the quietest whisper possible.[3]

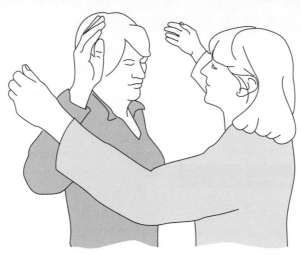

Fig. 24.1 Finger rub test. In this illustration the clinician is testing the patient's right ear, and the patient indicates by raising the right arm that the sound of the finger rub is perceived (i.e., "test negative," defined as the patient *can* hear the finger rub). In the original study of this finding,[4] each ear was tested 3 times (with both faint and strong stimuli), and "cannot hear finger rub" was defined as failure to hear any of the three stimuli. Because the patient must raise the arm indicating the side the stimulus is heard, masking the untested ear is unnecessary (i.e., if the right ear is being tested in a patient with severe unilateral right hearing loss, the clinician will be able to detect that the unmasked left ear is detecting the sound because the left arm is raised).

B. FINGER RUB TEST

The clinician stands directly in front of the patient with outstretched arms and tests one ear at a time by rubbing thumbs against the distal fingers (Fig. 24.1).[4] During the test the patient has the eyes closed and is encouraged to listen carefully to indicate which side the rubbing is heard by raising the ipsilateral arm. A *strong* finger rub is as loud as the clinician can muster without snapping the fingers; a *faint* rub is the softest the clinician can still hear. *Inability* to hear the finger rub is "test positive."

C. TICKING WATCH TEST

The clinician positions a ticking watch 6 inches away from the patient's ear while the patient occludes the opposite ear. The test is repeated 6 times, and inability to hear the ticking sound during any of these trials is a positive test.[5] To prevent providing visual clues, the clinician should test the patient from behind or ask the patient to close his or her eyes.

D. TUNING FORK TESTS

1. Introduction

After hearing loss is identified, tuning forks tests distinguish neurosensory from conductive loss. All tuning fork tests are based on the same fundamental principle, discovered almost 500 years ago,* that sound conducts preferentially through bone to ears with disease causing conductive

---

*The Italian physician Capivacci made this discovery after connecting his subject's teeth to a zither and then plucking the zither's strings.[6]

hearing loss. Tuning fork tests were introduced into clinical otology in the early 1800s, and at one time there were over 15 distinct tuning fork tests.[7] After introduction of audiometry, however, enthusiasm for tuning fork tests waned, and now only two are commonly used, the Weber and Rinne test.

2. The Frequency of the Tuning Fork

Most authorities recommend using the 512-Hz tuning fork for tuning fork tests,[8] because frequencies above 512-Hz detect conductive hearing loss less well and because frequencies of 128-Hz or lower generate so many vibrations that even patients without hearing can sense them.[9–11] The 512-Hz fork is preferred to the 256-Hz fork, because the 256-Hz fork produces more false-positive results in some studies.[12,13]

3. Method of Striking the Fork

Most authorities recommend striking the fork against a soft surface, such as a rubber pad or the muscles of the forearm.[8] The principal tone produced is the same whether the tines are struck on a soft or harder surface, but the harder surface generates multiple overtones that may confound interpretation by the patient.[7,14] Weights, sometimes added to the tines to minimize overtones, also shorten the time of vibration and are not recommended.

4. Weber Test

In the Weber test, the clinician strikes the fork, places it in the middle of the patient's vertex, forehead, or bridge of nose, and asks "Where do you hear the sound?" (Fig. 24.2). In patients *with unilateral hearing loss*, the sound is preferentially heard in the *good* ear if the loss is neurosensory and in the *bad* ear if the hearing loss is conductive.[8,15] Weber himself recommended placing the vibrating fork on the incisors,[16] and subsequent studies do show that this is the most sensitive technique,[17] although concerns of transmitting infectious diseases now prohibit this method.

According to traditional teachings, persons with normal hearing perceive the sound in the midline or inside their head, but studies show that up to 40% of normal-hearing persons also lateralize the Weber test.[11] Therefore, the Weber test should be interpreted only in patients with hearing loss.

The **hum test** is often used to simulate the Weber test, particularly when clinicians are concerned about a unilateral conductive hearing loss and tuning forks are unavailable (e.g., the clinician may be discussing symptoms with a patient over the telephone).[18] The patient is asked to hum a sustained pitch for a few seconds and then note whether the sound is more pronounced on the right or left side or perceived equally. In patients with conductive loss, the sound should be more pronounced in the bad ear.[†]

5. Rinne Test

In the Rinne (pronounced "RIN-neh") test, the clinician tests each ear individually to determine whether that ear detects sound better through air or bone (Fig. 24.2). Air conduction (AC) is tested by holding the vibrating fork about 2.5 cm away from the ear, traditionally with the axis joining the tips of the tines in line with the axis through both external auditory canals. Bone conduction (BC) is tested by holding the stem of the vibrating fork against the mastoid (excessive force should be avoided because it diminishes the test's specificity).[19] There are two methods for comparing AC and BC: (1) loudness comparison technique, in which the fork is held about 2 seconds in each position and the patient indicates which position is louder, and (2) threshold technique, in which the clinician uses a stopwatch to time how long the patient

---

[†] Clinicians can simulate this by plugging one of their own ears with a finger (thus creating a conductive hearing loss) and then humming a sustained pitch. The sound will be more pronounced in the plugged ear.

WEBER TEST   RINNE TEST

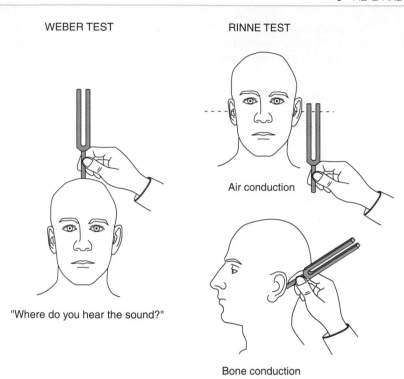

Air conduction

"Where do you hear the sound?"

Bone conduction

Fig. 24.2 **Weber and Rinne tuning fork tests.** In the Weber test (*left*), the clinician holds the vibrating tuning fork in the midline against the patient's vertex, forehead, or bridge of nose and asks "Where do you hear the sound?" In the Rinne test (*right*), the clinician tests one ear at a time, comparing perception of sound conducted through air (*top right*) to perception of sound conducted through bone (*bottom right*). When testing air conduction, the tuning fork is held so that an axis through both external auditory canals (*dashed line*) passes through both tines of the fork. When testing bone conduction, the stem of the vibrating fork is held against the mastoid.

hears the sound, from the moment the fork is struck to when the sound disappears, first for AC and then BC.[8]

Patients with normal hearing or neurosensory hearing loss perceive sound better (i.e., louder or longer) through AC than through BC, whereas those with conductive hearing loss perceive it better through BC. According to a confusing tradition, the finding of *BC better than AC* is recorded "Rinne negative," although it is more explicit to record "BC > AC" for the abnormal result.

The orientation of the tines of the fork affects the performance of the air conduction portion of the Rinne test. Traditionally, the tuning fork is held so that an axis through both ears passes through both tines of the fork ("parallel orientation"; Fig. 24.2), although a "perpendicular orientation" is also commonly used.[20] The parallel orientation produces a louder sound than does the perpendicular orientation,[20] but as long as a consistent technique is employed the accuracy of the Rinne test is the same whether a parallel or perpendicular orientation is used.[21] In contrast, oblique orientations of the tines should be avoided, because sound waves emanate in two directions from the fork, one direction parallel to the axis of the tines and the other perpendicular to it. If the tines are held at an oblique angle, these sound waves may actually cancel each other out and markedly diminish the sound.[7] (Clinicians can easily convince themselves of this by rotating the stem of a vibrating fork near their own ear, noting that the sound intermittently disappears.)

Table 24.1 presents examples of different Weber and Rinne test results and possible interpretations.

TABLE 24.1 ■ Tuning Fork Tests - Traditional Interpretation

Weber Test	Rinne Test	Possible Interpretations
Midline	AC > BC, bilateral	1) Normal hearing, bilateral 2) Neurosensory loss, bilateral
Louder in left	BC > AC, left AC > BC, right	1) Conductive loss, left
Louder in left	AC > BC, bilateral	1) Normal hearing, bilateral 2) Neurosensory loss, worse on right
Louder in right	BC > AC, bilateral	1) Conductive loss, bilateral but worse on right 2) Conductive loss on right and severe neurosensory loss on left[†]

[†]Some patients with severe neurosensory loss have the finding BC > AC because the BC stimulus is cross-heard by the better cochlea on the nontest side.
AC, Air conduction; *BC,* bone conduction.
From British Society of Audiology. Recommended procedure for Rinne and Weber tuning-fork tests. *Br J Audiol.* 1987;21(3):229–230.

III. Clinical Significance

A. PATIENT'S PERCEPTIONS OF HEARING LOSS

The patient is a poor judge of personal hearing loss. When compared to pure tone audiometry, the question "do you feel you have any difficulty hearing?" has limited accuracy (sensitivity of 60% to 89%; specificity of 41% to 86%; positive likelihood ratio [LR] not significant; negative LR = 0.4).[4,22]

B. WHISPERED VOICE TEST

EBM Box 24.1 reveals that the abnormal whispered voice test increases probability of significant hearing loss (i.e., >20–30 dB; LR = 6.7), whereas the normal test decreases it (LR = 0.1).

C. FINGER RUB TEST

In a study of 221 outpatients to a neurology clinic, the *inability* to hear the *strong* finger rub is pathognomonic for hearing loss (LR = 355.4), whereas the *ability* to hear the *faint* finger rub indicates normal hearing (LR = 0.02).

D. TICKING WATCH TEST

In one study of 107 patients, the inability to hear the ticking watch was a compelling argument for hearing loss (LR = 105.7).

E. TUNING FORK TESTS

Using the loudness comparison technique, the Rinne test accurately detects conductive hearing loss. The finding of "BC > AC" increases the probability of an audiometric air-bone gap of 20 dB or more (LR = 27.6, EBM Box 24.1); the finding of "AC > BC" decreases the probability of an air-bone gap this large (LR = 0.3). The larger the patient's air-bone gap on audiometry, the more likely the Rinne test will reveal "BC > AC" (for comparison, the mean air-bone gap in otosclerosis and otitis media is 21 to 27 dB).[13,25,27]

| EBM BOX 24.1 | Hearing Tests* | | | |

| Finding (Reference)[†] | Sensitivity (%) | Specificity (%) | Likelihood Ratio[‡] if Finding Is | |
			Present	Absent
Hearing tests				
Abnormal whispered voice test[2,3,22–24]	79–99	80–92	**6.7**	**0.1**
Unable to hear *strong* finger rub[4]	61	100	**355.4**	0.4
Unable to hear *faint* finger rub[4]	98	75	**3.9**	**0.02**
Unable to hear ticking watch[5]	44	100	**105.7**	0.6
Tuning fork tests (patients with unilateral hearing loss)				
Rinne test, detecting conductive hearing loss[9,13,25–27]	55–89	95–99	**27.6**	0.3
Weber test lateralizes to good ear, detecting neurosensory loss[11,26]	4–58	78–98	2.5	NS
Weber test lateralizes to bad ear, detecting conductive loss[11,26]	53–62	88–99	NS	0.5

*Diagnostic standard: for *hearing loss*, mean pure tone threshold >20 dB.[24] >25 dB,[4,5,22] or >30 dB[2,3,23] on audiometry; for *conductive hearing loss (Rinne test)*, air-bone gap on audiometry >15 dB[26] or >20 dB.[9,13,25,27]

[†]Definition of findings: for *abnormal whispered voice test* and *finger rub test*, see text; for *Rinne test*, bone conduction (BC) greater than air conduction (AC), using the loudness comparison technique; all tuning fork tests used a 512 Hz tuning fork except one study,[26] which used 256 Hz tuning fork.

[‡]Likelihood ratio (LR) if finding present = positive LR; LR if finding absent = negative LR.
NS, Not significant.

SIGNIFICANT HEARING LOSS

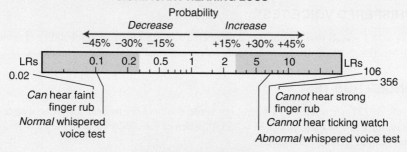

Probability

Decrease | Increase

−45% −30% −15%   +15% +30% +45%

LRs 0.02 0.1 0.2 0.5 1 2 5 10 LRs 106
356

Can hear faint finger rub
Normal whispered voice test

Cannot hear strong finger rub
Cannot hear ticking watch
Abnormal whispered voice test

TUNING FORK TESTS

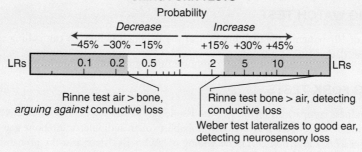

Probability

Decrease | Increase

−45% −30% −15%   +15% +30% +45%

LRs 0.1 0.2 0.5 1 2 5 10 LRs

Rinne test air > bone, *arguing against* conductive loss

Rinne test bone > air, detecting conductive loss

Weber test lateralizes to good ear, detecting neurosensory loss

On the other hand, the Weber test is less accurate. When the sound lateralizes to the good ear in patients with unilateral hearing loss, the probability of neurosensory hearing loss increases only small amount (LR = 2.5). The Weber test performs poorly because many patients with unilateral hearing loss, whether neurosensory or conductive, localize the tuning fork sound in the midline.[11]

Tuning fork tests cannot distinguish normal hearing from bilateral neurosensory losses (see Table 24.1) and thus should always be performed after hearing tests. Moreover, tuning fork tests cannot distinguish a pure conductive loss from a mixed conductive and neurosensory defect (see Table 24.1).

References may be accessed online at *Elsevier eBooks for Practicing Clinicians*.

Thyroid and Its Disorders

- The normal thyroid has a constant relationship with two prominent landmarks of the neck, the laryngeal prominence (of the thyroid cartilage) and the cricoid cartilage. The best definition of goiter is enlarged thyroid lobes (e.g., each larger than the distal phalanx of the patient's thumb), apparent by both inspection and palpation (without extending the neck).
- Seventy-five percent to 90% patients with substernal goiters also have *cervical* goiters. One-third of patients with substernal goiters have a displaced trachea. Some develop congestion of the face when they elevate their arms (Pemberton sign).
- In patients with thyroid nodules or goiters, the presence of cervical adenopathy, vocal cord paralysis, or fixation to adjacent tissues greatly increases probability of carcinoma.
- In patients with suspected thyroid disease, the findings that increase probability of hypothyroidism the most are hypothyroid speech; cool, dry, and coarse skin; bradycardia; and delayed ankle reflexes.
- In patients with suspected thyroid disease, the findings that increase the probability of hyperthyroidism the most are eyelid retraction, eyelid lag, fine finger tremor, moist and warm skin, and tachycardia.

GOITER

I. Introduction

In industrialized areas of the world, goiter (i.e., enlarged thyroid) occurs in up to 10% of women and 2% of men, with the usual causes being multinodular goiter, Hashimoto thyroiditis, or Graves disease (the most common cause world-wide is endemic goiter, largely from inadequate iodine intake).[1] About 80% of patients with goiter are clinically euthyroid, 10% are hypothyroid, and 10% are hyperthyroid. Most patients with goiter are asymptomatic or present for evaluation of a neck mass. A few patients, especially those with substernal goiters, present with dyspnea, stridor, hoarseness, or dysphagia (see the section on substernal goiters).

Endemic goiter has been described for millennia, although it is unclear whether early clinicians distinguished goiter from other causes of neck swelling such as tuberculous lymphadenitis. The first person to clearly differentiate cystic goiter from cervical lymphadenopathy was Celsus, the Roman physician writing in AD 30.[2]

II. Technique

A. NORMAL THYROID[3]

The important landmarks for locating the thyroid gland are the V-shaped protrusion at the top of the thyroid cartilage (the *laryngeal prominence*) and the cricoid cartilage (Fig. 25.1). These two structures, which are usually 3 cm apart, are the most conspicuous structures in the midline of the neck. The isthmus of the normal thyroid lies just below the cricoid cartilage and is usually 1.5 cm wide, covering the second through fourth tracheal rings. Each lateral lobe of the thyroid is 4 to 5 cm long and hugs the trachea tightly, extending from the middle of the thyroid cartilage down to the fifth or sixth tracheal rings. A pyramidal lobe is found in up to 50% of anatomic dissections, usually on the left side, and is palpable in 10% of nontoxic goiters but seldom in normal-sized glands.

The thyroid has a constant relationship with the laryngeal prominence (which is approximately 4 cm above the thyroid isthmus) and the cricoid cartilage (which is just above the isthmus), but the position of these structures in the neck (and thus of the thyroid in the neck) varies considerably among patients (Fig. 25.1).[4] If the laryngeal prominence and suprasternal notch of the manubrium are far apart (separated by more than 10 cm), the patient may have a conspicuous *high-lying thyroid*, which resembles a goiter even though it is normal-sized (see the section on pseudogoiter later). If the laryngeal prominence is close to the suprasternal notch (separated by less than 5 cm), the patient has a *low-lying thyroid*, which often is concealed behind the sternocleidomastoid muscles and clavicles, making complete palpation of the gland impossible.[4,5] Low-lying thyroids are more common in elderly patients.

In areas of the world with iodine-replete diets, the normal thyroid is less than 20 mL in volume.[6]

B. EXAMINATION FOR GOITER

1. Inspection

Two maneuvers make the thyroid more conspicuous: (1) extending the patient's neck, which lifts the trachea (and thyroid) approximately 3 cm away from the suprasternal notch and stretches the skin against the thyroid, and (2) inspecting the patient's neck from the side. In patients with normal- or high-lying thyroids, the line between the cricoid prominence and suprasternal notch, when viewed from the side, should be straight. Anterior bowing of this line suggests a goiter (Fig. 25.2).[7]

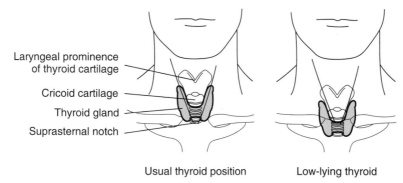

Laryngeal prominence
of thyroid cartilage

Cricoid cartilage

Thyroid gland

Suprasternal notch

Usual thyroid position   Low-lying thyroid

Fig. 25.1   The normal thyroid. The thyroid gland has a constant relationship with the two most prominent landmarks of the middle of the neck—the laryngeal prominence of the thyroid cartilage and the cricoid cartilage. On the *left* is the usual position of the thyroid gland. On the *right* is a *low-lying thyroid*, most of which is hidden behind the clavicles and sternum, inaccessible to palpation.

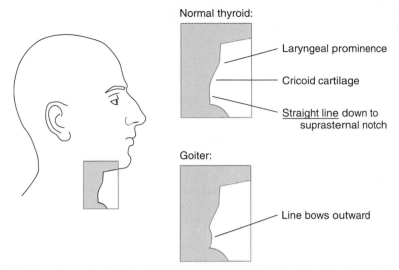

Fig. 25.2   Neck contour and goiter. The shaded profile of the neck (*left*) is enlarged on the right, to contrast the normal thyroid contour with that of a goiter. Below the cricoid cartilage, the contour of the normal neck in the midline (*top right*) is a straight line downward to the suprasternal notch. In patients with goiter, this line bows outward (*bottom right*) because of enlargement of the thyroid isthmus. This line is visible only in patients with normal-lying and high-lying thyroids, not low-lying thyroids (see Fig. 25.1).

2. Palpation

Palpation of the thyroid may proceed from the patient's front or back, whichever is most comfortable and effective for the clinician, because studies fail to show either method to be superior.[8] The patient's neck should be slightly flexed (to relax the sternocleidomastoid and sternohyoid muscles), and a firm technique should be used. The following features should be noted: thyroid size, consistency (i.e., soft, firm, or hard; a "soft" thyroid has the consistency of the surrounding tissue in the neck), texture (diffuse or nodular), tenderness, tracheal deviation (a clue to asymmetric goiter), and lymphadenopathy.

3. Observing the Patient Swallow[9]

Because the thyroid and trachea are firmly attached by ligaments and must move together, observation as the patient swallows helps distinguish the thyroid tissue from other neck structures. During a normal swallow, both the thyroid and trachea make an initial upward movement of 1.5 to 3.5 cm; the larger the oral bolus, the greater the movement. The thyroid and trachea then hesitate 0.2 to 0.7 s before returning to their original position.

Therefore a neck mass is probably *not* in the thyroid if one of the following is detected: (1) the mass is immobile during a swallow or moves less than does the thyroid cartilage; (2) the mass does not hesitate before descending to its original position; or (3) the mass returns to its original position before complete descent of the thyroid cartilage.

III. The Findings

A. CERVICAL GOITER

Common definitions of goiter include the following: **(1) Rule of thumb**. This states that a lateral lobe is enlarged if it is larger than the distal phalanx of the patient's thumb. **(2) Estimates of thyroid volume by palpation**. For example, a thyroid whose lateral lobes each measure 3 cm wide,

2 cm deep, and 5 cm long would have an estimated volume of 60 mL (i.e., $2 \times 3 \times 2 \times 5 = 60$). Any estimate more than 20 mL is classified as a goiter (i.e., each lateral lobe is normally 10 mL or less). **(3) Epidemiologic definitions of goiter**. These definitions are designed for clinicians who survey large numbers of persons rapidly in areas of endemic goiter (some clinicians examine 150 to 200 patients per hour). The revised World Health Organization definition has three grades: grade 0, no palpable or visible goiter; grade 1, goiter that is palpable *but not visible* with the head in the normal position; and grade 2, a goiter that is palpable *and* clearly visible when the neck is in a normal position.[10]

B. SUBSTERNAL AND RETROCLAVICULAR GOITERS

Large goiters may extend from the neck to the superior mediastinum, passing through the inflexible thoracic inlet (i.e., the bony ring formed by the upper sternum, first ribs, and first thoracic vertebral body). At the thoracic inlet, such goiters may compress the trachea, esophagus, or neck veins and thus produce dyspnea, dysphagia, facial plethora, cough, and hoarseness. Sometimes, when these patients flex or elevate the arms, the thoracic inlet is pulled up into the cervical goiter, just as if the thyroid were a cork and the thoracic inlet were the neck of a bottle. This causes the characteristic **Pemberton sign**, which is congestion of the face, cyanosis, and eventual distress induced by arm elevation (Fig. 25.3).[11–13] The exact frequency of Pemberton sign is unknown because reports vary greatly; two small series of patients with substernal goiter claim the sign is present in every patient,[14,15] while two other large series

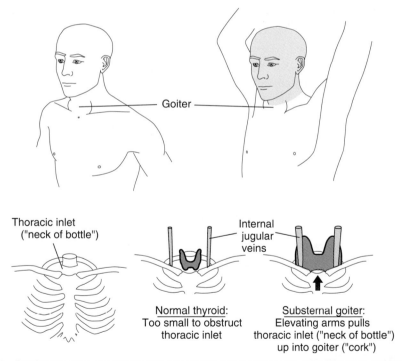

Fig. 25.3   Pemberton sign. If a patient with retrosternal goiter elevates his arms (*top row*), dramatic facial congestion may occur (i.e., positive Pemberton sign). This occurs because the thoracic inlet ("neck of bottle," *bottom left*) is an inflexible bony ring formed by the first thoracic vertebra, first ribs, and upper sternum (its outline is approximately the same size and shape as the patient's kidney). A normal-sized thyroid (*bottom middle*) is too small to obstruct the thoracic inlet. In contrast, a goiter of sufficient size (*bottom right*) may obstruct the thoracic inlet, especially if the goiter extends below the sternum and the patient elevates his arms (which pulls the thoracic inlet, or "neck of bottle," up into the goiter, or "cork," *arrow*).

fail to mention the sign at all,[16,17] and another series of 72 patients reports that Pemberton sign is present in 44%.[18]

In patients with substernal goiters, associated findings include cervical goiter (i.e., palpable goiter above the thoracic inlet, 75% to 90% of patients), tracheal deviation (33% by palpation, 75% by chest radiograph), distended neck veins (5% to 20%), and stridor (7% to 16%).[16–19]

C. THYROGLOSSAL CYST[20]

Thyroglossal cysts are cystic swellings of the thyroglossal duct, an epithelium-lined remnant marking the embryologic descent of thyroid tissue from the base of the tongue to its final location anterior to the larynx. Thyroglossal cysts present at any age, appearing as tense, nontender, mobile, nonlobulated round tumors, usually at the level of the hyoid bone or just below it (the hyoid bone is *above* the thyroid cartilage). Pain and tenderness may follow infection or acute hemorrhage into the capsule. The cysts are in the midline of the neck, unless they are so low they lie to one side of the thyroid cartilage. Despite their cystic structure, they do not usually transilluminate. If the cyst remains attached to the base of the tongue or hyoid bone, a characteristic physical sign of thyroglossal cysts is upward movement when the patient protrudes the tongue, just as if the two structures were connected by a string. Thyroglossal cysts account for three-quarters of congenital neck masses, the other one-quarter being branchial cleft cysts, which are located more laterally, usually anterior to the sternocleidomastoid muscle at the level of the hyoid bone.[21,22]

D. PSEUDOGOITER

Pseudogoiter refers to thyroid glands that appear enlarged even though they are normal-sized. There are three causes: **(1) High-lying thyroid gland**, which, although normal-sized, lies so high in the neck it is unusually conspicuous after neck extension. In these patients, the laryngeal prominence is 10 cm or more above the suprasternal notch and both thyroid lobes are smaller than the distal phalanx of the patient's thumb. In one study, high-lying but normal-sized thyroids accounted for 8% of suspected goiters referred to an endocrinology service.[4] **(2) Other cervical masses**, such as adipose tissue, cervical lymphadenopathy, branchial cleft cysts, and pharyngeal diverticula (see Chapter 27). Observation during swallowing helps identify these lesions. **(3) Modigliani syndrome**, which describes a normal-sized thyroid lying in front of an exaggerated cervical spine lordosis,[23] named after the painter Amedeo Modigliani, whose portraits had subjects with long, curved necks.

E. THE DELPHIAN NODE

The Delphian node, a lymph node that drains the thyroid gland and larynx, lies directly anterior to the cricothyroid ligament (just cephalad to the thyroid isthmus, see Fig. 25.4). When enlarged, the node is readily palpable because of its superficial location in front of the unyielding trachea. The node is called *Delphian* because it is the first one exposed during surgery, and its appearance often foretells what the surgeon will find in the thyroid (e.g., carcinoma), just as the oracle at Delphi foretold the future.* The Delphian node enlarges in some patients with thyroid cancer, Hashimoto thyroiditis, or laryngeal cancer. Its involvement in both laryngeal and thyroid cancer is associated with a poorer prognosis.[25–27]

---

*The word *Delphian* was originally suggested by Raymond Randall, a fourth year medical student attending the thyroid clinic at The Massachusetts General Hospital.[24]

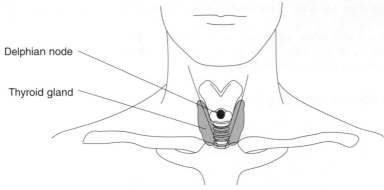

Fig. 25.4   The Delphian node. The Delphian node lies in midline of the neck, just above the thyroid isthmus and in front of the cricothyroid ligament, where it can easily be palpated against the unyielding cricoid cartilage.

IV. Clinical Significance

A. DETECTING GOITER

The findings listed in EBM Box 25.1 are categorized into three levels; (1) no goiter by palpation or inspection (including inspection of the extended neck); (2) goiter by palpation, but the gland is not conspicuous until the patient's neck is extended; and (3) goiter by palpation and inspection with the neck in the normal position. The first finding, absence of goiter by inspection and palpation, decreases modestly the probability of an enlarged thyroid (likelihood ratio [LR] = 0.4; see EBM Box 25.1). Although up to half of patients with enlarged glands by ultrasonography have this finding, these goiters are presumably small. The intermediate finding (i.e., goiter by palpation but visible only after neck extension) fails to distinguish goiter from normal-sized glands (LR not significant), suggesting that subtle enlargement by palpation without a visible goiter (in the normal neck position) is an unreliable sign of goiter. A gland that is both enlarged by palpation and visible when the patient's neck in the normal position greatly increases the probability of an enlarged thyroid (LR = 26.3).

B. ETIOLOGY OF GOITER

In clinically euthyroid patients with goiter, the most common causes are multinodular goiter or Hashimoto thyroiditis. In hypothyroid patients it is Hashimoto thyroiditis, and in hyperthyroid patients it is Graves disease or multinodular goiter. The associated finding of ophthalmopathy (tearing, diplopia, proptosis) or dermopathy (pretibial myxedema) indicates Graves disease (see the section on Graves ophthalmopathy).

Although thyroid cancer can also cause a goiter, cancer usually presents instead as a thyroid nodule (see the section on thyroid nodule). Three findings increase the probability that a goiter contains carcinoma: cervical adenopathy (LR = 15.4, see EBM Box 25.2), vocal cord paralysis (LR = 11.3), and fixation of the goiter to surrounding tissues (LR = 10.5).

Silent and postpartum lymphocytic thyroiditis may also produce a goiter, but it is rarely prominent, and the clinician's attention is instead directed toward the findings of hyperthyroidism or hypothyroidism.[37] The finding of a painful or tender thyroid gland, sometimes mimicking pharyngitis, suggests subacute thyroiditis[38] or hemorrhage into a cyst or nodule (although most thyroid

EBM BOX 25.1	Goiter*		

Finding (Reference)	Sensitivity (%)	Specificity (%)	Likelihood Ratio† if Finding Is Present
No goiter by palpation or inspection[7,28-32]	5–57	0–40	0.4
Goiter by palpation, visible only after neck extension[28]	13	...	NS
Goiter by palpation and inspection with neck in normal position[28-30,32]	43–82	88–100	**26.3**

*Diagnostic standard: for *goiter*, ultrasound volume >20 mL,[28,30,32] ultrasound volume >18 ml (women) or >25 ml (men),[31] or surgical weight >23 g.[7]
†Likelihood ratio (LR) if finding present = positive LR; LR if finding absent = negative LR.
NS, Not significant.

GOITER
Probability

Decrease	Increase
−45% −30% −15%	+15% +30% +45%

LRs | 0.1 0.2 0.5 | 1 | 2 5 10 | LRs

No goiter by palpation or inspection

Goiter by palpation *and* inspection

hemorrhage is painless).[39] In subacute thyroiditis, the thyroid is modestly enlarged, usually 1.5 to 3 times the normal size.

THYROID NODULES

I. Introduction[40]

Palpable thyroid nodules occur in approximately 5% of women and 1% of men, most of whom are clinically euthyroid. Although thyroid nodules raise concerns about thyroid cancer, over 95% of nodules reflect benign disorders, such as colloid cysts, adenomas, or dominant nodules of a multinodular gland.

II. Occult Nodules ("Incidentalomas")

Because thyroid nodules are palpable in only 1% to 5% of persons yet are discovered in up to 50% of patients during ultrasound or autopsy surveys,[41] it is obvious that most thyroid nodules are *occult* (i.e., detectable by clinical imaging but not by palpation). Furthermore, when the clinician feels a single *palpable* nodule in the patient's thyroid gland, ultrasonography reveals multiple nodules half the time.[42] Occult nodules are not palpable either because the patient's neck is too short or thick,[43] the nodules are buried in the posterior parts of the gland,[44] or the nodules are too small (i.e., the mean diameter of a *palpable* nodule is 3 cm; palpation fails to detect 50% of nodules less than 2 cm in diameter and over 90% of nodules less than 1 cm in diameter).[43]

EBM BOX 25.2	Goiter and Thyroid Nodules - Findings Predicting Carcinoma*

Finding (Reference)[†]	Sensitivity (%)	Specificity (%)	Likelihood Ratio[‡] if Finding Is Present	Absent
Goiter				
Cervical adenopathy[33]	45	97	**15.4**	0.6
Vocal cord paralysis[17,33]	24–44	94–99	**11.3**	0.7
Fixation to surrounding tissues[33]	60	94	**10.5**	0.4
Goiter nodular (vs. diffuse)[33]	78	49	1.5	0.5
Pyramidal lobe present[33]	2	90	NS	NS
Thyroid Nodule				
Vocal cord paralysis[34,35]	5–14	99–100	**17.9**	NS
Fixation to surrounding tissues[34,36]	13–37	95–98	**7.8**	NS
Cervical adenopathy[34,35]	24–31	96–97	**7.2**	0.8
Diameter ≥4 cm[36]	66	66	1.9	0.5
Very firm nodule[34]	3	99	NS	NS

*Diagnostic standard: for *carcinoma*, pathologic examination of tissue.[33–36]
[†]Definition of findings: for *vocal cord paralysis*, visualization of vocal cords[33–35] or symptomatic dysphonia.[17]
[‡]Likelihood ratio (LR) if finding present = positive LR; LR if finding absent = negative LR.
NS, Not significant.

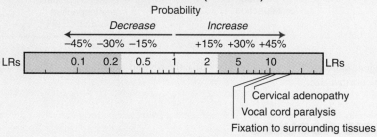

THYROID CARCINOMA (IF GOITER)

Cervical adenopathy
Vocal cord paralysis
Fixation to surrounding tissues

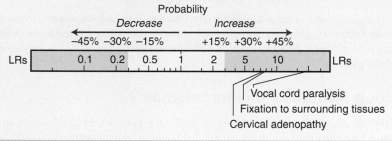

THYROID CARCINOMA (IF THYROID NODULE)

Vocal cord paralysis
Fixation to surrounding tissues
Cervical adenopathy

III. Clinical Significance

The most important diagnostic tests for thyroid nodules (whether palpable or nonpalpable) are thyroid function testing, ultrasonography, and, if indicated, fine needle aspiration. Nonetheless, a few signs, if present, increase the probability of carcinoma in thyroid nodules (EBM Box 25.2):

vocal cord paralysis (LR = 17.9), fixation of the nodule to surrounding tissues (LR = 7.8), and cervical adenopathy (LR = 7.2). All of these findings, however, are insensitive, with fewer than one of three patients with carcinomatous nodules having any of these findings.

HYPOTHYROIDISM (MYXEDEMA)

I. Introduction

Hypothyroidism is a clinical syndrome that results from diminished levels of thyroid hormone, which reduces the patient's metabolic rate, slows neuromuscular reactions, and causes mucopolysaccharides to accumulate in the skin and other tissues throughout the body. In areas of the industrialized world with iodine-replete diets, hypothyroidism affects 9% of women and 1% of men.[1] The usual cause is disease in the thyroid gland itself (primary hypothyroidism), most often from Hashimoto thyroiditis (60% to 70% of cases) or previous radioiodine treatment for Graves disease (20% to 30% of cases).[1]

The diagnosis of hypothyroidism relies on laboratory tests, which have been available for over one hundred years.[†] Nonetheless, bedside diagnosis is still essential for two reasons: (1) examination estimates the likelihood of thyroid disease, which then can be used to identify subgroups of patients with high or low probability of abnormal thyroid function, thus increasing the yield of laboratory testing; and (2) examination is essential when diagnosing subclinical hypothyroidism or sick euthyroid syndrome, conditions that, by definition, describe patients with abnormal laboratory tests but without bedside findings of thyroid disease.

All of the classic bedside findings of hypothyroidism—puffy skin, slow reflexes, thick speech, and sluggish thinking—were first described by William Gull and William Ord in the 1870s.[46,47]

II. Findings and Their Pathogenesis

A. SKIN AND SOFT TISSUE[48,49]

The nonpitting puffiness of hypothyroidism results from dermal accumulation of mucopolysaccharides (mostly hyaluronic acid and chondroitin sulfate), which freely bind water. These changes cause a "jelly-like swelling (and) overgrowth of mucus-yielding cement," which led Ord in 1877 to coin the term "myxedema."[47] Even after effective thyroid replacement, these changes may persist for months.

Some myxedematous patients also have a yellow tint to their skin, which occurs because of hypercarotenemia from diminished conversion of carotenoids to retinol. The apparent coolness of the skin is attributed to diminished dermal blood flow, and dryness results in part from decreased sebum production. The loss of hair from the lateral eyebrows occurs in some hypothyroid patients but is one of the least specific signs (see later).

B. THE ACHILLES REFLEX

The ankle jerk has been investigated more extensively than has any other physical finding of thyroid disease. By the 1970s, at least nine different instruments had been designed to precisely measure the duration of reflex to the nearest millisecond. Both the contraction and relaxation phase of the ankle jerk are prolonged in hypothyroidism, although prolonged relaxation seems most prominent to the human eye (and on many of the tracings of the reflex). In one study, the mean half-relaxation time

---

[†]The first thyroid test was the basal metabolic rate (BMR) (i.e., oxygen consumption), introduced in the 1890s; radioactive iodine uptake appeared in the 1940s; serum protein-bound iodide (PBI) in the 1950s; serum total thyroxine (T4) in the 1960s; and sensitive assays for thyroid stimulating hormone in the 1980s.[45]

(i.e., the time from the hammer tap to the moment the Achilles tendon has returned halfway to its original position) for hypothyroid patients was 460 ms (standard deviation [SD], 40 ms), compared to 310 ms (SD, 30 ms) for euthyroid patients.[50] Experiments in hypothyroid rats suggest that the prolongation results from diminished calcium transport by the sarcoplasmic reticulum and subsequent slowing of the interaction between actin and myosin.[51]

When testing for hypothyroidism, clinicians usually elicit the ankle jerk by tapping on the Achilles tendon with the patient kneeling on a chair‡. The force of the tap does not affect the duration of the reflex, although slightly more force is necessary in hypothyroid patients to generate a reflex than in hyperthyroid patients.

C. HYPOTHYROID SPEECH

Hypothyroid speech, seen in approximately one-third of patients with hypothyroidism, has a slow rate and rhythm and is characteristically deep, low-pitched, and hyponasal (i.e., as if the patient has a cold).[53] Some patients even slur their words slightly, leading one clinician to describe the hypothyroid voice as "a bad gramophone record of a drowsy, slightly intoxicated person with a bad cold and a plum in the mouth."[54] Biopsies of vocal cords have revealed deposition of mucinous material.

D. OBESITY

Obesity is no more common in hypothyroid patients than euthyroid patients.[55]

III. Clinical Significance

EBM Box 25.3 summarizes the diagnostic accuracy of physical signs associated with hypothyroidism, as applied to over 1500 patients with suspected thyroid disease. The **Billewicz scoring scheme**, which combines symptoms and signs, is fully described in Table 25.1.

In patients with suspected thyroid disease, the findings increasing the probability of hypothyroidism the most are hypothyroid speech (LR = 5.4, EBM Box 25.3), cool *and* dry skin (LR = 4.7), slow pulse rate (LR = 4.2), coarse skin (LR = 3.4), and delayed ankle reflexes (LR = 3.4)§. Hair loss of the eyebrows is one of the least compelling diagnostic signs (LR = 1.9), and the finding of *isolated* coolness or dryness of the palms is unhelpful (LR not significant). No individual finding, when present or absent, significantly decreases the probability of hypothyroidism (i.e., no LR has a value less than 0.6).

A Billewicz score of +30 points or higher greatly increases the probability of hypothyroidism (LR = 18.8), whereas a score of fewer than −15 points decreases the probability of hypothyroidism (LR = 0.1). The Billewicz score may perform less well in elderly patients, who, as a rule, have fewer findings than do younger patients.[63]

HYPERTHYROIDISM

I. Introduction

Hyperthyroidism is a clinical syndrome due to the increased production or release of thyroid hormone, which elevates the metabolic rate and causes the characteristic findings of the skin, thyroid,

---

‡ Other muscle stretch reflexes may also be delayed in hypothyroidism, such as the biceps reflex (as illustrated in an online video in reference 52).

§ Precise measurements of the ankle jerk using special instruments discriminate well between patients with and without hypothyroidism: the finding of a half-relaxation time >370–380 ms detects hypothyroidism with a sensitivity of 91% to 99%, specificity of 94% to 97%, positive LR=18.7, and negative LR=0.1.[50,56,62]

| EBM BOX 25.3 | Hypothyroidism* | | | |

Finding (Reference)†	Sensitivity (%)	Specificity (%)	Likelihood Ratio‡ if Finding Is Present	Absent
Skin				
Cool and dry skin[56]	16	97	**4.7**	0.9
Coarse skin[57,58]	29–61	74–95	**3.4**	0.7
Cold palms[57]	37	77	NS	NS
Dry palms[57]	42	73	NS	NS
Periorbital puffiness[57,58]	53–91	21–81	NS	0.6
Puffiness of wrists[57]	39	86	2.9	0.7
Hair loss of eyebrows[57]	29	85	1.9	NS
Pretibial edema[58]	78	31	NS	NS
Speech				
Hypothyroid speech[57]	37	93	**5.4**	0.7
Pulse				
Slow pulse rate[56,58,59]	29–43	89–98	**4.2**	0.7
Thyroid				
Enlarged thyroid[56]	46	84	2.8	0.6
Neurologic				
Delayed ankle reflexes[58]	48	86	**3.4**	0.6
Slow movements[58]	87	13	NS	NS
Billewicz score[60,61]				
Less than −15 points	3–4	28–68	**0.1**	...
−15 to +29 points	35–39	...	NS	...
+30 points or more	57–61	90–99	**18.8**	...

*Diagnostic standard: for *hypothyroidism*, low free thyroxine (T4) level and high thyroid-stimulating hormone,[58,59,61] or low protein-bound iodide (PBI) level.[56,57,60] The PBI level and total T4 level correlate closely, except in patients with thyroiditis or those who ingest exogenous iodides (e.g. radiocontrast dye, cough suppressants), diagnoses in which the PBI level may be falsely high. These diagnoses, however, were largely excluded from the studies reviewed here.
†Definition of findings: for *slow pulse rate*, <60 beats/min[58,59] or <70 beats/min[56]; for *delayed ankle reflexes*, assessment of contraction and relaxation of calf muscle by naked eye[58]; for *slow movements*, patients required more than 1 minute to fold a 2-meter-long bed sheet.[58]
‡Likelihood ratio (LR) if finding present = positive LR; LR if finding absent = negative LR.
NS, Not significant.

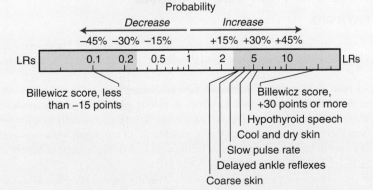

HYPOTHYROIDISM
Probability

TABLE 25.1 ■ Billewicz Diagnostic Index for Hypothyroidism

Finding*	Points Scored If Finding is:	
	Present	Absent
Symptoms		
Diminished sweating	+6	−2
Dry skin	+3	−6
Cold intolerance	+4	−5
Weight increase	+1	−1
Constipation	+2	−1
Hoarseness	+5	−6
Paresthesiae	+5	−4
Deafness	+2	0
Physical Signs		
Slow movements	+11	−3
Coarse skin	+7	−7
Cold skin	+3	−2
Periorbital puffiness	+4	−6
Pulse rate <75/min	+4	−4
Slow ankle jerk	+15	−6

*Definition of findings: for *weight increase*, recorded increase in weight or tightness in clothing; for *slow movements*, observations while patient removing and replacing a buttoned garment; for *coarse skin*, roughness and thickening of skin of hands, forearms, and elbows; for *slow ankle jerk*, reflex appears slow with patient kneeling on a chair, grasping its back.
Based upon reference 60.

eyes, and neuromuscular system. The most common causes of hyperthyroidism are Graves disease (60% to 90% of cases), toxic nodular goiter, thyroiditis (subacute, silent, or postpartum), and iatrogenic overtreatment with thyroid replacement.[64] Hyperthyroidism affects women (4% prevalence) more than men (0.2% prevalence).

Three clinicians—Caleb Parry, Robert Graves, and Adolf von Basedow—all writing between 1825 and 1840 independently described the classic physical signs associated with thyrotoxicosis. All three were especially impressed with the triad of goiter, prominent eyes, and forceful tachycardia.[65]

II. Findings and Their Pathogenesis

A. THE THYROID

A goiter is present in 70% to 93% of patients with hyperthyroidism.[66-68] The goiter is diffuse and symmetric in patients with Graves disease and thyroiditis, but nodular in those with toxic nodular goiter.[68]

A thyroid bruit is a common feature of Graves disease (73% of patients in one study).[69] Nonetheless, the finding was also noted in 30% of elderly patients with toxic nodular goiter,[70] suggesting that the finding is not as specific for Graves disease as classically taught. Bruits often radiate far from their source, and perhaps the "thyroid bruit" in the elderly with toxic nodular goiter is actually a carotid bruit made prominent by the increased cardiac output of hyperthyroidism.¶

¶The opposite phenomenon—a "carotid bruit" emanating from the superior thyroid artery—has also been described.[71]

B. EYE FINDINGS

Three distinct eye findings are associated with hyperthyroidism: lid lag (von Graefe sign, 1864), lid retraction (Dalrymple sign, 1849),[#] and Graves ophthalmopathy. Graves ophthalmopathy afflicts exclusively patients with Graves disease, whereas lid lag and lid retraction may occur in hyperthyroidism from any etiology.

1. Lid Lag

This sign describes the appearance of white sclera between the margin of the upper eyelid and corneal limbus as the patient looks downward. In von Graefe's words, "...as the cornea looks down, the upper eyelid does not follow."[65]

2. Lid Retraction

This sign describes a peculiar staring appearance of the eyes, caused by a widened palpebral fissure. As the patient looks straight ahead, the upper eyelid is positioned abnormally high, revealing white sclera between the lid margin and superior limbus. Normally the margin of the upper eyelid rests just below the edge of the corneal limbus and covers about 1 mm of the iris.[74]

Both lid lag and lid retraction are attributed in part to the sympathetic hyperactivity of hyperthyroidism, which causes excess contraction of the Müller muscle (the involuntary lid elevator whose paralysis causes the ptosis of Horner syndrome). Although the findings often improve after treatment with beta-blocking medications,[75] mechanisms other than sympathetic hyperactivity must contribute to the lid lag and retraction of some patients with Graves disease, because their lid findings may persist after the restoration of normal thyroid function and may be unilateral and associated with normal-sized pupils (the pupils should be dilated if sympathetic hyperactivity is the cause).[76,77] In these patients, lid findings may represent incipient Graves ophthalmopathy (even without exophthalmos or other findings of ophthalmopathy; see the section on Graves ophthalmopathy). One proposed mechanism implicates an overactive levator palpebrae muscle (thus elevating the eyelid); the levator's action is linked to that of that of the superior rectus muscle, which according to this theory is contracting excessively in attempts to vertically align the eye against a shortened and restricted *inferior* rectus muscle.[78]

Other common causes of lid retraction are contralateral ptosis, ipsilateral facial muscle weakness, previous eyelid surgery, and irritation from wearing contact lenses.[79] Ptosis causes contralateral lid retraction because attempts to elevate the weakened lid generate excessive neural signals to the motor neuron of the healthy lid, thus elevating it.[80] A simple test confirming ptosis as the cause is to occlude the eye that has ptosis, which then causes the lid retraction in the opposite eye to resolve. Facial weakness causes retraction of the ipsilateral eyelid because the lid elevators are no longer opposed by the orbicularis oculi muscle.[81]

3. Graves Ophthalmopathy

Graves ophthalmopathy is a constellation of findings, apparent in 25% to 50% of patients with Graves disease, which results from edema and lymphocytic infiltration of the orbital fat, connective tissue, and eye muscles.[82,83] Characteristic physical findings are lid edema, limitation of eye movements, conjunctival chemosis and injection, and exophthalmos (as measured with an exophthalmometer). Clinicians should suspect Graves ophthalmopathy when patients complain of gritty sensation in the eyes, tearing, eye discomfort, or diplopia. The orbital swelling of Graves ophthalmopathy may threaten the optic nerve and vision. The bedside findings best

---

[#]The British eye surgeon John Dalrymple (1803-52) apparently thought so little of his sign that he never published a description of it. Writing in 1849, W. White Cooper attributed the sign to his friend Dalrymple.[72] Albrecht von Graefe A (1828-70) described his sign in 1864.[65] Ruedemann coined the term *lid lag* in 1932.[73]

predicting incipient optic neuropathy are lid edema and limitation of eye movements—not, surprisingly, the degree of proptosis (proptosis does not predict incipient optic neuropathy perhaps because intraocular pressure is relieved in some patients by the outward protrusion).[77,84]

C. CARDIOVASCULAR FINDINGS

Hyperthyroidism may cause a fast heart rate, loud snapping first heart sounds, midsystolic flow murmurs, and supraventricular arrhythmias.[85] Rare patients with severe hyperthyroidism may develop the Means-Lerman scratch,[86] a systolic rub or murmur with a prominent rough or grating character that appears near the left second intercostal space. Its pathogenesis is unknown.

D. SKIN FINDINGS[48,49]

The skin of hyperthyroid patients is warm, moist, and smooth, probably because of increased sympathetic tone to sweat glands and increased dermal blood flow. These skin findings often resolve after treatment with beta-blocker medications.

Up to 4% of patients with Graves disease develop skin lesions with the confusing name **pretibial myxedema**, characterized by bilateral, asymmetric raised, firm plaques or nodules, which are pink to purple-brown in color and usually distributed over the anterior shins.[48,87]

E. NEUROMUSCULAR FINDINGS

The neuromuscular findings of hyperthyroidism are weakness and diminished exercise tolerance, tremor, and brisk ankle jerks. The diminished exercise tolerance (affecting 67% of patients) is due to an inability to increase cardiac output appropriately with exercise and also to proximal muscle wasting and weakness from accelerated protein catabolism.[68,85,88] The fine tremor of hyperthyroidism occurs because of increased sympathetic tone and resolves with beta-blocking medications. Brisk reflexes are noted at the bedside in only 25% of patients or fewer,[89] and even precise measurements of the half-relaxation time (see the section on hypothyroidism for definition) reveal considerable overlap between the normal (range, 230 to 420 ms) and hyperthyroid values (range, 200 to 300 ms).[50]

III. Clinical Significance

EBM Box 25.4 presents the diagnostic accuracy of physical signs for hyperthyroidism, as applied to over 1700 patients with suspected thyroid disease. The **Wayne index**, which combines symptoms and signs, is described fully in Table 25.2.

EBM BOX 25.4	Hyperthyroidism*			
Finding (Reference)	Sensitivity (%)	Specificity (%)	Likelihood Ratio if Finding Is	
			Present	Absent
Pulse				
Pulse ≥90 beats/min[68]	80	82	4.5	0.2
Skin				
Skin moist and warm[68]	34	95	6.8	0.7
Thyroid				
Enlarged thyroid[68]	93	59	2.3	0.1
Eyes				
Eyelid retraction[68]	34	99	33.2	0.7
Eyelid lag[68]	19	99	18.6	0.8

(Continued)

EBM BOX 25.4	Hyperthyroidism* —Cont'd

| Finding (Reference) | Sensitivity (%) | Specificity (%) | Likelihood Ratio if Finding Is | |
			Present	Absent
Neurologic				
Fine finger tremor[68]	69	94	**11.5**	0.3
Wayne index[90,91]				
<11 points	1–6	13–32	**0.04**	...
11–19 points	12–30	...	NS	...
≥20 points	66–88	92–99	**18.2**	...

*Diagnostic standard: for *hyperthyroidism*, high levels of protein-bound iodide (PBI) for patients evaluated in the 1960s, total thyroxine (T4) for those in the 1970s, and total T4 and thyroid stimulating hormone (TSH) for those in the 1980s and 1990s (see footnote to EBM Box 25.3 for discussion of PBI).
†Likelihood ratio (LR) if finding present = positive LR; LR if finding absent = negative LR.
NS, Not significant.

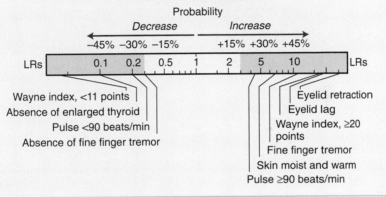

HYPERTHYROIDISM

TABLE 25.2 ■ Wayne Diagnostic Index for Hyperthyroidism

Symptoms of Recent Onset or Increased Severity	Present	Signs	Present	Absent
Dyspnea on effort	+1	Palpable thyroid	+3	−3
Palpitations	+2	Bruit over thyroid	+2	−2
Tiredness	+2	Exophthalmos	+2	
Preference for heat (irrespective of duration)	−5	Lid retraction	+2	
Preference for cold	+5	Lid lag	+1	
Excessive sweating	+3	Hyperkinetic movements	+4	−2
Nervousness	+2	Fine finger tremor	+1	
Appetite increased	+3	Hands:		
Appetite decreased	−3	Hot	+2	−2
Weight increased	−3	Moist	+1	−1
Weight decreased	+3	Casual pulse rate:		
		Atrial fibrillation	+4	
		<80, regular	−3	
		80–90, regular	0	
		>90, regular	+3	

Based up reference 90.

The findings that increase the probability of hyperthyroidism the most are lid retraction (LR = 33.2; see EBM Box 25.4), lid lag (LR = 18.6), fine finger tremor (LR = 11.5), moist and warm skin (LR = 6.8), and a pulse of 90 bpm or more (LR = 4.5). The findings that decrease the probability of hyperthyroidism the most are normal thyroid size (LR = 0.1), pulse less than 90 bpm (LR = 0.2), and absence of finger tremor (LR = 0.3).

A Wayne index score of 20 or higher increases the probability of hyperthyroidism (LR = 18.2) and one less than 11 decreases the probability of hyperthyroidism (LR = 0.04). Nonetheless, this index may be less useful in elderly patients,[92] who, as a rule, have less goiter and less tachycardia than younger patients.[93-96] In one study, 36% of elderly hyperthyroid patients had scores less than 11.[70] Elderly patients also have more atrial fibrillation than younger patients,[68,70,96-98] but the frequency of lid retraction and lid lag is the same.[68,70]

References may be accessed online at *Elsevier eBooks for Practicing Clinicians.*

Meninges

I. The Findings

The terms *meningeal signs* and *meningismus* refer to the physical findings that develop after meningeal irritation from inflammation, tumor, or hemorrhage. Those most widely known are neck stiffness (or *nuchal rigidity*), Kernig sign, and Brudzinski sign.

A. NECK STIFFNESS

Neck stiffness denotes involuntary resistance to neck flexion, which the clinician perceives when trying to bend the patient's neck, bringing the chin down to the chest. One specific definition of *neck stiffness* (from studies of patients with subarachnoid hemorrhage) is the inability to either touch the chin to the chest or lift the head 8 cm off the bed when supine.[1] Occasionally, the aggravated extensor tone of the neck and spine is so severe that the patient's entire spine is hyperextended, leaving the torso of the supine patient supported by only occiput and heels, an extreme posture called **opisthotonus**.

B. KERNIG SIGN

The Kernig sign was first described by Vladimir Kernig in 1882. With the patient's hip and knee flexed, Kernig sign is positive when the patient resists extension of the knee. Kernig called this a "contracture" of the hamstrings, because the knee would not extend beyond 135 degrees (with hip flexed), even though the knee extended fully if the hip was first positioned in the fully extended position (Fig. 26.1).[2] Most clinicians perform this test in the supine patient, although Kernig described the test being performed in the seated patient.

Kernig sign

Difficulty fully extending
knee if hip flexed

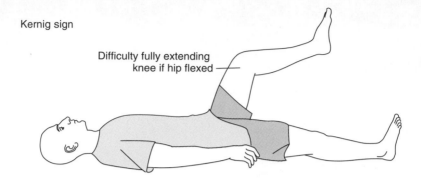

Brudzinski sign

Neck flexion causes knee flexion

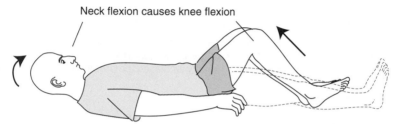

Fig. 26.1   Kernig and Brudzinski signs. In Kernig sign (*top*), the patient resists full extension of the knee when the knee and hip are first flexed (patient's left leg), although the knee extends normally if the hip is extended (patient's right leg). In Brudzinski sign (*bottom*), flexion of the patient's neck causes the hips and knees to flex, pulling both legs up toward the chest (see the text).

C. BRUDZINSKI SIGN

Jozef Brudzinski described several meningeal signs between 1909 and 1916. In his most popular sign, flexion of the supine patient's neck causes the patient to flex both hips and knees, thus retracting the legs toward the chest (see Fig. 26.1).[2]

D. JOLT ACCENTUATION HEADACHE

First proposed in 1991, jolt accentuation headache was felt to be a sensitive sign of meningitis in patients with headache and fever.[3] To perform the test, the clinician asks the patient to rotate the head side to side 2 to 3 times per second. Exacerbation of the patient's baseline headache is defined as the positive result.

II. Pathogenesis of Meningeal Signs

The basis for all meningeal signs is the patient's natural rejection of any movement that stretches spinal nerves, all of which pass through the irritated subarachnoid space. Experiments with cadavers show that flexion of the neck pulls the spinal cord toward the head, thus stretching spinal nerves, whereas flexion of the hips with knees extended pulls on the sciatic nerve, thus displacing the conus of the spinal cord downward toward the sacrum.[4] Flexion of the hips with knees flexed, in contrast, does not stretch the sciatic nerve.

These experiments explain why patients with meningeal irritation have neck stiffness and a positive Kernig sign, and they also show that Kernig sign does not differ from the straight leg raising test for sciatica (see Chapter 64). Brudzinski sign, however, is more difficult to understand. At first, it seems logical that patients with meningeal irritation would want to extend their hips and flex their knees when their neck is flexed. Although this position removes tension from the sciatic nerve, it stretches the femoral nerve,[4] explaining why Brudzinski test causes the patient to flex both hips and knees, thus relieving tension on both nerves.

III. Clinical Significance

A. ACUTE BACTERIAL MENINGITIS

Table 26.1 summarizes the frequency of individual findings of 3100 adults with acute bacterial meningitis (principally from *Streptococcus pneumoniae*, *Neisseria meningitidis*, and *Listeria monocytogenes*; cases of tuberculosis were excluded). This table reveals that the most frequent findings in bacterial meningitis are neck stiffness, fever, and altered mental status. Neck stiffness is a more frequent sign than Kernig or Brudzinski sign (sensitivity is 74% to 92% for neck stiffness vs. 61% for Kernig or Brudzinski sign), although this difference is not statistically significant and may reflect in part the clinician's diligence in looking for these findings. Of the patients with petechial rash, 73% to 92% have infection with *Neisseria meningitidis*.[6,8,13–15]

Nonetheless, the accuracy of these traditional physical signs is meager in studies of patients presenting with headache and fever. EBM Box 26.1 summarizes 8 studies of over 1500 patients. Neck stiffness, Kernig sign, Brudzinski sign, and jolt accentuation headache all have positive likelihood ratios (LRs) of only 1.5 to 2.4 (meningitis in these studies was defined as cerebrospinal

TABLE 26.1 ■ Acute Bacterial Meningitis and Subarachnoid Hemorrhage*

Finding	Frequency (%)†
Acute Bacterial Meningitis	
Neck stiffness	74–92
Fever	66–97
Altered mental status	55–95
Kernig or Brudzinski sign	61
Focal neurologic signs	9–37
Seizures	5–28
Petechial rash	3–52
Subarachnoid Hemorrhage	
Neck stiffness	21–86
Seizures	7–32
Altered mental status	29–64
Focal neurologic findings	10–36
Fever	6
Preretinal hemorrhages	4

Diagnostic standard: For *meningitis*, cerebrospinal fluid pleocytosis and microbiologic or postmortem data supporting bacterial meningitis; for *subarachnoid hemorrhage*, computed tomography or lumbar puncture.
*Data obtained from 3100 patients with meningitis from references 5–15. 692 patients with subarachnoid hemorrhage from references 16–19.
†Results are overall mean frequency or, if statistically heterogeneous, the range of values.

EBM BOX 26.1	Meningitis*

Finding (Reference)	Sensitivity (%)	Specificity (%)	Likelihood Ratio[†] if Finding Is Present	Absent
Neck stiffness[20-27]	13–78	56–80	1.5	0.7
Kernig sign[20-25,27]	2–56	73–97	2.1	NS
Brudzinski sign[20-25]	2–64	74–98	2.4	NS
Jolt accentuation headache[3,21-27]	6–97	33–99	1.8	0.7

*Diagnostic standard: for meningitis, cerebrospinal fluid pleocytosis ≥5 white blood cells per microliter.
[†]Likelihood ratio (LR) if finding present = positive LR; LR if finding absent = negative LR.
NS, Not significant.

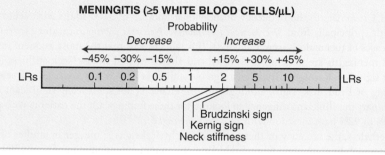

MENINGITIS (≥5 WHITE BLOOD CELLS/µL)

fluid white blood cell count [CSF WBC] ≥5/µL). Jolt accentuation headache turns out to have widely varying sensitivities (in one study, as low as 6%, EBM Box 26.1). No physical finding significantly decreases the probability of meningitis in patients with headache and fever. There are at least 2 explanations for the differences between the patients in Table 26.1 (where sensitivity of neck stiffness is 74% to 92%) and EBM Box 26.1 (sensitivity of neck stiffness is 13% to 78%): (1) relatively few of the patients in EBM Box 26.1 had bacterial meningitis (on average, only 1 of 6 with meningitis in these studies had bacterial meningitis; most had aseptic meningitis), and (2) almost all studies reviewed in EBM Box 26.1 excluded patients with altered mental status, which is one of the most prominent findings in observational studies of patients with bacterial meningitis (sensitivity 55% to 95%; Table 26.1). Even so, after applying a more rigorous definition of meningitis to the patients studied in EBM Box 26.1 (i.e., CSF WBC ≥100/µL instead of ≥5/µL), the diagnostic accuracy of the traditional meningeal signs is unchanged (neck stiffness, LR = 1.5; Kernig sign, LR = 2.5; Brudzinski sign, LR = 2.2).[20-22]

When present, Kernig sign should be symmetric. In one study of 51 consecutive comatose patients with Kernig sign, asymmetry of the sign indicated that the patient would have hemiparesis after awakening, the side with the less prominent Kernig sign indicating the side with subsequent paresis.[28]

B. SUBARACHNOID HEMORRHAGE AND INTRACEREBRAL HEMORRHAGE

Table 26.1 summarizes the findings of almost 700 patients with subarachnoid hemorrhage, 70% to 95% of whom presented with a severe precipitous headache. The most common physical finding in these patients was neck stiffness (sensitivity, 21% to 86%). In studies of more than 4000 patients presenting to emergency departments with acute atraumatic severe headache, the finding of neck stiffness significantly increased the probability of subarachnoid hemorrhage (LR = 6.7, EBM Box 26.2).

EBM BOX 26.2	Intracranial Hemorrhage*				

Finding (Reference)[†]	Sensitivity (%)	Specificity (%)	Likelihood Ratio[‡] if Finding Is	
			Present	Absent
Neck stiffness, detecting subarachnoid hemorrhage in patients with sudden atraumatic headache[1,29–31]	22–67	89–97	6.7	0.7
Neck stiffness, detecting intracranial hemorrhage in patients with stroke[32–37]	16–48	81–98	5.4	0.7

*Diagnostic standard: for *intracranial hemorrhage*, neuroimaging; for *subarachnoid hemorrhage*, neuroimaging, lumbar puncture, or both.
[†]Definition of findings: for *neck stiffness*, undefined or inability to touch chin to sternum or lift the head 8 cm.
[‡]Likelihood ratio (LR) if finding present = positive LR; LR if finding absent = negative LR.
NS, Not significant.

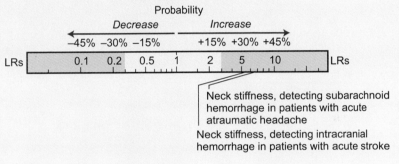

MENINGEAL SIGNS

Neck stiffness, detecting subarachnoid hemorrhage in patients with acute atraumatic headache

Neck stiffness, detecting intracranial hemorrhage in patients with acute stroke

Significant intracerebral hemorrhage may also produce subarachnoid bleeding and neck stiffness (i.e., intraventricular blood may pass through the median and lateral apertures of the fourth ventricle into the subarachnoid space at the base of the brain). In studies of almost 1000 patients presenting to emergency departments with stroke (i.e., acute neurologic deficits believed to be vascular in origin), the finding of neck stiffness increased the probability of intracranial blood, either subarachnoid or intracerebral hemorrhage (LR = 5.4). Subarachnoid hemorrhage was more likely in these patients if there were no focal findings (sensitivity of 64%, specificity of 89%, positive LR = 5.9).[18]

References may be accessed online at *Elsevier eBooks for Practicing Clinicians.*

Peripheral Lymphadenopathy

I. Introduction

Lymphatic vessels are located in all tissues and organs of the body except the central nervous system. These vessels collect extracellular tissue fluid (or lymph) and carry it to the systemic venous system, traversing along the way regional collections of bean-shaped structures called **lymph nodes**. As these lymph nodes slowly filter the lymph fluid, they may encounter microbes, malignant cells, particulate debris, or other substances to which they react, enlarge, and harden. Should such nodes enlarge or harden enough, they may become palpable, a problem called **peripheral lymphadenopathy**.

Ancient Greek and Roman physicians recognized peripheral lymphadenopathy as an important sign of tuberculosis (scrofula),[1,2] and for more than a century clinicians have known that lymphadenopathy may signify serious disorders such as carcinoma, lymphoma, leukemia, and certain infectious diseases (tuberculosis, syphilis, and plague, among others)[3]. How often adenopathy reflects one of these serious disorders in current practice depends on the clinical setting. In family practice clinics, peripheral lymphadenopathy is benign 99% of the time, sometimes reflecting known disorders (such as pharyngitis, dermatitis, or insect bites) but more often appearing and resolving without explanation.[4,5] In specialized lymph node clinics, however, 18% to 24% of referred patients are eventually diagnosed with malignancy (i.e., lymphoma or metastatic cancer) and up to 5% have a treatable infectious or granulomatous disorder (e.g., tuberculosis, human immunodeficiency virus [HIV] infection, sarcoidosis).[6-8] This chapter focuses on the physical findings that help discriminate these serious causes of lymphadenopathy from more benign causes.

II. Anatomy and Pathogenesis

A. INTRODUCTION

The lymphatic drainage of the body is subdivided into seven distinct regions, all of which converge and drain into the great veins near the base of the neck (Fig. 27.1). A normal adult has approximately 400 to 450 lymph nodes, although only about a quarter are in locations that could ever become palpable: 30 in the arm and axilla, 20 in the leg, and 60 to 70 in the head and neck (the remaining lymph nodes reside deep in the thorax and abdomen and are detectable only by clinical imaging).[9] Anatomists divide lymph nodes into **superficial nodes** and **deep nodes**, based on whether they accompany superficial or deep blood vessels. Superficial nodes lie just under the surface of the skin, accompany superficial veins, and often are visible when enlarged. Most palpable nodes are superficial nodes. The only deep nodes detectable by bedside examination are the deep cervical nodes (which accompany the carotid artery and internal jugular vein under the sternocleidomastoid muscle) and the axillary nodes (which surround the axillary vessels).

The fact that lymph nodes accompany blood vessels is helpful when searching for two nodal groups: (1) the epitrochlear nodes, which lie near the basilic vein, and (2) the vertical group of inguinal nodes, which surround the proximal saphenous vein (Fig. 27.2).

B. REGIONAL LYMPH NODE GROUPS

Maps of regional lymphatic drainage are based on older experiments in living humans and cadavers, in which injections of mercury, Prussian blue, radiocontrast materials, or other dyes were used to highlight normal lymph channels and regional nodes.[9–12] (Lymph vessels are otherwise difficult to distinguish from small veins during dissection.) These maps of lymph drainage are helpful because they allow clinicians to predict the spread of local infections or neoplasms and, when faced with isolated adenopathy, to focus the diagnostic search to a particular region. Nonetheless, clinical experience demonstrates that disease does not always spread in an orderly way through these channels and nodes. For example, infections and malignancy may occasionally skip one regional node group to travel to another (e.g., an infection of the ring finger may involve the axillary nodes and skip the epitrochlear nodes), and malignancy may sometimes travel in a retrograde direction between nodal groups (e.g., supraclavicular adenopathy, see the section on supraclavicular nodes).[11] In addition, despite the implication of these maps, isolated adenopathy does not necessarily reflect focal disease but instead may represent the sole sign of a generalized disorder (e.g., tuberculosis or lymphoma).

1. Cervical Nodes

All structures of the head and neck drain into the deep cervical nodes, either directly or via intermediary superficial nodes (Fig. 27.3). The skin of the face and neck drains into the superficial nodes in a predictable fashion (Fig. 27.3). The pharynx, nasal cavity, and sinuses usually drain to the upper deep cervical nodes; the mouth and teeth to the submandibular nodes and eventually the upper cervical nodes; and the larynx to both upper and lower cervical nodes. The tongue has the most diverse drainage: efferents travel to the submental, submandibular, upper deep cervical, and lower deep cervical nodes, and disease near the midline may travel to either side.[9,11,13,14]

2. Supraclavicular Nodes

Although supraclavicular nodes actually belong to the deep cervical nodes, they are considered separately because of their strategic location in the base of the neck, close to where all lymph drainage returns to the systemic venous system (see Fig. 27.1). Because of this location, supraclavicular adenopathy may signify serious disease located in the thoracic or abdominal cavities, regions where nodes are otherwise hidden from the examiner. The anatomy depicted in Fig. 27.1 predicts that right supraclavicular adenopathy would be associated with disorders of the right

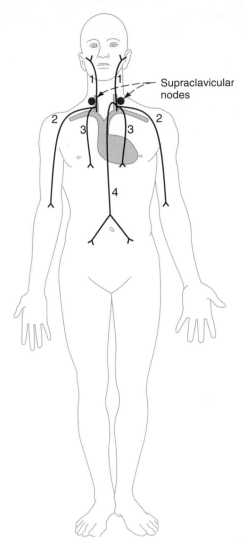

Supraclavicular
nodes

Fig. 27.1 The seven regions of lymphatic drainage. All lymphatic drainage of the body converges on the right and left junctions of the internal jugular and subclavian veins (shaded gray, along with the superior vena cava and heart). The great veins on the right side of the neck receive drainage from: the right head and neck (region 1, traversing cervical nodes); the right arm, chest wall, and breast (region 2, traversing axillary nodes); and the right lung and mediastinal structures (region 3, via mediastinal and tracheobronchial nodes but no peripheral nodes). The left great veins receive drainage from similar regions of the left upper body (regions 1 to 3) and, via the thoracic duct, drainage from all tissues below the diaphragm (region 4). Only the supraclavicular nodes are depicted, illustrating their strategic proximity to the confluence of these seven major lymph channels.

thorax, arm, and neck; and that the left supraclavicular adenopathy would be associated with disorders of the left thorax, arm, neck, and also the abdomen and pelvis.

Normally, lymph flows from supraclavicular nodes downward toward the confluence of lymph channels and great veins (see Fig. 27.1). Therefore, in order for intraabdominal or intrathoracic disorders to involve the supraclavicular nodes, disease must spread in a *retrograde* direction from the thoracic duct or bronchomediastinal lymphatic vessels through the cervical efferents leaving

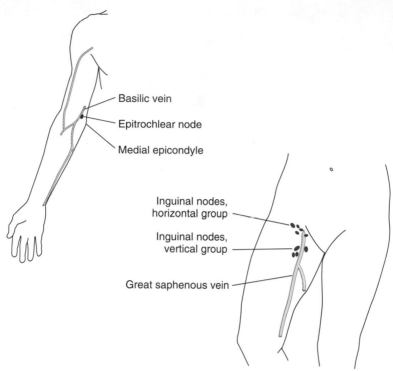

Fig. 27.2 Epitrochlear and inguinal nodes. The epitrochlear nodes (*left side of figure*) are located 2 to 3 cm above the medial epicondyle of the humerus, just medial to the basilic vein, which lies along the groove medial to the biceps muscle. The inguinal nodes (*right side of figure*) consist of a horizontal group and vertical group; the vertical group lies along the termination of the greater saphenous vein.

the supraclavicular nodes. Such retrograde spread easily occurs and does not imply obstruction of lymphatic channels. In one investigation of 92 patients undergoing lymphangiography of the lower limbs, radiopaque material appeared in the supraclavicular nodes within 48 hours in 55% of the patients.[15] As expected, the dye opacified exclusively the left supraclavicular nodes in 48 of 51 patients, but it opacified both right and left supraclavicular nodes in two patients and exclusively the right supraclavicular nodes in one patient, indicating normal anatomical variation in the connections between the thoracic duct and supraclavicular nodes.[15]

Supraclavicular adenopathy appears just behind the clavicle, underneath or posterior to the sternocleidomastoid muscle.[16] A Valsalva maneuver may make these nodes more prominent by pushing the apical pleural surface upward against the nodes and bringing them into view.[17] In 1848, Virchow first observed the association between abdominal malignancies and metastases to supraclavicular nodes.[15,18,19] Unaware of Virchow's description, the French clinician and pathologist Trosier described the same association in 1886, emphasizing the predisposition to the left side.[15,18,19] Left supraclavicular adenopathy has been therefore called **Virchow nodes, Trosier nodes, Virchow-Trosier nodes, sentinel nodes,** or **signal nodes.**[20]

3. Epitrochlear Nodes

Epitrochlear nodes (supratrochlear or cubital nodes, see Fig. 27.2) are superficial nodes, located on the anteromedial arm 2 to 3 cm above the medial epicondyle of the humerus. They drain the ulnar side of the forearm and hand (i.e., little and ring fingers) and send efferents to the axillary nodes.

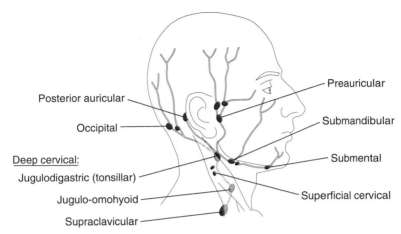

Fig. 27.3 Cervical lymph nodes. Superficial cervical nodes are named according to regional anatomy: occipital nodes, posterior auricular (or mastoid) nodes, preauricular (or parotid) nodes, submandibular nodes, submental nodes, and superficial cervical nodes. Deep cervical nodes lie along the carotid sheath and are mostly buried under the sternocleidomastoid muscle, although the uppermost nodes appear in front of this muscle and the lowermost posterior to it. Three deep cervical nodes have specific names because of their size and clinical importance: (1) the jugulodigastric node, an upper deep cervical node at the level of the hyoid bone that becomes tender and prominent in patients with pharyngitis (i.e., the tonsillar node), (2) the jugulo-omohyoid node, a lower deep cervical node located where the omohyoid muscle crosses the jugular vein (this node drains the tongue and may become enlarged in patients with tongue carcinoma), and (3) the supraclavicular nodes, which are the lowermost deep cervical nodes and are considered separately in the section on Supraclavicular nodes.

A common method for palpating these nodes is for the clinician to face the patient and reach across to shake the patient's hand on the side to be examined. The examiner then places his or her free hand behind the patient's arm, just proximal to the elbow, and uses his fingertips to palpate these nodes above and anterior to the medial epicondyle.

Although epitrochlear adenopathy may indicate infection or malignancy on the ulnar side of the forearm or hand, these nodes have historically been associated with conditions causing generalized lymphadenopathy, especially when they are enlarged bilaterally. (See the sections on epitrochlear adenopathy and detecting HIV infection in developing nations.) One hundred years ago, epitrochlear adenopathy was felt to be a compelling sign of secondary syphilis, occurring in 25% to 93% of cases.[21–23] Modern examples of this specific association, however, are scarce.

4. Axillary Nodes

Axillary nodes drain the ipsilateral arm, breast, and chest wall (see Fig. 27.4). To examine these nodes, the clinician should ensure that the patient's axillary skin is relaxed, by first supporting and adducting the patient's arm. Nodes are located in the posterior, anterior, or medial walls of the axillary fossa or in its apex. Efferent lymph vessels travel directly to the systemic veins at the root of the neck, although a few efferents pass first through the ipsilateral supraclavicular nodes (see Fig. 27.4).[9,11]

5. Inguinal Nodes

Inguinal nodes are superficial nodes that are organized into two groups: a proximal or *horizontal* group located just below the inguinal ligament, which drains the external genitalia, perineum, and lower anterior abdomen; and a distal or *vertical* group located at the termination of the great saphenous vein, which drains the leg (see Fig. 27.2).[9]

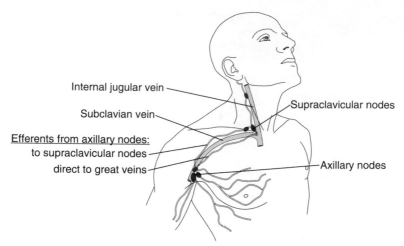

Fig. 27.4 Axillary nodes. The axillary nodes receive lymphatic drainage from the ipsilateral arm, breast, and chest wall. Efferent vessels travel to the great veins at the root of the neck, although a few vessels travel first through the supraclavicular nodal group.

III. The Finding

A. DESCRIBING ADENOPATHY

Important features to observe when describing adenopathy are location, size, number, hardness, and tenderness. *Fixed nodes* are immobile from attachments to adjacent structures, implying malignant invasion of these tissues. A *hard node* has the consistency of a rock, again implying malignant disease (the hardness presumably reflects the accompanying fibrosis induced by the tumor). *Shotty adenopathy* indicates multiple tiny superficial nodes, mimicking the sensation of buckshot under the skin, a finding sometimes observed in the inguinal region but without particular diagnostic significance.[24] The size of a particular node can be indicated by recording its maximal length and width or, as some investigators suggest, by recording the product of these two numbers (e.g., a node measuring 2.5 cm × 3 cm is "7.5 cm²").

B. GENERALIZED LYMPHADENOPATHY

Generalized adenopathy is defined as simultaneous enlargement of two or more regional lymph node groups.[25] Most affected patients have either combined cervical and inguinal adenopathy or combined cervical and axillary adenopathy.[26] Generalized lymphadenopathy implies a systemic disorder affecting lymph nodes, such as lymphoma or leukemia, specific infectious diseases (e.g., infectious mononucleosis, HIV infection, or syphilis), anticonvulsant hypersensitivity syndrome, sarcoidosis, or connective tissue disorders.[25]

C. "GLANDULAR" SYNDROMES

The term *glandular* refers to lymph nodes (e.g., *glandular fever* was the original name for infectious mononucleosis). Therefore, the **ulceroglandular syndrome** is the triad of fever, ulceration on the distal arm or leg (indicating the portal of entry of infectious agent), and regional adenopathy. The oculoglandular syndrome (**Parinaud syndrome***) describes the association of conjunctivitis with ipsilateral preauricular and submandibular adenopathy. Both ulceroglandular and oculoglandular syndromes have been associated with specific microbial agents. (See the sections on ulceroglandular and oculoglandular syndromes.)

Chapter 25 reviews the Delphian node and Chapter 50 discusses the Sister Mary Joseph nodule.

IV. Clinical Significance

A. DEFINITION OF DISEASE

EBM Box 27.1 reviews the diagnostic accuracy of physical examination in distinguishing serious causes of adenopathy from more benign disorders. All of the patients in these studies were referred to specialists because of persistent unexplained peripheral lymphadenopathy. Most patients (35% to 83%) presented with cervical adenopathy, 1% to 29% with supraclavicular adenopathy, 4% to 24% with axillary adenopathy, 3% to 16% with inguinal adenopathy, and 16% to 32% with generalized adenopathy.[4,6,8,26,28,32,33]

The etiology of lymphadenopathy in these studies was determined either by fine needle or excisional biopsy or, in a few low-risk patients who did not undergo biopsy, prolonged periods of observation.[7,8] Some of these studies defined a "serious disorder" (or "disease") as any disorder in which the biopsy results would imply specific treatment or prognosis. These studies therefore included both malignancy and granulomatous disease (e.g., tuberculosis or sarcoidosis) as "disease."[6,7,30–32,39,40] Other studies confined "disease" to the diagnosis of malignancy alone.[8,28,29,33,35] Both definitions of disease are combined in EBM Box 27.1, because analyzing the definitions separately revealed similar diagnostic accuracy, and because the overwhelming majority of patients in all studies had a malignant cause for their disease.

B. EXTRANODAL MIMICS OF LYMPH NODES

Up to 15% of patients referred for unexplained "lymphadenopathy" instead have extranodal explanations for their subcutaneous lumps.[8] Common mimics of lymphadenopathy at all locations are skin nodules such as lipomas or epidermoid cysts. In the cervical region, thyroglossal cysts, branchial cleft cysts, and prominent carotid sinuses may be mistaken for nodes (see Chapter 25). In the supraclavicular region, synovial cysts from rheumatoid arthritis of the shoulder,[41] cervical ribs, and abnormal articulations of the first rib[42,43] have all been mistaken for nodes.

C. INDIVIDUAL FINDINGS

In these studies, the symptom of generalized pruritus increased probability of serious disease, probably because of its association with lymphoma (sensitivity of 6% to 10%, specificity of 98% to 100%, likelihood ratio [LR] = 4.9).[6,7] According to the LRs in EBM Box 27.1, several physical findings also argue for serious disease: fixed lymph nodes (LR = 10.9), size of 9 cm^2 or more (i.e., the equivalent of 3 × 3 cm or larger, LR = 8.4), hard texture (LR = 3.2), supraclavicular adenopathy (LR = 2.9), weight loss (LR = 2.8), and age of 40 years or more (LR = 2.4).

Only three findings argue against serious disease, all of them reducing probability only modestly: age less than 40 years (LR = 0.4), lymph node size less than 4 cm^2 (i.e., 2 × 2 cm or smaller,

---

*Henri Parinaud, one of the world's first neuroophthalmologists, was recruited to Paris by Charcot in the late 1800s. He also described the pupillary and eye movement abnormalities of the pretectal syndrome (see Chapter 21).[27]

EBM BOX 27.1	Lymphadenopathy*			

Finding (Reference)[†]	Sensitivity (%)	Specificity (%)	Likelihood Ratio[‡] if Finding Is	
			Present	Absent
General and skin findings				
Male sex[6,7,28–30]	44–59	49–72	1.3	0.8
Age ≥40 years[6,7,28,29,31,32]	48–91	53–87	2.4	0.4
Weight loss[6,7,29,33,34]	19–28	71–95	2.8	0.8
Fever[6,7,30,33,34]	1–31	56–80	0.7	1.1
Distribution of adenopathy				
Head and neck nodes (excluding supraclavicular nodes)[6–8,28–30,32,33,35–38]	21–79	15–69	NS	NS
Supraclavicular nodes[6–8,29,32,33,35–38]	8–61	84–99	2.9	0.8
Axillary nodes[6–8,28–30,32,33,35–38]	6–52	30–94	0.8	NS
Inguinal nodes[6–8,28–30,32,33,35–38]	3–22	61–96	0.6	NS
Epitrochlear nodes[30]	2	97	NS	NS
Generalized lymphadenopathy[8,28,34,37–39]	15–48	31–95	NS	NS
Characteristics of adenopathy				
Lymph node size[6,7]				
<4 cm²	33–36	9–37	0.4	...
4 – 8.99 cm²	26–30	...	NS	...
≥9 cm²	37–38	91–98	**8.4**	...
Hard texture[6,7]	48–62	83–84	**3.2**	0.6
Lymph node tenderness[6,7,30,33,34]	3–18	50–86	0.4	1.3
Fixed lymph nodes[6,33]	12–56	97	**10.9**	NS
Other findings				
Rash[7,30]	4–8	85–95	NS	NS
Palpable spleen[6,7,30]	5–10	92–96	NS	NS
Palpable liver[7,30]	14–16	86–89	NS	NS
Lymph node score[6,7]				
−3 or less	1–3	42–72	**0.04**	...
−2 or −1	1–3	...	**0.1**	...
0 to 4	23	...	NS	...
5 or 6	17–26	...	**5.1**	...
7 or more	49–56	94–99	**21.9**	...

Diagnostic standard: for *diagnosis*, see text.
[†]*Definition of findings*: for *finding*, see text.
[‡]Likelihood ratio (LR) if finding present = positive LR; LR if finding absent = negative LR.
NS, Not significant.

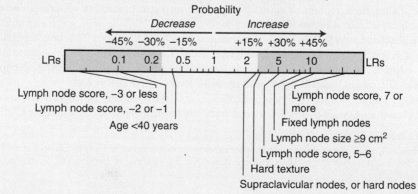

SERIOUS DISEASE (IF LYMPHADENOPATHY)
Probability

LR = 0.4), and lymph node tenderness (LR = 0.4). Tenderness may be less specific for benign disorders than expected because hemorrhage or necrosis into neoplastic nodes also causes discomfort mimicking acute inflammatory changes. The symptom of throat soreness also argues against serious disease (sensitivity of 3% to 14%, specificity of 23% to 89%, LR = 0.2).[6,7,40]

Findings that are unhelpful in distinguishing serious from benign disease include rash, regional distribution of nodes (other than supraclavicular location), fever, a palpable spleen, and a palpable liver (all LRs either not significant or very close to the value of 1).

The finding of generalized adenopathy, defined as involvement of two or more regional node groups, also lacks diagnostic value (LR not significant). Even when generalized lymphadenopathy is defined as involvement of four or more regional lymph node groups, it fails to discriminate serious from benign causes (LR not significant),[39] probably because this finding appears just as often in benign disorders (e.g., infectious mononucleosis) as in serious disorders (e.g., lymphoma).

D. COMBINED FINDINGS

Based on evaluation of more than 300 patients, Vassilakopoulos and others have identified six independent predictors of serious disease, creating a *lymph node score* that can easily be calculated at the bedside (Table 27.1).[7] According to this scoring scheme, a score of −3 or less virtually excludes serious disease (LR = 0.04, EBM Box 27.1), one of −2 or −1 argues *against* a serious cause (LR = 0.1), one of 5 or 6 argues *for* a serious disorder (LR = 5.1), and one of 7 or more is practically diagnostic *for* serious disease (LR = 21.9). Scores of 0 to 4 lack diagnostic significance.

E. LYMPH NODE SYNDROMES

1. Supraclavicular Adenopathy

In studies confined to patients undergoing biopsy of supraclavicular adenopathy, 54% to 87% of patients are discovered to have malignancy, mostly metastatic carcinoma (46% to 69% of all patients).[43-49] As expected, supradiaphragmatic carcinomas (e.g., lung or breast carcinoma) are equally distributed between the right and left sides. Most lung and breast cancers spread to the ipsilateral supraclavicular nodes, although examples of contralateral spread occur.[11,19,44-49]

TABLE 27.1 ■ **Lymph Node Score***

Finding	Points
Age >40 years	+5
Lymph node tenderness	−5
Lymph node size	
<1 cm²	0
1 – 3.99 cm²	+4
4 – 8.99 cm²	+8
≥9 cm²	+12
Generalized pruritus	+4
Supraclavicular nodes present	+3
Lymph node is hard	+2
Correction factor	– 6†

*From Vassilakopoulos TP, Pangalis GA. Application of a prediction rule to select which patients presenting with lymphadenopathy should undergo a lymph node biopsy. *Medicine*. 2000;79:338–347.
†Included in every patient's score. For example, a 55 year old asymptomatic patient with nontender but hard supraclavicular adenopathy measuring 6 cm² has a score of 12 (i.e., 5 + 8 + 3 + 2 – 6).

Surprisingly, infradiaphragmatic carcinomas do not always spread to the left supraclavicular nodes as would be predicted by normal anatomy (see Fig. 27.1) and implied by Virchow's and Trosier's eponym. On average, only three-quarters of infradiaphragmatic carcinomas metastatic to supraclavicular nodes go to the left side; one-quarter appear on the *right* side (range = 0% to 38%). Two proposed mechanisms for involvement of the right side by these tumors include the following: (1) some patients normally have anatomic connections between the thoracic duct and the right supraclavicular nodes (see the section on supraclavicular nodes), and (2) metastatic tumor first involves the mediastinal nodes, which via the right bronchomediastinal lymphatic vessels provide passage to the right neck. In support of the second explanation, one autopsy study of patients with infradiaphragmatic malignancies metastatic to the supraclavicular nodes documented that most patients also had mediastinal metastases.[19]

About 50% of patients whose supraclavicular node biopsies revealed malignancy were unaware of the diagnosis before biopsy,[19,46] illustrating the diagnostic importance of this node. In patients with metastases to the *right* supraclavicular node, the most common primary tumors by far are lung and breast cancer, followed by esophageal cancer and a medley of other tumors located above and below the diaphragm.[19,44–49] In those with metastases to the *left* side, lung, breast, gastric, and gynecologic primary tumors figure prominently in reported series of cases, although carcinoma of virtually any organ located in the thorax, abdomen, and pelvis has been associated with metastases to these nodes.[19,44–52]

2. Sore Throat and Adenopathy

The pharynx drains to the upper cervical nodes located *in front* of the sternocleidomastoid muscle (i.e., *anterior* cervical nodes, see tonsillar node in Fig. 27.3). Consequently, anterior cervical adenopathy is expected in patients with sore throat caused by localized bacterial pharyngitis (e.g., streptococcal pharyngitis). In contrast, when patients with sore throat present with adenopathy located at other lymph node sites, the clinician should consider infectious mononucleosis, a systemic viral infection that causes generalized adenopathy. In support of this, one study of 709 consecutive patients with sore throat demonstrated that the *presence* of adenopathy in the following locations increased probability of infectious mononucleosis (i.e., positive heterophile antibody): posterior cervical nodes (posterior cervical nodes are located *behind* the sternocleidomastoid muscle; LR = 3.1), posterior auricular nodes (LR = 11), axillary nodes (LR = 3), and inguinal nodes (LR = 3).[53] In this study, marked axillary adenopathy in a patient with sore throat greatly increased probability of infectious mononucleosis (LR = 19.8). Even so, the *absence* of adenopathy at any of these locations did not affect probability of infectious mononucleosis (i.e., all negative LRs not significant; sensitivity ranged from only 20% to 53%).

3. Epitrochlear Adenopathy

Epitrochlear nodes are a rare finding in normal individuals but are commonly observed in patients with disorders causing generalized lymphadenopathy. They are palpable in 25% to 30% of patients with sarcoidosis, lymphoma, and chronic lymphocytic leukemia, and up to 55% of patients with infectious mononucleosis.[21]

4. Identifying HIV Infection in Developing Nations

Adenopathy provides an important clue to HIV infection in patients from developing nations. In one study hospitalized patients in Zimbabwe, where HIV infection is prevalent, the finding of epitrochlear adenopathy (i.e., epitrochlear nodes > 0.5 cm diameter) distinguished patients with HIV seropositivity from those without it (sensitivity of 84%, specificity of 81%, positive LR = 4.5, negative LR = 0.2).[54] In studies from both Zimbabwe and India, the finding of axillary adenopathy in patients being treated for active tuberculosis increases probability of HIV coinfection (sensitivity of 26% to 43%, specificity of 93% to 95%, positive LR = 4.9).[54,55]

5. Fever of Unknown Origin (FUO)

The finding of peripheral lymphadenopathy in a patient with fever of unknown origin is a modest indicator that a bone marrow examination will be diagnostic (usually of a hematologic malignancy, LR = 1.9; see Chapter 18 and section on fever of unknown origin).[56–58]

6. Staging Patients with Known Cancer

The absence of regional adenopathy is often unhelpful when staging patients with known malignancies. For example, up to 50% of patients with head and neck tumors and negative nodes by examination have nodal metastases discovered during radical neck exploration.[59–61] In women with breast carcinoma, palpable axillary adenopathy does indicate metastatic nodal disease (sensitivity of 31% to 35%, specificity of 94% to 98%, positive LR = 9.3), but the absence of adenopathy is unhelpful (negative LR = 0.7; i.e., many patients with negative axillary examinations have axillary nodal metastases discovered at surgery).[62,63] Finally, up to one-quarter of patients with lung carcinoma and negative supraclavicular nodes have involvement of these nodes histologically.[64,65] Bedside examination is inaccurate because malignancy may involve regional nodes without changing their appearance. Even surgeons directly inspecting the physical characteristics of dissected nodes during staging operations often cannot distinguish metastatic nodes from normal ones.[59,61]

7. Ulceroglandular and Oculoglandular Syndromes

Common reported causes of the ulceroglandular syndrome are tularemia, rickettsial infections, and herpes simplex infections.[66] Important etiologies of the oculoglandular syndrome are cat-scratch disease, tularemia, and viral infections (especially enterovirus and adenovirus).[67,68]

References may be accessed online at *Elsevier eBooks for Practicing Clinicians*.

The Lungs

The Lungs

Inspection of the Chest

This chapter discusses the findings of clubbing, barrel chest, pursed lip breathing, accessory muscle use, and inspiratory white noise. Other relevant findings from inspection of the respiratory system include cyanosis (Chapter 9), abnormal respiratory rate, and abnormal breathing patterns (Chapter 19).

I. Clubbing (Acropachy, Hippocratic fingers)

A. INTRODUCTION

Clubbing is a painless focal enlargement of the connective tissue in the terminal phalanges of the digits.[1,2] Clubbing is usually symmetric, affecting fingers more prominently than toes. Although some persons have hereditary clubbing, the finding usually indicates serious underlying disease (see the section on clinical significance).

Hippocrates first described clubbing in the 3rd century BC. He noted it in patients with empyema, commenting that "the fingernails become curved and the fingers become warm, especially at their tips."[3]

B. THE FINDING

Precise definitions of clubbing were developed in the 1960s and 1970s, prompted by reports that clinicians of that time were using at least a dozen different definitions[4] and by the observation that clubbing regresses after effective treatment of the underlying disorder, thus making accurate measures of this physical finding an important endpoint to follow. There are three substantiated

235

definitions of clubbing (Fig. 28.1): (1) interphalangeal depth ratio greater than 1, (2) hyponychial angle greater than 190 degrees, and (3) positive Schamroth sign.

1. Interphalangeal Depth Ratio

Measurement of the interphalangeal depth ratio is described in Fig. 28.1. If this ratio exceeds 1, clubbing is present, a conclusion supported by two observations: (1) the interphalangeal depth ratio of normal persons is 0.895 ± 0.041, making the threshold of 1 more than 2.5 standard deviations (SDs) above normal,[5,6] and (2) a ratio of 1 distinguishes digits of healthy persons from those of patients with disorders traditionally associated with clubbing (such as cyanotic heart disease and cystic fibrosis). For example, studies demonstrate that 75% to 91% of patients with cystic fibrosis have an interphalangeal depth ratio exceeding 1, but only 0% to 1.5% of normal persons do.[5,6]

2. Hyponychial Angle

Measurement of the hyponychial angle is described in Fig. 28.1. If this angle exceeds 190 degrees, clubbing is present, a conclusion supported by three observations: (1) the normal hyponychial angle is 180 ± 4.2 degrees, and thus the 190 degree threshold is almost 2.5 standard deviations above normal,[5,7,8] (2) the hyponychial angle is the best parameter distinguishing plaster casts of

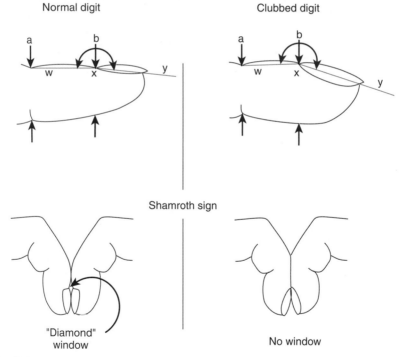

Fig 28.1   Clubbing. The normal digit is on the *left*: the clubbed one, on the *right*. The distal interphalangeal joint is denoted by *a*; the junction of the nail and skin at the midline is denoted by *b*. The interphalangeal depth ratio is the ratio of the digit's depth measured at *b* divided by that at *a*. The hyponychial angle is the angle *wxy*. In the figure, the depth ratio is 0.9 for the normal digit and 1.2 for the clubbed digit (a ratio >1 indicates clubbing), and the hyponychial angle is 185 degrees for the normal digit and 200 degrees for the clubbed digit (a hyponychial angle >190 degrees indicates clubbing). The Schamroth sign refers to the absence of the diamond-shaped window that normally appears when the terminal phalanges of similar digits are opposed to each other.

digits labeled "definitely clubbed" by experienced clinicians from those labeled "definitely normal",[9] and (3) studies show that 69% to 80% of patients with cystic fibrosis have hyponychial angles exceeding 190 degrees, whereas only 0% to 1.6% of normal persons have angles this large.[7,8]

A disadvantage of the hyponychial angle is the special equipment required for precise measurements. Historically, clinicians used an apparatus called the shadowgraph, an instrument projecting the silhouette of the finger against a screen fitted with a movable protractor.[10] Modern investigators measure the angle using digital photographs and computerized protractors.[8]

3. Schamroth Sign

In 1976, after watching his own clubbing come and go during an episode of endocarditis, the renown electrocardiographer Leo Schamroth[11] suggested that clinicians place the terminal phalanges of similar fingers back to back (especially ring fingers) and look for a small diamond-shaped window outlined by the bases of nail beds and nails. Clubbing is *absent* when this window appears; clubbing is *present* when this window is missing (Fig. 28.1). Schamroth suggested further study of his sign and, in 2010, investigators using the interphalangeal depth ratio as the diagnostic standard demonstrated that Schamroth sign had a sensitivity of 77% to 87%, specificity of 90%, positive likelihood ratio [LR] = 8, and negative LR = 0.2.[12]

4. Other Definitions

Parameters found to be less accurate definitions of clubbing (compared to the hyponychial angle and interphalangeal depth ratio) are the distal interphalangeal *width* ratio, the longitudinal curvature of nail, the transverse curvature of the nail, and the profile angle (i.e., the angle between line *wx* in Fig. 28.1 and a second line extending from *x* to a point on the top of nail about a third of the distance from nail fold to nail tip).[9,13]

C. CLINICAL SIGNIFICANCE

1. Etiology

In a study of 350 patients with clubbing, 80% had underlying respiratory disorders (e.g., lung tumor, bronchiectasis, lung abscess, empyema, interstitial fibrosis), 10% to 15% had miscellaneous disorders (congenital cyanotic heart disease, liver cirrhosis, chronic diarrhea, subacute endocarditis), and 5% to 10% had hereditary or idiopathic clubbing.[14]

2. Relationship of Clubbing to Hypertrophic Osteoarthropathy

Clubbing may be associated with hypertrophic osteoarthropathy, a painful condition causing swelling and arthritis of the distal arms and legs. Radiographs reveal periosteal elevation of the diaphysis of long bones.[15] The usual cause is intrathoracic neoplasm (e.g., lung cancer or mesothelioma).

3. Clubbing and Cystic Fibrosis

In patients with cystic fibrosis, clubbing (i.e., interphalangeal depth ratio >1) predicts significant hypoxemia (i.e., PaO_2 ≤88 mm Hg on room air) with a positive LR = 3.2 and negative LR = 0.1 (see EBM Box 28.1). After lung transplantation, the clubbing of cystic fibrosis regresses slowly over months.[26]

4. Clubbing and Endocarditis

In a study of almost 2000 patients undergoing evaluation for endocarditis,[16] the finding of clubbing increased the probability of definite endocarditis (LR = 5.1; see EBM Box 28.1).

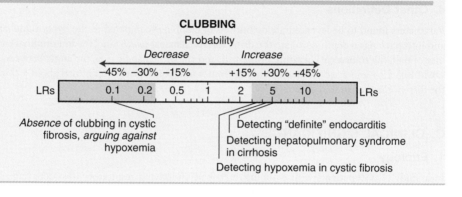

EBM BOX 28.1   Clubbing*

Finding (Reference)[†]	Sensitivity (%)	Specificity (%)	Likelihood Ratio[‡] if Finding Is	
			Present	Absent
Detecting hypoxemia (pO$_2$ ≤ 88 mm Hg) in patients with cystic fibrosis[6]	91	72	3.2	0.1
Detecting "definite" endocarditis[16]	6	99	5.1	NS
Detecting hepatopulmonary syndrome in patients with cirrhosis[17-25]	12–91	64–96	4.3	0.6

Diagnostic standard: for *definite endocarditis*, modified Duke criteria; for *hepatopulmonary syndrome*, triad of cirrhosis, intrapulmonary shunting by contrast echocardiography, and hypoxemia, defined as arterial pO$_2$ <70 mm Hg[25] or <80 mm Hg,[17,21] alveolar-arterial pO$_2$ gradient ≥15 mm Hg[20,22-24] or >20 mm Hg,[18] or *either* pO$_2$ <70 mm Hg or AapO$_2$ >20 mm Hg.[19]
[†]*Definition of findings*: for *clubbing*, interphalangeal depth ratio >1[6] or undefined (all other studies)
[‡]Likelihood ratio (LR) if finding present = positive LR; LR if finding absent = negative LR.
NS, Not significant.

CLUBBING
Probability

Decrease   *Increase*

-45% -30% -15%   +15% +30% +45%

LRs   0.1   0.2   0.5   1   2   5   10   LRs

Absence of clubbing in cystic fibrosis, *arguing against* hypoxemia

Detecting "definite" endocarditis
Detecting hepatopulmonary syndrome in cirrhosis
Detecting hypoxemia in cystic fibrosis

5. Clubbing and Hepatopulmonary Syndrome

In patients with liver cirrhosis, the finding of clubbing increases the probability of hepatopulmonary syndrome (LR = 4.3, EBM Box 28.1; see Chapter 8).

D. PATHOGENESIS

The increased volume of the clubbed digit is primarily due to increased amounts of vascular connective tissue,[27] although the cause of this fibrovascular proliferation is still debated. According to one hypothesis, clubbing results from large megakaryocytes and clumps of platelets that become trapped in the distal digits and then release growth factors, causing soft tissue growth.[28,29] Megakaryocytes do not normally appear in arterial blood but instead leave the bone marrow and travel in the systemic veins to the pulmonary capillaries, where they become trapped because of their large size (20 to 50 μm in diameter), eventually fragmenting into smaller platelets. In most patients with clubbing, the pulmonary capillaries are either damaged (e.g., as in many inflammatory and neoplastic pulmonary disorders) or a right-to-left shunt exists (e.g., as in congenital heart disease or the hepatopulmonary syndrome of cirrhosis), which allows the large megakaryocytes to travel freely through the lung into arterial blood and the distal digits, where they become wedged in the digital capillaries and release growth factors, causing fibrovascular proliferation and clubbing.

This hypothesis explains why clubbing accompanies endocarditis and why it is sometimes found unilaterally in the digits distal to an infected dialysis shunt. In both examples, platelet clumps are presumably released from the infected surface to travel to the digits, where they become embedded within capillaries and release growth factors.[28]

An alternative hypothesis (though not necessarily a contradictory one) proposes that clubbing stems from elevated levels of prostaglandin E2 (PGE_2). In families of patients with hereditary clubbing and osteoarthropathy, defective catabolism of PGE_2 causes high levels of PGE_2 to accumulate.[30]

II. Barrel Chest

A. THE FINDING

The normal chest is shaped like an oval cylinder, its anteroposterior diameter being less that its lateral diameter. The ratio of the anteroposterior to lateral diameter (called the *thoracic ratio*, *thoracic index*, or *chest index*) is normally about 0.70 to 0.75 in adults and increases as persons grow older. The upper normal limit is about 0.9.[31]

Barrel chest deformity refers to a chest whose transverse section is more round than oval. It is traditionally a finding of chronic obstructive lung disease (i.e, chronic bronchitis, emphysema). Most patients also have dorsal kyphosis, a prominent sternum, widened intercostal spaces, elevated clavicles, and a shortened neck.[31] According to traditional teachings, the thoracic ratio of these patients exceeds 0.9, presumably because overactive scalene and sternocleidomastoid muscles lift the upper ribs and sternum. (See the section on accessory muscle use.)

B. CLINICAL SIGNIFICANCE

Evidence linking the barrel chest deformity with chronic obstructive lung disease is conflicting. Two studies did find a significant correlation between the barrel chest deformity and more severe airflow obstruction,[32,33] although another two studies found no relationship between the two variables.[31,34] Additional problems with this physical sign are that the barrel chest is not specific for obstruction but also occurs in elderly persons without lung disease.[31] In some patients, the large anteroposterior dimension of the barrel chest is an illusion; the actual anteroposterior dimension is normal, but it appears to be abnormally large because it contrasts with an abnormally thin abdominal dimension caused by weight loss (see Fig. 28.2).[35]

In a single study, the presence of a barrel chest, defined either as clinician's global impression of barrel chest or more precisely as a thoracic ratio ≥0.9, modestly increased the probability of obstructive disease (LRs = 1.5 to 2.0, EBM Box 28.2).

III. Pursed Lip Breathing

A. THE FINDING

Many patients with chronic obstructive lung disease instinctively learn that pursing the lips during expiration reduces dyspnea. The exact cause of the relief of dyspnea is still debated. Pursed lip breathing significantly reduces the respiratory rate (from about 20 breaths/min to 12 to 15 breaths/min), increases tidal volume (by about 250 to 800 mL), decreases $PaCO_2$ (by 5%), and increases oxygen saturation (by 3%).[40-43] Dyspnea may diminish because there is less work of breathing (from slower rate), less expiratory airway collapse (the pressure drop across the lips,

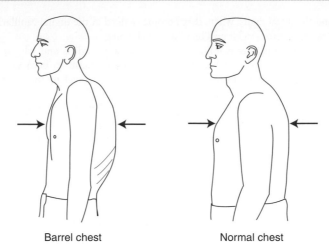

Barrel chest   Normal chest

Fig 28.2 Barrel chest deformity. In some patients, the "large" anteroposterior dimension of the barrel chest (*left*) is an illusion, because it is no bigger that the anteroposterior dimension of the normal chest (*right*). Instead, what strikes the clinician's eyes is the barrel chest's prominent dorsal kyphosis and marked contrast between the preserved anteroposterior chest dimension and the thin abdomen.

2 to 4 cm of water, provides continuous expiratory positive pressure), or recruitment of respiratory muscles in a way that is less fatiguing to the diaphragm.[40,41,44]

B. CLINICAL SIGNIFICANCE

In a study of 200 patients presenting for pulmonary function tests, the finding of pursed lip breathing increased the probability of chronic obstructive disease (LR = 2.7; EBM Box 28.2).

IV. Accessory Muscle Use

A. THE FINDING

The only muscle used in normal breathing is the diaphragm, which contracts during inspiration. Normal expiration is a passive process that relies on the elastic recoil of the lungs.[45] The term **accessory muscle use**, therefore, refers to the contraction of muscles other than the diaphragm during inspiration (usually the sternocleidomastoid and scalene muscles) or to the contraction of any muscle during expiration (primarily the abdominal oblique muscles). Accessory muscle use is a common finding in patients with chronic obstructive lung disease or respiratory muscle fatigue.

B. PATHOGENESIS

Contraction of the sternocleidomastoid and scalene muscles lifts the clavicles and first ribs, which helps expand the thorax of distressed patients, especially those with chronic obstructive lung disease whose flattened diaphragm generates only meager inspiratory movements. Contraction of the abdominal oblique muscles assists ventilation in two ways. In patients with obstructed airways, the abdominal muscles help expel air across the obstructed airways; in patients with respiratory muscle fatigue (e.g., amyotrophic lateral sclerosis), the abdominal muscles characteristically

| EBM BOX 28.2 | **Inspection of the Chest*** |

Finding (Reference)[†]	Sensitivity (%)	Specificity (%)	Likelihood Ratio[‡] if Finding Is Present	Absent
Chest wall appearance				
Barrel chest, detecting chronic obstructive lung disease[36]	65	58	1.5	0.6
AP/L chest diameter ratio ≥0.9, detecting chronic obstructive lung disease[36]	31	84	2.0	NS
Pursed lip breathing				
Pursed lip breathing, detecting chronic obstructive lung disease[36]	58	78	2.7	0.5
Accessory muscle use				
Scalene/sternocleidomastoid muscle use, detecting chronic obstructive lung disease (COPD)[36]	39	88	**3.3**	0.7
Scalene/sternocleidomastoid muscle use in patients with amyotrophic lateral sclerosis (ALS), detecting respiratory neuromuscular weakness[37]	81	83	NS	**0.2**
Accessory muscle use, detecting pulmonary embolism[38]	17	89	NS	NS
Retractions and nasal flaring				
Intercostal retractions, detecting acidosis[39]	58	74	2.2	0.6
Suprasternal retractions, detecting acidosis[39]	33	92	**4.0**	0.7
Nasal flaring, detecting acidosis[39]	58	87	**4.6**	0.5

**Diagnostic standard*: for *chronic obstructive lung disease*, FFV_1/FVC <0.7; for *respiratory neuromuscular weakness*, transdiaphragmatic sniff pressure <70 cm H_2O; for *pulmonary embolism*, pulmonary angiogram; for *acidosis*, pH <7.35 (most had respiratory acidosis).

[†]*Definition of findings*: for *accessory muscle use* in patients with amyotrophic lateral sclerosis, the patients were examined supine; for *retractions* and *nasal flaring*, see the text.

[‡]Likelihood ratio (LR) if finding present = positive LR; LR if finding absent = negative LR.

AP/lat, Ratio of anterior-posterior chest dimension to lateral dimension; FEV_1, forced expiratory volume in 1 second; *FVC*, forced vital capacity; *NS*, not significant.

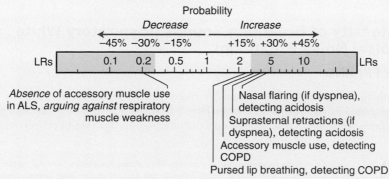

INSPECTION OF THE CHEST

Probability

Decrease — *Increase*

−45% −30% −15%   +15% +30% +45%

LRs   0.1   0.2   0.5   1   2   5   10   LRs

Absence of accessory muscle use in ALS, *arguing against* respiratory muscle weakness

Nasal flaring (if dyspnea), detecting acidosis
Suprasternal retractions (if dyspnea), detecting acidosis
Accessory muscle use, detecting COPD
Pursed lip breathing, detecting COPD

contract right at the moment expiration ends, to compress the lungs so that the early part of the subsequent inspiration can occur passively.[46]

C. CLINICAL SIGNIFICANCE

Accessory muscle use—defined as inspiratory contraction of the sternocleidomastoid and scalene muscles—is associated with severe obstructive disease.[32,34,47–49] Over 90% of patients hospitalized with acute exacerbations of chronic obstructive lung disease use accessory muscles, but by hospital day 5, less than half do.[50] In one study, patients whose clavicle lifted more than 5 mm during inspiration identified patients with more severe obstructive disease (mean forced expiratory volume in one second [FEV_1] = 0.6 L vs. 1.5 L, p < 0.001),[47] * and in patients referred for pulmonary function tests, accessory muscle use increases the probability of chronic obstructive disease (LR = 3.3, EBM Box 28.2).

Inspection of accessory muscles also provides useful information in patients with amyotrophic lateral sclerosis. When these patients are supine, the *absence* of sternocleidomastoid and scalene contractions decreases the probability of respiratory neuromuscular weakness (LR = 0.2).

Accessory muscle use is less specific in the evaluation of acute dyspnea, and in one study of patients with suspected pulmonary embolism, the finding had no diagnostic value (EBM Box 27.2).

V. Chest Wall Retractions and Nasal Flaring

A. THE FINDING

In patients with severe dyspnea, the accessory muscles may contract so vigorously during inspiration that the volume of the expanding bony chest exceeds the flow of air into the lungs, causing the softer parts of the chest wall to briefly draw inward, or "retract." Such inspiratory retractions are typically most conspicuous between the ribs (**intercostal retractions**) or just above the suprasternal notch (**suprasternal retractions**). In addition, some dyspneic patients have **nasal flaring**, an inspiratory widening of the nostrils, an action that presumably improves the flow of air.[39]

B. CLINICAL SIGNIFICANCE

In one study of 212 adults presenting to the emergency department with significant dyspnea, nasal flaring (LR = 4.6; EBM Box 28.2), suprasternal retractions (LR = 4), and intercostal retractions (LR = 2.2) all increased probability that the patient will have acidosis on arterial blood gas testing (arterial pH < 7.35). The acidosis in these patients was usually respiratory acidosis (with hypercapnia), a finding that eventually led to mechanical ventilation in 71% of acidotic patients.[39]

VI. Intensity of Breathing Sounds (Inspiratory White Noise; Noisy Breathing)

A. THE FINDING

The breathing of normal persons is inaudible more than a few centimeters from the mouth, unless the person is sighing, panting, or gasping.[52] In three clinical settings, breathing sometimes becomes very noisy and is easily heard a distance from the bedside: in patients with lower

---

*FEV_1 is forced expiratory volume in one second, a measure of ventilatory capacity. Normal values are 3 to 3.8 L.[51] The FEV_1 is abnormally low in obstructive lung disease and restrictive lung disease, dyspnea first appearing in these conditions when the FEV_1 falls below 2.5 L. An FEV_1 less than 1 L in chronic obstructive lung disease indicates severe disease.

airways obstruction, who may have audible *expiratory* wheezing (see Chapter 30), in patients with upper airway obstruction, who may have *inspiratory* stridor (see Chapter 30), and in patients with chronic bronchitis or asthma, who may have *inspiratory* white noise.[52]

White noise is an acoustical term. Unlike wheezing and stridor, white noise lacks a musical pitch and therefore resembles more the static of a radio tuned between stations. In patients with chronic bronchitis and asthma, the loud inspiratory white noise heard at the patient's bedside without the stethoscope often contrasts sharply with the quiet inspiratory sounds heard through the stethoscope during auscultation (see Chapter 30).

B. PATHOGENESIS

Inspiratory white noise results from air turbulence caused by narrowed central airways,[53] a conclusion based on the observation that the sounds diminish after the patient receives effective bronchodilator treatment (which increases the patient's FEV_1) or breathes a mixture oxygen and helium (a gas mixture that reduces turbulence).[53] Inspiratory white noise is not a feature of emphysema, presumably because the inspiratory caliber of the central airways in these patients is normal.[53]

C. CLINICAL SIGNIFICANCE

Inspiratory white noise is a feature of chronic bronchitis and asthma, not emphysema. The intensity of white noise in patients with asthma and chronic bronchitis correlates inversely with the patient's FEV_1 (r = −0.60 to −0.64).[53]

References may be accessed online at *Elsevier eBooks for Practicing Clinicians.*

Palpation and Percussion of the Chest

PALPATION

I. Introduction

Palpation of the chest is limited because the bony rib cage conceals many abnormalities of the underlying lungs. The traditional reasons to palpate the chest are to detect the following signs: (1) chest wall tenderness or masses, (2) pleural friction rubs, (3) bronchial fremitus, (4) abnormal respiratory excursion, and (5) asymmetric tactile fremitus. Bronchial fremitus is an inspiratory vibratory sensation felt in some patients with airway secretions. Respiratory excursion is assessed while the patient breathes in and out, either by simultaneously palpating symmetric areas of the chest or measuring the changing circumference with a tape measure. According to traditional teachings, chest excursion is reduced bilaterally in chronic airflow obstruction and neuromuscular disease (see Chapter 33) and unilaterally in pleural effusion or consolidation.

II. Tactile Fremitus

A. THE FINDING

Tactile fremitus (vocal fremitus) is the vibration felt by the clinician's hand resting on the chest wall of a patient who is speaking or singing.

B. TECHNIQUE

To elicit the sign, the patient usually says "one-two-three" or "ninety-nine" repeatedly and evenly while the clinician compares symmetric areas of the chest. Some early German physical diagnosticians used the word *neun-und-neuzig* (German for "ninety-nine") to elicit vocal fremitus, prompting modern English-speaking authors to suggest that the "oy" sound is necessary to elicit the finding (e.g., "toy boat" or "Toyota", to mimic the vowel sound in the German word *neun-und-neunzig*). This is incorrect, however, and the early German diagnosticians just as often used other words, such as "one, one, one" (*eins, eins, eins*) and "one, two, three" (*eins, zwei, drei*),[1-3] or had their patients sing or scream to elicit the finding.[3]

C. FINDING

Vocal fremitus is more prominent in men than women because men have lower-pitched voices, which conduct more easily though lung tissue than do higher-pitched voices. (See the section on pathogenesis of vocal resonance in Chapter 30.) Therefore, tactile fremitus may be absent in some healthy persons, especially those with high-pitched or soft voices or those with thick chest walls (which insulate the hand from the vibrating lung). Consequently, only *asymmetric* tactile fremitus is an abnormal finding. According to traditional teachings, fremitus is asymmetrically diminished whenever air, fluid, or tumor pushes the lung away from the chest wall (*unilateral* pneumothorax, pleural effusion, neoplasm) and is asymmetrically increased when there is consolidation of the underlying lung (i.e., *unilateral* pneumonia).

The pathogenesis of tactile fremitus is discussed in Chapter 30 (section on vocal resonance).

III. Clinical Significance

A. CHEST EXPANSION

Just as is traditionally taught, the finding of asymmetric chest wall expansion increases the probability of unilateral pneumonia in patients with cough and fever (the side with pneumonia moves less, likelihood ratio [LR] = 44.1, EBM Box 29.1), and it increases the probability of underlying pleural effusion in hospitalized patients with respiratory complaints (LR = 8.1). After intubation of a patient, asymmetric chest wall expansion increases the probability of right mainstem bronchus intubation (LR = 15.8).

Nonetheless, the opposite finding—*symmetric* chest expansion—does not change the probability of either pneumonia or endobronchial intubation, although it does decrease the probability of underlying pleural effusion (LR = 0.3). The physical examination should never be used as the sole tool confirming placement of an endotracheal tube after intubation.

B. TACTILE FREMITUS

In a study of 278 patients hospitalized with respiratory complaints, the finding of asymmetric diminished tactile fremitus significantly increased the probability of an underlying pleural effusion (LR = 5.7; EBM Box 29.1); symmetric fremitus decreased the probability of effusion (LR = 0.2).

C. CHEST WALL TENDERNESS

According to traditional teachings, the finding of chest wall tenderness in a patient with chest complaints suggests benign disease, commonly referred to as **costochondritis**. Even so, this conclusion is accurate only in patients with acute atraumatic chest pain, in whom chest wall

| EBM BOX 29.1 | Diagnostic Accuracy of Palpation of the Chest* |

Finding (Reference)	Sensitivity (%)	Specificity (%)	Likelihood Ratio[†] if Finding Is	
			Present	Absent
Asymmetric chest expansion				
Detecting pneumonia in patients with acute cough[4]	5	100	**44.1**	NS
Detecting pleural effusion in hospitalized patients with respiratory complaints[5]	74	91	**8.1**	0.3
Asymmetric chest wall movements after intubation, detecting right mainstem bronchus intubation[6,7]	32–50	98	**15.8**	0.6
Diminished tactile fremitus				
Detecting pleural effusion[5]	82	86	**5.7**	0.2
Chest wall tenderness				
Detecting pneumonia in patients with acute cough[8]	5	96	NS	NS
Detecting pulmonary embolism in patients with pleuritic chest pain[9,10]	11–17	79–80	NS	NS
Detecting coronary artery disease in outpatients with chronic chest pain[11–14]	1–69	16–97	0.8	NS
Detecting myocardial infarction in patients with acute nontraumatic chest pain[15–19]	3–15	51–83	**0.3**	1.2

*Diagnostic standard: For pleural effusion, chest radiograph, for pulmonary embolism, coronary artery disease, and myocardial infarction, see Chapters 34 and 49.
[†]Likelihood ratio (LR) if finding present = positive LR; LR if finding absent = negative LR.
NS, Not significant.

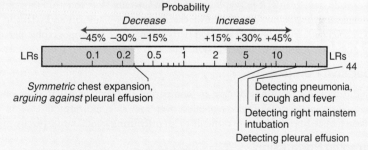

ASYMMETRIC CHEST EXPANSION

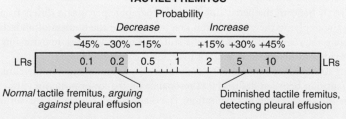

TACTILE FREMITUS

tenderness decreases the probability of myocardial infarction (LR = 0.3, EBM Box 29.1). In contrast, in studies of pneumonia, chronic coronary artery disease, and pulmonary embolism, the finding has little diagnostic value, occurring just as often in serious disease as in benign disorders (LRs 0.8 or not significant, EBM Box 29.1).

PERCUSSION

I. Introduction

In 1761, after studying patients and cadavers at the Spanish Hospital in Vienna for 7 years, Leopold Auenbrugger published a 95-page booklet containing the first detailed description of chest percussion.[20] His work was largely ignored for half a century, until Corvisart (physician to Napoleon) translated it into French and taught the technique to his students, including Laennec, the subsequent inventor of the stethoscope.[21] The discovery of percussion was a major diagnostic advance because, for the first time, clinicians could reliably distinguish empyema from tuberculosis and other pneumonias.[21] Until the discovery of roentgen rays in 1895, percussion and auscultation were the only methods to investigate and define diseases of the lungs during the patient's life.

II. Technique

A. DIRECT VS. INDIRECT METHOD

In the direct method, the percussion blow lands directly on the body wall (the method of Auenbrugger and Laennec). In the indirect method, the blow falls instead on an intervening substance, called a pleximeter, placed against the body wall. Historically, pleximeters were made of ivory or wood, or a coin was used, although today most clinicians use the middle finger of their left hand.

B. TYPES OF PERCUSSION

There are three ways to percuss the patient: (1) comparative percussion (the original method of Auenbrugger and Laennec), (2) topographic percussion (invented by Piorry of France in 1828),[22,23] and (3) auscultatory percussion (introduced by the Americans Camman and Clark in 1840).[21,24] Today, most clinicians use the indirect method with comparative and topographic percussion and the direct method with auscultatory percussion.

1. Comparative Percussion

Comparative percussion identifies disease by comparing the right and left sides of the chest. Prominent dullness or unusual hyperresonance over one side indicates disease in that part. Bilateral disease, by definition, is more difficult to identify using comparative percussion.

2. Topographic Percussion

Topographic percussion attributes any dullness in the chest or abdomen to airless intrathoracic tissue lying directly beneath the percussion blow. Topographic percussion differs from comparative percussion by implying the clinician can precisely outline the borders of underlying organs and then measure their span. The technique is still used today to measure excursion of the diaphragm (and to identify an enlarged heart or liver; see Chapters 37 and 51).

When using topographic percussion to determine diaphragm excursion, the clinician locates the point of transition between dullness and resonance on the lower posterior chest, first during full inspiration and then during full expiration. The diaphragm excursion is the vertical distance between these two points. The reported normal excursion of healthy persons ranges from 3 to 6 cm (for comparison, the corresponding excursion on the chest radiograph is about 5 to 7 cm in normal persons and 2 to 3 cm in patients with lung disease).[21,25,26]

3. Auscultatory Percussion

Auscultatory percussion was introduced to further refine the goals of topographic percussion.[24] Instead of listening to sounds as they resonate off the chest into the surrounding room, the clinician using auscultatory percussion places the stethoscope on the body wall and listens through it to the sounds transmitted by nearby percussive blows.

Since the mid-1800s, auscultatory percussion of the chest has repeatedly fallen out of favor and then resurfaced as a "new sign."[21] In the most recent version of auscultatory percussion of the chest, introduced in 1974, the clinician taps lightly over the manubrium and listens over the posterior part of the chest with the stethoscope.[27,28] Using this technique, the clinician should find identical sounds at corresponding locations of the two sides of the chest; a note of decreased intensity on one side supposedly indicates ipsilateral disease between the tapping finger and stethoscope.

The technique of using auscultatory percussion to detect pleural fluid, first developed in 1927,[29] is slightly different. The clinician places his stethoscope on the posterior chest of the seated patient, 3 cm below the twelfth rib, and percusses the posterior chest from apex to base. At some point the normal dull note changes to an unusually loud note: if this occurs with strokes above the twelfth rib, the test is abnormal, indicating pleural fluid.[30]

C. THE PERCUSSION BLOW

1. Force

Each percussion blow should strike the same part of the pleximeter with identical force, and the pleximeter finger should be applied with the same force and orientation when comparing right and left sides. Consistent technique is important because both the percussion force and the pleximeter govern the percussion sound produced. Lighter strokes produce sounds that are duller than those produced by stronger strokes. Lifting the pleximeter finger, even slightly, can transform a resonant note into a dull one.

Even though a consistent technique is important, the force and speed of percussion blows vary 3-fold among different clinicians,[31] which probably explains why interobserver agreement for topographic percussion is poor compared with that for other physical findings (see Chapter 5).

2. Rapid Withdrawal of Plexor

The traditional teaching is that the plexor finger should be promptly withdrawn after a blow, mimicking the action of a piano key striking a string. The only study of this found that clinicians could not distinguish the note created by a rapid withdrawal from one in which the plexor finger lightly rested on the pleximeter after the blow.[32]

III. The Finding

A. PERCUSSION SOUNDS

There are three percussion sounds—**tympany** (normally heard over the abdomen), **resonance** (heard over normal lung), and **dullness** (heard over the liver or thigh) (Fig. 29.1). Tympany differs from resonance and dullness because it contains vibrations of a dominant frequency, which allows the clinician to actually identify its musical pitch. Resonance and dullness, in contrast, are "noise" in an acoustical sense, consisting of a jumble of frequencies that prevent identification of

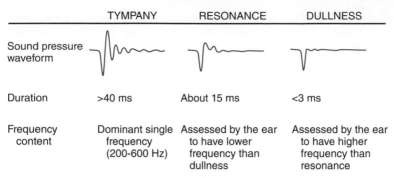

	TYMPANY	RESONANCE	DULLNESS
Sound pressure waveform			
Duration	>40 ms	About 15 ms	<3 ms
Frequency content	Dominant single frequency (200-600 Hz)	Assessed by the ear to have lower frequency than dullness	Assessed by the ear to have higher frequency than resonance

Fig. 29.1   The percussion sounds. In the older literature, synonyms for resonance were "full," "clear," "distinct"; synonyms for dullness were "empty," "not distinct," and "thigh" sound. Adapted from references 21 and 33.

a specific musical pitch. The three sound characteristics that distinguish resonance from dullness are intensity, duration, and frequency content: Resonance is louder and longer and contains more low-frequency energy.[21,33] Of these three sound characteristics, clinicians appreciate most easily that resonance is louder than dullness.

Some clinicians take advantage of resonance being louder than dullness and apply a technique called threshold percussion, in which percussion blows are so light that dull areas produce no sound. As the blows move along the body wall with precisely the same amount of force, a note abruptly appears the moment the blow encounters a resonant area. An old adage in percussion, attributed to Weil, is that it is much easier to distinguish "something from nothing" than to distinguish "more from less."[21]

B. SENSE OF RESISTANCE

All great teachers of percussion have emphasized that the tactile sense in the pleximeter finger provides as much information as the audible notes. Dull areas, according to these teachers, move less or offer more resistance than resonant areas (thus earning pleural effusion the descriptor "stony dullness"). Experiments using light-weight accelerometers taped to the pleximeter finger confirm that dull areas do move less than resonant areas.[34]

C. GLOSSARY OF ADDITIONAL PERCUSSION TERMS

Historically, the vocabulary of clinical percussion was diverse. Some of the more commonly used terms appear below.

1. Skodaic Resonance

Skodaic resonance is a hyperresonant note produced by percussion of the chest above a pleural effusion. The cause of this finding is unknown. Skodaic resonance was originally described by Josef Skoda,[35] a champion of topographic percussion and the first to apply the principles of physics to percussion.

2. Grocco Triangle

The **Grocco triangle** is a right-angled triangle of dullness found over the posterior region of the chest *opposite* a large pleural effusion. The horizontal side of the triangle follows the diaphragm for several centimeters; the vertical side lies over the spinous processes but usually ends below the top level of the effusion.[21] This finding was originally described by Koranyi (Hungary, 1897) and later by Grocco (Italy, 1902) and Rauchfuss (Germany, 1903).

3. Metallic Resonance (Amphoric Resonance; Coin Test)

Metallic resonance is a pure tympanitic sound containing very high frequencies, found over large superficial pulmonary cavities or pneumothoraces.[35,36] Flicking the tense cheek while holding the mouth open mimics the sound. The sound was best elicited with a hard plexor and pleximeter (e.g., 2 coins) and is best perceived through the stethoscope or with the examiner's ear near the patient's chest.[21]

4. Krönig Isthmus

Krönig isthmus is a narrow band of resonance over each lung apex that lies between the dullness from the neck and the dullness from the shoulder muscles. Diseases of the lung apex, such as tuberculosis, supposedly reduced the width of the band.[21] Georg Krönig (Germany) described the finding in 1889.[37]

5. Cracked-Pot Resonance

Cracked-pot resonance is a percussion sound over superficial tubercular cavities, mimicked by pressing the palms together and hitting the back of one hand against the knee.[35,38] To detect the sound in patients, the clinician delivers a strong percussion blow and listens near the patient's open mouth.[2,39] Although the sound was traditionally attributed to the sudden efflux of air through bronchi communicating with a tubercular cavity, the only published pathologic study found no bronchial communication in 11 patients with this sound.[40]

IV. Pathogenesis

A. TOPOGRAPHIC PERCUSSION VS. CAGE RESONANCE THEORY

From the earliest days of percussion, two opposing theories have explained the genesis of percussion sounds: the topographic percussion theory and the cage resonance theory. The topographic percussion theory argued that only the physical characteristics of the soft tissues directly beneath the percussion blow controlled whether resonance or dullness was produced. This theory emphasized that the body wall itself contributed little to the resulting sound but acted merely to convey the vibrations from the underlying tissues (much like a diaphragm in a microphone transmits the sound vibrations imparted to it). A fundamental tenet of the topographic percussion theory was the several centimeter rule, advanced by Weil in 1880,[41] which stated that the percussion stroke penetrated only the most superficial 4 to 6 cm of tissue, and only anatomic abnormalities in this layer influenced the sound produced.

In contrast, the cage resonance theory argued that the percussion sound reflected the ease with which the body wall vibrates, which in turn was influenced by many variables, including the strength of the stroke, the condition and state of the body wall, and the underlying organs. Advocates of the cage resonance theory argued that precise topographic percussion was impossible because underlying organs or disease could cause dullness to occur at distant sites.

The topographic percussion theory became very popular—largely through the persuasive efforts of renowned clinical teachers, including Piorry, Skoda, Mueller, and Mueller's pupil, Ralph Major, who wrote one of the most popular American physical diagnosis textbooks.[1] Nonetheless, the evidence cited to support this theory and the several centimeter rule was meager and of uncertain relevance[21]; it included only a few experiments with cadavers[41] and some sound recordings of exenterated lung slices as they were being percussed.[42]

In contrast, considerable evidence supports the cage resonance theory.

1. Analysis of Sound Recordings

The percussion sound contains more frequencies than can be explained by vibrations of just the area of the body wall percussed.[34,43–45] Areas of the body wall distant to the blow must also vibrate and contribute to the sound.

2. Condition and State of the Body Wall

External pressure on the chest—from a pillow, a stretcher, or an extra hand placed near the point of percussion—impedes chest wall motion and dampens the percussion note.[36,46]

Pressure against the inner wall of the chest of cadavers also causes dullness, even in areas of the body wall distant from where the pressure is applied.[36] The best clinical example of the distant effects of internal pressure is the Grocco triangle, a right-angled triangle of dullness found over the posterior region of the chest *opposite* a large pleural effusion (see earlier discussion on Grocco triangle). The Grocco triangle proves that pressure on the chest wall at one point (e.g., from pleural fluid) may cause dullness at sites distant to that pressure (i.e., over the opposite chest). Even in patients without pleural fluid, external pressure on one side of the posterior chest from a hand or water bottle will produce the Grocco triangle on the opposite chest.[47,48]

Heavier patients have larger liver spans than patients who weigh less,[49] not because the livers of heavier patients are larger, but instead because the excess subcutaneous fat influences the cage resonance and dampens the vibrations, resulting in more dullness and larger spans.

3. The Strength of the Percussion Blow

The strength of the blow influences whether resonance or dullness is produced, especially near areas of the body wall marking the transition between resonance and dullness. For example, in percussion of the liver, the span of the liver is about 3 cm smaller when using strong strokes than it is when using light strokes (see Chapter 51).[49–51] This occurs because the heavy stroke, when located near where the liver touches the body wall, more easily generates the vibrations necessary for the resonant note, whereas the light stroke is insufficient until further removed. These findings contradict the assertion of topographic percussionists, who taught that stronger blows penetrated tissues more deeply than softer ones; if this were true, percussion of the liver with heavy strokes should produce a larger span than with light strokes (because heavier strokes would detect the dome of the liver, which is removed from the body wall).

B. AUSCULTATORY PERCUSSION

The advocates of auscultatory percussion believe that sound waves travel directly from the tapping finger through the lung to the stethoscope and are altered along the way by diseased tissue. It is much more likely, however, that these sounds are conducted circumferentially in the chest wall, for several reasons. (1) The technique fails to detect the heart, which should render some notes of the left chest more dull if sound waves traveled directly to the stethoscope. (2) Sound recordings during auscultatory percussion are the same whether the patient breathes room air or a mixture of helium and oxygen.[52] Because sound characteristics depend on the gas density of the conducting medium, which is different for the two gas mixtures, it is unlikely sound travels through the lung. (3) The characteristics of the sound change during the Valsalva and Mueller maneuvers, which increase tension in the chest wall but do not alter the underlying lung.[52] (4) Contour maps reveal that the loudest sounds during auscultatory percussion appear over bony prominences, such as the scapula, indicating that the sound produced depends on the contour of the chest wall. The intervening lung contributes less to the sound heard because these sound maps do not change even when there is a large underlying tumor.[53]

V. Clinical Significance

A. COMPARATIVE PERCUSSION

EBM Box 29.2 shows that asymmetric dullness is a helpful though infrequent finding that increases the probability of pneumonia in patients with fever and cough (LR = 3.6), for underlying abnormalities on the chest radiograph of unselected patients (LR = 3), and for pleural effusion in hospitalized patients with respiratory complaints (LR = 4.8). In these studies, percussion detected all large pleural effusions (sensitivity 100%), but very few consolidations (sensitivity 0% to 15%) and no intraparenchymal nodules or granulomata. The presence of normal resonance decreases significantly the probability of underlying pleural effusion (LR = 0.1) but does not change the probability of other significant lung pathology.

In chronic smokers, hyperresonance of the chest is a valuable finding increasing the probability of chronic airflow obstruction (LR = 7.3, EBM Box 29.2).

B. TOPOGRAPHIC PERCUSSION OF THE DIAPHRAGM

In patients with lung disease, clinicians usually overestimate the actual movements of the diaphragm and differ from the chest film by 1 to 3 cm.[25,65] The correlation between actual and percussed movements is poor in the only study of this finding (r = 0.14 to 0.42, not significant half the time).[25] Another study showed that a percussed diaphragm excursion of less than 2 cm is an infrequent and unreliable diagnostic sign of chronic obstructive lung disease (LRs not significant, EBM Box 29.2).[63]

C. AUSCULTATORY PERCUSSION

Studies of auscultatory percussion have widely varying results, usually showing the technique has greater sensitivity than comparative percussion but also lower specificity. Overall, the pooled results show that this technique is an unreliable diagnostic sign (both positive and negative LRs not significant; see EBM Box 29.2).

Like conventional percussion, auscultatory percussion identifies most pleural effusions (sensitivity 58% to 96%, see EBM Box 29.2). A positive result (see the section on auscultatory percussion for definition of technique) significantly increases the probability of pleural effusion (LR = 8.3).

EBM BOX 29.2	Diagnostic Accuracy of Percussion of the Chest*			
	Sensitivity	Specificity	Likelihood Ratio‡ if Finding Is	
Finding (Reference)†	(%)	(%)	Present	Absent
Comparative percussion				
Percussion dullness				
Detecting pneumonia in patients with fever and cough[4,54-59]	4–26	82–99	3.6	NS
Detecting any abnormality on chest radiograph[60-62]	8–15	94–98	3.0	NS
Detecting pleural effusion in patients with respiratory complaints[5]	89	81	4.8	0.1
Hyperresonance				
Detecting chronic airflow obstruction[63,64]	21–33	94–98	7.3	0.8

Continued

| EBM BOX 29.2 | Diagnostic Accuracy of Percussion of the Chest*—Cont'd |

Finding (Reference)[†]	Sensitivity (%)	Specificity (%)	Likelihood Ratio[‡] if Finding Is	
			Present	Absent
Topographic percussion				
Diaphragm excursion <2 cm				
Detecting chronic airflow obstruction[63]	13	98	NS	NS
Auscultatory percussion				
Abnormal dullness				
Detecting any abnormality on chest radiograph[60–62]	16–69	74–88	NS	NS
Detecting pleural fluid[5,30]	58–96	85–95	**8.3**	NS

*Diagnostic standard: for *pneumonia* or *pleural effusion*, infiltrate or effusion on chest radiograph; for *chronic airflow obstruction*, FEV$_1$ <60% predicted or the FEV$_1$/FVC ratio <0.6–0.7.
†Definition of findings: for *abnormal dullness during auscultatory percussion for chest radiograph abnormalities*, asymmetric dullness, with stethoscope on posterior chest and while directly percussing sternum anteriorly; for *abnormal dullness during auscultatory percussion for pleural fluid*, transition to unusually loud note above 12th rib posteriorly in midclavicular line, with stethoscope 3 cm below 12th rib and while directly percussing posterior chest from apex to base.[30]
‡Likelihood ratio (LR) if finding present = positive LR; LR if finding absent = negative LR.
COPD, Chronic obstructive pulmonary disease; *FEV$_1$*, forced expiratory volume in 1 second; *FVC*, forced vital capacity; *NS*, not significant.

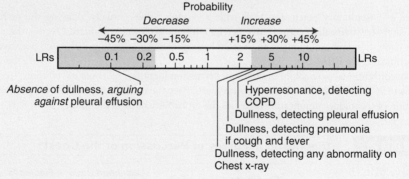

PERCUSSION OF THE CHEST

References may be accessed online at *Elsevier eBooks for Practicing Clinicians.*

Auscultation of the Lungs

- In patients with chronic dyspnea, *symmetric* diminished breath sounds increase probability of chronic obstructive lung disease. *Unilateral* diminished breath sounds increase probability of underlying pleural effusion or, in patients with cough and fever, pneumonia.
- In patients with cough and fever, egophony and bronchial breath sounds increase probability of pneumonia.
- Crackles increase probability of interstitial fibrosis in asbestos workers. In patients with cough and fever, crackles increase probability of pneumonia. Early inspiratory crackles are characteristic of severe chronic airflow obstructive disease.
- The absence of crackles decreases probability of "honeycombing" fibrosis on computed tomography.
- Unforced wheezing increases probability of obstructive lung disease, although the amplitude of wheezing correlates poorly with severity of obstruction.
- The inspiratory squawk increases probability of hypersensitivity pneumonitis.

The three categories of auscultatory findings of the lungs are breath sounds, vocal resonance (i.e., the sound of the patient's voice through the stethoscope), and adventitious sounds (i.e., sounds other than breath sounds or vocal resonance). Almost all of the findings discussed in this chapter were originally described in 1819 by Laennec, in his masterpiece *A Treatise on the Disease of the Chest.*[1]

I. Breath Sounds

A. FINDING

1. Vesicular Versus Bronchial Breath Sounds

There are two types of breath sounds: (1) vesicular breath sounds, which are normally heard over the posterior chest, and (2) bronchial breath sounds, which are normally heard over the trachea and right apex. These sounds are distinguished by their timing, intensity, and pitch (Fig. 30.1). Vesicular sounds are mostly inspiratory sounds that have a soft, breathy quality, which Laennec likened to the sound of leaves rustling in a gentle breeze. Bronchial sounds have a prominent expiratory component and much harsher quality, sounding like air blowing forcibly through a tube. (Hence, they are sometimes called tubular breath sounds.)

Bronchial breath sounds are abnormal when they occur over the posterior or lateral chest (especially the lower parts). According to traditional teachings, which in turn are based on postmortem examinations, bronchial breath sounds occur in these locations only if solid, collapsed

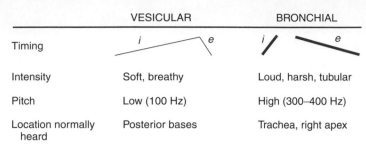

	VESICULAR	BRONCHIAL
Timing		
Intensity	Soft, breathy	Loud, harsh, tubular
Pitch	Low (100 Hz)	High (300–400 Hz)
Location normally heard	Posterior bases	Trachea, right apex

Fig. 30.1   Comparison of vesicular and bronchial breath sounds. In vesicular sounds (*left*), inspiration is longer than expiration, and there is no gap between inspiration and expiration. In bronchial sounds (*right*), expiration is longer than inspiration and there is a conspicuously audible gap between inspiration and expiration. Based upon references 2–6.

or consolidated lung is contiguous with the chest wall and extends some distance toward the hilum.[7-9] The usual causes are pneumonia and pleural effusion (large pleural effusions presumably compress the underlying lung just enough to alter its acoustic properties).[10]

2. Breath Sound Score

One important feature of vesicular breath sounds is their intensity, which can be graded using a scoring system developed by Pardee.[11] According to this system, the clinician listens sequentially over six locations on the patient's chest: bilaterally over the upper anterior portion of the chest, in the midaxillae, and at the posterior bases. At each site, the clinician grades the *inspiratory* sound as absent (0 points), barely audible (1 point), faint but definitely heard (2 points), normal (3 points), or louder than normal (4 points). The patient's total score may range from 0 (absent breath sounds) to 24 (very loud breath sounds at all 6 locations).

B. PATHOGENESIS

1. Vesicular Sounds

a. Origin

The *inspiratory* component of vesicular breath sounds originates in the peripheral portions of the lung near where the stethoscope is placed. It does not represent simple filtration of tracheal sounds by the intervening inflated lung. The *expiratory* component of vesicular sounds probably originates in more proximal, larger airways.[12] Several lines of evidence support these statements.

(1) In experiments performed with sheep's and calf's lungs over a century ago, Bullar kept the airways of both lungs patent but rhythmically inflated only one of the two lungs using negative pressure.[13] He showed that vesicular sounds occurred only if the lung contiguous to the stethoscope filled with air; if it remained airless, it simply transmitted the upper airway bronchial sounds.

(2) The intensity of the inspiratory component of breath sounds, corrected for flow rate at the mouth, is approximately proportional to regional ventilation.[14]

(3) The inspiratory component of vesicular sounds remains the same as the stethoscope is moved progressively from the upper to lower posterior chest, although the expiratory component becomes softer.[15]

(4) Vesicular sounds contain low-frequency components lacking in tracheal sounds. These low-frequency components cannot be reproduced in experiments interposing inflated lung between the trachea and stethoscope.[2-4]

b. Intensity

The intensity of vesicular sounds is proportional to the flow rate of air at the mouth, which in turn depends on the patient's effort and ventilatory capacity.[11,16,17] Breath sounds are thus louder if a normal person breathes hard after exercise, and they are faint if obstructive lung disease diminishes flow rates.[18] Breath sounds are also reduced when air or fluid is interposed between the chest wall and lung, as in patients with pneumothorax or pleural effusion.

2. Bronchial Sounds

Bronchial breath sounds originate in larger, proximal airways. They are normally heard over the right upper chest posteriorly but not over the left upper chest, because the trachea is contiguous with the right lung near the upper thoracic vertebrae but separated from the left lung by most of the mediastinum.[19] The glottis is not necessary to the sound, because bronchial sounds may occur in patients after laryngectomy or after intubation.[20] The pathogenesis of bronchial breath sounds in pneumonia and pleural effusion is discussed later in the section "pathogenesis" (of vocal resonance).

C. CLINICAL SIGNIFICANCE

1. Breath Sound Intensity

A breath sound score of 9 or less greatly increases the probability of chronic airflow obstruction (likelihood ratio [LR] = 10.2, EBM Box 30.1) and a score of 16 or more greatly decreases the probability (LR = 0.1). The breath sound score is superior to the clinician's "overall impression" of breath sound intensity in diagnosing chronic airflow obstruction (LR = 3.5 for overall impression of "diminished" breath sounds and LR = 0.5 for "normal or increased" breath sounds, EBM Box 30.1).

EBM BOX 30.1	Breath Sounds and Vocal Resonance*			
			Likelihood Ratio[‡] if Finding Is	
Finding (Reference)[†]	Sensitivity (%)	Specificity (%)	Present	Absent
Breath sound score				
Detecting chronic airflow obstruction[11,16]				
≤9	23–46	96–97	10.2	...
10–12	34–63	...	3.6	...
13–15	11–16	...	NS	...
≥16	3–10	33–34	0.1	...
Diminished breath sounds				
Detecting chronic airflow obstruction[21–25]	29–82	63–96	3.5	0.5
Detecting pleural effusion in hospitalized patients[26]	88	83	5.2	0.1
Detecting underlying pleural effusion in mechanically ventilated patients[27,28]	34–42	84–90	3.0	0.7
Detecting asthma during methacholine challenge testing[29]	78	81	4.2	0.3
Detecting pneumonia in patients with cough and fever[30–39]	7–60	73–98	2.4	0.8
Asymmetric breath sounds after intubation				
Detecting right mainstem bronchus intubation[40–43]	28–83	88–98	12.8	0.5
Bronchial breath sounds				
Detecting pneumonia in patients with cough and fever[30,38]	14–19	94–96	3.3	0.9

(continued)

EBM BOX 30.1	Breath Sounds and Vocal Resonance*—Cont'd

Finding (Reference)[†]	Sensitivity (%)	Specificity (%)	Likelihood Ratio[‡] if Finding Is	
			Present	Absent
Egophony				
Detecting pneumonia in patients with cough and fever[30,32,44]	4–16	96–99	4.1	NS
Diminished vocal resonance				
Detecting pleural effusion in hospitalized patients[26]	76	88	6.5	0.3

*Diagnostic standard: for *chronic airflow obstruction*, FEV_1 <40% predicted (breath sound score) or FEV_1/FVC (%) ratio <0.6–0.7 (diminished breath sounds); for *underlying pleural effusion*, chest radiography or (in mechanically ventilated) computed tomography or ultrasonography; for *asthma*, FEV_1 decreases by ≥20% during methacholine challenge; for *pneumonia*, infiltrate on chest radiograph; for *right mainstem intubation*, chest radiograph[40] or direct endoscopic visualization.[41–43]

†Definition of findings: for *breath sound score*, see text; for *diminished vocal resonance intensity*, the transmitted sounds from the patient's voice when reciting numbers, as detected by a stethoscope on the patient's posterior chest, are reduced or absent.[26]

‡Likelihood ratio (LR) if finding present = positive LR; LR if finding absent = negative LR.
COPD, Chronic obstructive pulmonary disease; *NS*, not significant.

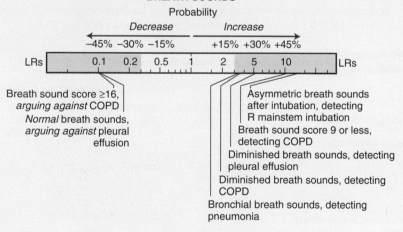

BREATH SOUNDS

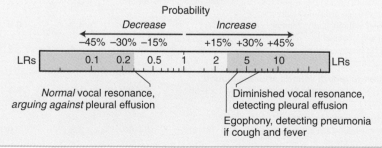

VOCAL RESONANCE

Unilaterally diminished breath sounds increases the probability of pleural effusion in hospitalized patients with respiratory complaints (LR = 5.2); in patients hospitalized in the intensive care unit (most of whom were receiving mechanical ventilation), the absence of breath sounds over a specific region of the chest also increases the probability of underlying pleural fluid (LR = 3). Also, the appearance of reduced breath sounds during methacholine challenge increases the probability of asthma (LR = 4.2) and, in patients with fever and cough, diminished breath sounds modestly increases the probability of pneumonia (LR = 2.4).

The presence of normal breath sound intensity greatly decreases the probability of underlying pleural effusion (LR = 0.1).

2. Asymmetric Breath Sounds After Intubation

If the endotracheal tube is placed too low during intubation of a patient, it risks intubating the right mainstem bronchus and leaving the left lung unventilated, a complication that logically would produce asymmetric breath sounds. In studies of patients after intubation, asymmetric breath sounds greatly increase probability of endobronchial intubation (LR = 12.8, EBM Box 30.1), but the converse is not true: the presence of symmetric breath sounds does not significantly decrease the probability of endobronchial intubation (LR = 0.5). Clinicians should always confirm appropriate tube placement by means other than physical examination.

3. Bronchial Breath Sounds

In patients with cough and fever, bronchial breath sounds increase the probability of pneumonia (LR = 3.3), although the sign is infrequent (sensitivity of 14% to 19%).

II. Vocal Resonance

A. THE FINDING

Vocal resonance refers to the sound of the patient's voice as detected through a stethoscope placed on the patient's chest. Normally, the voice sounds muffled, weak, and indistinct over most of the inferior and posterior chest, and words are unintelligible. Abnormal vocal resonance is classified as either *bronchophony*, *pectoriloquy*, or *egophony*, all terms originally introduced by Laennec.[1] Although these abnormalities have distinct definitions, the pathogenesis for all three is similar, and all may appear simultaneously in the same patient, frequently accompanied by bronchial breath sounds.

1. Bronchophony

Bronchophony describes a voice that is much louder than normal, as if the sounds were emitted directly into the stethoscope. The patient's words are not necessarily intelligible.

2. Pectoriloquy

Pectoriloquy implies that the patient's words are intelligible. Most clinicians test this by having the patient whisper words like "one-two-three"; intelligible whispered speech is called **whispered pectoriloquy**.

3. Egophony

Egophony is a peculiar nasal quality to the sound of the patient's voice, which Laennec likened to the "bleating of a goat."[1] Clinicians usually elicit the finding by having the patient vocalize the long vowel "EE" and then listening for the abnormal transformation of the sound into a loud nasal "AH" (the "AH" sound ranges from the "a" of the word hat to the "a" of the word cart; this finding is sometimes called **E-to-A change**).* Although all vowel sounds are altered by the lung (even healthy lung), what makes egophony distinctive is the intensity of the change and the suddenness with which it appears over a small area on *one* side of the chest.[47] Before concluding a patient has egophony, therefore, the clinician should confirm that a similar change of sound is absent over the identical location of the opposite chest.

B. PATHOGENESIS

Fig. 30.2 depicts the transmission of sound from the larynx to the chest wall in normal persons and in those with pneumonia or pleural effusion. Normal lung behaves like a low-pass filter, which means it easily transmits low frequency sounds (100 to 200 Hz) but filters out high frequency sounds (>300 Hz).[6,48–50] Because tactile fremitus (the palpable vibrations on the chest wall from the patient's voice) consists of low frequency vibrations (100 to 200 Hz), it is a normal finding when symmetric, although tactile fremitus is naturally more prominent in healthy men than healthy women (i.e., men's voices are lower pitched and therefore more likely to generate low frequency vibrations than women's voices). Tactile fremitus also diminishes as a healthy person sings an ascending scale, because the underlying lung resonates less well with higher pitches.

Abnormal vocal resonance (bronchophony, whispered pectoriloquy, and egophony) requires transmission of higher frequencies (>300 Hz) to the chest wall; understanding whispered speech requires the transmission of frequencies of more than 400 Hz (i.e., whispered pectoriloquy). The sound "AH" contains more high frequency energy than the sound "EE," and if the underlying lung preferentially amplifies the high frequency energy of a vocalized "EE," it may render it into a nasal

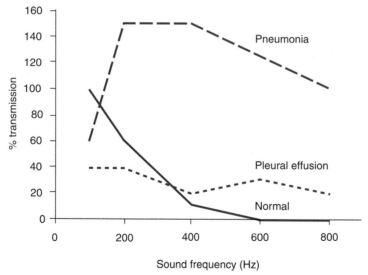

Fig 30.2 Transmission of sound to the chest wall. In this experiment, a speaker emitting pure musical tones of different frequencies was placed in the mouth of patients with normal lungs (solid line), pneumonia (*long dashes*), or pleural effusion (*short dashes*). Microphones on the chest wall recorded the transmission of each frequency (for purposes of comparison, 100% transmission is the transmission of 100 Hz in normal persons). Based upon reference 48.

The E-to-A change was simultaneously discovered in 1922 by Shibley[45] and Fröschel. [46] Shipley discovered it while testing for pectoriloquy in Chinese patients. He asked the patients to say "one-two-three" in the local dialect (*ee-er-san*), and he noted that the long "EE" of "one" acquired a loud nasal "AH" quality over areas of pneumonia or effusion.[45]

"AH" (i.e., egophony).[6,49] Because the normal lung does not transmit high frequency (>300 Hz) sounds well, especially to the lower posterior and lateral chest, egophony and bronchial breath sounds at these locations always indicate the presence of *abnormal* lung between the patient's vocal cords and clinician's stethoscope.

According to Fig. 30.2, consolidated lung transmits both high and low frequencies well, thus explaining why patients with pneumonia may simultaneously exhibit both increased tactile fremitus and abnormal vocal resonance (i.e., egophony). Moderate or large pleural effusion, in contrast, may *decrease* transmission of frequencies below 200 to 300 Hz but *augment* those greater than 400 Hz, compared to normal lung (Fig. 30.2).[6,10,48-50] This explains why some patients with pleural effusion exhibit both *decreased* tactile fremitus yet *abnormal* vocal resonance (i.e., egophony).

Nonetheless, the finding of egophony (abnormal vocal resonance) in patients with pleural effusion is an inconstant finding, and many patients instead demonstrate *reduced* or *absent* vocal resonance over the affected side (i.e., the patient's spoken voice is inaudible or markedly diminished and the nasal "AH" is absent). Laennec himself taught that egophony is not always present in pleural effusion but first appears when effusions are moderate in size, then *disappears* as effusions continue to grow larger, and finally *reappears* as effusions began to resolve.[1] The conventional explanation for these findings is that atelectatic lung, resting on top of an effusion, remains close enough to the chest wall to preferentially conduct enough high frequency sounds to produce abnormal vocal resonance (loudest near the angle of the scapula); as effusions continue to grow larger, the distance between compressed lung and chest wall increases and egophony thus disappears.

Nonetheless, this explanation has never been verified, and it remains a mystery why some patients with effusion have prominent egophony over large areas of the posterior chest wall yet others have diminished vocal resonance. The only study of this finding shows that pleural effusions producing abnormal vocal resonance (e.g., egophony) have higher positive intrapleural pressures than effusions without the finding.[10] From an acoustic standpoint, the variables responsible for abnormal vocal resonance might include not only the size of effusion and condition of the underlying compressed lung, but also the amount of air moving in and out of the underlying lung, the viscosity of the pleural fluid, and the condition of the underlying inflamed pleural surface and chest wall.

C. CLINICAL SIGNIFICANCE

Abnormal vocal resonance has the same significance (and pathogenesis) as bronchial breath sounds. In patients with cough and fever, the finding of egophony increases the probability of pneumonia (LR = 4.1, EBM Box 30.1), and in hospitalized patients with a variety of respiratory complaints, the finding of diminished vocal resonance (i.e., diminished intensity of patient's voice when reciting numbers) increases the probability of an underlying pleural effusion (LR = 6.5).

According to traditional teachings, an obstructed bronchus should diminish vocal resonance, although this teaching is probably incorrect, based on the observation that some patients with egophony and pneumonia have obstructed bronchi from tumors[49] and on experiments showing that sound conducts down the substance of the porous lung itself to the chest wall, not down the airway ducts.[51,†]

III. Adventitious Sounds

A. INTRODUCTION

Adventitious sounds are all sounds heard during auscultation other than breath sounds or vocal resonance. The common adventitious sounds are crackles, rubs, wheezes, rhonchi, and stridor.

---

†The acoustic characteristics of the transmitted sound are the same whether the patient breathes air or a mixture of oxygen and helium. If sound were conducted down the airways, its characteristics would change with different gas mixtures.[51]

Adventitious sounds have the most ambiguous and confusing nomenclature in all of physical diagnosis, and studies show clinicians use up to 16 different terms in scientific publications to describe similar sounds.[52] This confusion stems from the earliest days of auscultation and the writings of Laennec, who, in the first edition of his treatise, identified five adventitious sounds but called them all *rales*, distinguishing them further only by adding adjectives (e.g., "moist crepitus rale" for a crackling sound or "dry sibilus rale" for a whistling sound).[1,53] In later editions, Laennec substituted *rhonchus* for *rale* because he became worried that patients hearing *rale* would misinterpret it for the death rattle (*rale* means rattle). In 1831, a British editor introduced the Anglo-Saxon term *wheeze*, again to refer to all lung sounds.[53] Finally, Robertson in 1957 proposed using *crackling sounds* for discontinuous sounds and *wheeze* for continuous, musical sounds, and suggested eliminating *rale* and *rhonchus* altogether.[54]

The recommended terms for lung sounds, based on their acoustic characteristics, are **crackle** for discontinuous sounds and **wheeze** or **rhonchus** for continuous sounds (Table 30.1).[12,55]

B. THE FINDING

1. Crackles

Crackles are discontinuous sounds, resembling the sound produced by rubbing strands of hair together in front of the ear or by pulling apart strips of Velcro. There are **coarse crackles**, which are loud, low-pitched, and fewer in number per breath, and **fine crackles**, which are soft, higher-pitched, and greater in number per breath. Crackles that appear early during inspiration and do not continue beyond mid-inspiration are called **early inspiratory** crackles; those that continue into the second half of inspiration are called **late inspiratory** crackles.[59] Many American clinicians still use the word *rale* as a synonym for crackle, although British clinicians more often use crackle.[60,61]

The finding **posturally-induced crackles**, which may have significance after myocardial infarction (see subsequent section on clinical significance) describes crackles that appear in the supine position but disappear in the sitting position. To elicit the finding, the clinician listens to the lower chest wall near the posterior axillary line with the patient in three sequential positions: sitting, supine, and supine with legs elevated 30 degrees.[62] The clinician listens only after the patient has been in each position for 3 minutes. If crackles are absent when upright but appear either when supine or with legs elevated, the test is positive (i.e., the patient has posturally-induced crackles).

TABLE 30.1 ■ Terminology for Lung Sounds

Recommended ATS Term	Acoustic Characteristics	Terms in Some Textbooks	British Usage
Coarse crackle	Discontinuous sound: loud, low in pitch	Coarse rale	Crackle
Fine crackle	Discontinuous sound: soft, higher pitch, shorter duration	Fine rale	Crackle
Wheeze	Continuous sound: high-pitched, dominant frequency ≥400 Hz	Sibilant rhonchus	High-pitched wheeze
Rhonchus	Continuous sound: low-pitched, dominant frequency ≤200 Hz	Sonorous rhonchus	Low-pitched wheeze

Adapted from references 55–58.
ATS, American Thoracic Society.

2. Wheezes and Rhonchi

According to the American Thoracic Society, a wheeze is a high-pitched, continuous musical sound and a rhonchus is a low-pitched one (Table 30.1). This distinction may be superfluous because both sounds have the same pathophysiology and there is no proven clinical importance to separating them. The term *rhonchus* is probably best avoided, not only for these reasons but because many use the term to refer to the coarse discontinuous sounds heard in patients with excess airway secretions.[60]

3. Stridor

Stridor is a loud, musical sound of definite and constant pitch (usually about 400 Hz) that indicates upper airway obstruction.[50,57] It is identical acoustically to wheezing in every way except for two characteristics: (1) stridor is confined to inspiration whereas wheezing is either confined entirely to expiration (30% to 60% of patients) or occurs during both expiration and inspiration (40% to 70% of patients)[63,64]; (2) stridor is always louder over the neck, whereas wheezing is always louder over the chest.[64]

In some patients with upper airway obstruction, stridor does not appear until the patient breathes rapidly through an open mouth.[65]

4. Pleural Rub

Pleural rubs are loud grating or rubbing sounds associated with breathing that occur in patients with pleural disease. Sometimes, a pleural rub has a crackling character (**pleural crackling rub**) and acoustically resembles the crackles heard in patients with parenchymal disease.[66,67] The timing of the crackling sound best distinguishes the pleural crackling rub from parenchymal crackles: the pleural crackling rub is predominately *expiratory* (i.e., 65% of crackling sound occurs during expiration), but parenchymal crackles are predominately *inspiratory* (i.e., only 10% of crackling sound occurs during expiration).[68]

5. Inspiratory Squawk

The **squawk** is a short, late-inspiratory musical sound associated with parenchymal crackles in patients with interstitial lung disease,[69] although the sound has also been described in pneumonia.[70] It is best heard over the upper anterior chest when the patient is semirecumbent and breathing deeply. Because the sound is sometimes found in patients with bird-fancier's lung (a cause of hypersensitivity pneumonitis), the synonym **chirping rale** has been proposed.[71]

In patients with hypersensitivity pneumonitis, the squawk tends to be shorter, higher-pitched, and later in inspiration than the squawk of patients with diffuse pulmonary fibrosis.[69]

C. PATHOGENESIS

1. Crackles[50,59,66,72–74]

Crackles were initially attributed by Laennec and early auscultators to air bubbling through airway secretions. Although some crackles result from secretions, these promptly clear after the patient coughs. All remaining crackling sounds are felt to represent the sounds of distal airways, collapsed from the previous exhalation, as they abruptly open during inspiration. Several lines of evidence support this conclusion: (1) crackles are predominantly heard during inspiration, whereas air bubbling though secretions would cause both inspiratory and expiratory sounds; (2) the number of crackles has no relationship to the amount of sputum the patient produces (the disease with the most crackles, interstitial fibrosis, produces scant sputum or no sputum at all)[75]; (3) crackles have a stereotypic pattern with each respiratory cycle (i.e., in a single patient at a single location on the chest, they are always early-, late-, or paninspiratory, and individual crackles occur at the same esophageal (transpulmonary) pressure in consecutive respiratory cycles;[76] and (4) crackles are loudest in the lower portions of the chest, even when the lung disease is distributed diffusely.

Course crackles are felt to originate in larger, more proximal airways than fine crackles, based on the observations that distinct patterns of coarse crackles (identified by their fingerprint of identical timing and number) radiate to a larger area of the chest wall than do distinct patterns of fine crackles.[77,78]

2. Wheezes

Wheezes are caused by vibrations of the opposing walls of narrowed airways.[66,72,79,80] They are not due to resonance of air in the airways (i.e., like the sound of a flute or pipe organ) for the following reasons: (1) if they were due to resonance of air in a hollow pipe, the length of pipe for some low-pitched wheezes would be several feet, far exceeding the length of human airways; (2) the pitch of a wheeze may change between inspiration and expiration; and (3) the pitch of the wheeze remains the same when inspired air is replaced with a gas mixture of oxygen and helium. (If due to resonance of air, the pitch should change.)

D. CLINICAL SIGNIFICANCE

1. Crackles

The crackles discussed below refer only to crackling sounds that persist after the patient coughs.

a. Normal Persons

Crackles are rare in healthy persons during normal tidal breathing.[81,82] Fine crackling sounds, however, may appear in up to 60% of healthy persons, especially over the anterior chest, if the person first exhales as much as possible and breathes in from residual volume instead of functional residual capacity.[81,82]

b. Crackles and Disease

(1) Presence of Crackles. EBM Box 30.2 indicates that the finding of crackles increases the probability of pulmonary fibrosis in asbestos workers (LR = 5.9), of pneumonia in patients with cough and fever (LR = 2.8), of elevated left atrial pressure in patients with known heart disease (LR = 2.1), and of myocardial infarction in patients with chest pain (LR = 2.1). In the evaluation of patients for either pulmonary embolism or pleural effusion, the finding of crackles is unhelpful (LRs not significant; see Chapters 34 and 35).

In one study of 132 patients being evaluated in interstitial lung disease clinics, the *absence* of bilateral "Velcro" crackles markedly *decreased* the probability of "honeycombing" fibrosis on computed tomography (LR = 0.04; EBM Box 30.2). Amongst patients with interstitial lung disease, virtually all patients with idiopathic pulmonary fibrosis have crackles whereas a smaller number of patients with fibrosis from sarcoidosis and cryptogenic organizing pneumonia have crackles, probably because sarcoidosis and organizing pneumonia are more centrally located than idiopathic pulmonary fibrosis and tend to spare the subpleural area near the chest wall.[75,84,94]

Although the finding of posturally-induced crackles after myocardial infarction has been associated with higher pulmonary capillary wedge pressures and worse survival,[62] it is clear that any crackles in patients with acute coronary syndromes portends a worse prognosis. In one study of patients with acute sustained ischemic chest pain, crackles predicted 30-day mortality with a sensitivity of 36%, specificity of 92%, and a positive LR of 4.5.[95] The extent of crackles in patients with newly diagnosed congestive heart failure also predicts future cardiovascular mortality.[96]

(2) Characteristics of Crackles.[68,93,97–99] Table 30.2 describes the characteristic number, timing, and type of crackles in common crackling disorders, such as pulmonary fibrosis, congestive heart

EBM BOX 30.2	Crackles*			

Finding (Reference)	Sensitivity (%)	Specificity (%)	Likelihood Ratio[†] if Finding Is Present	Absent
Crackles				
Detecting pulmonary fibrosis in asbestos workers[83]	81	86	**5.9**	0.2
Detecting "honeycombing" fibrosis (on computed tomography) in patients attending interstitial lung disease clinic[84]	98	45	1.8	**0.04**
Detecting elevated left atrial pressure in patients with cardiomyopathy[85–88]	15–64	82–94	2.1	NS
Detecting myocardial infarction in patients with chest pain[89,90]	20–38	82–91	2.1	NS
Detecting pneumonia in patients with cough and fever[30–37,39,44,91,92]	19–67	36–97	2.8	0.8
Early inspiratory crackles				
Detecting chronic airflow obstruction in patients with crackles[59,93]	25–77	97–98	**14.6**	NS
Detecting severe disease in patients with chronic airflow obstruction[59]	90	96	**20.8**	0.1

*Diagnostic standard: for *pulmonary fibrosis*, fibrosis on high resolution computed tomography; for *elevated left atrial pressure*, pulmonary capillary wedge pressure >20 mm Hg[86,87] or >22 mm Hg;[85,88] for *myocardial infarction*, development of new electrocardiographic Q waves, elevations of cardiac biomarkers (CK-MB or troponin), or both; for *pneumonia*, infiltrate on chest radiograph; for *chronic airflow obstruction*, FEV_1/FVC <0.75[59] or less than lower 95% confidence interval for age, gender and height.[93]
[†]Likelihood ratio (LR) if finding present = positive LR; LR if finding absent = negative LR.
COPD, Chronic obstructive pulmonary disease; *NS,* not significant.

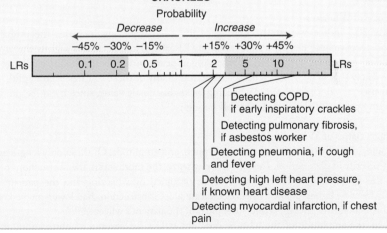

CRACKLES
Probability

Decrease   *Increase*

−45% −30% −15%   +15% +30% +45%

LRs   0.1   0.2   0.5   1   2   5   10   LRs

Detecting COPD, if early inspiratory crackles

Detecting pulmonary fibrosis, if asbestos worker

Detecting pneumonia, if cough and fever

Detecting high left heart pressure, if known heart disease

Detecting myocardial infarction, if chest pain

TABLE 30.2 ▪ **Characteristics of Crackles in Various Disorders***

Diagnosis	Number of Crackles per Inspiration	Timing of Crackle	Type of Crackle
Pulmonary fibrosis	6–14	Late inspiratory (0.5 → 0.9)	Fine
Congestive heart failure	4–9	Late or paninspiratory (0.4 → 0.8)	Coarse or fine
Pneumonia	3–7	Paninspiratory (0.3 → 0.7)	Coarse
Chronic airflow obstruction	1–4	Early inspiratory (0.3 → 0.5)	Coarse or fine

*Number of crackles is mean number of crackles ± 1 standard deviation, after the patient first coughs to clear airway secretions. The descriptors *early inspiratory, late inspiratory, paninspiratory, coarse,* and *fine* are observations made by clinicians listening with the stethoscope; the numbers under *timing* refer to when crackles begin and end during a full inspiration (e.g., 0.5 à 0.9 means that crackles first appear at midinspiration [0.5] and end when the patient has reached 90% of full inspiration [0.9]). Based on references 68,93,97.

failure, pneumonia, and chronic obstructive lung disease. The crackles of interstitial fibrosis are characteristically fine, have a large number of individual crackling sounds each inspiration, and persist to the end of inspiration (i.e., they are late inspiratory crackles). Crackles of chronic airflow obstruction are coarse or fine, have the smallest number of crackling sounds, and are confined to the first half of inspiration (early inspiratory crackles). The crackles of heart failure and pneumonia lie between these extremes; with treatment, the crackles of pneumonia become finer and move toward the end of inspiration.[98,99]

EBM Box 30.2 indicates the finding of early inspiratory crackles greatly increases the probability of chronic obstructive lung disease (LR = 14.6). Most patients with these crackles have severe obstruction (LR = 20.8).

2. Wheezes

a. Presence of Wheezes

EBM Box 30.3 indicates that the finding of unforced wheezing increases the probability of chronic obstructive lung disease a small amount (LR = 2.6) and decreases slightly the probability of pulmonary embolism (LR = 0.4). If wheezing appears during methacholine challenge testing, asthma is likely (LR = 6). The absence of wheezing in any of these settings is unhelpful.

In contrast, the finding of *forced* wheezing lacks diagnostic value, since it can be produced by most healthy persons if they exhale forcibly enough.[100,109]

b. Characteristics of Wheezing

The characteristics of wheezes are their length, pitch, and amplitude. Of these, only length and pitch vary with severity of obstruction. The longer the wheeze, the more severe the obstruction (r = −0.89 between the proportion of the respiratory cycle occupied by wheezing and the patient's FEV_1,[‡] p < 0.001).[63,110,111] Higher-pitched wheezes indicate worse obstruction than lower-pitched ones, and effective bronchodilator therapy reduces the pitch of the patient's wheeze.[63,110]

Even so, the amplitude of the wheeze does not reflect the severity of obstruction, principally because many patients with severe obstruction have faint or no wheezes.[63,100,110,111] This finding supports the old adage that, in a patient with asthma, the quiet chest is not necessarily a favorable sign but may instead indicate a tiring patient who is unable to push air across the obstructed airways.

---

‡See Chapter 28 for definition of FEV_1.

| EBM BOX 30.3 | **Wheezes, Rubs, and Squawks*** |

Finding (Reference)	Sensitivity (%)	Specificity (%)	Likelihood Ratio[†] if Finding Is Present	Absent
Unforced wheezing				
Detecting chronic airflow obstruction[21,23,25,100–103]	13–56	86–99	2.6	0.8
Detecting pneumonia in patients with cough and fever[30–34,36,39,91,92]	4–36	50–96	0.8	NS
Detecting pulmonary embolism[104–106]	3–31	68–91	0.4	NS
Wheezing during methacholine challenge testing				
Detecting asthma[29]	44	93	**6.0**	0.6
Pleural rub				
Detecting pulmonary embolism[106,107]	1–14	91–99	NS	NS
Detecting pleural effusion[26]	5	99	NS	NS
Inspiratory Squawk				
Hypersensitivity pneumonitis in patients with interstitial lung disease[108]	11	97	**3.2**	NS

*Diagnostic standard: for *chronic airflow obstruction*, FEV_1/FVC <0.6, [21]<0.7, [23,25,100]or less than lower 95% confidence interval for age, gender, and height;[101–103] for *pulmonary embolism*, see Chapter 34; for *asthma*, FEV_1 decrease ≥20% during methacholine challenge;[29] for *pleural effusion*, chest radiograph; and for *hypersensitivity pneumonitis*, clinical consensus using standard criteria.
†Likelihood ratio (LR) if finding present = positive LR; LR if finding absent = negative LR.
COPD, Chronic obstructive pulmonary disease; *NS,* not significant.

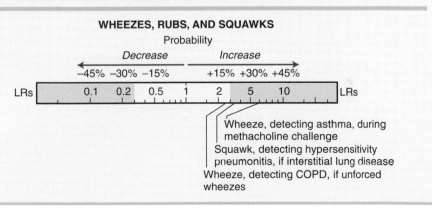

WHEEZES, RUBS, AND SQUAWKS

Wheeze, detecting asthma, during methacholine challenge
Squawk, detecting hypersensitivity pneumonitis, if interstitial lung disease
Wheeze, detecting COPD, if unforced wheezes

The **slide whistle sound,** a unique wheezing sound whose pitch rises during inspiration and falls during expiration, has been described in a patient with a spherical tumor arising from the carina that nearly completely obstructed the trachea.[112]

3. Stridor

In patients with tracheal stenosis after tracheostomy, stridor is a late finding, usually appearing after symptoms like dyspnea, irritative cough, or difficulty clearing the throat.[65] Stridor indicates that the airway diameter is less than 5 mm.[65]

4. Pleural Rub

EBM Box 30.3 indicates that the presence or absence of a pleural rub does not change the probability of pulmonary embolism or pleural effusion.

5. Inspiratory Squawk

In patients presenting to pulmonary specialists with a variety of interstitial lung diseases, the presence of the inspiratory squawk increases the probability of hypersensitivity pneumonitis (LR = 3.2).

References may be accessed online at *Elsevier eBooks for Practicing Clinicians.*

Ancillary Tests

I. Forced Expiratory Time

A. TECHNIQUE

To measure the forced expiratory time, the clinician places the stethoscope bell over the trachea of the patient in the suprasternal notch and asks the patient to take a deep breath and blow it all out as fast as possible.[1] Using a stopwatch, the duration of the audible expiratory sound is determined to the nearest half second.

Rosenblatt introduced this test in 1962 as a test of obstructive lung disease.[2]

B. PATHOGENESIS

The forced expiratory time should be prolonged in obstructive disease simply because, by definition, the ratio of FEV_1 to FVC (i.e., forced expiratory volume in 1 second divided by forced vital capacity, a measure of flow rate) is reduced in this disorder. Slower flow rates prolong expiratory times.

C. CLINICAL SIGNIFICANCE

EBM Box 31.1 summarizes the accuracy of this finding, showing that a forced expiratory time of 9 seconds or more increases the probability of obstructive disease (likelihood ratio [LR] = 3.9) and a time less than 3 seconds decreases probability (LR = 0.2).

The forced expiratory time is a specific test for obstructive lung disease. Patients with restrictive lung disease, despite having reductions in the FEV_1 similar to those seen in obstructive lung disease, usually have forced expiratory times of 4 seconds or less.[1,2]

EBM BOX 31.1	Ancillary Tests

Finding (Reference)*	Sensitivity (%)	Specificity (%)	Likelihood Ratio† if Finding Is Present	Likelihood Ratio† if Finding Is Absent
Forced expiratory time Detecting chronic airflow obstruction[1,3-5]				
≥9 seconds	5–50	86–99	3.9	...
3–9 seconds	42–94	...	NS	...
<3 seconds	1–10	26–89	0.2	...
Unable to blow out the match (Snider test) Detecting FEV_1 of ≤1.6L[6,7]	62–90	91–93	9.6	0.2

*Diagnostic standard: for *chronic airflow obstruction*, FEV_1/FVC[1,3] <0.7 or FEV_1/FVC below normal as predicted from equations based on the patient's age and height.[4,5]

†Likelihood ratio (LR) if finding present = positive LR; LR if finding absent = negative LR.

COPD, Chronic obstructive pulmonary disease; FEV_1, forced expiratory time in 1 second; *FVC*, forced vital capacity; *NS*, not significant; *s*, seconds.

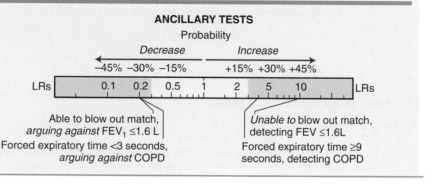

ANCILLARY TESTS
Probability

Decrease   *Increase*

−45% −30% −15%   +15% +30% +45%

LRs   0.1   0.2   0.5   1   2   5   10   LRs

Able to blow out match, *arguing against* FEV_1 ≤1.6 L
Forced expiratory time <3 seconds, *arguing against* COPD

Unable to blow out match, detecting FEV ≤1.6L
Forced expiratory time ≥9 seconds, detecting COPD

II. Blow-Out-The-Match Test

A. TECHNIQUE

The clinician lights a match and holds it 10 to 15 cm in front of the seated patient, who then attempts to extinguish it by blowing as forcibly as possible. It is important that the patient hold the mouth open and not purse the lips. Inability to extinguish the burning match is the positive finding.

The match test was introduced by Snider in 1959, who reasoned that the ability to extinguish a match was related to the velocity of exhaled air.[6] The test is often called the **Snider test**.

B. CLINICAL SIGNIFICANCE

EBM Box 31.1 indicates that a positive Snider test (i.e., inability to extinguish the match) greatly increases the probability that the patient's FEV_1 is at least moderately reduced to 1.6 L or less (LR = 9.6). Being able to extinguish the match argues against an FEV_1 this low (LR = 0.2). Unlike the forced expiratory time, the Snider test is abnormal in both obstructive and restrictive lung disease, which probably explains why the Snider test performs poorly in studies using it as a specific sign of obstructive disease.[8]

References may be accessed online at *Elsevier eBooks for Practicing Clinicians*.

Selected Pulmonary Disorders

Pneumonia

- Many of the classic physical findings of lobar consolidation—diminished chest excursion, dullness, diminished breath sounds, bronchial breath sounds, egophony, and crackles— are accurate signs of pneumonia in patients with cough and fever. Nonetheless, these findings appear in only the minority of patients with proven pneumonia; their *absence* is therefore diagnostically unhelpful.
- In patients with cough and fever, the *presence* of normal vital signs (i.e., temperature, pulse rate, respiratory rate) *decreases* probability of pneumonia.
- The Heckerling scoring scheme combines five independent findings of pneumonia (tachycardia, fever, crackles, diminished breath sounds, and *absence* of asthma) and greatly increases the clinician's diagnostic accuracy.
- The CURB-65 score, which combines five findings to accurately predict the prognosis of patients with pneumonia, provides essential information when making decisions about patient triage and care.

I. Introduction

Like most of the pulmonary examination, the traditional findings of lobar pneumonia were described in 1819 by Laennec, who wrote that clinicians using his newly invented stethoscope could detect acute pneumonia "in every possible case."[1] According to traditional teachings, the earliest findings of pneumonia are crackles and diminished breath sounds, followed by dullness to percussion, increased tactile fremitus and vocal resonance, and bronchial breath sounds.[2]

II. Clinical Significance

A. INDIVIDUAL FINDINGS

EBM Box 32.1 reviews the findings from over 12,000 patients presenting with acute fever, cough, sputum production, or dyspnea, all of whom underwent chest radiography (the diagnostic standard for pneumonia). The findings increasing probability of pneumonia, in descending order of their LRs, are asymmetric chest expansion (likelihood ratio [LR] = 44.1), egophony (LR = 4.1), cachexia (LR = 4), percussion dullness (LR = 3.6), bronchial breath sounds (LR = 3.3), oxygen saturation of less than 95% (LR = 3), crackles (LR = 2.8), respiratory rate greater than 28/min (LR = 2.7), temperature greater than 37.8°C (LR = 2.5), diminished breath sounds (LR = 2.4), heart rate greater than 100/min (LR = 2.1), and abnormal mental status (LR = 1.9).

EBM BOX 32.1   Pneumonia*

Finding (Reference)[†]	Sensitivity (%)	Specificity (%)	Likelihood Ratio[‡] if Finding Is Present	Absent
General appearance				
Cachexia[3]	10	97	**4.0**	NS
Abnormal mental status[4-6]	12–14	92–95	1.9	NS
Vital signs				
Heart rate >100/min[3-14]	12–65	60–96	2.1	0.8
Temperature >37.8°C[3-17]	16–75	44–95	2.5	0.7
Respiratory rate >28/min[5-7,16]	7–36	80–99	2.7	0.9
Oxygen saturation <95%[8,13,16,17]	32–52	80–99	**3.0**	0.7
All vital signs normal[5,8,11,13,18,19]	3–38	24–81	**0.3**	2.3
Lung findings				
Asymmetric chest expansion[3]	5	100	**44.1**	NS
Chest wall tenderness[15]	5	96	NS	NS
Percussion dullness[3-5,20-23]	4–26	82–99	**3.6**	NS
Diminished breath sounds[4,5,9,10,13,14,20-22,24]	7–60	73–98	2.4	0.8
Bronchial breath sounds[4,22]	14–19	94–96	**3.3**	0.9
Egophony[3-5]	4–16	96–99	**4.1**	NS
Crackles[3-6,9,10,13-15,20,21,24]	19–67	36–97	2.8	0.8
Wheezing[4-6,9,13,15,20,21,24]	4–36	50–96	0.8	NS
Diagnostic score (Heckerling et al)[4,18]				
0 or 1 findings	7–29	33–65	**0.3**	...
2 or 3 findings	48–55	...	NS	...
4 or 5 findings	38–41	92–97	**8.2**	...

*Diagnostic standard: for *pneumonia*, infiltrate on chest radiograph.
[†]Definition of findings: for *low oxygen saturation*, <93%[13] or <95% (all other studies); for *all vital signs normal*, most studies required 3 normal vital signs: temperature (<37.8°C), pulse (≤100/min), and respirations (<24/min[13] or ≤20 [all other studies]); Kahli[19] also required oxygen saturation >95%; for *Heckerling diagnostic score*, the clinician scores 1 point for each of the following 5 findings that are present: temperature >37.8°C, heart rate >100/min, crackles, diminished breath sounds, and *absence* of asthma.
[‡]Likelihood ratio (LR) if finding present = positive LR; LR if finding absent = negative LR.
NS, Not significant.

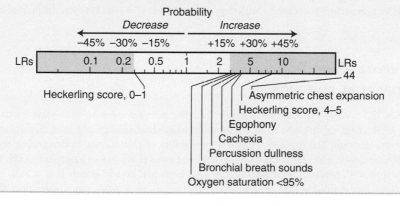

PNEUMONIA
Probability

Decrease   Increase

−45% −30% −15%   +15% +30% +45%

LRs   0.1   0.2   0.5   1   2   5   10   LRs
                                                 44

Heckerling score, 0–1

Asymmetric chest expansion
Heckerling score, 4–5
Egophony
Cachexia
Percussion dullness
Bronchial breath sounds
Oxygen saturation <95%

The only finding decreasing the probability of pneumonia was the finding that all vital signs were normal (LR = 0.3). In many studies, wheezing was found more often in patients *without* pneumonia, primarily because the cause of the acute respiratory complaints in these patients was asthma, not pneumonia.[4,5,20,21]

B. LAENNEC VS. MODERN STUDIES

There are three reasons why the studies in EBM Box 32.1 contradict Laennec's assertion that physical diagnosis is the perfect diagnostic tool: (1) Patients diagnosed with pneumonia today include those with more mild disease than in Laennec's time, when the only available diagnostic standard was postmortem examination (i.e., his conclusions were drawn only from patients dying from severe disease). (2) Many traditional findings appear only after several days of illness, times when the modern clinician, already familiar with the chest radiograph, often examines patients in a more cursory fashion. In contrast, Laennec examined each of his patients diligently day after day, concluding that bronchial breath sounds and bronchophony usually appeared only after 1 to 3 days of hospitalization, and dullness to percussion appeared only after day 4.[1,25] (3) Antimicrobial medications probably alter the course of the physical findings. For example, in the preantibiotic era, fever usually lasted 7 days in patients with lobar pneumonia[26]; in the antibiotic era it lasts usually only 3 or 4 days.[27,28]

Even so, many great clinicians of the past tempered Laennec's enthusiasm and taught that auscultation was an imperfect diagnostic tool. Writing just 20 years after Laennec's treatise, Thomas Addison* stated it was high time "to strip the stethoscope of the extravagant and meretricious pretensions thrust upon it...and to state fairly what it will not, as well as what it will do..."[29]

C. COMBINED FINDINGS

Combining findings improves the accuracy of bedside examination. One of the best models, validated in four different populations,[4,18] scores 1 point for each of the following five findings: (1) temperature greater than 37.8°C, (2) heart rate more than 100/min, (3) crackles, (4) diminished breath sounds, and (5) *absence* of asthma. EBM Box 32.1 shows that a score of 4 or 5 argues compellingly *for* pneumonia (LR = 8.2), whereas a score of 0 or 1 argues *against* pneumonia (LR = 0.3), which, in some groups of patients, may reduce the probability of pneumonia enough that a chest radiograph becomes unnecessary (e.g., in patients presenting to a community office with cough, in whom the probability of pneumonia is 10% or less, a score of 0 or 1 reduces the probability of pneumonia to 3% or less).

D. PNEUMONIA AND PROGNOSIS

In studies of immunocompetent adults hospitalized with community-acquired pneumonia, the 30 day mortality rate is 4% to 15%. Of the individual findings that predict an increased risk of death (EBM Box 32.2), the most compelling ones are hypotension (LR = 5.3), abnormal mental status (LR = 3.9), and hypothermia (LR = 3.5).

Several different scoring schemes combine bedside findings to predict mortality in patients with pneumonia. One of the best validated is the **Pneumonia Severity Index**,[68] which unfortunately has the disadvantage of requiring knowledge of 20 different clinical variables, making it difficult to recall and apply at the bedside. A much simpler rule is the CURB-65 score, based on five prognostic variables† identified decades ago by the British Thoracic Society[44]: (1) confusion, (2) blood urea nitrogen (BUN) levels over 19 mg/dL (>7 mmol/L), (3) respiratory rate of 30 breaths/min

---

*Thomas Addison, the discoverer of adrenal insufficiency, was also a recognized master of percussion and auscultation.
†CURB-65 is an acronym for Confusion, Urea, Respiratory rate, Blood pressure, and Age ≥65 years.

| EBM BOX 32.2 | **Pneumonia: Predictors of Hospital Mortality** |

| Finding* (Reference) | Sensitivity (%) | Specificity (%) | *Likelihood Ratio† if Finding Is* | |
			Present	Absent
General appearance				
Abnormal mental status[30-40]	11–65	70–98	**3.9**	0.8
Vital signs				
Heart rate >125/min[35,38,39]	6–33	86–98	2.6	NS
Systolic blood pressure <90 mm Hg[31,40-43]	11–47	87–99	**5.3**	0.7
Hypothermia[31,42]	14–43	93	**3.5**	NS
Respiratory rate >30/min[31,32,35-39,44-46]	9–85	63–99	2.4	0.9
Oxygen saturation <90%[47,48]	18–52	75–96	2.8	NS
"CURB-65" prognostic score [37,39,49-67]				
0 findings	0–16	41–92	**0.2**	...
1 finding	3–38	...	0.6	...
2 findings	17–51	...	1.3	...
3 findings	13–61	...	2.5	...
4 findings	4–35	...	**5.4**	...
5 findings	1–12	99–100	**8.4**	...

*Definition of findings: for *hypothermia*, body temperature <36.1°C[31] or <37.0°C[42]; for *CURB-65* prognostic score, the clinician scores 1 point for each of the following findings that are present: confusion; blood urea nitrogen >19 mg/dL; respiratory rate ≥30/min; low blood pressure (either systolic blood pressure ≤90 mm Hg or diastolic blood pressure ≤60 mm Hg); and age ≥65 years.
†Likelihood ratio (LR) if finding present = positive LR; LR if finding absent = negative LR.
NS, Not significant.

PNEUMONIA: PREDICTORS OF MORTALITY

or higher, (4) hypotension (i.e., diastolic blood pressure ≤60 mm Hg or systolic blood pressure ≤90 mm Hg), and (5) age 65 years or older. The presence of three or more of these CURB-65 variables is associated with increased hospital mortality (LR = 2.5 for three findings, LR = 5.4 for four findings, and LR = 8.4 for five findings, EBM Box 32.2), whereas the absence of all CURB-65 variables is associated with decreased hospital mortality (LR = 0.2 for 0 findings).

The CURB-65 score requires knowledge of the patient's blood urea nitrogen (BUN), which may not be immediately available to office-based clinicians. Related scores that omit laboratory values have also been developed, such as the "CRB-65" score, which is simply the CURB-65 without the BUN (thus creating possible scores of 0 to 4). Though less extensively studied than CURB-65, 10 studies of CRB-65 show it to be an accurate predictor of mortality (LR = 0.3 for a CRB-65 score of 0; 0.7 for 1 point; 1.9 for 2 points; 4.7 for 3 points; and 10.1 for 4 points).[35,36,50,54–57,66,69–71]

E. HOSPITAL COURSE

Among survivors of pneumonia, abnormalities of the vital signs—fever, tachycardia, tachypnea, and hypotension—usually become normal within 2 to 4 days.[27,28] Once this occurs, subsequent clinical deterioration is rare, and fewer than 1% of patients will require subsequent intensive care, coronary care, or telemetry monitoring.[27] If patients are discharged from the hospital before normalization of vital signs, there is an increased risk of readmission and death.[72–74]

References may be accessed online at *Elsevier eBooks for Practicing Clinicians.*

Chronic Obstructive Lung Disease

I. Introduction

Although descriptions of emphysema date to autopsy reports from the 1600s, it was Laennec who in 1819 recorded the clinical features associated with the disease, including dyspnea, hyperresonance, faint breath sounds, and wheezes.[1] Over the last 200 years, others have embellished Laennec's description, but the principal bedside findings are the same. Writing in 1892, Osler stated that emphysema could be recognized "at a glance" from its characteristic features, including rounded shoulders; barrel chest; prominent epigastric cardiac impulse; hyperresonant chest; loss of cardiac, liver, and splenic dullness; enfeebled breath sounds; and prolonged expiration.[2]

In the 1920s, clinicians began to recognize that these traditional physical signs had shortcomings.[3] In 1927, Cabot wrote that only about 5% of patients with emphysema at autopsy were recognized during life and that, of patients diagnosed with emphysema during life, only 25% actually had it at autopsy.[4] Spirometry, invented in 1846 and used in many forms (stethometers, pneumatometers, doppelstethograms) to supplement bedside diagnosis, gained favor because of these deficiencies and eventually became the favored diagnostic tool.[1]

This chapter compares the traditional physical signs with spirometry. As a general rule, the most accurate physical signs are also infrequent, occurring in fewer than 50% of affected patients, usually only those with the most severe disease.[5,6] For decades or longer, patients may harbor mild and moderate disease that is hidden from the eyes of the bedside examiner but is detectable by spirometry.

II. The Findings

Most of the traditional findings of chronic obstructive pulmonary disease (COPD) result from a hyperinflated chest and the great effort necessary to move air across obstructed airways. Some of these physical signs are discussed in other chapters: asynchronous breathing (Chapter 19); barrel chest, pursed-lip breathing, and accessory muscle use (Chapter 28); hyperresonance to percussion (Chapter 29); pulsus paradoxus (Chapter 15); diminished breath sounds and wheezing (Chapter 30), and prolonged forced expiratory times (Chapter 31).

Additional findings are discussed below.

A. INSPECTION

1. Inspiratory Recession of Supraclavicular Fossa and Intercostal Spaces

Some patients with respiratory distress from obstructive lung disease have recession or indrawing of the soft tissues of the intercostal spaces and supraclavicular fossa. This finding is attributed to vigorous breathing efforts and excess inspiratory resistance, which introduces a delay between the generation of large negative pleural pressures and subsequent increase in lung volume (see also Chapter 28).[7]

2. Costal Paradox (Hoover sign, Costal Margin Paradox)

The costal paradox is an abnormal movement of the costal angle, which is the angle formed by both costal margins as they approach the xiphoid process on the anterior body wall. The clinician assesses costal movements by placing his or her hands on each costal margin and observing how the hands move with respect to each other as the patient breathes. In a normal person, inspiration causes the lateral aspects of the lower ribs to move outward, like the handle of a bucket, and the clinician's hands separate as the costal angle widens. In patients with the costal paradox, in contrast, the hyperinflated chest can expand no further and the flattened diaphragm instead pulls the costal margins and the clinician's hands together. An excellent video of the Hoover sign appears in reference 8.

3. Leaning Forward on Arms Propped up on Knees[9,10]

Many patients with obstructive disease experience prompt relief of their dyspnea if they lean forward, which allows them to generate greater inspiratory force with fewer accessory muscles. This position probably diminishes dyspnea because it compresses the abdominal contents and pushes the diaphragm upward, helping restore the normal domed appearance necessary for efficient and strong inspiratory movements.

B. PALPATION: LARYNGEAL HEIGHT AND DESCENT

According to traditional teachings, the distance between the thyroid cartilage and suprasternal notch (*laryngeal height* or *tracheal length*) is shorter in obstructive lung disease than in normal persons, because the clavicles and sternum are positioned abnormally high. (See the section on Barrel Chest in Chapter 28.) Patients with severe obstruction also have more forceful diaphragmatic contractions that, although ineffective in moving large amounts of air, may pull the trachea abnormally downward during inspiration (*laryngeal descent*, *tracheal descent*, or *tracheal tug*).

III. Clinical Significance

A. INDIVIDUAL FINDINGS

EBM Box 33.1 shows that several findings increase the probability of obstructive lung disease: *early inspiratory* crackles (likelihood ratio [LR] = 14.6), absence of cardiac dullness (LR = 11.8), breath sound score of 9 or less (LR = 10.2), subxiphoid cardiac impulse (LR = 7.4), hyperresonance of the chest (LR = 7.3), forced expiratory time of 9 seconds or less (LR = 3.9), reduced breath sounds (i.e., overall impression without use of the breath sound score, LR = 3.5), use of the scalene or sternocleidomastoid muscles during inspiration (LR = 3.3), and pursed-lip breathing (LR = 2.7). Among patients with known obstructive lung disease, *early inspiratory* crackles imply that the disease is severe (i.e., forced expiratory volume in 1 sec [FEV_1]/forced vital capacity [FVC] < 0.44; LR = 20.8).[19] The simple presence of crackles without reference to their timing is diagnostically unhelpful (LR not significant).[6,14]

EBM BOX 33.1	Chronic Obstructive Pulmonary Disease*			
			Likelihood Ratio‡ if Finding Is	
Finding (Reference)†	**Sensitivity (%)**	**Specificity (%)**	**Present**	**Absent**
Barrel chest[11]	65	58	1.5	0.6
AP/L chest diameter ratio ≥0.9[11]	31	84	2.0	NS
Pursed-lip breathing[11]	58	78	2.7	0.5
Scalene/sternocleidomastoid muscle use[11]	39	88	3.3	0.7
Maximum laryngeal height ≤4 cm[12]	36	90	3.6	0.7
Laryngeal descent >3 cm[12]	17	80	NS	NS
Hoover sign[13]	58	86	4.2	0.5
Palpation				
Subxiphoid cardiac impulse[5,6]	4–27	97–99	7.4	NS
Percussion				
Absent cardiac dullness left lower sternal border[5]	15	99	11.8	NS
Hyperresonance of chest[5,14]	21–33	94–98	7.3	0.8
Diaphragm excursion percussed <2 cm[5]	13	98	NS	NS
Auscultation				
Reduced breath sounds[5,11,13–15]	29–82	63–96	3.5	0.5
Breath sound score[16,17]				
≤9	23–46	96–97	10.2	...
10–12	34–63	...	3.6	...
13–15	11–16	...	NS	...
≥16	3–10	33–34	0.1	...
Early inspiratory crackles[18,19]	25–77	97–98	14.6	NS
Any unforced wheeze[5,6,12–14,20,21]	13–56	86–99	2.6	0.8
Ancillary tests				
Forced expiratory time[21–24]				
≥9 seconds	5–50	86–99	3.9	...
3–9 seconds	42–94	...	NS	...
<3 seconds	1–10	26–89	0.2	...
Combined findings				
2 out of the following 3 findings present: (1) smoked 70 pack years or more; (2) self-reported history of chronic bronchitis or emphysema, (3) diminished breath sounds (5)	67	97	25.7	0.3

(continued)

EBM BOX 33.1 | **Chronic Obstructive Pulmonary Disease*–Cont'd**

Diagnostic standards: for *chronic obstructive lung disease*, FEV₁/FVC ratio <0.6–0.7 (palpation, percussion, diminished breath sounds, and combined findings), FEV₁/FVC <0.7–0.75 (inspection, crackles, wheezes, and forced expiratory time), or FEV₁ <40% predicted (breath sound score).
†*Definition of finding*: for *maximal laryngeal height*, distance between the top of the thyroid cartilage and suprasternal notch at the end of expiration; for *laryngeal descent*, difference in laryngeal height between end inspiration and end expiration; for *Hoover sign*, paradoxical indrawing of the lateral rib margin during inspiration, noted when the patient is standing; for *hyperresonance of chest*, upper right anterior chest⁵ or undefined location¹⁴; for *breath sound score*, see Chapter 30; for *forced expiratory time*, see Chapter 31.
‡Likelihood ratio (LR) if finding present = positive LR; LR if finding absent = negative LR.
AP/L, Anteroposterior/lateral; *cm*, centimeters; *FEV₁*, forced expiratory volume in 1 second; *FVC*, forced vital capacity; *NS*, not significant.

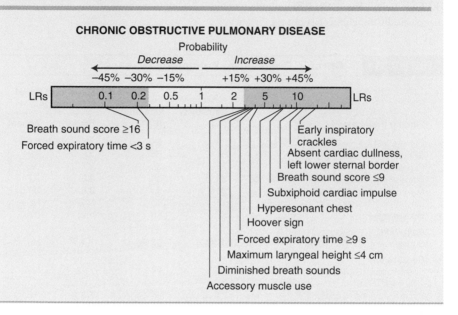

Only two findings significantly decrease the probability of obstructive disease: a breath sound score of 16 or more (LR = 0.1) and a forced expiratory time less than 3 seconds (LR = 0.2).

The evidence supporting the chest wall signs of obstructive lung disease is meager and conflicting. (See also the section on Barrel Chest in Chapter 28.) One study showed that indrawing of the soft tissues correlated with severity of obstruction,²⁵ while another did not.²⁶ Another study of adults presenting to the emergency department with significant dyspnea demonstrated that suprasternal retractions (LR = 4) and intercostal retractions (LR = 2.2) increased probability of hypercapnia and respiratory acidosis (but in this study only 57% had obstructive lung disease [see Chapter 28]).²⁷ In two studies, Hoover sign (LR = 4.2, EBM Box 33.1) and maximum laryngeal height of 4 cm or less (LR = 3.6) increased the probability of obstructive lung disease, but in two other studies these signs correlated poorly with measures of obstruction.²⁵,²⁸ A thoracic ratio of 0.9 or more increases probability of obstructive disease slightly (LR = 2). The degree of laryngeal descent is unhelpful (LR not significant).

The chest excursion of patients with obstructive disease (mean, 3 to 4 cm, measured as change in circumference between maximum inspiration and maximum expiration using a tape measure at the level of the fourth intercostal space) is less than that of normal persons (mean, 6 to 7 cm), but the lower limit observed in normal persons (2 to 3 cm) makes it impossible to draw significant conclusions in a single person.²⁸,²⁹

| EBM BOX 33.2 | Prognosis in COPD Exacerbation: the BAP-65 Score[30–32] |

| | | Mechanical ventilation or hospital mortality | |
BAP-65 Class	Definition*	%	Likelihood Ratio
1	0 BAP predictors present, age ≤65 years	1.6	0.3
2	0 BAP predictors present, age >65 years	2.6	0.4
3	1 BAP predictors present	6.1	NS
4	2 BAP predictors present	19.5	3.7
5	3 BAP predictors present	34.5	9.0

*"BAP predictors" include (1) Blood urea nitrogen >25 mg/dL, (2) Altered mental status (disoriented or Glasgow coma scale <14), and (3) Pulse ≥110 beats/min.
COPD, Chronic obstructive pulmonary disease; *NS*, not significant.

PROGNOSIS IN COPD: BAP-65 SCORE

B. COMBINED FINDINGS

Of the many successful diagnostic schemes that combine findings,[15,21] one of the simplest asks just three questions: (1) Has the patient smoked more than 70 pack-years? (2) Has the patient been previously diagnosed with chronic bronchitis or emphysema? and (3) Are breath sounds diminished in intensity? Answering "yes" to two or three of these questions is a compelling argument for obstructive disease (LR = 25.7, EBM Box 33.1).

Although using the self-reported history of emphysema as a diagnostic indicator seems to be a circular argument, the specificity of this question is only 74%, which means that 26% of patients *without* obstructive lung disease actually remembered such a history. This question is more discriminatory than other symptoms (i.e., dyspnea, sputum production, age, or use of theophylline, steroids, inhalers, or home oxygen) and many other findings (i.e., hyperresonant chest, absence of cardiac dullness, and wheezes).[5]

C. PROGNOSIS IN COPD EXACERBATION (BAP-65 SCORE)

In studies of more than 120,000 patients hospitalized with COPD exacerbation, three clinical findings accurately predict the risk of mechanical ventilation or hospital mortality (overall risk for these complications was 3% to 11%): (1) Blood urea nitrogen of more than 25 mg/dL, (2) Altered mental status, and (3) Pulse of 110/min or higher (the mnemonic "BAP"* helps clinicians recall these findings).[30] Based on the number of these findings and the patient's age, the patient can be classified into one of five prognostic groups, as defined in EBM Box 33.2. This class, in turn, stratifies the patient's risk of mortality or mechanical ventilation from 1.6% to 34.5% (LRs 0.3 to 9; see EBM Box 33.2).

Despite its similarities to the CURB-65 score (see Chapter 32), the BAP-65 score is slightly more accurate in predicting need for mechanical ventilation in patients with COPD exacerbations than the CURB-65 score.[33]

References may be accessed online at *Elsevier eBooks for Practicing Clinicians.*

BAP is an acronym for Blood urea nitrogen, Altered mental status, and Pulse.

CHAPTER 34

Pulmonary Embolism

KEY TEACHING POINTS

- In patients with suspected pulmonary embolism the principal role of bedside examination is to identify the patient's overall probability of disease.
- Some *individual* physical findings increase probability of pulmonary embolism—respiratory rate >30/min, unilateral calf swelling, and parasternal heave—but these findings are infrequent and the increase in probability is modest.
- By using well-validated scores (e.g., Wells Score, revised Geneva score), clinicians can combine risk factors and clinical findings to accurately distinguish patients with low, intermediate, or high probability of pulmonary embolism. This information, combined with quantitative D-dimer measurements or other structured rules, identifies which patients require definitive testing using computed tomography (or ventilation-perfusion lung scanning).

I. Introduction

The diagnosis of pulmonary embolism is a difficult challenge that has frustrated clinicians for over a century. In up to half of hospitalized patients who die of pulmonary embolism, for example, the diagnosis is not even considered.[1,2] When pulmonary embolism is suspected, the principal role of bedside examination is to determine the patient's overall probability of disease (i.e., low, intermediate, or high probability). This information, in turn, often combined with quantitative D-dimer levels or other structured rules, is used to select which patients should undergo definitive diagnostic testing for thromboembolism by computed tomography (CT) angiography, compression venous ultrasonography, or ventilation-perfusion lung scanning.

II. The Findings

Patients with pulmonary embolism present with dyspnea (61% to 83% of patients), pleuritic chest pain (40% to 48% of patients), hemoptysis (5% to 22% of patients), or syncope (4% to 26% of patients).[3-10] Syncope is more common (affecting 20% to 80% of patients) when pulmonary embolism is *massive*, meaning that it obstructs more than half of the pulmonary circulation.[11-13] Ten percent to 35% of patients report a prior history of thromboembolism, and 33% to 42% report calf or thigh pain.[3,5-9]

In recent years, several investigators using multivariate analysis have identified combinations of bedside findings that best identify a patient's overall probability of pulmonary embolism. Two widely studied scores are the **Wells Score** (Table 34.1)[14] and the **revised Geneva score** (Table 34.2).[15]* For each of these scores, the clinician simply adds the points corresponding to

---

*The original Geneva score[8] was later revised (i.e., "revised Geneva score") to remove the arterial blood gas analysis, which is often unavailable. Another *simplified* Geneva score[45] that has been developed with the same variables has the revised score but only 1 point applied to each variable; this simplified score is less well studied.

TABLE 34.1 ■ Wells Score for Pulmonary Embolism

Characteristic	Points
Risk factors	
Previous pulmonary embolism or deep venous thrombosis	1.5
Immobilization or surgery in the previous 4 weeks	1.5
Cancer	1
Clinical findings	
Hemoptysis	1
Heart rate >100/min	1.5
Clinical signs of deep venous thrombosis	3
Other	
Alternative diagnosis is less likely than pulmonary embolism	3

Based upon reference 14.
Interpretation of total score: 0–1 points, low probability; 2–6 points, moderate probability; 7 or more points, high probability.

TABLE 34.2 ■ Revised Geneva Score for Pulmonary Embolism

Characteristic	Points
Risk factors	
Age >65 years	1
Previous pulmonary embolism or deep venous thrombosis	3
Surgery (under general anesthesia) or fracture (of lower limbs) within 1 month	2
Cancer (active or considered cured <1 year)	2
Clinical findings	
Unilateral leg pain	3
Hemoptysis	2
Heart rate	
75–94 beats/min	3
≥95 beats/min	5
Pain on palpation of lower-limb deep veins and unilateral edema	4

Based upon reference 15.
Interpretation of total score: 0–3 points, low probability; 4–10 points, moderate probability; ≥11 points, high probability.

each of the independent predictors that are present. The total score determines overall probability, as defined in the footnotes to Tables 34.1 and 34.2. Both scores combine similar risk factors (prior thromboembolism, immobilization, surgery, and cancer) and clinical findings (hemoptysis, tachycardia, and signs of deep venous thrombosis) to arrive at overall clinical probability, although the Wells score also considers whether an alternative diagnosis is less likely than pulmonary embolism.

III. Clinical Significance

A. INDIVIDUAL FINDINGS

The studies included in EBM Box 34.1 enrolled over 5000 patients with suspected pulmonary embolism referred to centers having considerable experience with venous thromboembolism. In these studies, only 1 of 5 patients suspected of pulmonary embolism actually had the diagnosis.

EBM BOX 34.1	Pulmonary Embolism*

Finding (Reference)[†]	Sensitivity (%)	Specificity (%)	Likelihood Ratio[‡] if Finding Is Present	Absent
Individual findings				
General description				
Diaphoresis[9]	4	94	NS	NS
Cyanosis[4,9]	1–3	97–100	NS	NS
Vital signs				
Pulse >100/min[6–10,16–18]	22–43	66–91	1.4	NS
Systolic blood pressure ≤100 mm Hg[8]	8	95	1.9	NS
Temperature >38°C[4,6–9]	1–9	78–98	0.5	NS
Respiratory rate >30/min[8]	21	90	2.0	0.9
Lung				
Accessory muscle use[4]	17	89	NS	NS
Crackles[3,9,19]	21–59	45–82	NS	NS
Wheezes[6,9,19]	3–31	68–91	0.4	NS
Pleural friction rub[4,9]	1–14	91–99	NS	NS
Heart				
Elevated neck veins[4,9,19]	3–14	92–96	1.7	NS
Left parasternal heave[4,9]	1–5	98–99	2.4	NS
Loud P_2[3,9]	15–19	84–95	NS	NS
New gallop (S_3 or S_4)[3]	30	89	NS	NS
Other				
Chest wall tenderness[4,20]	11–17	79–80	NS	NS
Unilateral calf pain or swelling[5–7,9,10,17–19,21]	9–52	77–99	2.9	0.8
Combined findings				
Wells score[7,17,22–31]				
Low probability, 0–1 points	6–53	27–54	**0.3**	...
Moderate probability, 2–6 points	38–72	...	1.6	...
High probability, 7 or more points	7–54	90–100	**8.2**	...
Revised Geneva Score[15,17,26–29,32]				
Low probability, 0–3 points	1–27	43–85	0.4	...
Moderate probability, 4–10 points	57–69	...	NS	...
High probability, ≥11 points	10–42	92–99	**5.9**	...

*Diagnostic standard: for *pulmonary embolism*, pulmonary angiography, computed tomographic angiography, or ventilation-perfusion scanning (± compression venous ultrasonography). In 11 studies[15,17,18,20,22,23,25,27,29,30,32] some patients with low clinical risk and negative quantitative D-dimer tests were not fully tested but instead followed for at least 3 months without anticoagulation.
[†]Definition of findings: for *Wells Score and Revised Geneva Score*, see Tables 34.1 and 34.2.
[‡]Likelihood ratio (LR) if finding present = positive LR; LR if finding absent = negative LR.
NS, Not significant.

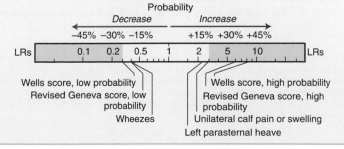

PULMONARY EMBOLISM

Probability

Decrease ← | → Increase

−45% −30% −15% | +15% +30% +45%

LRs | 0.1 0.2 0.5 1 2 5 10 | LRs

Wells score, low probability
Revised Geneva score, low probability
Wheezes

Wells score, high probability
Revised Geneva score, high probability
Unilateral calf pain or swelling
Left parasternal heave

Very few individual findings help the clinician distinguish patients with pulmonary embolism from those without it. The only individual symptoms *increasing* probability of pulmonary embolism are *sudden* dyspnea (likelihood ratio [LR] = 2.4),[6,7] syncope (LR = 2),[4–6] and hemoptysis (LR = 1.9)[3–10,17,18†]

The individual physical findings that increase the probability of pulmonary embolism are unilateral calf pain or swelling (LR = 2.9; see EBM Box 34.1), left parasternal heave (LR = 2.4), respiratory rate of more than 30 breaths/min (LR = 2), and systolic blood pressure 100 mm Hg or less (LR = 1.9). The presence of wheezes (LR = 0.4) and fever higher than 38°C (LR = 0.5) modestly decrease the probability of pulmonary embolism. The presence or absence of a pulse rate of more than 100/min as an isolated finding is unhelpful (LR = 1.4), although in one study the finding of a pulse less than 90/min decreased probability of pulmonary embolism (LR = 0.3).[3]

Other individual findings are unhelpful. Chest wall tenderness is found in 11% to 17% of patients in pulmonary embolism and has an LR that is not significant, emphasizing that this sign is not diagnostic of costochondritis (see Chapter 29). The presence of hypoxemia, defined either as room air pO_2 less than 80 mm Hg or as increased alveolar-arterial gradient, is also diagnostically unhelpful (both LRs not significant).[3,8,9,33]

B. COMBINING FINDINGS TO DETERMINE CLINICAL PROBABILITY OF EMBOLISM

In contrast to the modest accuracy of individual findings, EBM Box 34.1 indicates that a determination of "high probability" by either the Wells score (LR = 8.2) or revised Geneva score (LR = 5.9) markedly increases the probability of pulmonary embolism, whereas a determination of "low probability" by either score decreases it (LRs = 0.3 to 0.4).

Both scores emphasize that accurate assessment of a patient's probability combines both risk factors and clinical findings. The probability of embolism is high if the patient has typical signs (e.g., tachycardia, leg swelling) and risk factors (e.g., cancer, immobilization) and lacks an alternative diagnosis. The probability is low if the presentation is atypical, there are no risk factors, and there *is* a likely alternative diagnosis (e.g., angina, congestive heart failure). Many studies have shown that the probability of pulmonary embolism in patients presenting with both low clinical probability (using either score) and normal D-dimer levels is so low that further imaging is unnecessary and anticoagulation can safely be withheld.[15,23,25,27,34,35]

Nonetheless, the D-dimer measurement is a nonspecific test, resulting in many false positives that prompt further diagnostic testing in low clinical probability patients. Such testing is expensive, exposes patients to radiation, and could lead to overdiagnosis. In 2004, Kline proposed the Pulmonary Embolism Rule-out Criteria (i.e., the "PERC" rule) to further identify patients at such low risk of pulmonary embolism that no further testing (including D-dimer measurements) is necessary.[36] Importantly, to satisfy the rule, patients must be *both* low clinical probability (using a structured rule [e.g., Tables 34.1 or 34.2] or gestalt) and must meet 8 objective criteria: (1) age <50 years, (2) pulse <100 beats/min, (3) initial oxygen saturation >94% on room air, (4) no unilateral leg swelling, (5) no hemoptysis, (6) no recent trauma or surgery, (7) no prior pulmonary embolism or deep venous thrombosis, and (8) no exogenous estrogen use (patients meeting all 8 criteria are called "PERC negative"). If a patient is both low clinical probability *and* PERC

---

†In these studies, the following risk factors and symptoms were found just as frequently in patients with embolism as in those without it: female sex, older age, previous heart disease, previous lung disease, estrogen use, recent trauma, dyspnea, chest pain (pleuritic or nonpleuritic), and cough. A few individual risk factors have LRs between 1.4 and 2 and thus increase probability a small amount: cancer, recent immobilization, recent surgery, and prior venous thromboembolism.

negative, the probability of pulmonary embolism is only 0.93%, a risk regarded to be lower than the risk of further testing.[36-42] (The corresponding LR for combined low clinical probability and PERC negative is 0.1.)[37,39,40,42] Clinicians appropriately applying the PERC rule to low probability patients can safely reduce the number of diagnostic tests performed (both D-dimer measurements and computed tomography), shorten the time patients spend in emergency departments, and reduce hospitalizations.[43,44]

References may be accessed online at *Elsevier eBooks for Practicing Clinicians.*

CHAPTER 35

Pleural Effusion

KEY TEACHING POINTS

- In patients with dyspnea, the following findings increase probability of pleural effusion: abnormal auscultatory percussion, asymmetric chest expansion, diminished vocal resonance, reduced tactile fremitus, diminished breath sound intensity, and percussion dullness.
- The presence of *normal* breath sound intensity or *normal* resonance during percussion significantly decreases the possibility of underlying pleural effusion. Indeed, the diagnosis of pleural effusion is one of the main reasons students should still learn how to percuss the chest.

I. Introduction

Although ancient Greek physicians routinely recognized and treated empyema, the modern diagnostic signs of pleural effusion date to two physicians: Auenbrugger, who described the pathologic dullness and diminished chest expansion of effusions[1]; and Laennec, who described the uniform absence of breath sounds and, in some patients, the appearance of bronchial breath sounds and abnormal vocal resonance.[2] The introduction of percussion into 19th century medicine allowed clinicians to approach patients with chronic respiratory complaints and confidently distinguish empyema from tuberculosis.[3]

The most common causes of pleural effusions in the United States are congestive heart failure, pneumonia, and cancer.[4]

II. The Findings

Accumulation of pleural fluid, if large enough, expands the hemithorax (and collapses the underlying lung), which may create the appearance of an asymmetrically enlarged hemithorax with flattening or even bulging of the normally concave intercostal spaces. Because pleura fluid reduces transmission of low frequency vibrations (see Fig. 30.2), tactile fremitus is diminished on the involved side. All patients have diminished breath sounds, especially in the lower chest, from the combined effects of reduced flow rates (the underlying lung is collapsed) and diminished transmission of the low-frequency vesicular breath sounds through the fluid.

Nonetheless, testing of vocal resonance (i.e., sound of the patient's voice through the clinician's stethoscope) may produce either of two distinct findings: (1) diminished or absent vocal resonance (the patient's voice is muted compared to the uninvolved sign) or (2) "abnormal" vocal resonance with egophony, bronchophony, whispered pectoriloquy, and often, bronchial breath sounds. Chapter 30 discusses further these paradoxical findings (in the section on vocal resonance).

III. Clinical Significance

Several findings increase the probability of pleural effusion: abnormal auscultatory percussion (likelihood ratio [LR] = 8.3, EBM Box 35.1), asymmetric chest expansion (LR = 8.1), diminished vocal resonance (LR = 6.5), reduced tactile fremitus (LR = 5.7), diminished or absent breath sounds (LR = 5.2), and asymmetric percussion dullness (LR = 4.8). Findings that *decrease* the probability of pleural effusion include normal breath sound intensity (LR = 0.1), normal percussion resonance (LR = 0.1), normal tactile fremitus (LR = 0.2), symmetric chest expansion (LR = 0.3), and normal vocal resonance (LR = 0.3).

In two studies of patients in the intensive care unit, most of whom were mechanically ventilated, the absence of breath sounds over a region of the chest increased the probability of underlying pleural fluid (sensitivity of 34% to 42%, specificity of 84% to 90%, LR = 3).[5,6]

| **EBM BOX 35.1** | **Pleural Effusion*** | | | | |

Finding (Reference)[†]	Sensitivity (%)	Specificity (%)	Likelihood Ratio[‡] if Finding Is Present	Likelihood Ratio[‡] if Finding Is Absent
Inspection				
Asymmetric chest expansion[8]	74	91	**8.1**	0.3
Palpation				
Reduced tactile fremitus[8]	82	86	**5.7**	0.2
Percussion				
Dullness by conventional percussion[8]	89	81	**4.8**	0.1
Abnormal auscultatory percussion (method of Guarino)[7,8]	58–96	85–95	**8.3**	NS
Auscultation				
Diminished or absent breath sounds[8]	88	83	**5.2**	0.1
Diminished vocal resonance[8]	76	88	**6.5**	0.3
Crackles[8]	44	38	NS	1.5
Pleural rub[8]	5	99	NS	NS

*Diagnostic standard: for *pleural effusion*, chest radiograph.
[†]Definition of findings: for *abnormal auscultatory percussion*, the method of Guarino[7] (see the section on auscultatory percussion in Chapter 29); for *diminished vocal resonance intensity*, reduction or absence of transmitted sounds from the patient's voice when reciting numbers, as detected by a stethoscope on the patient's posterior chest;[8] for all other findings, see Chapters 28 to 30.
[‡]Likelihood ratio (LR) if finding present = positive LR; LR if finding absent = negative LR.
NS, Not significant.

PLEURAL EFFUSION
Probability

Decrease	Increase
−45% −30% −15%	+15% +30% +45%

LRs   0.1   0.2   0.5   1   2   5   10   LRs

Absence of dullness by conventional percussion
Normal breath sound intensity
Normal tactile fremitus
Symmetric chest expansion
Normal vocal resonance

Abnormal auscultatory percussion
Asymmetric chest expansion
Diminished vocal resonance
Reduced tactile fremitus
Diminished or absent breath sounds
Dullness by conventional percussion

References may be accessed online at *Elsevier eBooks for Practicing Clinicians.*

The Heart

Inspection of the Neck Veins

- In patients with dyspnea, ascites, or edema, determination of venous pressure at the bedside is essential. If venous pressure is elevated, the patient has cardiopulmonary disease; if venous pressure is normal, liver or kidney disease is likely.
- Bedside estimates of venous pressure are accurate when compared to measured values.
- In patients with chest pain or dyspnea, elevated neck veins increase probability of elevated left heart pressure and depressed ejection fraction.
- The most important feature that distinguishes the internal jugular venous waveform from arterial movements is its conspicuous *inward* movement (arterial movements have a conspicuous *outward* movement).
- Kussmaul sign and the positive abdominojugular test often appear together. They appear in constrictive pericarditis and right ventricular infarction and in some patients with severe heart failure. In heart failure, Kussmaul sign is associated with an unfavorable prognosis.

I. Introduction

Clinicians should inspect the neck veins for the following reasons: (1) to detect elevated central venous pressure (CVP) and (2) to detect specific abnormalities of venous waveforms, which are characteristic of certain arrhythmias and some valvular, pericardial, and myocardial disorders.

Clinicians first associated conspicuous neck veins with heart disease approximately 3 centuries ago.[1,2] In the late 1800s Sir James Mackenzie described venous waveforms of arrhythmias and various heart disorders, using a mechanical polygraph applied over the patient's neck or liver. His labels for the venous waveforms—A, C, and V waves—are still used today.[3,4] Clinician began to estimate venous pressure at the bedside routinely in the 1920s, after the introduction of the glass manometer and after Starling's experiments linking venous pressure to cardiac output.[5]

II. Venous Pressure

A. DEFINITIONS

1. Central Venous Pressure

Central venous pressure (CVP) is the mean vena caval or right atrial pressure, which, in the absence of tricuspid stenosis, equals the right ventricular end-diastolic pressure. Disorders that increase diastolic pressures of the right side of the heart—left heart disease, lung disease, primary pulmonary hypertension, and pulmonic stenosis—all increase the CVP and make the neck veins abnormally conspicuous. CVP is expressed in millimeters of mercury (mm Hg) or centimeters (cm) of water above atmospheric pressure (1.36 cm water = 1.0 mm Hg).

Estimations of CVP are most helpful in patients with ascites or edema, in whom an elevated CVP indicates heart or lung disease and a normal CVP suggests alternative diagnoses, such as chronic liver disease. Despite the prevailing opinion, the CVP is normal in patients with liver disease (without associated cardiopulmonary disease); the edema in patients with isolated liver disease results from hypoalbuminemia and the weight of ascites compressing veins to the legs.[6–9]

2. Physiologic Zero Point

Physiologists have long assumed that a location in the cardiovascular system (presumed to be the right atrium in humans) tightly regulates venous pressure so that it remains the same even when the person changes position.[5,10–12] All measurements of the CVP—whether by clinicians inspecting neck veins or by catheters in intensive care units—attempt to identify the pressure at this zero point (e.g., if a manometer connected to a systemic vein supports a column of saline 8 cm above the zero point, with the top of the manometer open to atmosphere, the recorded pressure in that vein is 8 cm water). Estimates of CVP are related to the zero point because interpretation of this value does not need to consider the hydrostatic effects of different patient positions, and any abnormal value thus indicates disease.

3. External Reference Point

Clinicians require some external reference point to reliably locate the level of the zero point. Of the many such reference points that have been proposed over the last century,[5] only two are commonly used today: the sternal angle and the phlebostatic axis.

a. Sternal Angle
In 1930 Sir Thomas Lewis, a pupil of Mackenzie, proposed a simple bedside method for measuring venous pressure designed to replace the manometer, which he found too burdensome for general use.[13] He observed that the top of the jugular veins of normal persons (and the top of the fluid in the manometer) always came to lie within 1 to 2 cm of vertical distance from the sternal angle, whether the person was supine, semiupright, or upright (an observation since confirmed by others).[14] If the top level of the neck veins was more than 3 cm above the sternal angle, Lewis concluded the venous pressure was elevated.

Others have modified this method, stating that the CVP equals the vertical distance between the top of the neck veins and a point 5 cm below the sternal angle (Fig. 36.1).[15] This variation is commonly called the **method of Lewis**, although Lewis himself never made such a claim.

b. Phlebostatic Axis
The phlebostatic axis is the midpoint between the anterior and posterior surfaces of the chest at the level of the fourth intercostal space. This reference point, the most common landmark used in intensive care units and cardiac catheterization laboratories, was originally proposed in the 1940s, when studies showed that using it as the zero point minimized variation in venous pressure of normal persons as they changed position between 0 and 90 degrees.[11]

c. Relative Merits of Sternal Angle and Phlebostatic Axis
Obviously, the measurement of venous pressure is only as good as the reference point used. The phlebostatic axis locates a point in the right atrium several centimeters posterior to the point identified by the method of Lewis (i.e., the zero point using the phlebostatic axis is 9 to 10 cm posterior to the sternal angle; that using the method of Lewis is 5 cm below the sternal angle).[16,17] This means that clinicians using the phlebostatic axis will estimate the CVP to be several cm of water higher than those using the method of Lewis, even if these clinicians completely agree on the location of the neck veins.

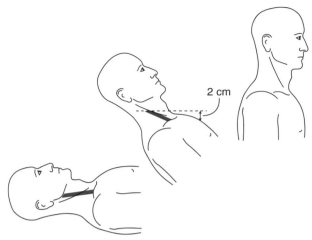

Fig. 36.1 Measurement of venous pressure. The clinician should vary the patient's position until the top of the neck veins become visible. In this patient, who has normal central venous pressure (CVP), the neck veins are fully distended when supine and completely collapsed when upright. A semiupright position, therefore, is used to estimate pressure. In this position, the top of the neck veins is 2 cm above the sternal angle, and according to the method of Lewis, the patient's CVP is 2+5 = 7 cm water.

The sternal angle is a better reference point for bedside examination, simply because clinicians can reproducibly locate it more easily than the phlebostatic axis. Even using standard patient positions and flexible right-angle triangles or laser levels, experienced observers trying to locate a point similar to the phlebostatic axis disagreed by several centimeters in both horizontal and vertical directions.[18,19]

B. ELEVATED VENOUS PRESSURE

1. Technique

To measure the patient's venous pressure, the clinician should examine the veins on the right side of the patient's neck, because these veins have a direct route to the heart. Veins in the left side of the neck reach the heart by crossing the mediastinum, where the normal aorta may compress them, causing left jugular venous pressure to be sometimes elevated even when CVP and right venous pressure are normal.[20,21]

The patient should be positioned at whichever angle between the supine and upright position best reveals the top of the neck veins (see Fig. 36.1). The top of the neck veins is indicated by the point above which the subcutaneous conduit of the external jugular vein disappears or above which the pulsating waveforms of the internal jugular vein become imperceptible.

2. External vs. Internal Jugular Veins

Either the external or internal jugular veins may be used to estimate pressure, because measurements in both are similar.[22] Traditionally clinicians have been taught to use only the internal jugular vein because the external jugular vein contains valves that purportedly interfere with the development of a hydrostatic column necessary to measure pressure. This teaching is erroneous for two reasons: (1) The internal jugular vein also contains valves, a fact known to anatomists for centuries.[23–25] These valves are essential during cardiopulmonary resuscitation, preventing blood from flowing backward during chest compression[26]; (2) Valves in the jugular veins do not interfere with pressure measurements because flow is normally toward the heart. In fact, valves probably act like a transducer membrane (e.g., the diaphragm of a speaker), which amplify right atrial pressure pulsations and make the venous waveforms easier to see.[23]

3. Definition of Elevated CVP

After locating the top of the external or internal jugular veins, the clinician should measure the vertical distance between the top of the veins and one of the external reference points discussed above (see Fig. 36.1). The venous pressure is abnormally elevated if (1) the top of the neck veins are more than 3 cm above the sternal angle, (2) the CVP exceeds 8 cm water using the method of Lewis (i.e., >3 cm above the sternal angle + 5 cm), or (3) the CVP is greater than 12 cm water using the phlebostatic axis.

C. BEDSIDE ESTIMATES OF VENOUS PRESSURE VS. CATHETER MEASUREMENTS

1. Diagnostic Accuracy*

In studies employing a standardized reference point, bedside estimates of CVP are within 4 cm water of catheter measurements 85% of the time.[22,30,31] According to these studies, the finding of an elevated CVP (i.e., top of neck veins >3 cm water above sternal angle or >8 cm water using method of Lewis) greatly increases the probability that catheter measurements are elevated (likelihood ratio [LR] = 8.9, EBM Box 36.1). The finding of a normal CVP on examination (< 8 cm using the method of Lewis) decreases significantly the probability of a measured CVP > 12 cm water (LR = 0.2; see EBM Box 36.1). If disease is defined instead as measured CVP > 8 cm, the finding of normal venous pressure on examination is slightly less compelling (LR = 0.3), indicating that some patients with normal venous pressure on examination have modestly elevated measured values (between 8 and 12 cm water[†]).

This tendency to slightly underestimate the measured values, which is elucidated further in the following section, explains why estimates made during expiration are slightly more accurate than are those made during inspiration: during expiration, the neck veins move upward in the neck, increasing the bedside estimate and minimizing the error.[22]

2. Why Clinicians Underestimate Measured Values

Of the many reasons why clinicians tend to underestimate the measured values of CVP, the most important one is that the vertical distance between the sternal angle and physiologic zero point varies as the patient shifts position (see Fig. 36.2).[5,47] Catheter measurements of the venous pressure are always made while the patient is lying supine, whether the venous pressure is high or low. Bedside estimates of the venous pressure, however, must be made in the semiupright or upright positions if the venous pressure is high, because only these positions reveal the top of the distended neck veins. Fig. 36.2 shows that the semiupright position increases the vertical distance between the right atrium and sternal angle by approximately 3 cm, compared with the supine position, which effectively lowers the bedside estimate by the same amount. The significance of this is that patients with a mildly elevated CVP by catheter measurements (i.e., 8 to 12 cm), whose neck veins are interpretable only in more upright positions, may have bedside estimates that are normal (i.e., <8 cm water).

In support of this, even catheter measurements using the sternal angle as reference point are approximately 3 cm lower when the patient is in the semiupright position than when the patient is supine.[48-50]

---

*Studies that test the diagnostic accuracy of bedside estimates of CVP are difficult to summarize because they often fail to standardize which external reference point was used.[27-29]

†For purposes of comparison, "measured pressure" here is in centimeters water using the method of Lewis. Most catheterization laboratories measure pressure in mm Hg using the phlebostatic axis as the reference point.

| EBM BOX 36.1 | Inspection of the Neck Veins* | | | |

Finding (Reference)[†]	Sensitivity (%)	Specificity (%)	Likelihood Ratio[‡] if Finding Is	
			Present	Absent
Estimated venous pressure elevated				
Detecting measured CVP >8 cm water[22,30-33]	47–92	83–96	8.9	0.3
Detecting measured CVP >12 cm water[22,30,31]	78–95	67–93	6.6	0.2
Detecting elevated left heart diastolic pressures[34-36]	10–58	96–97	3.9	NS
Detecting low LV ejection fraction[37-39]	7–25	96–98	6.3	NS
Detecting myocardial infarction (if chest pain)[40]	10	96	2.4	NS
Detecting pulmonary hypertension[41]	70	72	2.5	0.4
Predicting postoperative pulmonary edema[42,43]	19	98	11.3	NS
Predicting postoperative MI or cardiac death[42,43]	17	98	9.4	NS
Estimated venous pressure low				
Detecting measured CVP ≤5 cm water[33]	90	89	8.4	0.1
Positive abdominojugular test				
Detecting elevated left heart diastolic pressures[34,44,45]	55–84	83–98	8.0	0.3
Early systolic outward movement (CV wave)				
Detecting moderate-to-severe tricuspid regurgitation[46]	37	97	10.9	0.7

*Diagnostic standard: for *measured CVP*, measurement by catheter in supine patient using method of Lewis[22,30,32,33] or unknown;[31] for *elevated left heart diastolic pressures* or *low ejection fracture*, see Chapter 48; for *pulmonary hypertension*, measured mean pulmonary artery pressure ≥25 mm Hg; for *myocardial infarction*, see Chapter 49.

[†]Definition of findings: for *elevated venous pressure*, bedside estimate >8 cm water using method of Lewis,[22,30,31,41] >12 cm water using phlebostatic axis,[42,43] or unknown method;[34-37] for *low venous pressure*, estimate CVP ≤ 5 cm water using method of Lewis;[33] and for *positive abdominojugular test*, see the text.

[‡]Likelihood ratio (LR) if finding present = positive LR; LR if finding absent = negative LR.

CVP, Central venous pressure; LV, left ventricular; MI, myocardial infarction; NS, not significant.

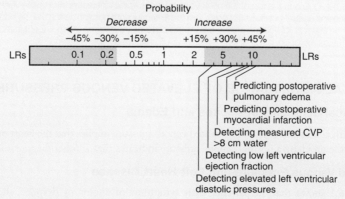

ELEVATED VENOUS PRESSURE
Probability

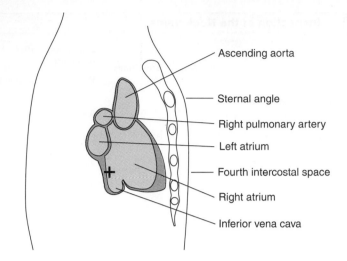

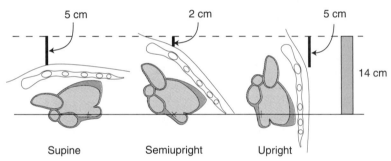

Fig. 36.2 Central venous pressure and position of patient. The *top half* of the figure shows the sagittal section of a 43-year old man, just to the right of the midsternal line, demonstrating the relationship between the sternal angle, right atrium, and phlebostatic axis (indicated by the *black cross* in the posterior right atrium). The *bottom half* of the figure illustrates the changing vertical distance between the phlebostatic axis *(solid horizontal line)* and sternal angle in the supine (0 degrees), semiupright (45 degrees), and upright (90 degrees) positions. The venous pressure is the same in each position (14 cm above the phlebostatic axis, *gray bar on right*), but the vertical distance between the sternal angle and the top of the neck veins changes in the different positions: the vertical distance is 5 cm in the supine and upright positions but only 2 cm in the semiupright position. Using the method of Lewis (see text), therefore, the estimate of venous pressure from the semiupright position (7 cm = 2+5) is 3 cm *lower* than estimates from the supine or upright positions (10 cm = 5+5 cm). Based upon reference 5.

D. CLINICAL SIGNIFICANCE OF ELEVATED VENOUS PRESSURE

1. Differential Diagnosis of Ascites and Edema

In patients with ascites and edema, an elevated venous pressure implies that the heart or pulmonary circulation is the problem; a normal venous pressure indicates that another diagnosis is the cause.

2. Elevated Venous Pressure and Left Heart Disease

EBM Box 36.1 shows that, in patients with symptoms of angina or dyspnea, the finding of elevated venous pressure increases the probability of elevated left atrial pressure (LR = 3.9, see

EBM Box 36.1)[‡] and depressed ejection fraction (LR = 6.3). The opposite finding (normal neck veins) provides no diagnostic information about the left heart pressure or function (negative LRs not significant, see EBM Box 36.1). In patients presenting to emergency departments with sustained chest pain, the finding of elevated venous pressure increases the probability of myocardial infarction (LR = 2.4).

3. Elevated Venous Pressure and Pulmonary Hypertension

In a study of 116 patients seeing pulmonary hypertension specialists, the finding of elevated venous pressure detected a measured mean pulmonary artery pressure ≥25 mm Hg with a positive LR = 2.5 and negative LR = 0.4 (see EBM Box 36.1).

4. Elevated Venous Pressure during Preoperative Consultation

The finding of elevated venous pressure during preoperative consultation predicts that the patient—without diuresis or other treatment—will develop postoperative pulmonary edema (LR = 11.3; see EBM Box 36.1) or myocardial infarction (LR = 9.4).

5. Elevated Venous Pressure and Pericardial Disease

Elevated venous pressure is a cardinal finding of cardiac tamponade (100% of cases) and constrictive pericarditis (94% of cases). Therefore, the absence of elevated neck veins is a compelling argument against these diagnoses. In every patient with elevated neck veins, the clinician should search for other findings of tamponade (i.e., pulsus paradoxus; prominent x′ descent but absent y descent in venous waveforms) and constrictive pericarditis (pericardial knock, prominent x′ and y descents in venous waveforms) (see Chapter 47).

6. Unilateral Elevation of Venous Pressure

Distention of the left jugular veins with normal right jugular veins sometimes occurs because of kinking of the left innominate vein by a tortuous aorta.[20,21] In these patients the elevation often disappears after a deep inspiration.

Persistent unilateral elevation of the neck veins usually indicates local obstruction by a mediastinal lesion, such as aortic aneurysm or intrathoracic goiter.[53]

E. CLINICAL SIGNIFICANCE OF LOW ESTIMATED VENOUS PRESSURE

Few studies have addressed whether clinicians can accurately detect *low* venous pressure, a potentially difficult issue because *normal* venous pressure is often defined as less than 8 cm water (i.e., the *low* and *normal* measurements overlap). Nonetheless, in one study of 38 patients in the intensive care unit (approximately half of whom received mechanical ventilation), the clinician's estimate of a CVP of 5 cm water or less accurately detected a measured value of 5 cm water or less (positive LR = 8.4), an important finding if the clinician is contemplating whether or not fluid challenge is indicated.

F. USING HAND VEINS TO DETERMINE CENTRAL VENOUS PRESSURE

If a saline-filled manometer (open to the atmosphere) is connected to a central vein, the height of the saline column above the patient's zero point is equal to the patient's CVP (see the earlier section on physiologic zero point). Clinicians have long wondered whether the patient's own hand

---

[‡]During cardiac catheterization, a measured right atrial pressure ≥10 mm Hg detects a measured pulmonary capillary wedge pressures of ≥22 mm Hg with an LR of 3.5, similar to bedside examination (LR = 3.9).[51,52]

veins could substitute for the manometer. According to this theory, the hand veins should fill and be distended when the hand is held below the point corresponding to the top of the saline column in a manometer but should collapse the moment the hand is higher than this point.

In a commonly used technique, the clinician takes the supine patient's hand and first moves it below the patient's body level to guarantee the filling of the hand veins. Then, the clinician slowly lifts the hand, closely observing the most visible vein on the back of the patient's hand and marking precisely the point when the vein collapses. The vertical distance between this point and the patient's zero point (using either method of Lewis or phlebostatic axis) is the estimated CVP.

In one study of 82 intensive care unit patients, this technique detected an elevated CVP (catheter measurement >12 mm Hg above the phlebostatic axis) with a sensitivity of 29%, specificity of 94%, positive LR = 4.9, and negative LR = 0.8. Similarly, the technique detected a low CVP (<7 mm Hg above the phlebostatic axis) with a sensitivity of 93%, specificity of 60%, positive LR = 2.3, and negative LR = 0.1).[54] In one of three patients, however, this technique could not be used because of the presence of hand edema or venous catheters.

III. Abdominojugular Test

A. THE FINDING

During the abdominojugular test, the clinician observes the neck veins while pressing firmly over the patient's mid-abdomen for 10 seconds, a maneuver that probably increases the venous return by displacing the splanchnic venous blood toward the heart.[45] The CVP of healthy persons usually remains unchanged during this maneuver or rises for a beat or two before returning to normal or below normal.[30,44,45,55,56] If the CVP rises by more than 4 cm water and remains elevated for the entire 10 seconds, the abdominojugular test is positive.[34,45] Most clinicians recognize the positive response by observing the neck veins at the moment the abdominal pressure is released, regarding a *fall* of more than 4 cm as positive.

The earliest version of the abdominojugular test was the **hepatojugular reflux**, introduced by Pasteur in 1885 as a pathognomonic sign of tricuspid regurgitation.[57] In 1898, Rondot discovered that patients with normal tricuspid valves could develop the sign, and by 1925, clinicians realized that pressure anywhere over the abdomen, not just over the liver, would elicit the sign.[55] Several investigators have contributed to the current definition of the abdominojugular test.[30,45,58]

B. CLINICAL SIGNIFICANCE

In patients presenting for cardiac catheterization (presumably because of chest pain or dyspnea), a positive abdominojugular test is an accurate sign of elevated left atrial pressure (i.e., ≥15 mm Hg, LR = 8, see EBM Box 36.1). Therefore, a positive abdominojugular test is an important finding in patients with dyspnea, indicating that at least some of the dyspnea is due to disease in the left side of the heart. A negative abdominojugular test decreases the probability of left atrial hypertension (LR = 0.3, EBM Box 36.1).

In patients with severe heart failure, the finding of a positive abdominojugular test is associated with increased 6-month mortality (27% in those with a positive abdominojugular test compared to 14% without the finding, p = 0.004).[59]

IV. Kussmaul Sign

The Kussmaul sign is the paradoxical elevation of the CVP during inspiration. In healthy persons the venous pressure falls during inspiration, because the pressures in the right heart decrease as the intrathoracic pressures fall. The Kussmaul sign is classically associated with constrictive pericarditis, but occurs in only a minority of patients with constriction[60,61] and is found in other disorders such as severe heart failure,[61-63] pulmonary embolus,[64] and right ventricular infarction.[65-68]

An excellent video of the Kussmaul sign is available at reference 69.

A. PATHOGENESIS OF ELEVATED VENOUS PRESSURE, ABDOMINOJUGULAR TEST, AND KUSSMAUL SIGN

The peripheral veins of healthy persons are distensible vessels that contain approximately two-thirds of the total blood volume and can accept or donate blood with relatively little change in pressure. In contrast, the peripheral veins of patients with heart failure are abnormally constricted from tissue edema and intense sympathetic stimulation, a change that reduces the extremity blood volume and increases the central blood volume. Because constricted veins are less compliant, the added central blood volume causes the CVP to be abnormally increased.[5]

In addition to causing an elevated CVP, venoconstriction probably also contributes to the positive abdominojugular test and Kussmaul sign, two signs that often occur together. Most patients with constrictive pericarditis and the Kussmaul sign also have a markedly positive abdominojugular test; many patients with severe heart failure and a markedly positive abdominojugular test also have the Kussmaul sign.[61] The venous pressure of these patients, unlike that of healthy persons, is very susceptible to changes in the venous return. Maneuvers that increase the venous return—exercise, leg elevation, or abdominal pressure—increase the venous pressure of patients with the abdominojugular test and Kussmaul sign, but not that of healthy persons.[5] The Kussmaul sign may be nothing more than an inspiratory abdominojugular test, with the downward movement of the diaphragm compressing the abdomen and increasing venous return.[70]

Even so, an abnormal right ventricle probably also contributes to the Kussmaul sign, because all of the disorders associated with the Kussmaul sign are characterized by a right ventricle that is unable to accommodate more blood during inspiration (i.e., in constrictive pericarditis the normal ventricle is constrained by the diseased pericardium, and in severe heart failure, acute cor pulmonale, or right ventricular infarction, the dilated right ventricle is constrained by the normal pericardium). A right side of the heart thus constrained only exaggerates the inspiratory increments of CVP, making the Kussmaul sign more prominent.[5]

B. CLINICAL SIGNIFICANCE OF KUSSMAUL SIGN

In addition to serving as an important clue to the diagnoses of constrictive pericarditis and right ventricular infarction, the Kussmaul sign is associated with an adverse prognosis when found in patients with severe heart failure (LR = 3.5 for 1-year mortality).[63]

V. Venous Waveforms

A. IDENTIFYING THE INTERNAL JUGULAR VEIN

Venous waveforms are usually only conspicuous in the internal jugular vein, which lies under the sternocleidomastoid muscle and therefore becomes evident by causing pulsating movements of the soft tissues of the neck (i.e., it does not resemble a subcutaneous vein). Since the carotid artery also pulsates in the neck, the clinician must learn to distinguish the carotid artery from the internal jugular vein, using the principles outlined in Table 36.1.

Of the distinguishing features listed in Table 36.1, the most conspicuous one is the character of the movement. Venous pulsations have a prominent *inward* or *descending* movement, the outward one being slower and more diffuse. Arterial pulsations, in contrast, have a prominent *ascending* or *outward* movement, the inward one being slow and diffuse.

TABLE 36.1 ▪ Distinguishing Internal Jugular Waveforms from Carotid Pulses*

Characteristic	Internal Jugular Vein	Carotid Artery
Character of movement	Descending movement most prominent	Ascending movement most prominent
Number of pulsations per ventricular systole	Two, usually	One
Palpability of pulsations	Not palpable or only slight undulation	Easily palpable
Change with respiration	During inspiration, pulsations become more prominent but drop lower in neck	No change
Change with position	Pulsations lower in neck as patient sits up	No change
Change with abdominal pressure	Pulsations may temporarily become more prominent and move higher in neck	No change
Change with pressure applied to the neck just below pulsations	Pulsations become less prominent	No change

*Based on references 71–74.

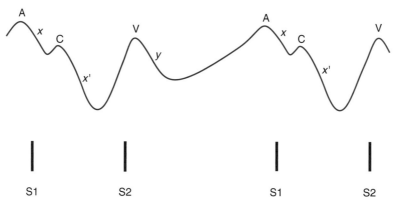

Fig. 36.3 Venous waveforms on pressure tracings. There are three positive waves (A, C, and V) and three negative waves (x, x', and y descents). The A wave represents right atrial contraction; the x descent, right atrial relaxation. The C wave—named "C" because Mackenzie originally thought it was a carotid artifact—probably instead represents right ventricular contraction and closure of the tricuspid valve, which then bulges upward toward the neck veins.[75,76] The x' descent occurs because the floor of the right atrium (i.e., the A-V valve ring) moves downward, pulling away from the jugular veins, as the right ventricle contracts (physiologists call this movement the "descent of the base").[77] The V wave represents right atrial filling, which eventually overcomes the descent of the base and causes venous pressure to rise (most atrial filling normally occurs during ventricular systole, not diastole). The y descent begins the moment the tricuspid valve opens at the beginning of diastole, causing the atrium to empty into the ventricle and venous pressure to abruptly fall.

B. COMPONENTS OF VENOUS WAVEFORMS

Although venous pressure tracings reveal three positive and negative waves (Fig. 36.3), the clinician at the bedside usually sees only two descents, namely, a more prominent x' descent and a less prominent y descent (Fig. 36.4). Fig. 36.3 outlines the physiology of these waveforms.

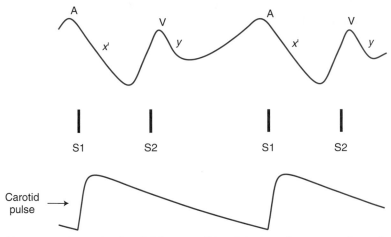

Fig. 36.4 Venous waveform: what the clinician sees. Although tracings of venous waveforms display three positive and three negative waves (see Fig. 36.3), the C wave is usually too small to see. Instead, the clinician sees two descents per cardiac cycle: the first represents merging of the x and x′ descents and is usually referred to as the x′ descent (i.e., "x-prime" descent). The second is the y descent, which is smaller than the x′ descent in normal persons. The clinician identifies the descents by timing them with the heart tones or carotid pulsation (see text).

C. TIMING THE X′ AND Y DESCENTS

The best way to identify the individual venous waveforms is to time their *descents*, by simultaneously listening to the heart tones or palpating the carotid pulsation (Fig. 36.4).

1. Using Heart Tones

The x′ descent ends just *before* S_2, as if it were a collapsing hill that slides into S_2 lying at the bottom. In contrast, the y descent begins just *after* S_2.

2. Using the Carotid Artery

The x′ descent is a systolic movement that coincides with the tap from the carotid pulsation. The y descent is a diastolic movement beginning after the carotid tap, with a delay approximately equivalent to the interval between the patient's S_1 and S_2.[73,78]

D. CLINICAL SIGNIFICANCE

The normal venous waveform has a prominent x′ descent and a small or absent y descent; there are no abrupt outward movements.[78]

Abnormalities of the venous waveforms become conspicuous at the bedside for one of two reasons: (1) the descents are abnormal or (2) there is a sudden outward movement in the neck veins.

1. Abnormal Descents

There are three abnormal patterns: **(1) The W or M pattern** (x′ = y pattern). The y descent becomes unusually prominent, which, along with the normal x′ descent, creates two prominent descents per systole and traces a W or M pattern in the soft tissues of the neck; **(2) The diminished X′ descent pattern** (x′ < y pattern). The x′ descent diminishes or disappears, making the y descent most prominent. This is the most common abnormal pattern, occurring both in atrial fibrillation (loss of A wave) and many different cardiomyopathies (more sluggish "descent of the base,"

TABLE 36.2 **Venous Waveforms**

Finding	Etiology (ref)
Abnormal Descents	
W or M pattern (x′ = y)	Constrictive pericarditis[72,79]*
	Atrial septal defect[80-82]
Diminished x′ descent (x′ < y)	Atrial fibrillation
	Cardiomyopathy[78]
	Mild tricuspid regurgitation
Absent y descent[†]	Cardiac tamponade[72]
	Tricuspid stenosis[83]
Abnormally Prominent Outward Waves	
Giant A wave (presystolic wave)	Pulmonary hypertension[72]
	Pulmonic stenosis[72]
	Tricuspid stenosis[83,84]
Systolic wave	Tricuspid regurgitation[46,85-87]
	Cannon A waves[72]

*The prominent Y descent of constrictive pericarditis is sometimes called *Friedreich's diastolic collapse of the cervical veins* (after Nikolaus Friedreich, 1825–1882).
†If venous pressure is normal, the absence of a y descent is a normal finding; if venous pressure is elevated, however, the absence of the y descent is abnormal and suggests impaired early diastolic filling.

which is defined in Fig. 36.3), and **(3) The absent y descent pattern**. This pattern is only relevant in patients with elevated venous pressure, because healthy persons with normal CVP also have a diminutive y descent.

The etiologies of each of these patterns are presented in Table 36.2.

2. Abnormally Prominent Outward Waves

If the clinician detects an abnormally abrupt and conspicuous outward movement in the neck veins, the clinician should determine if the outward movement begins just before S_1 (presystolic giant A waves) or after S_1 (tricuspid regurgitation and cannon A waves).

a. Giant A Waves (Abrupt Presystolic Outward Waves)

Giant A waves have two requirements: (1) sinus rhythm and (2) some obstruction to right atrial or ventricular emptying, usually from pulmonary hypertension, pulmonic stenosis, or tricuspid stenosis.[71,72,84] Nonetheless, many patients with severe pulmonary hypertension lack this finding, because their atria contract too feebly or at a time in the cardiac cycle when the venous pressures are falling.[82,88]

Some patients with giant A waves have an accompanying abrupt presystolic sound that is heard with the stethoscope over the jugular veins.[89]

b. Systolic Waves

(1). Tricuspid Regurgitation. In patients with tricuspid regurgitation and pulmonary hypertension, the neck veins are elevated (over 90% of patients) and consist of a single outward systolic movement that coincides with the carotid pulsation and collapses after S_2 (i.e, prominent y descent).[85-87] Some patients have an accompanying midsystolic clicking sound over the jugular veins.[90] Because the jugular valves often become incompetent in chronic tricuspid regurgitation, the arm and leg veins also may pulsate with each systolic regurgitant wave (see Chapter 46).

The finding of early systolic outward venous waveforms (CV wave) greatly increases the probability of moderate-to-severe tricuspid regurgitation (LR = 10.9, EBM Box 36.1). An excellent video of this finding appears in reference 91.

(2). Cannon A Waves. Cannon A waves represent an atrial contraction that occurs just after ventricular contraction, when the tricuspid valve is closed.[§] Instead of ejecting blood into the right ventricle, the contraction forces blood upward into the jugular veins. Cannon A waves may be regular (i.e., with every arterial pulse) or intermittent.

(a). *Regular Cannon A Waves.* This finding occurs in many paroxysmal supraventricular tachycardias (fast heart rates) and junctional rhythms (normal heart rates), both of which have retrograde P waves buried within or just after the QRS complex.[72] An excellent video of regular cannon A waves in a patient with pacemaker syndrome and retrograde conduction of P waves from ventricular pacing appears in reference 92.

(b). *Intermittent cannon A waves.* If the arterial pulse is regular but cannon A waves are intermittent, only one mechanism is possible: atrioventricular dissociation (see Chapter 16).[93] In patients with ventricular tachycardia, the finding of intermittently appearing cannon A waves detects atrioventricular dissociation with a sensitivity of 96%, specificity of 75%, positive LR of 3.8, and negative LR of 0.1[94] (see Chapter 16).

If the arterial pulse is irregular, intermittent cannon A waves have less importance because they commonly accompany ventricular premature contractions, and less commonly, atrial premature contractions (see Chapter 16).

References may be accessed online at *Elsevier eBooks for Practicing Clinicians.*

[§]The electrocardiographic correlate of the cannon A wave is a P wave (atrial contraction) falling between the QRS and T waves (ventricular systole).

Percussion of the Heart

I. Introduction

Percussion of the heart has its roots in the 1820s, when a student of Laennec, Pierre Piorry, enthusiastically introduced topographic percussion, a technique purportedly allowing clinicians to precisely outline the borders of the underlying organs, including those of the heart.[1-3] Although many of Piorry's claims seem extraordinary today (e.g., he declared that he could outline pulmonary cavities, the spleen, hydatid cysts, and even individual heart chambers), many of his innovations persist, including indirect percussion, the pleximeter (Piorry used an ivory plate, but most clinicians now use the left middle finger), and the current practice of using percussion to locate the border of the diaphragm on the posterior chest or the span of the liver on the anterior body wall.[4]

In 1899, only 4 years after the discovery of roentgen rays, Williams challenged the accuracy of cardiac percussion, showing that many patients with moderately large hearts (autopsy weight of 350 to 500 grams) had normal findings during cardiac percussion.[5] Cardiac percussion suffered another setback in 1907, when Moritz published the composite outlines of cardiac dullness according to various authorities, showing that these authorities not only disagreed with each other but also with the true roentgenographic outline.[4,6] By the 1930s, many leading clinicians began to regard percussion of the heart as unreliable and often inaccurate.[4,7]

II. Clinical Significance

Studies of cardiac percussion have several limitations, the most important of which is selectively enrolling only healthy patients lacking chest deformities or emphysema. Nonetheless, even these studies show that the percussed outline of the heart correlates only moderately with the true cardiac border. Whether the patient is supine or upright, the average error in locating the cardiac border is 1 to 2 cm (the standard deviation of this error is about 1 cm). The clinician usually overestimates the left border by placing it too far lateral and underestimates the right border by placing it too near the sternum (these errors tend to cancel each other if the study's endpoint is total transverse diameter of the heart).[8-11] In patients with emphysema, the errors are even greater.[12]

The traditional sign of an enlarged heart by percussion is cardiac dullness that extends too far laterally. The findings of either cardiac dullness extending beyond the midclavicular line or more than 10.5 cm from the midsternal line modestly increase the probability of an enlarged cardiothoracic ratio (likelihood ratio [LR] = 2.4 to 2.5; EBM Box 37.1). If cardiac dullness does not

EBM BOX 37.1   **Percussion of the Heart***

Finding (Reference)	Sensitivity (%)	Specificity (%)	Likelihood Ratio† if Finding Is	
			Present	Absent
Dullness extends more than 10.5cm from midsternal line, patient supine				
Detecting cardiothoracic ratio >0.5[13]	97	61	2.5	0.05
Detecting increased left ventricular end-diastolic volume[14]	94	32	1.4	NS
Dullness extends beyond midclavicular line, patient upright				
Detecting cardiothoracic ratio >0.5[8]	97	60	2.4	0.1

*Diagnostic standard: for *cardiothoracic ratio*, maximal transverse diameter of heart on chest radiography divided by maximal transverse diameter of thoracic cage; for *increased left ventricular end-diastolic volume*, >186mL by ultrafast computed tomography.[14]
†Likelihood ratio (LR) if finding present = positive LR; LR if finding absent = negative LR.
NS, Not significant.

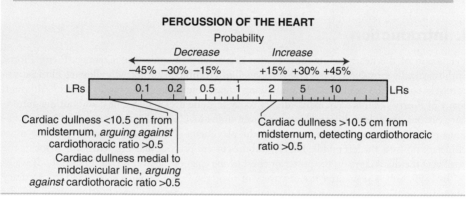

PERCUSSION OF THE HEART

Probability

Decrease   *Increase*

−45% −30% −15%   +15% +30% +45%

LRs   0.1   0.2   0.5   1   2   5   10   LRs

Cardiac dullness <10.5 cm from midsternum, *arguing against* cardiothoracic ratio >0.5
Cardiac dullness medial to midclavicular line, *arguing against* cardiothoracic ratio >0.5

Cardiac dullness >10.5 cm from midsternum, detecting cardiothoracic ratio >0.5

extend beyond these points, the patient probably does not have an enlarged cardiothoracic ratio (LRs = 0.05 to 0.1; EBM Box 37.1). Nonetheless, it is unlikely that this information is clinically useful since the cardiothoracic ratio has uncertain clinical significance.[15]

References may be accessed online at *Elsevier eBooks for Practicing Clinicians*.

Palpation of the Heart

I. Introduction

Much of the science of heart palpation is based on impulse cardiography and kinetocardiography, research tools from the 1960s that precisely timed normal and abnormal precordial movements and compared them with hemodynamic data and angiograms of the right ventricle and left ventricle. These precise and sensitive instruments could detect very small movements of the body wall, many of which are inconspicuous to the clinician's hand. Although this chapter refers to these studies to make certain points, only those movements easily palpable at the bedside are discussed.

Palpation of the heart is among the oldest physical examination technique, having been recorded as early as 1550 BC by ancient Egyptian physicians (along with palpation of the peripheral pulses).[1] In the early 19th century, Jean-Nicolas Corvisart, personal physician to Napoleon and teacher of Laennec, was the first to correlate cardiac palpation with postmortem findings and distinguish right ventricular enlargement from left ventricular enlargement.[2-4] During animal experiments performed in 1830, James Hope proved that the cause of the apical impulse was ventricular contraction, which threw the heart up against the chest wall.[5]

II. Technique

When palpating the chest, the clinician should describe the location, size, timing, and type of precordial movements.[6]

A. PATIENT POSITION

The clinician should first palpate the heart when the patient is lying supine and again with the patient lying on his or her left side. The supine position is used to locate all precordial movements and to identify whether these movements are abnormally hyperkinetic, sustained, or retracting (see later). The left lateral decubitus position is used to measure the diameter of the apical impulse and to detect additional abnormal diastolic filling movements (i.e., palpable third or fourth heart sounds).[7]

Because the left lateral decubitus position distorts the systolic apical movement, including those of healthy subjects (i.e., up to half of healthy patients have abnormally sustained movements in the lateral decubitus position), only the supine position should be used to characterize the timing of the precordial movement.[8]

B. LOCATION OF ABNORMAL MOVEMENTS

Complete palpation of the heart includes four areas on the chest wall (Fig. 38.1).[1,6,9–12]

1. Apex Beat

The **apex beat** or **apical impulse** is the palpable cardiac impulse farthest away from the sternum and farthest down on the chest wall, usually caused by the left ventricle and located near the midclavicular line (MCL) in the fifth intercostal space. The clinician should also palpate the areas above and medial to the apex beat, where ventricular aneurysms sometimes become palpable.

2. Left Lower Sternal Area (Fourth Intercostal Space Near Left Edge of Sternum)

Abnormal right ventricular and left atrial movements appear at this location.

3. Left Base (Second Intercostal Space Near the Left Sternum)

Abnormal pulmonary artery movements or a palpable P_2 appear at this location.

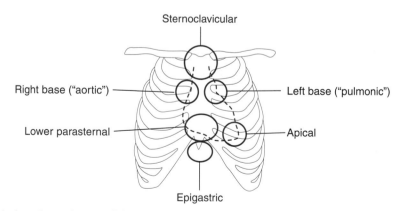

Fig. 38.1 Locations of precordial movements. The principal areas of precordial pulsations are the apical area, lower parasternal area, left base (i.e., second left intercostal parasternal space, "pulmonic area"), right base (i.e., second right intercostal parasternal space, "aortic area"), and sternoclavicular areas. In some patients, especially those with chronic lung disease, right ventricular movements may appear in the epigastric area. The best external landmark is the sternal angle, which is where the second rib joins the sternum.

4. Right Base (Second Intercostal Space Near Right Edge of Sternum) and Sternoclavicular Joint

Movements from an ascending aortic aneurysm may become palpable here.

C. MAKING PRECORDIAL MOVEMENTS MORE CONSPICUOUS

Two teaching techniques are often used to bring out precordial movements and make them easier to time and characterize. In the first technique, the clinician puts a dot of ink on the area of interest, whose direction and timing then become easy to see. In the second technique, the clinician holds a cotton-tipped applicator stick (or wooden coffee stirrer) against the chest wall, with the end of the stick just off the center of the area of interest (the stick should be several inches long). The stick becomes a lever and the pulsating chest wall a fulcrum, causing the free end of the stick to trace in the air a magnified replica of the precordial movement.[13] A folded paper stick-on note may substitute for the applicator stick.[14]

III. The Findings

Precordial movements are timed by simultaneously listening to the heart tones and noting the relationship between outward movements on the chest wall and the first and second heart sounds. There are four types of systolic movement: normal, hyperkinetic, sustained, and retracting.[1,6,9–11]

A. NORMAL

The normal systolic movement is a small outward movement that begins with S_1, ends by mid systole, and then retracts inward, returning to its original position long before S_2.

The normal apical impulse is caused by a brisk early systolic anterior motion of the anteroseptal wall of the left ventricle against the ribs.[15] Despite its name, the apex beat bears no consistent relationship to the anatomic apex of the left ventricle.[15] In the supine position, the apex beat is palpable in only 25% to 40% of adults.[16–19] In the lateral decubitus position, it is palpable in 50% to 73% of adults.[16,20,21] The apex beat is more likely to be palpable in patients who have less body fat and who weigh less.[22] Some studies show that the apical impulse is more likely to be present in women than men, but this difference disappears after controlling for the participant's weights.[18]

B. HYPERKINETIC

The hyperkinetic (or overacting) systolic movement is a movement identical in timing to the normal movement, although its amplitude is exaggerated. Distinguishing normal from hyperkinetic amplitude is a subjective process, even on precise tracings from impulse cardiography. This probably explains why the finding has minimal diagnostic value, appearing both in patients with volume overload of the left ventricle (e.g., aortic regurgitation, ventricular septal defect) and in some normal persons who have thin chests or increased cardiac output.

C. SUSTAINED

The sustained movement is an abnormal outward movement that begins at S_1 but, unlike normal and hyperkinetic movements, extends to S_2 or even past it before beginning to descend to its original position. The amplitude of the sustained movement may be normal or increased. Sustained apical movements are always abnormal, indicating either pressure overload of the left ventricle (e.g., aortic stenosis, severe hypertension), volume overload (e.g., aortic regurgitation, ventricular septal defect), a combination of pressure and volume overload (combined aortic stenosis and regurgitation), severe cardiomyopathy, or ventricular aneurysm.

D. RETRACTING

In the retracting movement, inward motion begins at S_1 and outward motion does not start until early diastole. Because retracting movements are sometimes identical to normal movements in every characteristic except for timing, they are easily overlooked unless the clinician listens to the heart tones when palpating the chest. Only two diagnoses cause the retracting impulse, constrictive pericarditis and severe tricuspid regurgitation.[1,8,11]

E. HEAVES, LIFTS, AND THRUSTS

The words *heave* and *lift* sometimes refer to sustained movements, and *thrust* to hyperkinetic ones, but these terms, often used imprecisely, are best avoided.[1,9–11]

IV. Clinical Significance

A. APEX BEAT

1. Location

A traditional sign of an enlarged heart is an abnormally displaced apical impulse, which means it is located lateral to some external reference point. The three traditional reference points are (1) the MCL, (2) a set distance from the midsternal line (the traditional upper limit of normal is 10 cm), and (3) the nipple line.

Of these three landmarks, the MCL is the best, as long as the clinician locates it precisely by palpating the acromioclavicular and sternoclavicular joints and marking the midpoint between them with a ruler.[23,24] In the supine patient, an apical impulse located outside the midclavicular line increases the probability that the heart is enlarged on the chest radiograph (likelihood ratio [LR] = 3.4; see EBM Box 38.1), the ejection fraction is reduced (LR = 10.3), the left ventricular end-diastolic volume is increased (LR = 5.1), and the pulmonary capillary wedge pressure is increased (LR = 5.8). Other studies confirm the relationship between the displaced apical impulse and depressed ejection fraction.[32]

Using a point 10 cm from the midsternal line to define the displaced impulse is not a useful predictor of the enlarged heart (positive LR not significant, negative LR = 0.5; see EBM Box 38.1), probably because the 10 cm threshold is set too low (the MCL usually lies 10.5 to 11.5 cm from the midsternal line).[23] Finally, the nipple line is the least reliable of the three landmarks, bearing no consistent relationship to the apical impulse or to the size of the chest, even in men. The distance of the nipple line from the midsternum or midclavicular line varies greatly[33]

2. Diameter of the Apical Impulse

As measured in the left lateral decubitus position at 45 degrees, an apical impulse with a diameter of 4 cm or more increases the probability that the patient has a dilated heart (LR = 4.7 for increased left ventricular end-diastolic volume; see EBM Box 38.1). Smaller thresholds (e.g., 3 cm) discriminate between dilated and normal hearts in some studies, but not in others.[20,31]

3. Abnormal Movements

a. Hyperkinetic Apical Movements

The hyperkinetic apical movement is an important finding in one setting. In patients with mitral stenosis, left ventricular filling is impaired, causing the apical impulse to be normal or even

EBM BOX 38.1	Size and Position of Palpable Apical Impulse*

Finding (Reference)[†]	Sensitivity (%)	Specificity (%)	Likelihood Ratio[‡] if Finding Is	
			Present	Absent
Position of Apical Beat				
Supine apical impulse lateral to MCL				
Detecting cardiothoracic ratio >0.5[19,22,25]	39–60	76–93	3.4	0.6
Detecting low ejection fraction[26–29]	5–66	93–99	10.3	0.7
Detecting increased left ventricular end-diastolic volume[21,30]	33–34	92–96	5.1	0.7
Detecting pulmonary capillary wedge pressure >12 mm Hg[30]	42	93	5.8	NS
Supine apical impulse >10 cm from midsternal line				
Detecting cardiothoracic ratio >0.5[17,22,25]	61–80	28–97	NS	0.5
Size of Apical Beat				
Apical beat diameter ≥4 cm in left lateral decubitus position at 45 degrees				
Detecting increased left ventricular end-diastolic volume[20,31]	48–85	79–96	4.7	NS

*Diagnostic standard: for *cardiothoracic ratio*, maximal transverse diameter of heart on chest radiography divided by maximal transverse diameter of thoracic cage; for *low ejection fraction*, LV ejection fraction <0.50 or <0.53 by scintigraphy,[26,27] <0.5 by echocardiography,[29] or LV fractional shortening <25% by echocardiography[28]; for *increased LV end-diastolic volume*:[30] >90 ml/M² or >138 mL (echocardiography,[31] >109.2 ml/M² (computed tomography),[21] or upper 5th percentile of normal (echocardiography).[20]

†Definition of findings: except for "apical beat diameter," these data apply to all patients, whether or not an apical beat is palpable (i.e., nonpalpable apical beat = test "negative"). The only exception is the data for "apical beat diameter," which applies only to patients who have a measurable apical beat in the left lateral decubitus position (i.e., apical beat diameter ≥4 cm = test positive; <4 cm = test negative; unable to measure diameter = unable to evaluate using these data).

‡Likelihood ratio (LR) if finding present = positive LR; LR if finding absent = negative LR.

LV, Left ventricle; *MCL*, midclavicular line; *NS*, not significant.

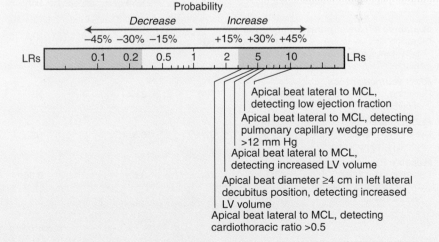

SIZE AND POSITION OF PALPABLE APICAL IMPULSE

reduced.[34] Therefore, if patients with the murmur of mitral stenosis also have a hyperkinetic apical impulse, an abnormality other than isolated mitral stenosis must be present, such as mitral regurgitation or aortic regurgitation (LR = 11.2; see EBM Box 38.2).

b. Sustained Apical Movements

A sustained or double apical movement (*double* refers to the combination of palpable S_4 and apical movement, see Chapter 41) increases the probability of left ventricular hypertrophy (LR = 5.6). In patients with aortic flow murmurs, the finding of a sustained apical impulse increases the probability of severe aortic stenosis (LR = 4.1; see EBM Box 38.2). In patients with the early diastolic murmur of aortic regurgitation, the sustained impulse is less helpful (LR = 2.4 for significant regurgitation), although the finding of a normal or absent apical impulse (i.e., not sustained or

EBM BOX 38.2	Abnormal Palpable Movements*			
			Likelihood Ratio‡ if Finding Is	
Finding (Reference)†	Sensitivity (%)	Specificity (%)	Present	Absent
Hyperkinetic apical movement				
Detecting associated mitral regurgitation or aortic valve disease in patients with mitral stenosis[34]	74	93	**11.2**	0.3
Sustained or double apical movement				
Detecting left ventricular hypertrophy[21]	57	90	**5.6**	0.5
Sustained apical movement				
Detecting severe aortic stenosis in patients with aortic flow murmurs[35]	78	81	**4.1**	0.3
Detecting moderate-to-severe aortic regurgitation in patients with basal early diastolic murmurs[36]	97	60	2.4	0.1
Lower sternal pulsations				
Detecting moderate-to-severe tricuspid regurgitation[37]	17	99	**12.5**	0.8
Sustained left lower parasternal movement				
Detecting right ventricular peak pressure ≥50 mm Hg[38]	71	80	**3.6**	0.4
Right ventricular rock				
Detecting moderate-to-severe tricuspid regurgitation[37]	5	100	**31.4**	NS
Pulsatile liver				
Detecting moderate-to-severe tricuspid regurgitation[37,39]	12–30	92–99	**6.5**	NS
Palpable P_2				
Detecting pulmonary hypertension in patients with mitral stenosis[40]	96	73	**3.6**	0.05

continued

*Diagnostic standard: for *LV hypertrophy*, computed tomographic LV mass index >104 g/M²;[21] for *severe aortic stenosis* and *moderate-to-severe aortic regurgitation*, see EBM Boxes in Chapters 44 and 45; for *moderate-to-severe tricuspid regurgitation*, 3+ or 4+ by angiography[39] or as assessed visually from echocardiography,[37] and; for *pulmonary hypertension*, mean pulmonary artery pressure ≥50mm Hg.[40]
†Definition of findings: for *abnormal apical movement*, "apical impulse heave or enlarged,"[36] "sustained,"[35] or "thrust"[34]; for *sustained or double apical movement*, apical movement extending beyond S_2 or combination of palpable S_4 + LV apical movement[21]; for *abnormal parasternal movement*, "movement extending to or past S_2."[38]; for *right ventricular rock*, see text; for *palpable P_2* "palpable late systolic tap in second left intercostal space next to sternum, which frequently followed parasternal lift."[40]
‡Likelihood ratio (LR) if finding present = positive LR; LR if finding absent = negative LR.
LV, Left ventricle; *NS*, not significant.

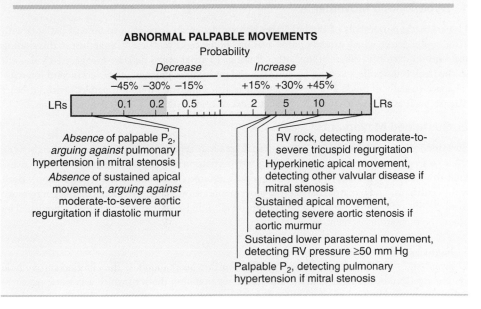

ABNORMAL PALPABLE MOVEMENTS
Probability

Decrease — *Increase*

−45% −30% −15%   +15% +30% +45%

LRs   0.1   0.2   0.5   1   2   5   10   LRs

Absence of palpable P_2, *arguing against* pulmonary hypertension in mitral stenosis

Absence of sustained apical movement, *arguing against* moderate-to-severe aortic regurgitation if diastolic murmur

RV rock, detecting moderate-to-severe tricuspid regurgitation

Hyperkinetic apical movement, detecting other valvular disease if mitral stenosis

Sustained apical movement, detecting severe aortic stenosis if aortic murmur

Sustained lower parasternal movement, detecting RV pressure ≥50 mm Hg

Palpable P_2, detecting pulmonary hypertension if mitral stenosis

hyperkinetic) in these patients *decreases* significantly the probability of moderate-to-severe aortic regurgitation (LR = 0.1; see EBM Box 38.2).

c. Retracting Apical Impulse

(1). Constrictive Pericarditis. In up to 90% of patients with constrictive pericarditis, the apical impulse retracts during systole (sometimes accompanied by systolic retraction of the left parasternal area).[8,41] In these patients, the diseased pericardium prevents the normal outward systolic movement of the ventricles but allows rapid and prominent early diastolic filling of the ventricle. The prominent diastolic filling causes a palpable diastolic outward movement, which contributes to the overall impression that the apical impulse retracts during systole (see Chapter 47).

The first clinician to recognize the retracting apical impulse as a sign of "adhesive" pericarditis was Skoda in 1852.[42]

(2). Tricuspid Regurgitation. In severe tricuspid regurgitation, a dilated right ventricle, occupying the apex, ejects blood into a dilated right atrium and liver, located nearer the sternum.[8] This causes a characteristic rocking motion (or **right ventricular rock**), the apical area retracting inward during systole and the lower left or right parasternal area moving outward during systole,[43] often accompanied by a pulsatile liver. All three findings increase

the probability of moderate-to-severe tricuspid regurgitation (LR = 31.4 for right ventricular rock, LR = 12.5 for lower sternal pulsations, and LR = 6.5 for pulsatile liver, see EBM Box 38.2).

B. LEFT LOWER PARASTERNAL MOVEMENTS

In normal persons, the clinician either palpates no movement or only a tiny inward one during systole at this location. Abnormal movements at this location are classified as hyperkinetic or sustained, depending on their relationship to S_2.

1. Hyperkinetic Movements

Hyperkinetic movements of the left lower parasternal area occur in up to 50% of patients with atrial septal defect, which causes volume overload of the right ventricle.[44] Nonetheless, this finding has limited diagnosis value without other findings of atrial septal defect—exaggerated y descent in the neck veins, wide and fixed S_2 splitting, and midsystolic murmur at the left second intercostal space (usually of grade 2 of 6)—because it is also sometimes found in patients without heart disease, such as those with thin chests, pectus excavatum, fever, or other high output states.[38,44]

2. Sustained Movements

Sustained movements of the left lower sternal area may represent either an abnormal right ventricle (e.g., pressure overload from pulmonary hypertension or pulmonic stenosis or volume overload from atrial septal defect) or an enlarged left atrium (e.g., severe mitral regurgitation). Both right ventricular and left atrial parasternal movements are outward movements that begin to move inward only at S_2 or just after it and therefore are classified as sustained; they are distinguished by when the outward movement *begins*.

a. Right Ventricle

Outward right ventricular movements begin at the first heart sound. If the clinician can exclude volume overload of the right ventricle and mitral regurgitation (both of which also cause parasternal movements), the finding of a sustained left parasternal movement is a modest sign of pulmonary hypertension (often accompanied by tricuspid regurgitation; see earlier). In patients with mitral stenosis, the duration of the sustained lower parasternal movement correlates well with pulmonary pressures.[34] In patients with a wide variety of valvular and congenital heart lesions (excluding mitral regurgitation), the sustained lower left parasternal movement is a modest discriminator between those with peak right ventricular pressures >50 mm Hg and those with lower pressures (positive LR = 3.6, negative LR 0.4; see EBM Box 38.2). In patients with chronic liver disease undergoing evaluation for liver transplantation, the right ventricular heave increases probability of pulmonary hypertension (i.e., mean pulmonary artery pressures ≥25 mm Hg, LR = 8.8; see Chapter 8).[45] Even so, in patients seeing pulmonary hypertension specialists, the right ventricular heave was not an accurate sign of pulmonary hypertension (defined as mean pulmonary artery pressure ≥25 mm Hg; sensitivity = 42%, specificity = 84%, LR not significant).[46] Up to 30% of patients with atrial septal defect, whether or not there is associated pulmonary hypertension, also have sustained lower left parasternal movements.[44]

b. Left Atrium and Mitral Regurgitation

In patients with severe mitral regurgitation, ventricular contraction forces blood backwards into a dilated left atrium, which lies on the posterior surface of the heart and acts like an expanding cushion to lift up the heart, including the left parasternal area. This sustained movement, most easily palpated in the 4th or 5th intercostal space near the sternum,[47,48] differs from those caused by the right ventricle, because outward movement begins in the second half of systole (it parallels the V wave on the left atrial pressure tracing).

In patients with isolated mitral regurgitation, the degree of the late systolic outward movement at the lower sternal edge correlates well with the severity of mitral regurgitation (r = 0.93, p <0.01; the correlation is much worse if there is associated mitral stenosis, which may cause parasternal movements from pulmonary hypertension).[47,48] In pure mitral regurgitation, as in atrial septal defect, the parasternal movement has no relationship to right ventricular pressures.[49]

C. ANEURYSMS

In one study of consecutive patients with ventricular aneurysms identified by angiography, 33% had abnormal precordial movements.[50] Typical findings were (1) a double cardiac impulse, the first component representing the normal apical outward movement and second the bulging of the aneurysm during peak ventricular pressures later in systole,[51,52] and (2) a sustained impulse that extended superiorly or medially from the usual location of the apical impulse.[50] If detectable by palpation, the aneurysm originates in the anterior wall or apex of the left ventricle; aneurysms originating from the inferior or lateral wall are too distant from the anterior chest wall to be detectable by palpation.[50]

D. DIFFUSE PRECORDIAL MOVEMENTS

Diffuse outward movements of the entire precordium, from the apex to lower parasternal area, may result from (1) right ventricular enlargement (which dilates to occupy the apical area), (2) left ventricular enlargement (which rotates to occupy the lower parasternal area), or (3) biventricular enlargement.[11] Palpation alone cannot distinguish these different etiologies—even sensitive recordings from impulse cardiography or kinetocardiography could not do this—and the clinician must rely on other findings to determine which chamber is most likely causing the diffuse movement.

E. RIGHT LOWER PARASTERNAL MOVEMENTS

Abnormal systolic outward movements appear in the right lower parasternal area from tricuspid regurgitation (ejection of blood into the right atrium and liver that lies under the right side of the sternum) or from mitral regurgitation (ejection of blood in a dilated left atrium).[11,43,53]

F. PALPABLE P$_2$

A palpable P$_2$ (i.e., the pulmonic component of second heart sound) is a sharp, brief snapping sensation felt over the left base, coincident with S$_2$. It is much briefer than other precordial movements. In patients with mitral stenosis, a palpable P$_2$ increases the probability of pulmonary hypertension (LR = 3.6 for mean pulmonary pressure >50 mm Hg). More importantly, the absence of a palpable P$_2$ in these patients *decreases* the probability of a pulmonary pressure this high (LR = 0.05; see EBM Box 38.2). Nonetheless, in other settings, such as pulmonary hypertension clinics, the palpable P$_2$ did not accurately identify pulmonary hypertension (defined as mean pulmonary artery pressure ≥25 mm Hg; LR not significant).[46]

G. PALPABLE THIRD AND FOURTH HEART SOUNDS

Some patients with rapid early ventricular filling (e.g., mitral regurgitation) have a palpable early diastolic movement at the apex. Other patients with strong atrial contractions into stiff ventricles (e.g., hypertensive or ischemic heart disease) have palpable presystolic apical movements. These movements have the same significance as their audible counterparts, the third and fourth heart sound (i.e., S_3 and S_4, see Chapter 41). They are usually called *palpable S_3* and *palpable S_4*.

The S_4 is much more likely to be palpable than the S_3, and both are more likely to be felt when the patient is in the lateral decubitus position.[7,9,10] The palpable S_4 causes either a double outward impulse near S_1 (a common analogy is the grace note in music, see *double apical movement* in EBM Box 38.2) or single outward movement, consisting of the palpable S_4 and apical beat together, which is distinguished from the apical beat alone because the outward movement begins slightly before S_1.[10,11] An excellent video of a palpable S_4 (double apical movement), made visible with use of a wooden coffee stirrer, appears in the reference by Phan.[13]

References may be accessed online at *Elsevier eBooks for Practicing Clinicians*.

CHAPTER 39

Auscultation of the Heart: General Principles

- Careful auscultation of the heart requires a quiet examination room. The clinician should systematically inch the stethoscope from apex to base (or in the opposite direction, from base to apex). At each location, the clinician should focus sequentially on the different elements of the cardiac cycle (i.e., S_1, S_2, systole, and diastole).
- The bell of the stethoscope is used to identify low-frequency sounds; the diaphragm is used to listen to high-frequency sounds.
- The best way to distinguish systole from diastole is by the cadence of heart tones (systole is shorter than diastole if the heart rate is normal) or by identifying S_2 at the second left parasternal space, where it is the louder, snappier heart sound.

I. Characteristics of Heart Sounds and Murmurs

Different heart sounds and murmurs are distinguished by four characteristics: (1) timing (i.e., systolic or diastolic), (2) intensity (i.e., loud or soft), (3) duration (i.e., long or short), and (4) pitch (i.e., low or high frequency). A fifth characteristic, the sound's quality, is also sometimes included in descriptions of sounds (e.g., it may be described as "musical," a "whoop," or a "honk"). Almost all heart sounds contain a mixture of frequencies (i.e., they are not musical in the acoustical sense, but instead are "noise," like the static of a radio tuned between stations). Therefore, the descriptors *low-frequency* and *high-frequency* do not indicate that a sound has a pure musical tone of a certain low or high pitch, but instead that the bulk of the sound's energy is within the low or high range.

Although the human ear can hear sounds with frequencies from 20 to 20,000 cycles per second (Hz), the principal frequencies of heart sounds and murmurs are at the lower end of this range, from 20 to 500 Hz.[1,2] **Low-frequency sounds**, therefore, are those whose dominant frequencies are less than 100 Hz, such as third and fourth heart sounds and the diastolic murmur of mitral stenosis. These sounds are usually difficult to hear because the human ear perceives lower frequencies relatively less well than higher frequencies. The murmur containing the highest frequency sound is aortic regurgitation, whose dominant frequencies are about 400 Hz. The principal frequencies of other sounds and murmurs are between 100 and 400 Hz.

II. The Stethoscope

A. BELL AND DIAPHRAGM

The traditional stethoscope has two different heads to receive sound, the bell and the diaphragm. The bell is used to detect low-frequency sounds and the diaphragm to detect high-frequency sounds.

The traditional explanation that the bell selectively transmits low-frequency sounds and the diaphragm selectively filters out low-frequency sounds is probably incorrect. Actually, the bell transmits all frequencies well, but in some patients with high-frequency murmurs (e.g., aortic regurgitation), any additional low-frequency sound may mask high-frequency sound and make high-frequency murmurs more difficult to detect.[3] The diaphragm does not selectively filter out low-frequency sounds, but instead attenuates all frequencies equally, thus dropping the barely audible low-frequency ones below the threshold of human hearing.[3]

B. PERFORMANCE OF DIFFERENT STETHOSCOPE MODELS

Many studies have examined the acoustics of stethoscopes, but the clinical relevance of this research has never been formally tested. In general, these studies show that shallow bells transmit sound as well as deeper bells and that double tube stethoscopes are equivalent to single tube models.[3] The optimal internal bore of a stethoscope is somewhere between one-eighth and three-sixteenths of an inch, because smaller bores diminish transmission of the higher frequency sounds.[1,4,5] Compared with shorter lengths of stethoscope tubing, longer tubes impair the conduction of high-frequency sounds.[1]

Most modern stethoscopes, however, transmit sound equally well, the differences among various models for single frequencies being very small.[3] The most important source of poor acoustic performance is an air leak, which typically results from poorly fitting ear pieces. Even a tiny air leak with a diameter of only 0.015 inch will diminish transmission of sound by as much as 20 dB,* particularly for those sounds less than 100 Hz.[6]

III. Use of the Stethoscope

Between the 1950s and late 1970s, cardiac auscultation was at its peak.[†] During this time cardiologists perfected their skills by routinely comparing bedside findings to the patient's phonocardiogram, angiogram, and surgical findings, which allowed clinicians to make precise and accurate diagnoses from bedside findings alone. The principles of bedside diagnosis used by these clinicians are included elsewhere in this book. How these clinicians specifically used the stethoscope to examine the patient is presented below.

A. EXAMINATION ROOM

Many faint heart sounds and murmurs are inaudible unless there is complete silence in the room. The clinician should close the door to the examination room, turn off the television and radio, and ask that all conversation stop.

[†]*Decibels* describe relative intensity (or loudness) on a logarithmic scale.
[†]In the late 1970s, two events initiated the decline of cardiac auscultation: the widespread introduction of echocardiography and the decision by insurance companies to no longer make reimbursements for phonocardiography.

B. BELL PRESSURE

To detect low-frequency sounds, the stethoscope bell should be applied to the body wall with only enough pressure to create an air seal and exclude ambient noise. Excessive pressure with the bell stretches the skin, which then acts like a diaphragm and makes low-frequency sounds more difficult to hear. By selectively varying the pressure on the stethoscope bell, the clinician can easily distinguish low- from high-frequency sounds: if a sound is audible with the bell using light pressure but disappears with firm pressure, it is a low-frequency sound. This technique is frequently used to confirm that an early diastolic sound is indeed a third heart sound (i.e., third heart sounds are low-frequency sounds, whereas other early diastolic sounds like the pericardial knock are high-frequency sounds) and to distinguish the combined fourth and first heart sounds (S_4-S_1) from the split S_1 (the S_4 is a low-frequency sound but the S_1 is not; firm pressure renders the S_4-S_1 into a single sound but does not affect the double sound of the split S_1).

C. PATIENT POSITION

The clinician should listen to the patient's heart with the patient in three positions: supine, left lateral decubitus, and seated upright. The lateral decubitus position is best for detection of the third and fourth heart sounds and the diastolic murmur of mitral stenosis (to detect these sounds, the clinician places the bell lightly over the apical impulse or just medial to the apical impulse).[7] The seated upright position is necessary to further evaluate audible expiratory splitting of S_2 (see Chapter 40) and to detect some pericardial rubs and murmurs of aortic regurgitation (see Chapters 45 and 47).

D. ORDER OF EXAMINATION

Routine auscultation of the heart should include the right upper sternal area, the entire left sternal border, and the apex. Some cardiologists recommend proceeding from base to apex[2]; others from apex to base.[8] The diaphragm of the stethoscope should be applied to all areas, especially at the upper left sternal area to detect S_2 splitting and at all areas to detect other murmurs and sounds. After using the diaphragm to listen to the lower left sternal area and apex, the bell should also be applied to these areas to detect diastolic filling sounds (S_3 and S_4) and diastolic rumbling murmurs (e.g., mitral stenosis).

In selected patients, the clinician should also listen over the carotid arteries and axilla (in patients with systolic murmurs, to clarify radiation of the murmur), the lower right sternal area (in patients with diastolic murmur of aortic regurgitation, to detect aortic root disease), the back (in young patients with hypertension, to detect the continuous murmur of coarctation), or other thoracic sites (in patients with central cyanosis, to detect the continuous murmur of pulmonary arteriovenous fistulas).

E. DESCRIBING THE LOCATION OF SOUNDS

When describing heart sounds and murmurs, the clinician should identify where on the chest wall the sound is loudest. Traditionally, the second right intercostal space next to the sternum is called the *aortic area* or *right base*; the second left intercostal space next to the sternum, the *pulmonary area* or *left base*; the fourth or fifth left parasternal space, the *tricuspid area* or *left lower sternal border*; and the most lateral point of the palpable cardiac impulse, the *mitral area* or *apex* (see Fig. 38.1 in Chapter 38).

Even so, the terms *aortic area, pulmonary area, tricuspid area,* and *mitral area* are ambiguous and are best avoided. Many patients with aortic stenosis have murmurs loudest in the mitral area, and some with mitral regurgitation have murmurs in the pulmonary or aortic area. A more precise way to describe the location of sounds is to use the apex and the parasternal areas as reference points, the parasternal location being further specified by the intercostal space (first, second, or third intercostal space; or lower sternal border) and whether it is the right or left edge of the sternum. For example, a sound might be loudest at the "apex," the "second left intercostal space" (i.e., next to the left sternal edge in the 2nd intercostal space), or "between the apex and left lower sternal border."

F. TECHNIQUE OF FOCUSING

The human brain has an uncanny ability to isolate and focus on one type of sensory information by repressing awareness of all other sensations. A common example of this phenomenon is the person reading a book in a room in which a clock is ticking: the person may read long passages of the book without even hearing the clock but hears the ticking clock immediately after putting the book down. When listening to the heart, the clinician's attention is quickly drawn to the most prominent sounds, but this occurs at the expense of detecting the fainter sounds. Therefore, to avoid missing these fainter sounds or subtle splitting, the clinician should concentrate sequentially on each part of the cardiac cycle, asking the following questions at each location: (1) Is S_1 soft or loud? (2) Is S_2 split and, if so, how is it split? (3) Are there are any extra sounds or murmurs during systole? and (4) Are there are any extra sounds or murmurs during diastole?

G. IDENTIFYING SYSTOLE AND DIASTOLE

Because all auscultatory findings are characterized by their timing, distinguishing systole from diastole accurately is essential. Three principles help the clinician distinguish these events.

1. Systole is Shorter than Diastole

If the heart rate is normal or slow, systole can be easily distinguished from diastole because systole is much shorter. The normal cadence of the heart tones, therefore, is

lub dup   *lub dup*   *lub dup*   *lub dup*

(*lub* is S_1 and *dup* is S_2). When the heart rate accelerates, however, diastole shortens and, at a rate of 100 or more, the cadence of S_1 and S_2 resembles the following "tic toc" rhythm:

lub dup lub dup lub dup lub dup lub dup lub dup

In these patients, other techniques are necessary to distinguish systole from diastole.

2. Characteristics of the First and Second Heart Sounds

At the second left intercostal space, S_2 is generally louder, shorter, and sharper than S_1 (S_2 has more high-frequency energy than S_1, which is why *dup*, a snappier sound than *lub*, is used to character- ize S_2). If the timing of extra heart sounds and murmurs is confusing at the lower sternal edge or apex (as it often is in patients with fast heart rhythms), the clinician can return the stethoscope to the second left intercostal space, identify S_2 by its louder and sharper sound, and then inch slowly back to the area of interest, keeping track of S_2 along the way.

3. Carotid Impulse

The palpable impulse from the carotid usually occurs just after S_1, which the clinician detects by simultaneously listening to the heart tones and palpating the carotid artery. In elderly patients with tachycardia, however, this rule is sometimes misleading because the carotid impulse seems to fall closer to S_2, although even in these patients the carotid impulse still falls between S_1 and S_2.

References may be accessed online at *Elsevier eBooks for Practicing Clinicians*.

The First and Second Heart Sounds

The first and second heart sounds (S_1 and S_2) define systole and diastole and therefore form the framework for analyzing all other auscultatory physical signs, including the third and fourth heart sounds, clicks and ejection sounds, knocks and opening snaps, and systolic and diastolic murmurs. In his classic treatise describing the discovery of the circulatory system, written in 1628, Harvey described both S_1 and S_2, comparing them to the gulping sound made by a horse drinking water.[1] The first person to state that S_1 and S_2 were the sounds of closing heart valves was Rouanet of France, who wrote in his 1832 MD thesis that S_1 occurred when the atrioventricular (i.e., mitral and tricuspid) valves closed, and S_2 occurred when the semilunar (i.e., aortic and pulmonic) valves closed.[2]

THE FIRST HEART SOUND (S_1)

I. The Finding

S_1 is heard well across the entire precordium, both with the bell and diaphragm of the stethoscope. It is usually loudest at or near the apex and contains more low frequency energy than does S_2, which explains why, when mimicking the sound, the term *lub* is used for S_1 and the sharper term *dup* for S_2.*

---

*It was Williams in 1840 who invented the *lub dup* onomatopoeia.[3]

II. Pathogenesis

A. CAUSE OF S₁

The precise cause of S_1 has been debated for decades. Although its two recordable components coincide with closure of the mitral and tricuspid valves, the force of valve closure itself is insufficient to generate sound.[4] Instead, their closure probably causes moving columns of blood to abruptly decelerate, which sets up vibrations in the chordae tendineae, ventricles, and blood as a unit (i.e., **cardiohemic system**).[4,5]

B. INTENSITY OF S₁

The most important abnormalities of S_1 relate to its intensity: The sound can be abnormally loud, abnormally faint, or vary in intensity abnormally from beat to beat. The primary variables governing intensity of S_1 are strength of ventricular contraction and the position of the atrioventricular leaflets at the onset of ventricular systole.

1. Ventricular Contractility

The stronger the ventricular contraction, the louder the S_1. Strong contractions, which have a high dP/dT (i.e., large increase in pressure with respect to time), intensify S_1 because the valves close with more force and generate more vibrations in the cardiohemic system.[6-8]

2. Position of the Valve Leaflets at Onset of Ventricular Systole

If the mitral valve is wide open at the onset of ventricular systole, it will take longer to close completely than if it had been barely open. Even this small delay in closure intensifies S_1, because closure occurs on a later and steeper portion of the left ventricular (LV) pressure curve (i.e., dP/dT is greater).[9]

The PR interval is the main variable determining the position of the valves at the beginning of ventricular systole. If the PR interval is short, ventricular systole immediately follows atrial systole (i.e., the R wave immediately follows the P wave). Because atrial systole kicks the valve open, a short PR guarantees that the valve will be wide open at the onset of ventricular systole. In contrast, a long PR interval allows time for the cusps of the atrioventricular valves to float back together before ventricular systole occurs. Studies show that, with PR intervals less than 0.20 seconds, the intensity of S_1 varies inversely with the PR interval (the shorter the PR interval, the louder the sound). With PR intervals greater than 0.20 seconds, S_1 is faint or absent.[8-10]

III. Clinical Significance

A. LOUD S₁

S_1 may be abnormally loud because of unusually vigorous ventricular contractions or because of delayed closure of the mitral valve.

1. Vigorous Ventricular Contractions

Vigorous contractions, such as those occurring from fever and sympathetic stimulation (e.g., beta-adrenergic inhalers, thyrotoxicosis), increase dP/dT and intensify S_1.[6]

2. Delayed Closure of the Mitral Valve

a. Prolapsed Mitral Valve

In patients with the murmur of mitral regurgitation, a loud S_1 is a clue to the diagnosis of early prolapse of the mitral valve (many patients with mitral regurgitation have a normal or soft S_1).[11,12]

S_1 is loud in these patients because the prolapsing leaflets stop moving and tense later than normal, when dP/dT in the ventricle is greater.[11]

b. Mitral Stenosis

Ninety percent of patients with pure uncomplicated mitral stenosis have a loud S_1.[13] Because the murmur of mitral stenosis is often difficult to hear, a traditional teaching is that clinicians should suspect mitral stenosis in any patient with an unexplained loud S_1 and listen carefully for the murmur with the patient lying on the left side.

Mitral stenosis delays closure of the mitral valve because the pressure gradient between the left atrium and left ventricle keeps the leaflets open until the moment of ventricular systole. After successful valvuloplasty, the loud S_1 becomes softer.[13]

c. Left Atrial Myxoma

Many patients with left atrial myxoma (7 of 9 in one series) also have a loud S_1 because the tumor falling into the mitral orifice during diastole delays closure of the valve.[14]

B. FAINT OR ABSENT S_1

S_1 is unusually faint if ventricular contractions are weak or if the mitral valve is already closed when ventricular systole occurs.

1. Weak Ventricular Contractions (Low dP/dT)

Common examples of weak contractions causing a faint S_1 are myocardial infarction and left bundle branch block.[15]

2. Early Closure of the Mitral Valve

Common causes of early mitral closure causing the faint S_1 include the following:

a. Long PR Interval (>0.20 seconds)

See the section on intensity of S_1.

b. Acute Aortic Regurgitation

In patients with the murmur of aortic regurgitation, the faint or absent S_1 is an important clue that the regurgitation is acute (e.g., endocarditis) and not chronic. Patients with acute aortic regurgitation have much higher LV end diastolic pressures than those with chronic regurgitation, because the acutely failing valve has not allowed time for the ventricle to enlarge, as it does to compensate for chronic regurgitation. The high pressures in the ventricle eventually exceed diastolic left atrial pressures, closing the mitral valve before ventricular systole and thus making S_1 faint or absent.[16]

C. VARYING INTENSITY OF S_1

If the arterial pulse rhythm is *regular* but S_1 varies in intensity, the only possible explanation is that the PR interval is changing from beat to beat, which means the patient has atrioventricular dissociation. In contrast, in patients with *irregular* rhythms, changing intensity of S_1 has no diagnostic significance, because ventricular filling and dP/dT—and therefore S_1 intensity—depend completely on cycle length.

In patients with pacer-induced regular rhythms, an S_1 that varies in intensity is compelling evidence for atrioventricular dissociation (likelihood ratio [LR] = 24.4; see EBM Box 40.1). Presumably, the finding is also as accurate in patients with native rhythms. In patients with complete heart block, S_1 intensity is predictable, varying inversely with the PR interval for intervals

EBM BOX 40.1   The First and Second Heart Sounds*

Finding (Reference)[†]	Sensitivity (%)	Specificity (%)	Likelihood Ratio[‡] if Finding Is	
			Present	Absent
First heart sound				
Varying intensity S₁				
Detecting atrioventricular dissociation[17]	58	98	**24.4**	0.4
Second heart sound				
Fixed wide splitting				
Detecting atrial septal defect[18]	92	65	2.6	**0.1**
Paradoxic splitting				
Detecting significant aortic stenosis[19]	50	79	NS	NS
Loud P₂				
Detecting pulmonary hypertension in patients with mitral stenosis[20,21]	58–96	19–46	NS	NS
Detecting pulmonary hypertension in patients with cirrhosis[22]	38	98	**17.6**	NS
Palpable P₂				
Detecting pulmonary hypertension in mitral stenosis[20]	96	73	**3.6**	0.05
Absent or diminished S₂				
Detecting significant aortic stenosis in patients with aortic flow murmurs[19,23-27]	44–90	63–98	**3.8**	0.4

*Diagnostic standard: for *atrioventricular dissociation*, ventricles were paced independently of atria; for *atrial septal defect*, right heart catheterization; for *severe aortic stenosis*, aortic valve area <0.75 cm², <0.8 cm²;[22,25] peak gradient >50 mm Hg;[19,25] or peak velocity of aortic flow >3.6 m/sec[24] or ≥4 m/sec;[26] for *pulmonary hypertension*, mean pulmonary arterial pressure ≥50 mm Hg[20,21] or ≥25 mm Hg.[22]
[†]Definition of findings: for *loud P₂*, splitting heard with loud second component[20] or S₂ louder at left second interspace than right second interspace[21]; the figures for fixed splitting of S₂ apply only to patients having audible expiratory splitting.
[‡]Likelihood ratio (LR) if finding present = positive LR; LR if finding absent = negative LR.
AV, Atrioventricular; *NS*, not significant.

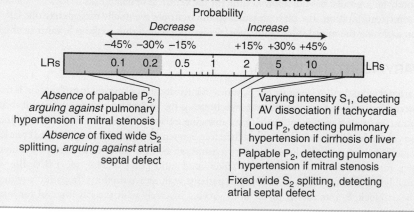

FIRST AND SECOND HEART SOUNDS

less than 0.2 seconds, becoming inaudible for intervals 0.2 to 0.5 seconds, and becoming louder again with intervals more than 0.5 seconds (because the mitral valve reopens).[10]

D. PROMINENT SPLITTING OF S_1

Any delay in the closure of the tricuspid valve, the second component of S_1, accentuates splitting of S_1. This finding therefore occurs in patients with right bundle branch block (RBBB) or in LV ectopic or paced beats, all of which delay the onset of right ventricular (RV) systole and also cause wide physiologic splitting of S_2 (see later).[5,28]

How to distinguish the split S_1 from other double sounds occurring around S_1, such as $S_4 + S_1$ and S_1 + ejection sound, is discussed in Chapter 41.

THE SECOND HEART SOUND (S_2)

I. Introduction

The most important diagnostic feature of S_2 is its "splitting," which refers to how the aortic and pulmonic components of S_2 vary in timing during the respiratory cycle. The intensity of S_2 has less diagnostic importance. (This contrasts with S_1, in which intensity is more important than splitting.) Splitting of S_2 was first recognized by Potain in 1865, and its importance to cardiac auscultation was described by Leatham in the 1950s, who called S_2 the "key to auscultation of the heart."[29,30] The correct explanation for normal splitting—increased "hangout" in the pulmonary circulation—was discovered in the 1970s.[31,32]

II. Normal Splitting of S_2

A. THE FINDING

In normal persons, the first component of S_2 is caused by closure of the aortic valve (A_2); the second, by closure of the pulmonic valve (P_2). During inspiration the interval separating A_2 and P_2 increases by about 20 to 30 milliseconds (ms) (Fig. 40.1).[18,30,32]

Although the phonocardiogram almost always records both components of S_2, the human ear perceives them as a single sound *during expiration* in over 90% of normal persons.[33] In normal persons *during inspiration*, the human ear either perceives two components (physiologic splitting, heard in 65% to 75% of normal adults; see Fig. 40.1)[†] or still perceives a single component (single S_2, heard in 25% to 35% of normal adults). The older the person, the more likely S_2 will be single instead of physiologic.[33,34]

In a minority of normal persons, expiratory splitting is heard in the supine position, although S_2 becomes single during expiration in these patients when they sit up.[37]

B. LOCATION OF SOUND

S_2 splitting is usually heard only in the second or third intercostal space, next to the left sternum.[34] It is sometimes heard at a slightly lower location, especially in patients with chronic pulmonary disease, and at a slightly higher location in those who are obese.[34] Splitting is not normally heard at other locations because P_2 is too faint.

[†]These two components are very close together, bordering the threshold of being perceived as a single sound. Harvey suggests mimicking the normal expiratory sound by striking a single knuckle against a tabletop and mimicking inspiratory physiologic splitting by striking two knuckles almost simultaneously.[35] Constant suggests mimicking inspiratory splitting by rolling the tongue as in a Spanish *dr* or *tr* or by saying *pa–da* as quickly and sharply as possible.[36]

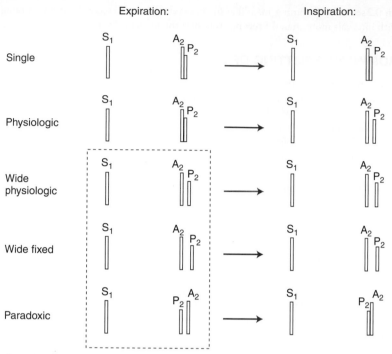

Fig. 40.1 S₂ splitting. Splitting refers to the separation of the aortic component (A_2) and the pulmonic component (P_2) during expiration (*left column*) and inspiration (*right column*). There are two normal patterns (single and physiologic) and three abnormal patterns (wide physiologic, wide fixed, and paradoxic). The *dotted lines* indicate that all three abnormal forms of splitting are distinguished by having audible expiratory splitting. See text.

C. TECHNIQUE

It is important that the patient breathe regularly in and out when evaluating S_2 splitting, because held inspiration or held expiration tends to make the two components drift apart, thus making it impossible to interpret the sound.[18]

D. PHYSIOLOGY OF SPLITTING

The normal delay in P_2 results from a long "hangout" interval in the normal pulmonary circulation. (It is not because RV systole ends later than LV systole; they actually end at the same moment, see Fig. 40.2.) *Hangout* means that the pulmonary circulation offers so little resistance to blood flow that flow continues for a short period even after completion of RV mechanical systole.[31,32] At the aortic valve, there is little hangout, causing flow to cease and the valve to close immediately after completion of LV contraction.

A_2 and P_2 move apart during inspiration, primarily because inspiration delays P_2 even more. About half of the inspiratory augmentation of the A_2-P_2 interval is due to a further increase in the hangout interval in the pulmonary circulation. About 25% of inspiratory augmentation is due to lengthening of RV systole (from increased filling of the right side of the heart during inspiration), and the remaining 25% is due to shortening of LV systole (from a reduction of filling of the left side of the heart during inspiration).[32]

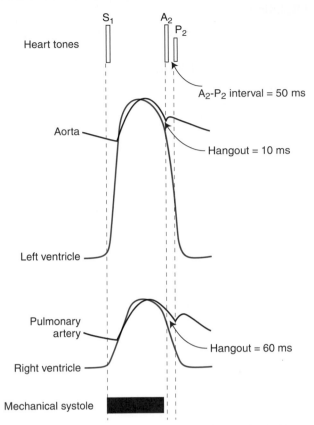

Fig. 40.2   Mechanism of S₂ splitting. The timing of heart tones (*top*) is correlated with pressure tracings from the left side of the heart (i.e., aorta and left ventricle, *top pressure tracings*) and right side of the heart (i.e., pulmonary artery and right ventricle, *bottom pressure tracings*). The *solid rectangle* at the bottom of the figure depicts the duration of mechanical systole, which is the same for the right and left ventricles. A_2 coincides with the incisura (i.e., notch) on the aorta tracing, P_2 coincides with the incisura on the pulmonary artery tracing, and both sounds occur a short interval after completion of mechanical systole (the interval between the end of mechanical systole and valve closure is called hangout). On the left side of the heart, hangout is very short (10 ms, i.e., the aortic valve closes almost immediately after completion of mechanical systole). On the right side of the heart, however, hangout is longer (60 ms) because the compliant pulmonary circulation offers so little resistance to continued forward flow. The difference between these numbers explains why P_2 normally occurs after A_2 (i.e., A_2P_2 interval in this patient = 60 − 10 = 50 ms). Changes in hangout also explain in part why splitting normally increases during inspiration, and why most patients with pulmonary hypertension have a single S_2. See the text.

III. Abnormal Splitting of S₂

A. THE FINDING

There are three abnormalities of S_2 splitting (Fig. 40.1):

1. Wide Physiologic Splitting

Wide physiologic splitting means that splitting occurs during inspiration and expiration, though the A_2P_2 interval widens further during inspiration.

2. Wide Fixed Splitting

Wide fixed splitting means that splitting occurs during inspiration and expiration, but the A_2P_2 interval remains constant.

3. Paradoxic Splitting (Reversed Splitting)

Paradoxic splitting means that audible expiratory splitting narrows or melds into a single sound during inspiration. Paradoxic splitting occurs because the order of the S_2 components has reversed: A_2 now follows P_2, and as P_2 is delayed during inspiration, the sounds move together.

B. SCREENING FOR ABNORMAL SPLITTING OF S$_2$

Fig. 40.1 reveals that all three abnormal second heart sounds—wide physiologic, fixed, and paradoxic—have audible splitting *during expiration* (dotted lines in Fig. 40.1). Therefore, the best screening tool for the abnormal S_2 is audible expiratory splitting that persists when the patient sits up.[37-40]

C. CLINICAL SIGNIFICANCE AND PATHOGENESIS

Table 40.1 lists the common causes of abnormal S_2 splitting.

1. Wide Physiologic Splitting

Wide physiologic splitting may result from P_2 appearing too late or A_2 too early (Table 40.1).[18,38] The most common cause is RBBB.

In pulmonic stenosis, the A_2P_2 interval correlates well with severity of stenosis (gauged by the RV systolic pressure, r = 0.87, p <0.001),[41] although in many patients the clinician must listen at the third interspace to hear splitting because the murmur is too loud at the second interspace.

TABLE 40.1 ■ Abnormal S$_2$ Splitting

Splitting and Pathogenesis	Etiology
WIDE PHYSIOLOGIC	
P$_2$ late	
Electrical delay of RV systole	RBBB
	LV paced or ectopic beats
Prolongation of RV systole	Pulmonic stenosis
	Acute cor pulmonale
Increased hangout interval	Dilation of pulmonary artery
A$_2$ Early	
Shortening of LV systole	Mitral regurgitation
WIDE AND FIXED	
Increased hangout interval or prolongation of RV systole	Atrial septal defect
Prolongation of RV systole	Right ventricular failure
PARADOXIC	
A$_2$ late	
Electrical delay of LV systole	LBBB
	RV paced or ectopic beats
Prolongation of LV systole	Aortic stenosis
	Ischemic heart disease

LBBB, Left bundle branch block; *LV,* left ventricular; *RBBB,* right bundle branch block; *RV,* right ventricular; *RV systole* and *LV systole* refer to the duration of right and left ventricular contraction.

In most patients with pulmonary hypertension, the normal hangout interval disappears and S_2 is single. S_2 becomes wide in these patients only if there is associated severe RV dysfunction and prolonged RV systole.[31,32,42] Most patients with pulmonary hypertension and a wide S_2 have either long-standing severe pulmonary hypertension[31,32,42] or massive pulmonary embolism (the wide S_2 of pulmonary embolism is temporary, usually lasting hours to days).[43]

2. Wide and Fixed Splitting

Patients with atrial septal defect have wide fixed splitting of S_2, although this is true only when their pulse is regular (if the patient has atrial fibrillation or frequent extrasystoles, the degree of splitting varies directly with the preceding cycle length).[30,44] The reason S_2 is wide is not the same in every patient: in some patients, hangout is increased; in others, RV mechanical systole is prolonged.[44] S_2 is fixed because hangout remains constant during respiration[44] and because the presence of a common left and right atrial chamber interrupts the normal respiratory variation of RV filling.[30]

In patients with audible expiratory splitting (and regular rhythm), the *absence* of fixed splitting significantly *decreases* the probability of atrial septal defect (LR = 0.1; see EBM Box 40.1), whereas the presence of fixed splitting increases the probability of atrial septal defect only modestly (LR = 2.6; see EBM Box 40.1). Patients with false-positive results (i.e., fixed splitting without atrial septal defect) commonly have the combination of RV failure and audible expiratory splitting from bundle branch block or some other cause.[18]

3. Paradoxic Splitting

In elderly adults with aortic flow murmurs, the finding of paradoxic splitting does not distinguish significant aortic stenosis from less severe disease (EBM Box 40.1).

D. S_2 SPLITTING VS. OTHER DOUBLE SOUNDS[40]

Other double sounds that mimic S_2 splitting include the following (see also Chapter 42):

1. S_2-Opening Snap

In contrast to the split S_2, the S_2-opening snap interval is slightly wider, the opening snap is loudest at the apex, and the opening snap ushers in the diastolic rumble of mitral stenosis at the apex. Patients with S_2-opening snap sometimes have a triple sound (split S_2 + opening snap) during inspiration at the upper sternal border.

2. S_2-Pericardial Knock

In contrast to the split S_2, the S_2-knock interval is slightly wider, the pericardial knock is loudest at or near apex, and the knock is always accompanied by elevated neck veins.

3. S_2-Third Heart Sound

In contrast to the split S_2, the S_2-S_3 interval is two to three times wider, and S_3 is a low frequency sound heard best with the bell.

4. Late Systolic Click-S_2

Clicks are loudest at or near apex and are often multiple. Their timing changes with maneuvers (see Chapter 46).

IV. Intensity of S_2

Traditionally, a loud P_2 has been regarded a reliable sign of pulmonary hypertension, but attempts to confirm this teaching have been largely unsuccessful. For example, in mitral stenosis patients, the loud P_2 defined either as an S_2 that is louder at the left side of the upper sternum compared with the right side[21] or as a split S_2 with a louder second component (i.e., $P_2 > A_2$)[20] did not discriminate between patients with pulmonary hypertension and those without it (see EBM Box 40.1). Furthermore, in patients with interstitial lung disease[45] or those attending pulmonary hypertension clinics,[46] the finding of $P_2 > A_2$ was not an accurate sign of pulmonary hypertension. Even when A_2 and P_2 were precisely identified by phonocardiography (e.g., A_2 corresponds to aortic incisura on simultaneous aortic pressure tracing), the relative intensities of the two components did not correlate well with pulmonary pressures.[45,47] Others have suggested that audible splitting at the apex indicates pulmonary hypertension (because P_2 should not be heard at the apex, and any splitting at that location indicated that P_2 was abnormally loud),[33] but even this finding correlates better with the etiology of heart disease—it is common in atrial septal defect and primary pulmonary hypertension—than it does with measurements of pulmonary pressure.[42,45,47]

Nonetheless, one study of patients with cirrhosis did demonstrate that the loud P_2 increased probability of pulmonary hypertension (i.e., porto-pulmonary hypertension, LR = 17.6; EBM Box 40.1, see Chapter 8). Also, the *palpable* S_2 in patients with mitral stenosis accurately detects pulmonary arterial pressures ≥50 mm Hg (positive LR = 3.6, negative LR = 0.05; see EBM Box 40.1). In this study, the palpable P_2 was defined as an abrupt tapping sensation coincident with S_2 at the second left intercostal space.

In patients with aortic flow murmurs, an absent or diminished S_2 increases the probability of significant aortic stenosis (LR = 3.8, see Chapter 44).

References may be accessed online at *Elsevier eBooks for Practicing Clinicians*.

The Third and Fourth Heart Sounds

KEY TEACHING POINTS

- The third and fourth heart sounds (S_3 and S_4) both originate from rapid diastolic filling of ventricles. They are collectively called *gallops*. The S_3 differs from the S_4 in timing and clinical significance.
- *Right ventricular gallops* appear at the left lower sternal border, intensify with inspiration, and are associated with abnormalities of the jugular venous waveforms. *Left ventricular gallops* appear at the apex and diminish in intensity during inspiration. All gallops are best heard with the bell of the stethoscope.
- The S_3 is an early diastolic sound. It is associated with a dilated ventricle, systolic dysfunction, and elevated filling pressures. The S_3 often disappears after the patient is treated with diuretic medications.
- The S_4 is a presystolic sound. It is associated with a stiff ventricle caused by ischemic, hypertensive, or hypertrophic cardiomyopathy. Once heard, the S_4 usually persists unless the patient develops atrial fibrillation. Unlike the S_3, the S_4 does not predict the patient's hemodynamic findings.

I. Introduction

Although the third and fourth heart sounds (S_3 and S_4) are both sounds that originate in the ventricle from rapid diastolic filling, they differ in timing and clinical significance. S_3 appears in early diastole and, if the patient is older than 40 years of age, the sound indicates severe systolic dysfunction or valvular regurgitation. In persons younger than 40 years of age, S_3 may be a normal finding (i.e., the *physiologic S_3*).[1] S_4 appears in late diastole, immediately before S_1, indicating that the patient's ventricle is abnormally stiff from hypertrophy or fibrosis. If discovered in persons of any age, the S_4 is an abnormal finding.

In the late 19th century, the great French clinician Potain accurately described most features of S_3 and S_4, their pathogenesis, and their distinction from other double sounds such as the split S_1 or split S_2.[2] In his writings he called them *gallops*, a term he attributed to his teacher Bouillard.[2,3]

II. Definitions

Several different terms have been used to describe these diastolic sounds.

A. GALLOP

A gallop is a triple rhythm with an extra sound in diastole (either S_3, S_4, or their summation). The term refers only to pathologic sounds (i.e., it excludes physiologic S_3) and, despite its connotation, a patient may have a gallop whether the heart rate is fast or slow.[2,4]

B. THIRD HEART SOUND (S_3)

The third heart sound is sometimes called the **ventricular gallop** or **protodiastolic gallop**.[2] It appears in early diastole, 120 to 180 ms after S_2.[5] To mimic the sound, the clinician should first establish the cadence of the normal S_1 (*lub*) and S_2 (*dup*):

        lub   *dup*   *lub*   *dup*   *lub*   *dup*

And then add an early diastolic sound (bub)*:

        lub   *du bub*   *lub*   *du bub*   *lub*   *du bub*

The overall cadence of the S_3 gallop (lub du bub) is similar to the cadence of the word Kentucky.

C. FOURTH HEART SOUND (S_4)

The fourth heart sound is sometimes called the **atrial gallop** or **presystolic gallop**.[2] To mimic the sound, the clinician establishes the cadence of S_1 and S_2 (*lub dup*) and then adds a presystolic sound (*be*):

        be lub   *dup*   *be lub*   *dup*   *be lub*   *dup*

The cadence of S_4 gallop (be lub dup) is similar to the cadence of the word Tennessee[†].

D. SUMMATION GALLOP

The summation gallop is a loud gallop that occurs in patients with tachycardia. In fast heart rhythms, diastole shortens, causing the events that produce S_3 (rapid early diastolic filling) to coincide with those producing S_4 (atrial systole). The resulting sound sometimes is louder than the patient's S_1 or S_2.

Not all gallop rhythms in patients with tachycardia are summation gallops. The only way to confirm the finding is to observe the patient after the heart rate slows. (In the past, slowing was often induced by carotid artery massage, although in elderly patients this is no longer recommended. See Chapter 16). If slowing causes the gallop to disappear or evolve into two distinct but fainter sounds (i.e., S_3 and S_4), it was a genuine summation gallop. If the sound evolves instead into a single S_3 or single S_4, it was not a summation gallop.[4,7]

---

*To pronounce the S_3 gallop with correct timing, the "p" of *dup* (S_2) must be dropped. In most patients the accent is on S_2 (*lub **du** bub*), although in others it falls on S_1 or S_3. The clinician can practice all three versions, always maintaining the same cadence, to become familiar with the varying sounds of S_3.

†Canadian teachers have suggested different mnemonics for the timing of S_3 and S_4: *Montreal* (pronounced MON TRE al) for S_3 and *Toronto* (tor ON to) for S_4.[6]

E. QUADRUPLE RHYTHM

The quadruple rhythm consists of S_1, S_2, and both S_3 and S_4.[4] It is an uncommon finding, usually only evident in patients with slow heart rates. It is sometimes called the **train wheel rhythm**, because the sound resembles that produced by the two pairs of wheels from adjacent train cars as they cross the coupling of a railroad track.[3,7]

be lub   du bub   be lub   du bub   be lub   du bub

III. Technique

A. LOCATION OF SOUND AND USE OF STETHOSCOPE

S_3 and S_4 are both low frequency sounds (20 to 70 Hz), bordering on the threshold of human hearing.[8] Therefore, they are best heard with the bell of the stethoscope, applied lightly to the body wall with only enough force to create an air seal.[2,5] Gallops that originate in the left ventricle are best heard with the bell over the apical impulse or just medial to it. They are sometimes only audible with the patient lying in the left lateral decubitus position.[9] Gallops from the right ventricle are best heard with the bell over the left lower sternal border or, in patients with chronic lung disease, the subxiphoid area.[2,5]

B. RIGHT VERSUS LEFT VENTRICULAR GALLOPS

Aside from their different locations, other distinguishing features of right and left ventricular gallops are their response to respirations and association with other findings in the neck veins and precordium. Right ventricular (RV) gallops become louder during inspiration; left ventricular (LV) gallops become softer during inspiration.[10] The RV S_4 may be associated with giant A waves in the neck veins and sometimes a loud presystolic jugular sound (see Chapter 36).[11] The LV S_4 may be associated with a palpable presystolic movement of the apical impulse (see Chapter 38).

C. DISTINGUISHING THE S_4-S_1 SOUND FROM OTHER SOUNDS

Three combinations of heart sounds produce a double sound around S_1: (1) the S_4-S_1 sound, (2) the split S_1, and (3) the S_1-ejection sound. The following characteristics distinguish these sounds[10]:

1. Use of the Bell

The S_4 is a low frequency sound, best heard with the bell. Firm pressure with the bell on the skin—which tends to remove low frequency sounds—will cause the S_4-S_1 combination to evolve into a single sound, in contrast to the split S_1 and the S_1-ejection sound, which remain double.

2. Location

The S_4-S_1 sound is heard best at the apex, left lower sternal border, or subxiphoid area (see the section on location of sound and use of stethoscope). The split S_1 is loudest from the apex to lower sternal border, but sometimes is also heard well over the upper left sternal area. The aortic ejection sound is heard from the apex to the upper right sternal border. The pulmonary ejection sound is restricted to the upper left sternal area.[12]

3. Effect of Respiration

Although the S_4 may become louder (RV S_4) or softer (LV S_4) during inspiration, respiration does not affect the interval between S_4 and S_1. In contrast, the split S_1 interval varies with respiration in up to one third of patients.

Expiration makes the pulmonary ejection sound louder.[12] The aortic ejection sound does not vary with respiration.[13]

4. Palpation

Only the S_4-S_1 sound is accompanied by a presystolic apical impulse (see Chapter 38). The intensity of the S_4 (i.e., by auscultation) correlates moderately with the amplitude of the presystolic impulse on apexcardiography (r = 0.46, p <0.01); similarly, the palpability of the presystolic impulse correlates roughly with the amplitude of S_4 on phonocardiography (r = 0.52, p <0.01).[14]

IV. Pathogenesis

A. NORMAL VENTRICULAR FILLING CURVES

Filling of the right and left ventricles during diastole is divided into three distinct phases (Fig. 41.1). The first phase, the rapid filling phase, begins immediately after opening of the atrioventricular valves. During this phase, blood stored in the atria rapidly empties into the ventricles. The second phase, the plateau phase (diastasis), begins at the moment the ventricles are unable to relax passively any further. Very little filling occurs during this phase. The third phase, atrial systole, begins with the atrial contraction, which expands the ventricle further just before the next S_1.

B. VENTRICULAR FILLING AND SOUND

Both S_3 and S_4 occur at those times during diastole when blood flow entering the ventricles temporarily stops, that is, the S_3 appears at the end of the rapid filling phase, and the S_4 toward the peak of atrial systole (Fig. 41.1). Sounds become audible if the blood *decelerates abruptly* enough, which transmits sufficient energy to the ventricular walls and causes them to vibrate (an analogy is the tensing of a handkerchief between two hands: abrupt tensing produces sound, whereas slow tensing is silent).[15-21] Two variables govern the suddenness of this deceleration, and therefore whether gallops become audible: (1) the flow rate during entry and (2) the stiffness of the ventricle. The greater the flow rate, the *louder* the sound. The stiffer the ventricle, the *higher the frequency* of the sound.[22] Since gallops consist of low frequencies that are difficult to hear (around 20 to 50 Hz), anything increasing their frequency content (i.e., stiff ventricles) makes the sound more likely to be heard.

Even though S_3 and S_4 both result from rapid flow rates into stiff ventricles, the diseases causing them differ completely.

C. THE THIRD HEART SOUND (S_3)

The S_3 gallop appears when early diastolic filling is exaggerated, which occurs in two types of cardiac disorders:

1. Congestive Heart Failure

The most common cause of the S_3 gallop is congestive heart failure from systolic dysfunction. In these patients, the S_3 indicates that atrial pressure is abnormally elevated, an especially important finding in patients with dyspnea, implying that heart disease is the principal cause of the shortness of breath. In addition to elevated atrial pressure, these patients typically have a dilated cardiomyopathy and low cardiac output.[23,24] Although both high atrial pressure (causing rapid flow rates) and cardiomyopathy (causing stiff ventricles) contribute to the sound, atrial pressure is the more important clinical variable, because the sound disappears as soon as atrial pressure decreases with diuresis.

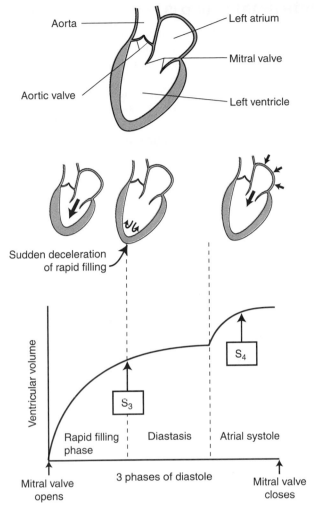

Fig. 41.1 Timing of third and fourth heart sounds. The figure depicts the three phases of diastolic filling of the left ventricle (y-axis on graph, ventricular volume; x-axis, time). The S_3 occurs at the end of the rapid filling phase, when passive filling suddenly decelerates. The S_4 occurs during atrial systole. Similar events on the right side of the heart may produce a right ventricular S_3 or S_4. See text.

2. Regurgitation and Shunts

Patients with valvular regurgitation or left-to-right cardiac shunts also may develop an S_3 gallop, whether or not atrial pressure is high, because these disorders all cause excess flow over the atrioventricular valves. Patients with mitral regurgitation, ventricular septal defect, or patent ductus arteriosus may develop a LV S_3 from excess diastolic flow over the mitral valve into the left ventricle (in mitral regurgitation, the excess diastolic flow simply represents the diastolic return of the regurgitant flow). Patients with atrial septal defect may develop a RV S_3 from excess flow over the tricuspid valve into the right ventricle.

D. THE FOURTH HEART SOUND (S₄)

The S_4 gallop occurs in patients with hypertension, ischemic cardiomyopathy, hypertrophic cardiomyopathy, or aortic stenosis—all disorders characterized by ventricles stiffened from hypertrophy or fibrosis.[2,23-25] Patients with the sound must be in sinus rhythm and have strong atrial contractions, and most have normal atrial pressures, normal cardiac output, and normal ventricular chamber size. Unlike the S_3, the S_4 is a durable finding that does not wax and wane unless the patient develops atrial fibrillation (and thus loses the atrial contraction).

E. SUMMATION GALLOP AND QUADRUPLE RHYTHM

The summation gallop occurs because fast heart rates shorten diastole, primarily by eliminating the plateau phase (Fig. 41.1), which brings the events causing S_3 close to those causing S_4. Diastolic filling is concentrated into a single moment, thus causing a very loud sound.

The quadruple rhythm typically occurs in patients who have had a long-standing S_4 gallop from ischemic or hypertensive heart disease but who then develop cardiac decompensation, high filling pressures, and a S_3.[7]

Rarely, an intermittent summation gallop may appear in patients with slow heart rates due to complete heart block (or VVI pacing).[26] The gallop appears only during those moments of atrioventricular dissociation when atrial systole and early diastole coincide (i.e., the P wave on the electrocardiogram falls just after the QRS). Although the sound is technically a summation gallop, the clinician perceives what sounds like an intermittent S_3. A similar mechanism has been invoked to explain intermittent early diastolic sounds in patients with Wenckebach heart block.[27]

F. PHYSIOLOGIC S₃

Persons younger than 40 years of age with normal hearts may also have a S_3 sound (i.e., physiologic S_3), because normal early filling can sometimes be so rapid that it ends abruptly and causes the ventricular walls to vibrate and produce sound. Compared with healthy persons lacking the sound, those with the physiologic S_3 are leaner and have more rapid early diastolic filling.[1] The physiologic S_3 disappears by age 40, because normal aging slows ventricular relaxation and shifts filling later in diastole, thus diminishing the rate of early diastolic filling and making the sound disappear.[28]

V. Clinical Significance

A. THE THIRD HEART SOUND

1. Congestive Heart Failure

EBM Box 41.1 shows that the presence of the S_3 gallop is a significant finding indicating depressed ejection fraction (likelihood ratio [LR] = 3.4 to 4.1; see EBM Box 41.1), elevated left atrial pressures (LR = 3.9), and elevated B-type natriuretic peptide (BNP) levels (LR = 10.1). Other studies confirm its value as a predictor of poor systolic function.[36,45] The *absence* of the S_3 gallop argues that the patient's ejection fraction is greater than 30% (i.e., negative LR = 0.3 for detecting ejection fraction <30%; see EBM Box 41.1).

In patients with a history of congestive heart failure, the S_3 predicts responsiveness to digoxin[46] and overall mortality.[47]

| EBM BOX 41.1 | **The Third and Fourth Heart Sounds*** |

Finding (Reference)	Sensitivity (%)	Specificity (%)	Likelihood Ratio[†] if Finding Is	
			Present	**Absent**
The third heart sound				
Detecting ejection fraction <0.5[20,29–32]	11–51	85–98	**3.4**	0.7
Detecting ejection fraction <0.3[30,31]	68–78	80–88	**4.1**	**0.3**
Detecting elevated left heart filling pressures[32–35]	12–37	85–96	**3.9**	0.8
Detecting elevated BNP level[36,37]	41–65	93–97	**10.1**	0.5
Detecting myocardial infarction in patients with acute chest pain[38]	16	95	**3.2**	NS
Predicting postoperative pulmonary edema[39,40]	17	99	**14.6**	NS
Predicting postoperative myocardial infarction or cardiac death[39,40]	11	99	**8.0**	NS
The fourth heart sound				
Detecting elevated left heart filling pressures[34,41]	35–71	50–70	NS	NS
Detecting severe aortic stenosis[42,43]	29–50	57–63	NS	NS
Predicting 5-year mortality in patients after myocardial infarction[44]	29	91	**3.2**	NS

*Diagnostic standard: for *ejection fraction*, left ventricular ejection fraction <0.5 or <0.3 (as indicated above) by scintigraphy or echocardiography (see Chapter 48); for *elevated left heart filling pressures*, pulmonary capillary wedge pressure >12 mm Hg[33] or left ventricular end diastolic pressure >15 mm Hg[32,34,35,41]; for *elevated BNP level*, ≥100 pg/mL[36] or >1525 pg/mL[37]; for *myocardial infarction*, development of new electrocardiographic Q waves, elevations of creatine kinase MB, or both; for *severe aortic stenosis*, peak gradient >50 mm Hg[42] or valve area <0.75 cm[2],[43]

[†]Likelihood ratio (LR) if finding present = positive LR; LR if finding absent = negative LR.
BNP, B type natriuretic peptide; *NS*, not significant.

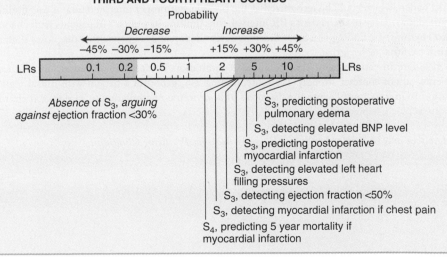

THIRD AND FOURTH HEART SOUNDS

Probability

Decrease   *Increase*

−45% −30% −15%   +15% +30% +45%

LRs   0.1   0.2   0.5   1   2   5   10   LRs

Absence of S_3, *arguing against* ejection fraction <30%

S_3, predicting postoperative pulmonary edema

S_3, detecting elevated BNP level

S_3, predicting postoperative myocardial infarction

S_3, detecting elevated left heart filling pressures

S_3, detecting ejection fraction <50%

S_3, detecting myocardial infarction if chest pain

S_4, predicting 5 year mortality if myocardial infarction

2. Valvular Heart Disease

In patients with mitral regurgitation, the S_3 is a poor predictor of elevated filling pressure (LR not significant) and depressed ejection fraction (LR = 1.9).[48] Some studies correlate the sound with the severity of mitral regurgitation,[20] whereas others do not.[48]

In contrast, the S_3 is a helpful finding in patients with aortic valve disease. In patients with aortic stenosis, the S_3 detects both elevated filling pressures (LR = 2.3 for pulmonary capillary wedge pressures ≥12 mm Hg) and a depressed ejection fraction (LR = 5.7 for EF <50%).[48] In patients with aortic regurgitation, the S_3 detects both severity of regurgitation (LR = 5.9 for regurgitant fraction ≥40%, see Chapter 45) and ejection fraction <50% (LR = 8.3).[20]

3. Patients with Acute Chest Pain

In patients with acute chest pain presenting to emergency departments, the finding of an S_3 increases the probability of myocardial infarction (LR = 3.2; EBM Box 41.1).

4. Preoperative Consultation

During preoperative consultation, the finding of S_3 is ominous, indicating that the patient, without any other intervention, has an increased risk of perioperative pulmonary edema (LR = 14.6) and myocardial infarction or cardiac death (LR = 8).[39]

B. THE FOURTH HEART SOUND

The finding of the S_4 gallop has less diagnostic value, simply because the disorders causing stiff ventricles are so diverse and because the S_4 does not predict the patient's hemodynamic findings. The finding does not predict ejection fraction, left heart filling pressures, or postoperative cardiac complications.[23,24,34,39,40] It also does not predict significant aortic stenosis in elderly patients with aortic flow murmurs, presumably because many patients with mild stenosis have the finding for other reasons, such as ischemic heart disease.[42,43]

Nonetheless, when detected one month after myocardial infarction, the S_4 is a modest predictor of 5 year cardiac mortality (LR = 3.2; see EBM Box 41.1). Experienced auscultators in the past did show that clinical deterioration in patients with ischemic disease caused the S_4-S_1 interval to widen, which could be recognized at the bedside, but proper interpretation of this finding required knowledge of the patient's PR interval, thus limiting its utility.[49] In patients with chaotic heart rhythms, the finding of a S_4 excludes atrial fibrillation and suggests other diagnoses such as multifocal atrial tachycardia.

S_4 is rare in patients with chronic mitral regurgitation, because the dilated atrium of these patients cannot contract strongly. Therefore, finding a S_4 gallop in a patient with mitral regurgitation is an important clue to the diagnosis of *acute* mitral regurgitation (e.g., ruptured chorda tendineae; see Chapter 46).[50-52]

References may be accessed online at *Elsevier eBooks for Practicing Clinicians.*

Miscellaneous Heart Sounds

In addition to the first, second, third, and fourth heart sounds, several other discrete, short sounds may occur (Fig. 42.1). These sounds include early systolic sounds (e.g., the aortic or pulmonary ejection sound), midsystolic or late systolic sounds (e.g., systolic click of mitral valve prolapse), early diastolic sounds (e.g., opening snap of mitral stenosis, pericardial knock of constrictive pericarditis, and tumor plop of atrial myxoma), and prosthetic valve sounds. All are high frequency sounds best heard with the diaphragm of the stethoscope.

EJECTION SOUNDS

I. The Finding and Pathogenesis

The ejection sound is the most common early systolic sound. It results from abnormal sudden halting of the semilunar cusps as they open during early systole.[1,2] Patients with aortic ejection sounds typically have aortic stenosis, a bicuspid aortic valve, or a dilated aortic root.[1,2] Those with pulmonary ejection sounds have pulmonary stenosis, pulmonary hypertension, or a dilated pulmonary trunk.[2,3]

Aortic and pulmonary ejection sounds are distinguished by their location, associated murmurs, and how they vary during respiration. An aortic ejection sound is a loud high-frequency sounds (often louder than S_1) best heard at the apex, although commonly also audible at the upper right sternal border.[4] It does not vary with respiration. Pulmonary ejection sounds are confined to the sternal edge at the second or third intercostal space; they often diminish in intensity during inspiration. Ejection sounds associated with aortic or pulmonic stenosis occur immediately before the onset of the systolic murmur.[4,5]

Chapter 41 describes how to distinguish ejection sounds from other double sounds around S_1, including the combination of S_4-S_1 and the split S_1.

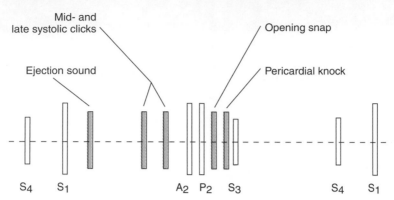

Fig. 42.1 Miscellaneous heart sounds. The figure shows the timing of the miscellaneous systolic sounds (ejection sounds and mid-to-late systolic clicks) and diastolic sounds (opening snap and pericardial knock), in relation to the principal heart sounds (first, second, third, and fourth heart sounds). The tumor plop of atrial myxoma, not depicted in the figure, has variable timing, ranging from 80 ms after A_2 (i.e., timing of the opening snap) to 150 ms after A_2 (i.e., timing of the third heart sound).[25]

II. Clinical Significance

The primary importance of these sounds is their etiologic associations. In patients with aortic stenosis, the ejection sound implies that the stenosis is at the valvular level and that there is some mobility to the valve. Elderly patients with calcific aortic stenosis usually do not have ejection sounds, because the calcific degeneration makes the valve leaflets inflexible. Children with noncalcific aortic stenosis, in contrast, usually have the ejection sound. In one consecutive series of 118 patients with aortic stenosis, the ejection sound was audible in 100% of patients with noncalcific valvular stenosis, in 32% with calcific valvular stenosis, and in none with subvalvular or supravalvular stenosis.[4]

MID-TO-LATE SYSTOLIC CLICKS

I. The Finding and Pathogenesis

Mid-to-late systolic clicks occur in patients with mitral valve prolapse. These sounds, which are sometimes multiple, are caused by sudden deceleration of the billowing mitral leaflet as it prolapses backward into the left atrium during systole.[6] The click is loudest at the apex or left lower sternal border and is frequently associated with a late systolic murmur.[7]

The hallmark of the click of mitral valve prolapse (and also of the associated murmur) is that its timing shifts during maneuvers that change venous return. For example, the straining phase of the Valsalva maneuver or the squat-to-stand maneuver, both of which decrease venous return, causes the mitral leaflets to prolapse earlier in systole, thus shifting the click (and murmur) closer to S_1 (see Fig. 46.1 in Chapter 46).[7,8]

Clicks have been heard by clinicians for over a century, although they were ascribed to pleuropericardial adhesions or other extracardiac causes[9] until the 1960s, when Barlow demonstrated the sound coincided with systolic prolapse of the posterior mitral leaflet.[10]

II. Clinical Significance

The presence of the characteristic click or murmur alone is sufficient grounds for the diagnosis of mitral valve prolapse.[11,12] Chapter 46 discusses these findings further.

OPENING SNAP

I. The Finding and Pathogenesis

The opening snap is an early diastolic sound heard in patients with mitral stenosis.* The sound occurs because the stenotic mitral leaflets (although fused, they are mobile) billow like a large sail into the ventricle during early diastole but then abruptly decelerate as they meet the limits of movement.[1,6] The abrupt deceleration causes a loud, medium-to-high frequency sound, which is then followed by the mid-diastolic rumbling murmur of mitral stenosis. The opening snap is best heard between the apex and left lower sternal border.

The clinician can mimic the sound of snap and murmur together by first setting up the cadence of S_1, S_2, and opening snap (RUP = S_1; bu = S_2; DUP = opening snap):

RUP   bu DUP   RUP   bu DUP   RUP   bu DUP

and then adding the murmur:

RUP   bu DUPʀʀʀRRRRRUP   bu DUPʀʀʀRRRRRUP   bu DUP

In some patients the opening snap is so loud it is easily heard at the second left intercostal space, where it then mimics a widely split S_2. Careful attention to inspiration in these patients, however, may reveal a *triple* sound (split S_2 and opening snap) at this location, confirming the last sound to be the opening snap.

The opening snap of mitral stenosis was first described by Bouillard in 1835.[1]

II. Clinical Significance

According to traditional teachings, the opening snap is inaudible in patients with mitral stenosis whose valve leaflets have become so thickened and inflexible they cannot create sound.[6,13] There is an inverse correlation between the opening snap amplitude and degree of calcification of the mitral valve ($r = -0.675$, $p<0.01$).[14]

The interval between the A_2 component of S_2 and the opening snap (A_2-OS interval) has been used to gauge the severity of mitral stenosis. Patients with more severe obstruction tend to have a narrower A_2-OS interval than those with milder disease. This occurs because the mitral valve opens when the pressure in the relaxing ventricle falls below the atrial pressure; the more severe the obstruction, the higher the atrial pressure and the sooner this crossover occurs. Nonetheless, determining the A_2-OS interval is primarily a phonocardiographic exercise, not an auscultatory one.[15] Furthermore, the A_2-OS interval also depends on variables other than severity of stenosis, such as ventricular relaxation time and heart rate, which further complicates interpreting it accurately at the bedside.[15]

The opening snap does indicate that the accompanying diastolic murmur represents mitral stenosis and not a flow rumble from increased flow over a nonstenotic valve (see Chapter 46 for discussion of flow rumbles).

PERICARDIAL KNOCK

The pericardial knock is a loud early diastolic sound heard in 20% to 94% of patients with constrictive pericarditis (see Chapter 47). It is heard over a wide area between the apex and left lower

---

*Patients with tricuspid stenosis also may have an opening snap, but all of these patients also have mitral stenosis and the mitral opening snap. Differentiating tricuspid and mitral opening snaps by auscultation is difficult.

sternal border. Compared with the third heart sound, the pericardial knock is a higher frequency sound (easily detected with the diaphragm of the stethoscope), appears over a wider area of the precordium, and occurs slightly earlier (although still later than the opening snap or widely split second heart sound).[16]

The pericardial knock results from the sudden deceleration of the filling ventricle as it meets the borders of the rigid pericardial sac.[16,17] In this way, it is similar to the third heart sound, although the more abrupt deceleration of constriction is what probably makes the pericardial knock higher-pitched and louder than the third heart sound (see Chapter 41).

TUMOR PLOP

The tumor plop is an early diastolic sound representing prolapse of the pedunculated tumor from the atrium over the mitral (or tricuspid) valve into the ventricle[18] In two large series of patients with myxoma (283 patients), it was detected in 15% to 50% of patients.[19,20] Characteristically, the intensity and timing of the tumor plop vary between examinations: the plop may occur as early as the timing of an opening snap, or as late as that of the third heart sound. It is often associated with a diastolic murmur that mimics the rumbling sound of mitral stenosis.[19]

An audio recording of a pansystolic murmur and tumor plop sound from a patient with a mitral valve myxoma can be found in reference by Doshi.[21]

PROSTHETIC HEART SOUNDS

I. Introduction

Abnormal prosthetic heart sounds may be the only clue explaining the patient's dyspnea, syncope, or chest pain. To recognize these abnormal sounds simply and quickly, the clinician must first understand the normal prosthetic heart sounds. This section focuses on rigid mechanical valves, such as caged-ball valves (Starr-Edwards)[†] single tilting-disc valves (Bjork-Shiley, Medtronic-Hall), and bileaflet tilting-disc valves (St. Jude Medical).[22–24]

II. Principles

The important observations are (1) timing and intensity of opening and closing sounds, which typically have a clicking or metallic quality and are often audible without a stethoscope, and (2) associated murmurs. Any new or changing sound or murmur requires investigation.

A. OPENING AND CLOSING SOUNDS

In patients with caged-ball valves, the opening sound is louder than the closing sound. In patients with tilting-disc valves (both single disc and bileaflet), the closing sounds are loud and the opening sounds are only faint or inaudible (Fig. 42.2).

1. Caged-Ball Valves

In the aortic position, the caged-ball valve produces a loud opening sound, which is an extra systolic sound occurring just after S_1 with timing identical to the aortic ejection sound (i.e., instead of just S_1 and S_2, *lub dup...lub dup*, the clinician hears *ledup dup...ledup dup*). Caged-ball valves

---

[†]The Starr-Edwards valve is no longer manufactured, although it is still in use.

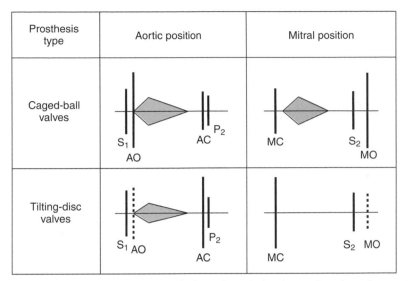

Fig. 42.2 Prosthetic valve sounds. The normal findings of prosthetic valves are based on references 22–24. *AC,* Closure sound of aortic prosthesis; *AO,* opening sound of aortic prosthesis; *MC,* closure sound of mitral prosthesis; *MO,* opening sound of mitral prosthesis; P_2, pulmonary component of second heart sound; S_1, first heart sound; S_2, second heart sound. See the text.

in the mitral position produce an extra diastolic sound when they open, with timing identical to that of the opening snap (i.e., instead of S_1 and S_2, *lub bup...lub bup*, it is *lub budup...lub budup*). These opening sounds should always be louder than the corresponding closing sound (i.e., closing sounds are coincident with S_2 in aortic prostheses and with S_1 in mitral prostheses). The finding of an inaudible or abnormally soft opening sound indicates something is interfering with excursion of the ball, such as thrombus.

2. Tilting-Disc Valves

These valves produce distinct, metallic closing sounds coincident with S_1 (mitral position) or S_2 (aortic position). Patients whose closing sounds are abnormally quiet may have significant valve dysfunction.

B. MURMURS

In the aortic position, all rigid valves (caged-ball and tilting-disc) typically produce short mid-systolic murmurs that are best heard at the base and sometimes radiate to the neck. Diastolic murmurs in these patients suggest perivalvular regurgitation and require investigation.[22–24]

In patients with rigid valves in the mitral position, any holosystolic murmur suggests perival-vular regurgitation and requires investigation. A normal finding in patients with the caged-ball valve in the mitral position (but not tilting-disc valves) is an early-to-midsystolic murmur at the left sternal border. This murmur does not indicate regurgitation but instead represents turbulence caused by the cage of the valve projecting into the left ventricular outflow tract.[22,24]

References may be accessed online at *Elsevier eBooks for Practicing Clinicians.*

Heart Murmurs: General Principles

I. Introduction

Since the 1830s, the understanding of heart murmurs has evolved in three distinct stages.[1] In the first stage, brilliant clinicians—James Hope (1801–1841), Austin Flint (1812–1886), and Graham Steell (1851–1942)— attentively observed patients at the bedside and correlated the timing and quality of murmurs to the patients' clinical course and post-mortem findings.[2] In the second stage, during the 1950s and 1960s, cardiac catheterization and phonocardiography helped clinicians understand the hemodynamics responsible for heart murmurs,[3-5] and the introduction of cardiac surgery increased the stakes of cardiac auscultation, stimulating clinicians to be as precise and accurate as possible. Finally, in the 1970s and 1980s, the introduction of echocardiography solved many of the remaining mysteries about murmurs, including the cause of ejection sounds in aortic stenosis and late systolic murmurs and clicks in mitral valve prolapse.

This chapter covers the principles of describing and diagnosing murmurs. Specific cardiac disorders and their associated murmurs are further discussed in Chapters 44 to 46.

II. The Findings

The important characteristics of heart murmurs are location (both where it's loudest and which direction the sound travels, or *radiates*), timing, intensity, and frequency (or *pitch*, which is high, low, or a mixture of high and low frequencies).[6] The terms *rough*, *rumbling*, *blowing*, *coarse*, and *musical* are also sometimes used to describe the specific tonal quality of murmurs.

Murmurs frequently vary in intensity during the respiratory cycle, but loud murmur-like sounds that completely disappear during inspiration or expiration are likely pericardial rubs, not murmurs.[7]

A. BASIC CLASSIFICATION OF MURMURS

Murmurs are broadly classified as systolic, diastolic, and continuous (Table 43.1).[6] **Systolic murmurs** occur during the time between S_1 and S_2. **Diastolic murmurs** occur at any time from S_2 to the next S_1. **Continuous murmurs** begin in systole but extend beyond S_2 into diastole, indicating they do not respect the confines of systole and diastole and thus arise *outside* the four heart chambers. Despite the name, continuous murmurs do not necessarily occupy all of systole and diastole.

TABLE 43.1 ■ Classification of Murmurs by Timing and Location

Systolic murmurs	Location Where Loudest
Abnormal flow over outflow tract or semilunar valve	
Aortic stenosis	R base, LLSB, and apex
Pulmonic stenosis	L base
Atrial septal defect*	L base
Hypertrophic cardiomyopathy with obstruction	LLSB
Regurgitation from high pressure chamber into low pressure chamber	
Mitral regurgitation	Apex
Tricuspid regurgitation	LLSB
Ventricular septal defect	LLSB
Diastolic murmurs	
Backward flow across leaking semilunar valve	
Aortic regurgitation	LLSB
Pulmonic regurgitation	L base
Abnormal forward flow over an atrioventricular valve	
Mitral stenosis	Apex
Tricuspid stenosis	LLSB
Continuous murmurs	
Abnormal connections between artery and vein	
Patent ductus arteriosus	L base
Arteriovenous fistula	Over fistula
Abnormal flow in veins	
Venous hum	Above head of clavicle
Mammary soufflé†	Between breast and sternum
Stenosis in peripheral artery	
Coarctation of the aorta	Over back

Apex, Point of apical impulse; *L base*, second left intercostal space next to sternum; *LLSB*, fourth and fifth left intercostal space next to sternum; *R base*, second right intercostal space next to sternum.
*The murmur of atrial septal defect is due to excess flow of blood over the pulmonic valve (from left-to-right shunting), not from flow through the defect itself.
†"Soufflé" (Fr. sound or murmur) is pronounced *SOO-ful*.

1. Systolic Murmurs

a. Etiology

There are two causes of systolic murmurs.

(1) Abnormal Flow over an Outflow Tract or Semilunar Valve. One cause is abnormal flow over an outflow tract or semilunar valve (i.e., aortic or pulmonic valve), such as (1) forward flow across an obstruction (e.g., aortic stenosis, pulmonic stenosis, or hypertrophic cardiomyopathy) or (2) increased flow across a normal semilunar valve (e.g., atrial septal defect or the flow murmurs of anemia, fever, pregnancy, or thyrotoxicosis).

(2) Regurgitation from a Ventricle into a Low Pressure Chamber. Examples are mitral regurgitation (leak between left ventricle and left atrium), tricuspid regurgitation (leak between right ventricle and right atrium), and ventricular septal defect (leak between left and right ventricles).

b. Older Classifications of Systolic Murmurs: "Ejection" and "Regurgitation" Murmurs

In 1958 Leatham divided all systolic murmurs into "ejection murmurs" and "regurgitant murmurs," based entirely on their relationship to S_2.[3,4] According to his classification, ejection murmurs begin after S_1, have a crescendo-decrescendo shape, and always end before S_2*. Ejection murmurs represent abnormal flow across the aortic or pulmonic valve. In contrast, regurgitant murmurs (e.g., mitral and tricuspid regurgitation) begin with S1, have a plateau shape, and extend up to S_2 or even slightly past it (thus obliterating S_2).

Leatham's classification is no longer widely used for several reasons: (1) It relies entirely on phonocardiography and does not always correspond to what clinicians hear at the bedside.[8] (2) It depends entirely on the audibility of the aortic and pulmonary components of S_2, sounds that sometimes are inaudible. (3) It assumes all ejection murmurs result from ejection over a semilunar valve, although experience has shown many are due to regurgitant lesions. (4) Its fundamental premise, that the intensity of a murmur depends on pressure gradients, is not always true (e.g., the murmur of mitral valve prolapse is loudest during late systole, when gradients are decreasing).

Instead, systolic murmurs are more easily classified using onomatopoeia as either midsystolic, early systolic, long systolic, holosystolic, and late systolic, based only on whether the murmur obscures S_1, S_2, or both sounds (see the section on timing and quality of murmurs using onomatopoeia).[1]

2. Diastolic Murmurs

There are two causes of diastolic murmurs: (1) abnormal backward flow across a leaking semilunar valve (e.g., aortic or pulmonic regurgitation) or (2) abnormal forward flow across an atrioventricular valve (e.g., mitral stenosis, tricuspid stenosis, and flow rumbles†).

3. Continuous Murmurs

Continuous murmurs result from any of the following disorders: (1) abnormal connections between the aorta and pulmonary trunk (e.g., patent ductus arteriosus), (2) abnormal connections between arteries and veins (e.g., arteriovenous fistulas) (see Chapter 54), (3) abnormal flow in veins (e.g., venous hum and mammary souffle), or (4) abnormal flow in arteries (e.g., coarctation of the aorta, renal artery stenosis).

---

*More precisely, "ejection" murmurs end before the S_2 component belonging to the side of the heart generating the murmur. For example, the murmur of aortic stenosis ends before A_2; the murmur of pulmonic stenosis ends before P_2.

†Flow rumbles are short low-frequency diastolic murmurs that result from increased flow over a nonobstructed atrioventricular valve. Atrial septal defects and tricuspid regurgitation increase diastolic flow over the tricuspid valve and may cause tricuspid flow rumbles (which resemble the murmur of tricuspid stenosis). Mitral regurgitation and ventricular septal defect increase diastolic flow over the mitral valve and may produce mitral flow rumbles (which resemble the murmur of mitral stenosis).

B. LOCATION ON THE CHEST WALL

The usual locations of conventional murmurs are described in Table 43.1. Nonetheless, in patients with systolic murmurs, one of the most helpful diagnostic signs is the distribution of the sound on the chest wall with reference to the third left parasternal space, a landmark that lies directly over both the aortic and mitral valves and distinguishes systolic murmurs into one of six possible patterns: (1) broad apical-base pattern; (2) small apical-base pattern; (3) left lower sternal pattern; (4) broad apical pattern; (5) isolated apical pattern; and (6) isolated base pattern (definitions of these patterns appear in Fig. 43.1).[7]

Inspection of the boundary surrounding all six patterns suggests the primary determinant of a murmur's radiation is not necessarily the direction of blood flow but instead the orientation of bony thorax, specifically the left lower ribs, sternum, and clavicles (Fig. 43.2). Increased flow across a semilunar valve or through a regurgitant leak generates vibrations in the ventricles, great arteries, or both, which—depending on their location, amplitude, and ease of conduction to the bones of the body wall—produce one of the six different murmur patterns. Indeed, one of the best arguments that bone conduction—and not direction of blood flow—governs distribution of sound is the murmur of mitral regurgitation: in this lesion blood flows from the left ventricle *rightward* (i.e., patient's "rightward," toward the midline) and *upward* to the left atrium, yet the murmur radiates almost perpendicular to this, along the left lower ribs to the axilla.[7]

The diagnostic significance of these six systolic murmur patterns is discussed in the section on differential diagnosis of systolic murmurs.

C. SPECIFIC TIMING AND QUALITY OF MURMURS USING ONOMATOPOEIA

Fig. 43.3 presents traditional diagrams of various heart murmurs, which in turn are based on phonocardiographic tracings. Because murmurs are sounds, however, diagrams such as these often fail to convey the precise cadence and tonal qualities that distinguish the various murmurs. Throughout the history of cardiac auscultation, clinicians have used onomatopoeia to mimic heart sounds and murmurs, finding this to be an effective teaching tool allowing clinicians to rapidly recognize the patterns of different sounds.[2,9,10]

The system described here is based on the published work of Feinstein[11] and Adolph.[12–15] High-frequency murmurs are mimicked by sounds from the front of the mouth; low-frequency murmurs are mimicked by sounds from the back of the throat. The high-frequency murmur of mitral and tricuspid regurgitation is mimicked by saying SHSHSHSH. The high-frequency murmur of aortic regurgitation is mimicked by blowing air out through slightly pursed lips, or whispering PHEWEWEWEWEW or AHAHAHAHAH (hence the "blowing" descriptor). The low-frequency murmurs of tricuspid or mitral stenosis are mimicked by the "RRRRR" portion of a growl (hence the "rumbling" descriptor). Murmurs containing a mixture of low and high frequencies, such as aortic stenosis, are mimicked by the sound made when clearing the throat (common descriptors are "coarse" or "harsh").

The clinician should first establish the normal cadence of S_1 and S_2 (*lub* is S_1 and *dup* is S_2):

| *lub* | *dup* | | *lub* | *dup* | | *lub* | *dup* |

Then, the murmur is added at the appropriate time. For example, the high frequency late systolic murmur of mitral valve prolapse preserves S_1 but obscures S_2 (i.e., "dup" is replaced by SHSHP):

| *lub SHSHP* | | *lub SHSHP* | | *lub SHSHP* |

Table 43.2 describes how to label the timing of systolic murmurs, and Fig. 43.4 shows how onomatopoeia can mimic many common murmurs.

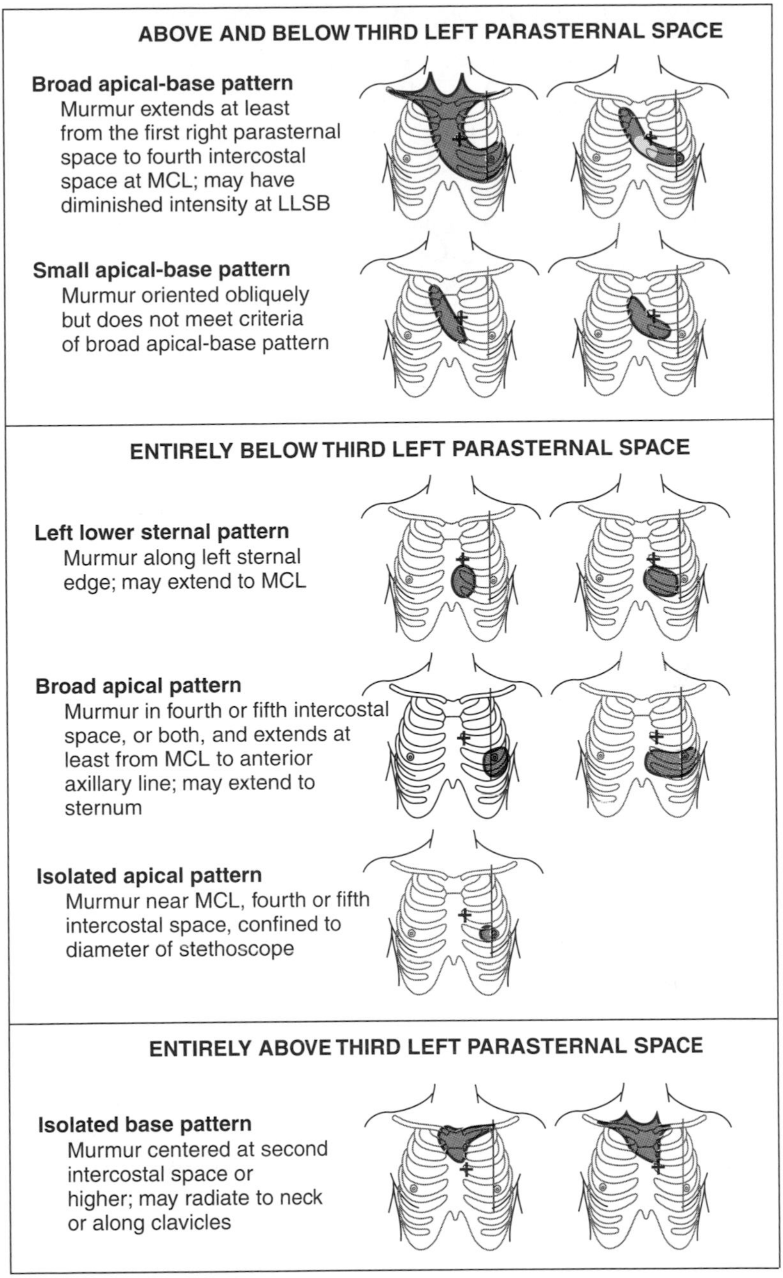

ABOVE AND BELOW THIRD LEFT PARASTERNAL SPACE

Broad apical-base pattern
Murmur extends at least
from the first right parasternal
space to fourth intercostal
space at MCL; may have
diminished intensity at LLSB

Small apical-base pattern
Murmur oriented obliquely
but does not meet criteria
of broad apical-base pattern

ENTIRELY BELOW THIRD LEFT PARASTERNAL SPACE

Left lower sternal pattern
Murmur along left sternal
edge; may extend to MCL

Broad apical pattern
Murmur in fourth or fifth intercostal
space, or both, and extends at
least from MCL to anterior
axillary line; may extend to
sternum

Isolated apical pattern
Murmur near MCL, fourth or fifth
intercostal space, confined to
diameter of stethoscope

ENTIRELY ABOVE THIRD LEFT PARASTERNAL SPACE

Isolated base pattern
Murmur centered at second
intercostal space or
higher; may radiate to neck
or along clavicles

Fig. 43.1 Six systolic murmur patterns. Each of the six topographic patterns are distinguished by their distribution with reference to the third left parasternal space (indicated by "+" symbol in each drawing). This landmark is easily identified by first identifying the sternal angle, where the second rib articulates, and then counting down to the second ICS, third rib, and then the third parasternal space. Two of the patterns traverse above and below this landmark (*broad apical-base* and *small apical base* patterns); three are confined below this landmark (*left lower sternal*, *broad apical*, and *isolated apical* patterns); and one is confined entirely above the landmark (*isolated base* pattern). *ICS*, Intercostal space; *LLSB*, left lower sternal border; *MCL*, midclavicular line. Adapted from McGee.[7]

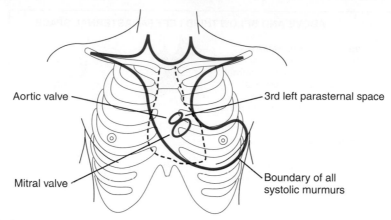

Aortic valve

3rd left parasternal space

Mitral valve

Boundary of all
systolic murmurs

Fig. 43.2 Boundary of systolic murmur patterns. The third left parasternal space overlies both the aortic and mitral valves. If the ventricles vibrate sufficiently to produce sound, murmurs are generated below this landmark. Vibrations of the right ventricle produce the *left lower sternal* pattern, whereas those of the left ventricle produce the *isolated apical* pattern or *broad apical* pattern. Should the great arteries vibrate sufficiently to make sound, the bones above this landmark vibrate and murmurs radiate from the upper sternum to clavicles and neck (*isolated base* pattern). With increased velocity across the aortic valve, both the left ventricle (lower ribs) and great arteries (upper sternum and clavicles) vibrate, causing the *apical-base pattern* and its variations. Adapted from McGee.[7]

By using onomatopoeia, clinicians can quickly learn the cadence of murmurs, which sometimes leads to rapid recognition of complicated sounds without first having to sort out the location of S_1 and S_2. For example, if auscultation reveals a cadence consisting of a single murmur and no heart sounds

SHSHSHP   *SHSHSHP*   *SHSHSHP*

the only possible diagnosis is a holosystolic murmur.

If auscultation reveals murmurs in both systole and diastole, there are three possible causes: (1) a true continuous murmur, (2) a to-fro murmur, or (3) combined mitral stenosis and regurgitation. In **true continuous murmurs**, the cadence is uninterrupted by the cardiac cycles ("*SHSHSHSHSHSHSHSHSHSH*"). **To-fro murmurs** consist of two high frequency murmurs, one in systole and another in diastole ("*SHSHSHSHP PHEWEWEWEWEW*"). To-fro murmurs result from isolated severe aortic regurgitation (the diastolic component representing aortic regurgitation and the systolic one representing increased systolic flow over the aortic valve) or aortic regurgitation combined with another systolic murmur, such as aortic stenosis, mitral regurgitation, or ventricular septal defect. In combined mitral stenosis and regurgitation, a high-frequency murmur is combined with a low-frequency one ("*PUSHSHSHSHP DUPRRRRRRRRUP*")

D. GRADING THE INTENSITY OF MURMURS

The intensity of murmurs is graded on a 1 to 6 scale, based on the work of Freeman and Levine, which was later modified by Constant and Lippschutz (their work is now collectively referred to as **Levine grading system**).[16–18] Although this system was devised for systolic murmurs, it is often applied to all murmurs.

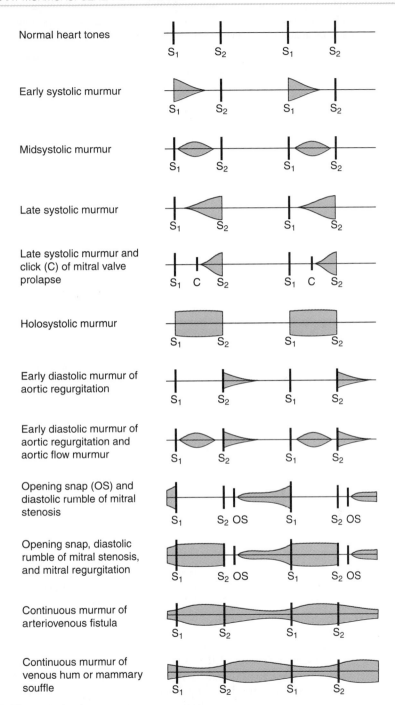

Fig. 43.3 Diagrams of various murmurs.

TABLE 43.2 ■ Using Onomatopoeia to Identify Systolic Murmur Timing

Onomatopoeia	Definition	Timing of Murmur
Lub shsh dup	Both S1 (lub) and S2 (dup) distinct:	Midsystolic
Shshsh dup	S_1 indistinct, S_2 distinct; gap before S_2	Early Systolic
Pushsh dup		
Shshshshdup	S_1 indistinct, S_2 distinct; no gap before S_2	Long Systolic
Pushshshdup		
Shshshshshsh	S_1 and S_2 indistinct	Holosystolic
ShshshshshshP		
Pushshshshsh		
PushshshshshP		
Lub shshshP	S_1 distinct, S_2 indistinct	Late systolic

Adapted from reference 7.

The six categories are as follows: **(1) grade 1 murmurs** are so faint they can be heard only with special effort. **(2) Grade 2 murmurs** can be recognized readily after placing the stethoscope on the chest wall. **(3) Grade 3 murmurs** are very loud. (Murmurs of grades 1 through 3 all lack thrills, which are palpable vibrations on the body wall resembling the purr of a cat. Murmurs of grades 4 through 6 have associated thrills.) **(4) Grade 4 murmurs** are very loud, although the stethoscope must be in complete contact with the skin to hear them. **(5) Grade 5 murmurs** are very loud and still audible if only the edge of the stethoscope is in contact with the skin; they are not audible after complete removal of the stethoscope from the chest wall. **(6) Grade 6 murmurs** are exceptionally loud and audible even when the stethoscope is just removed from the chest wall.

III. Clinical Significance

A. DETECTING VALVULAR HEART DISEASE

In EBM Box 43.1, a *characteristic* murmur refers to the expected murmur of the specific lesion (as described in Table 43.1 and Chapters 44 to Chapter 46). For example, in the detection of aortic regurgitation, a characteristic murmur refers to an early diastolic high-frequency murmur along the lower sternal border, not just any diastolic murmur. In these studies, trivial regurgitation (a common finding at echocardiography of no clinical significance) was classified as "no regurgitation" (i.e., "no disease").

For most of the lesions in EBM Box 43.1, the finding of the characteristic murmur is a conclusive argument that that lesion is present: aortic stenosis (likelihood ratio [LR] = 10.5, see EBM Box 43.1), pulmonic stenosis (LR = 55.4), tricuspid regurgitation (LR = 10.1), ventricular septal defect (LR = 28.1), mitral valve prolapse (LR = 12.1), aortic regurgitation (LR = 10.1), pulmonic regurgitation (LR = 17.4), and mitral stenosis (LR = 31.2). For mitral regurgitation, the positive LRs is less compelling (LRs = 5.5).

The *absence* of the characteristic murmur *decreases* the probability of some left-sided lesions—such as significant aortic stenosis (negative LR = 0.1), ventricular septal defect (LR = 0.1), and moderate-to-severe aortic regurgitation (negative LR = 0.1)—but does not exclude significant right-sided valvular lesions (the negative LRs for pulmonic stenosis, tricuspid regurgitation, and pulmonic regurgitation are not significant), probably because pressures on the right side of the heart are lower and thus generate less turbulence and sound than left-sided pressures. Many patients with *mild* mitral regurgitation or *mild* aortic regurgitation also lack murmurs.

Normal heart tones	**Lub**	**Dup**	**Lub**	**Dup**
	S_1	S_2	S_1	S_2

Early systolic murmur	**L**SHSHSH	**Dup**	**L**SHSHSH	**Dup**
	S_1	S_2	S_1	S_2

Midsystolic murmur	**Lub** SHSH **Dup**		**Lub** SHSH **Dup**	
	S_1	S_2	S_1	S_2

Late systolic murmur	**Lub**	SHSH**P**	**Lub**	SHSH**P**
	S_1	S_2	S_1	S_2

Late systolic murmur and click (C) of mitral valve prolapse	**Lub** **K**SHSH**P**		**Lub** **K**SHSH**P**	
	S_1 C	S_2	S_1 C	S_2

Holosystolic murmur	SHSHSHSHSH		SHSHSHSHSH	
	S_1	S_2	S_1	S_2

Early diastolic murmur of aortic regurgitation	**Lub**	**P**EWWWww	**Lub**	**P**EWWWww
	S_1	S_2	S_1	S_2

Early diastolic murmur of aortic regurgitation and aortic flow murmur	**Lub** SHSH **P**EWWWww		**Lub** SHSH **P**EWWWww	
	S_1	S_2	S_1	S_2

Opening snap (OS) and diastolic rumble of mitral stenosis	R**UP**	bu **DUP**RRRRR**RUP**	bu **DUP**RRRRR**RUP**	
	S_1	S_2 OS	S_1	S_2 OS

Opening snap, diastolic rumble of mitral stenosis, and mitral regurgitation	R**UP**SHSHSHS**P**	**DUP**RRRRR**RUP**SHSHSHS**P**	**DUP**RRRRR**RUP**	
	S_1	S_2 OS	S_1	S_2 OS

Continuous murmur of arteriovenous fistula	**Pu**SHSHSH**P**u**SH**SHSHSHSH **Pu**SHSH**P**u**SH**SHSHSHSH			
	S_1	S_2	S_1	S_2

Continuous murmur of venous hum or mammary souffle	**Pu**SHSHSHS**Pu**SHSH**SH**SHSH**Pu**SHSHSHS**Pu**SHSH**SH**SHSH			
	S_1	S_2	S_1	S_2

Fig. 43.4   Murmurs and onomatopoeia.

B. DIFFERENTIAL DIAGNOSIS OF SYSTOLIC MURMURS

Systolic murmurs are common bedside findings, occurring in 5% to 52% of young adults and 29% to 60% of older persons.[36] Over 90% of younger adults and over half of older adults with systolic murmurs have normal echocardiograms, which means the murmur is "innocent" or "functional."[36]

1. The Functional Murmur

Functional murmurs are short, early or midsystolic murmurs of grade 2/6 or less that are well-localized to the area of the left sternal border and diminish in intensity when the patient stands, sits up, or strains during the Valsalva maneuver. Patients with functional murmurs have normal neck veins, apical impulse, arterial pulse, and heart tones. The finding of a murmur that meets these characteristics (i.e., "functional murmur") increases the probability that the echocardiogram is normal (LR = 5.4, EBM Box 43.1).

2. Identifying the Cause of Systolic Murmurs

In patients with abnormal systolic murmurs (i.e., murmurs that are not functional) the most important causes are increased aortic velocity (from aortic stenosis or increased flow over an unobstructed valve), mitral regurgitation, and tricuspid regurgitation. In patients with abnormal

EBM BOX 43.1	**Murmurs and Valvular Heart Disease***			
Finding (Reference)[†]	Sensitivity (%)	Specificity (%)	Likelihood Ratio[‡] if Finding Is Present	Absent
Functional murmur				
Detecting normal findings on echocardiography[19–22]	66–99	69–95	5.4	0.1
Characteristic systolic murmur				
Detecting mild or worse aortic stenosis[7,23]	79–90	85–97	10.5	0.1
Detecting severe aortic stenosis[7,24,25]	83–98	71–76	3.5	0.1
Detecting pulmonic stenosis[23]	57	99	55.4	NS
Detecting mild mitral regurgitation or worse[23,26,27]	51–75	89–93	5.5	0.5
Detecting moderate-to-severe mitral regurgitation[7,26–28]	60–93	61–97	3.8	0.4
Detecting mild tricuspid regurgitation or worse[23,27]	23–63	93–98	10.1	NS
Detecting moderate-to-severe tricuspid regurgitation[7,27,28]	20–62	94–98	10.3	0.7
Detecting ventricular septal defect[20,23]	89–90	96–97	28.1	0.1
Detecting mitral valve prolapse[20]	55	96	12.1	0.5
Characteristic diastolic murmur				
Detecting mild aortic regurgitation or worse[23,27,29–35]	38–87	75–98	10.1	0.3

(continued)

EBM BOX 43.1 | **Murmurs and Valvular Heart Disease*—Cont'd**

Finding (Reference)[†]	Sensitivity (%)	Specificity (%)	Likelihood Ratio[‡] if Finding Is Present	Likelihood Ratio[‡] if Finding Is Absent
Detecting moderate-to-severe aortic regurgitation[27,33–35]	88–98	52–88	4.3	0.1
Detecting pulmonic regurgitation[27]	15	99	17.4	NS
Detecting mitral stenosis[23]	88	97	31.2	0.1

*Diagnostic standard: for all *valvular lesions*, Doppler echocardiography,[7,19–23,27,28,33]angiography,[25,26,29–31,34,35]or surgery.[24,32]Echocardiographic trivial regurgitation is classified as "absent regurgitation" (i.e., no disease).

[†]Definition of findings: for *functional murmur*, see text; for all other *murmurs*, the murmur characteristic in quality, location, and timing for that specific diagnosis. For example, the positive LR of 10.1 for aortic regurgitation refers to an early diastolic high-frequency blowing decrescendo murmur at the lower left sternal border, not any diastolic murmur.

[‡]Likelihood ratio (LR) if finding present = positive LR; LR if finding absent = negative LR.

NS, Not significant.

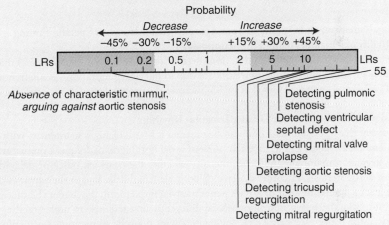

CHARACTERISTIC SYSTOLIC MURMUR

Probability

Decrease | Increase

−45% −30% −15% | +15% +30% +45%

LRs | 0.1 0.2 0.5 1 2 5 10 | LRs 55

Absence of characteristic murmur, *arguing against* aortic stenosis

Detecting pulmonic stenosis
Detecting ventricular septal defect
Detecting mitral valve prolapse
Detecting aortic stenosis
Detecting tricuspid regurgitation
Detecting mitral regurgitation

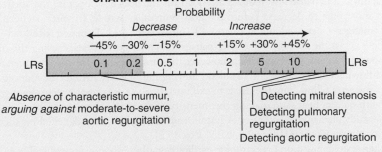

CHARACTERISTIC DIASTOLIC MURMUR

Probability

Decrease | Increase

−45% −30% −15% | +15% +30% +45%

LRs | 0.1 0.2 0.5 1 2 5 10 | LRs

Absence of characteristic murmur, *arguing against* moderate-to-severe aortic regurgitation

Detecting mitral stenosis
Detecting pulmonary regurgitation
Detecting aortic regurgitation

systolic murmurs, the most important features are distribution of sound on the chest wall (i.e., murmur pattern); intensity of S_1 and S_2; timing, radiation, and quality of sound; murmur intensity during irregular rhythms; and response to maneuvers.

a. Distribution of Murmur (Murmur Pattern, see Fig. 43.1)

EBM Box 43.2 indicates the one of the most important diagnostic signs is the distribution of sound on the chest wall. The broad apical-base pattern increases the probability of aortic stenosis (LR = 9.7, EBM Box 43.2), the broad apical pattern increases the probability of mitral regurgitation (LR = 6.8), and the left lower sternal pattern increases probability of tricuspid regurgitation (LR = 8.4).

In one study, the small apical-base pattern was due to mildly increased aortic velocity (but aortic stenosis was rare); the isolated base pattern usually stemmed from increased flow in the great arteries, not the heart (e.g., anemia, hemodialysis fistula, or subclavian stenosis); and the isolated apical pattern was nondiagnostic.[7]

b. Intensity of S_1 and S_2

If S_1 intensity is determined at the apex and S_2 intensity at the left 2nd parasternal space, and intensity is divided into four levels—inaudible, soft, normal, or loud—the finding of an inaudible S_1 (LR = 5.1, EBM Box 43.2) or inaudible S2 (LR = 12.7) in patients with systolic murmurs increases probability of aortic stenosis, whereas the finding of a loud S_2 increases the probability of mitral regurgitation (LR = 4.7).

c. Timing, Radiation, and Quality of Sound (see also the Section on Specific Timing and Quality of Murmurs using Onomatopoeia)

Pathologic murmurs have longer duration (long systolic or holosystolic, LRs 1.7 to 2.2) than nonpathologic ones. Most late systolic murmurs are due to mitral regurgitation.[7] Radiation into the neck (LR = 2.4) and coarse quality (LR = 3.3) increase the probability of aortic stenosis.

d. Intensity of Systolic Murmur During Irregular Rhythms

One important clue to the etiology of a systolic murmur is how it changes in intensity with changing cycle lengths, as occurs in the irregular pulse of atrial fibrillation or frequent premature beats. Mitral regurgitation maintains the same intensity whether the beats are quick or delayed.[37] The intensity of aortic stenosis, in contrast, depends on cycle length: the longer the previous diastole (e.g., beat after a premature beat or after a pause in atrial fibrillation), the louder the murmur.[37,38]

Explaining why these two murmurs behave differently first requires an understanding of the physiology of the pause (see Fig. 43.5). The pause causes diastolic filling and contractility to be greater for the next beat than it would have been if the cycle had been quicker (contractility is increased because of Starling forces and, in the case of extrasystoles, postextrasystolic accentuation of contractility). The pause also reduces afterload for the next beat, because the aortic pressures have had more time to decrease before the next ventricular systole. In aortic stenosis, all three of these changes—increased filling, increased contractility, and decreased afterload—promote greater flow across the stenotic valve after pauses than after quick beats, causing the murmur to become louder.[39] In mitral regurgitation, however, the stroke volume is divided between two paths: (1) blood flowing out the aorta and (2) blood flowing into the left atrium. The reduced afterload promotes the extra filling from the pause to exit into the aorta, leaving the regurgitant volume the same as with quicker beats and making the intensity of the murmur independent of cycle length.

In one study, unchanging intensity of systolic murmurs during irregular rhythms increased the probability of regurgitation (LR = 2.5, EBM Box 43.2).

Another systolic murmur, hypertrophic cardiomyopathy, responds unpredictably to changing cycle lengths: the long pause may make the murmur louder or softer or may not change it at all.[38]

EBM BOX 43.2	**Differential Diagnosis of Systolic Murmurs in Adults***		

Likelihood Ratio for Detecting

Finding†	Aortic Stenosis	Mitral Regurgitation	Tricuspid Regurgitation
Murmur pattern			
Broad apical-base pattern	9.7	NS	NS
Broad apical pattern	0.2	6.8	2.5
LLSB pattern	NS	NS	8.4
Heart tones			
S_1 inaudible, apex	5.1	NS	NS
S_2 inaudible	12.7	NS	NS
S_2 loud	NS	4.7	3.6
Murmur quality, timing, and intensity			
Radiation to neck	2.4	0.6	0.6
Timing mid-systolic or early-systolic	0.4	0.4	0.5
Timing long systolic or holosystolic	2.2	1.9	1.7
Coarse quality	3.3	0.5	0.5
If pulse irregular, murmur intensity same in beat after a pause	0.4	2.5	2.3

*Diagnostic standard: for *aortic stenosis*, AV peak velocity ≥2.5 m/sec by Doppler echocardiography (i.e., aortic stenosis is mild or worse); for *mitral* and *tricuspid regurgitation*, regurgitation is moderate or worse by Doppler echocardiography.[7]
Definition of findings: for *murmur pattern*, see Fig. 43.1; for *heart tones*, S_1 intensity is determined at the apex, S_2 intensity is determined at the left 2nd parasternal space, and intensity graded into four levels, as inaudible, soft, normal, or loud; for *quality* and *timing*, see the section "Specific Timing and Quality of Murmurs Using Onomatopoeia in text and Table 43.2.
AS, Aortic stenosis; *LLSB,* left lower sternal border; *TR,* tricuspid regurgitation; *MR,* mitral regurgitation; *NS,* Not significant.

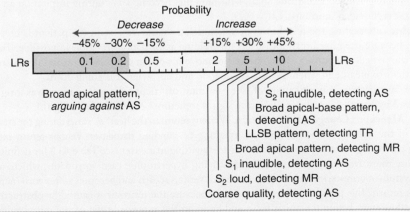

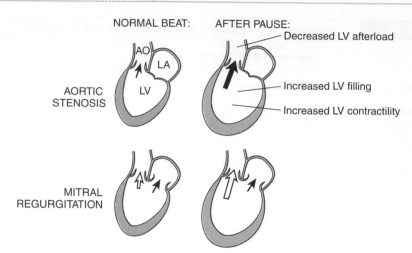

Fig. 43.5 **Intensity of systolic murmurs and irregular rhythms.** The figure depicts blood flow and intensity of systolic murmurs during normal beats (*left column*) and after pauses in the heart rhythm (from extrasystoles or atrial fibrillation, *right column*). In each drawing, the *size of the arrow* indicates the volume of blood flow: *black arrows* depict flow *causing* sound, whereas *open arrows* depict flow *not generating* sound. After the pause (*right column*), there is increased LV filling and contractility but *decreased* LV afterload. In aortic stenosis (*top row*), these changes all favor increased flow across the aortic valve and a louder murmur (i.e., dark arrow is larger after the pause). In mitral regurgitation (bottom row), these same forces again favor increased flow across the aortic valve (open arrow), but since this flow is not generating sound, the regurgitant volume (dark arrow) and murmur intensity remains unchanged. See text. *Ao,* Aorta; *LA,* left atrium; *LV,* left ventricle.

e. Maneuvers

Several maneuvers help differentiate systolic murmurs (Table 43.3). They are classified into respiratory maneuvers, maneuvers that change venous return (e.g., Valsalva maneuver, squatting-to-standing, standing-to-squatting, passive leg elevation), and maneuvers that primarily change systemic vascular resistance (isometric hand grip, transient arterial occlusion, and inhalation of amyl nitrite).

(1) Respiration. Inspiration increases venous return to the right side of the heart and decreases it to the left side of the heart[‡]. Therefore, murmurs that intensify during inspiration characteristically originate in the right side of the heart (e.g., tricuspid regurgitation or pulmonic stenosis; LR = 7.8; see EBM Box 43.3). Murmurs that become *softer* during inspiration are most likely *not* right-sided murmurs (LR = 0.2).

Before interpreting the test, however, the clinician should be certain the patient is breathing evenly, because irregular breathing or breath-holding makes interpretation impossible. To help direct the patient's breathing, the clinician can move his or her arm slowly up and down and ask the patient to breathe in when the arm is going up and out when it is going down.

The inspiratory intensification of the murmur of tricuspid regurgitation was originally described by Rivero-Carvallo in 1946 (the sign is sometimes called **Carvallo sign**).[48]

(2) Maneuvers Changing Venous Return. Venous return to the heart *decreases* during the straining phase of the Valsalva maneuver and the squatting-to-standing maneuver. Venous return *increases* during passive leg elevation and the standing-to-squatting maneuver (see Table 43.3 for definitions).

These maneuvers are most useful in identifying hypertrophic cardiomyopathy, which, unlike most systolic murmurs, intensifies with decreased venous return and becomes softer with increased venous return. This paradoxical response occurs because the murmur is caused by obstruction in the outflow tract, below the aortic valve and between the anterior leaflet of the mitral valve and

---

[‡]This occurs because pressures in the right side of the heart diminish with intrathoracic pressures during inspiration, increasing the pressure gradient between the right side of the heart and systemic veins and causing filling to increase to the right side of the heart. In contrast, inspiration increases the capacitance of pulmonary veins, thus reducing flow to the left side of the heart during inspiration.

TABLE 43.3 ■ Maneuvers and Heart Murmurs

Maneuver*	Technique	When to Note Change in Murmur
Respiration	The patient breathes normally in and out	During inspiration and expiration
Maneuvers affecting venous return		
Decrease venous return		
Valsalva maneuver	The patient exhales against closed glottis for 20 s	At end of the strain phase (i.e., at 20 s)
Squatting-to-standing	The patient squats for at least 30 s and then rapidly stands up	Immediately after standing
Increase venous return		
Standing-to-squatting	The patient squats rapidly from the standing position, while breathing normally to avoid a Valsalva maneuver	Immediately after squatting
Passive leg elevation	The patient's legs are passively elevated to 45 degrees while the patient is supine	15–20 s after leg elevation
Maneuvers affecting systemic vascular resistance (afterload)		
Increase afterload		
Isometric handgrip exercise	The patient uses one hand to squeeze the examiner's index and middle fingers together tightly[†]	After one minute of maximal contraction
Transient arterial occlusion	The examiner places blood pressure cuffs around both upper arms of patient and inflates them to pressures above the patient's systolic blood pressure	20 s after cuff inflation
Decrease Afterload		
Amyl nitrite	The patient takes three rapid deep breaths from a opened amyl nitrite capsule	15–30 s after inhalation

From information cited in references 39–43.
*Squatting-to-standing also decreases systemic vascular resistance, and amyl nitrite also diminishes pulmonary vascular resistance a small amount.
†In clinical studies, a hand dynamometer was used to confirm that at least 75% of maximal hand grip strength was sustained for 1 minute.[40]

EBM BOX 43.3   **Systolic Murmurs and Maneuvers***

Finding (Reference)[†]	Sensitivity (%)	Specificity (%)	Likelihood Ratio[‡] if Finding Is Present	Absent
Respiration				
Louder during inspiration				
Detecting right-sided murmurs (tricuspid regurgitation or pulmonic stenosis)[42,44]	78–95	87–97	7.8	0.2
Changing venous return				
Louder with Valsalva strain				
Detecting hypertrophic cardiomyopathy[42]	70	95	14.0	0.3
Louder with squatting-to-standing				
Detecting hypertrophic cardiomyopathy[42]	95	84	6.0	0.1

(continued)

| EBM BOX 43.3 | Systolic Murmurs and Maneuvers*—Cont'd |

Finding (Reference)[†]	Sensitivity (%)	Specificity (%)	Likelihood Ratio[‡] if Finding Is	
			Present	Absent
Softer with standing-to-squatting				
Detecting hypertrophic cardiomyopathy[42,45]	88–95	84–97	7.6	0.1
Softer with passive leg elevation				
Detecting hypertrophic cardiomyopathy[42]	90	90	9.0	0.1
Changing systemic vascular resistance (afterload)				
Softer with isometric hand grip				
Detecting hypertrophic cardiomyopathy[42]	90	75	3.6	0.1
Louder with isometric hand grip				
Detecting mitral regurgitation (MR) or ventricular septal defect (VSD)[40,42]	70–76	78–93	5.8	0.3
Louder with transient arterial occlusion				
Detecting mitral regurgitation or ventricular septal defect[42]	79	98	48.7	0.2
Softer with amyl nitrite inhalation				
Detecting mitral regurgitation or ventricular septal defect[40,42,46,47]	41–95	89–95	10.5	0.2

*Diagnostic standard: Doppler echocardiography or angiography.
[†]Definition of findings: see text; for *amyl nitrite inhalation*, the test was interpretable only if it induced tachycardia.
[‡]Likelihood ratio (LR) if finding present = positive LR; LR if finding absent = negative LR.

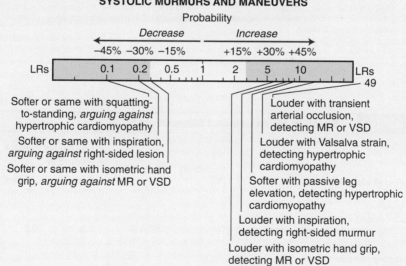

SYSTOLIC MURMURS AND MANEUVERS

the hypertrophied interventricular septum. Decreased venous return brings the mitral leaflet and septum closer together and aggravates the obstruction; increased return moves them apart and relieves the obstruction.

All four venous return maneuvers are useful in diagnosing hypertrophic cardiomyopathy (LRs = 6 to 14; see EBM Box 43.3), although intensification of the murmur during Valsalva strain increases probability the most (LR = 14). For three of the maneuvers (squatting-to-standing, standing-to-squatting, passive leg elevation), the *absence* of the characteristic response greatly decreases the probability of hypertrophic cardiomyopathy (LR = 0.1). Of these four maneuvers, only passive leg elevation can be easily performed in frail patients.

One other systolic murmur, mitral valve prolapse, may intensify during squatting-to-standing, although it does not become louder during Valsalva strain. This paradoxical finding, which is further discussed in Chapter 46, may explain why there are more false positives for squatting-to-standing (specificity = 84%) than Valsalva strain (specificity = 95%).

(3) Maneuvers Changing Systemic Vascular Resistance (or Afterload). Before employing maneuvers that change afterload in diagnosing systolic murmurs, the clinician has already addressed the possibility of right-sided murmurs (respiratory maneuver) and hypertrophic cardiomyopathy (venous return maneuvers). The primary remaining diagnostic possibilities are murmurs generated by flow over the aortic valve (e.g., aortic stenosis or increased aortic flow without stenosis) and murmurs from left-sided regurgitant lesions (e.g., mitral regurgitation, ventricular septal defect).

Changing afterload may distinguish these lesions. The murmurs of mitral regurgitation and ventricular septal defect intensify with increased afterload, because blood leaving the ventricle, having two paths to potentially follow, encounters more resistance in the aorta and therefore flows more readily through the regurgitant lesion. Similarly, these murmurs become softer when afterload is decreased, because enhanced aortic flow reduces the regurgitant volume.

The common techniques of manipulating afterload at the bedside are isometric hand grip and transient arterial occlusion (Table 43.3), both of which increase afterload. The finding of a systolic murmur that intensifies with either maneuver increases the probability of mitral regurgitation or ventricular septal defect (LR = 5.8 for isometric hand grip and 48.7 for transient arterial occlusion, EBM Box 43.3). Another maneuver that reduces afterload, amyl nitrite inhalation, was used commonly 40 to 50 years ago but is rarely used today.

References may be accessed online at *Elsevier eBooks for Practicing Clinicians.*

Selected Cardiac Disorders

Aortic Stenosis

I. Introduction

Aortic stenosis is any disorder of the aortic valve that obstructs the ejection of blood from the left ventricle into the aorta. Its characteristic findings are a systolic murmur, abnormal carotid pulse, and sustained apical impulse.

The pathology of aortic stenosis was recognized in the 1600s, but it was James Hope who in 1832 first clearly described the characteristic murmur.[1,2]

II. The Findings

A. THE MURMUR

The murmur of aortic stenosis is early systolic, midsystolic, or holosystolic. Although it may be loudest at the right second intercostal space (i.e., the classic "aortic" area), most aortic stenosis radiates above and below the third left parasternal space, obliquely and upwards towards the right clavicle and downward toward the apex, a distribution mimicked by placing a sash over the patient's right shoulder. Radiation of sound in the neck first appears on the right side (clavicle and neck), but as the stenosis worsens the sound appears on *both* sides of the neck and over both clavicles. In contrast, isolated radiation a murmur to just the *left* clavicle or *left* neck is not characteristic of aortic stenosis alone and suggests stenosis of a great artery (see Chapter 43).

In calcific aortic stenosis, the most common modern etiology, the murmur at the upper sternal borders contains both high- and low-frequency vibrations, giving it a harsh or rough sound, like that of a person clearing the throat. At the apex the murmur of calcific aortic stenosis sometimes loses low frequency components and instead consists of a narrow band of high frequency sound, thus making it sound like mitral regurgitation. This harmonic distortion of sound—the loss of low frequency components of sound when the stethoscope is moved "upstream" toward the apex—is called the **Gallavardin phenomenon**.[3]

B. ASSOCIATED CARDIAC SIGNS

Other traditional findings of severe aortic stenosis are the following: (1) a carotid pulse that is abnormally small in volume and delayed (**pulsus parvus et tardus**); (2) a palpable apical impulse that is abnormally sustained (see Chapter 38 for definition of sustained impulse) and (3) reduced intensity of the second heart sound, which occurs because the inflexible aortic leaflets close with less force than normal. Another traditional finding is a prominent A wave in the neck veins (i.e., the **Bernheim phenomenon**), although this wave is more often seen on pressure tracings than at the bedside. Its mechanism is disputed.[4]

III. Clinical Significance

A. DETECTING AORTIC STENOSIS

The presence of the characteristic aortic systolic murmur increases the probability of aortic stenosis (likelihood ratio [LR] = 10.5 for mild or worse aortic stenosis, see EBM Box 44.1); most false positives (i.e., patients with a characteristic aortic murmur but no aortic stenosis) have increased aortic flow without obstruction (e.g., from fever, anemia, pregnancy, or turbulence due to

---

EBM BOX 44.1	**Aortic Stenosis Murmur***			
Finding (Reference)[†]	**Sensitivity (%)**	**Specificity (%)**	**Likelihood Ratio[‡] if Finding Is**	
			Present	**Absent**
Aortic systolic murmur, detecting mild or worse aortic stenosis[5,6]	79–90	85–87	10.5	0.1
Aortic systolic murmur, detecting severe aortic stenosis[5,7,8]	83–98	71–76	3.5	0.1

*Diagnostic standard: for *mild or worse aortic stenosis*, peak aortic velocity ≥2.5 m/sec[5] or unstated echocardiographic parameter[6]; for *severe aortic stenosis*, maximal inter-aortic cusp distance 8 mm,[7] peak aortic velocity ≥4 m/sec,[5] or peak aortic gradient > 64 mm Hg.[8]
[†]Definition of findings: for *aortic systolic murmur*, either the broad apical-base pattern or small apical base pattern (see Chapter 43).
[‡]Likelihood ratio (LR) if finding present = positive LR; LR if finding absent = negative LR.

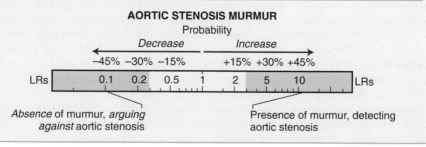

AORTIC STENOSIS MURMUR
Probability

Absence of murmur, *arguing against* aortic stenosis

Presence of murmur, detecting aortic stenosis

nonobstructing calcification). Most importantly, the *absence* of the aortic flow murmur decreases considerably the probability of aortic stenosis (LR = 0.1 for stenosis of any severity). Chapter 43 discusses further the differential diagnosis of systolic murmurs, and how the clinician—by observing the location of sound, the second heart sound, the quality of the murmur, and how the murmur responds to irregular heart beats and different maneuvers—can be more confident a systolic murmur indeed represents aortic stenosis and not another valvular lesion.

B. SEVERITY OF AORTIC STENOSIS

Once clinicians are confident a murmur represents an aortic flow murmur, they must decide whether or not the patient has significant aortic stenosis. Significant aortic stenosis refers to those lesions with such severe obstruction that valvular replacement is indicated if the patient has symptoms of angina, syncope, or dyspnea. (The footnotes of EBM Box 44.2 define severe stenosis.)

Many of the traditional teachings about aortic stenosis originated during a time when congenital and rheumatic disease were more common than they are today. Because the primary cause of aortic stenosis today is calcific aortic stenosis, some of these teachings may not be as relevant as they were in the past. In comparison to congenital and rheumatic disease, calcific aortic stenosis affects older patients, who commonly have aortic flow murmurs *without* stenosis (i.e., aortic sclerosis) and who often have ischemic heart disease, a disorder complicating the bedside evaluation because patients then have two possible explanations (i.e., severe aortic stenosis or ischemic heart disease) for symptoms of angina or dyspnea.

The patients whose clinical signs are summarized in EBM Box 44.2 (over 700 patients in all) were all elderly. Importantly, *all had aortic flow murmurs*, and the bedside question was whether or not the murmur represented *severe* aortic stenosis. Although some had mild aortic regurgitation, other significant valvular disease was excluded from most of these studies. In these studies, syncope was the only classic aortic stenosis symptom that increased the probability of severe aortic stenosis (LR = 3.1; the LRs for the other two classic aortic stenosis symptoms, angina and dyspnea, were not significant).[10,18,19]

1. Individual Findings

The following findings, in descending order of diagnostic accuracy (EBM Box 44.2), increase the probability of severe aortic stenosis in patients with aortic flow murmurs: sustained apical impulse (LR = 4.1), absent or diminished S_2 (LR = 3.8), late peaking murmur (LR = 3.7), delayed carotid artery upstroke (i.e., pulsus tardus, LR = 3.5), prolonged murmur (LR = 3), apical-carotid delay (i.e., a palpable delay between the apical impulse and carotid impulse, LR = 2.6), brachioradial delay (i.e., a palpable delay between the brachial and radial artery pulses, LR = 2.5), reduced carotid artery volume (i.e., pulsus parvus, LR = 2.3), and a murmur with an added humming quality (LR = 2.1).

The findings that *decrease* the probability of severe aortic stenosis in patients with aortic flow murmurs are absence of brachioradial delay (LR = 0.04; see EBM Box 44.2), absence of an apical-carotid delay (LR = 0.05), early systolic timing (LR = 0.1), blowing quality throughout (LR = 0.1), lack of radiation to the neck (LR = 0.1), and short duration of the murmur (LR = 0.2). Brachioradial delay and apical-carotid delay were each investigated in only single studies and thus require confirmation by others.

Two additional bedside findings are chest radiography (CXR) and electrocardiography (ECG). The finding of calcification of the aortic valve on CXR detects severe stenosis with a sensitivity of 31% to 81%, specificity of 63% to 96%, positive LR = 3.9, and negative LR = 0.5.[11,16,18,19] Left ventricular hypertrophy on ECG detects severe stenosis with a sensitivity of 49% to 94%, specificity of 57% to 86%, positive LR = 2.1, and negative LR = 0.5.[9,11,15,16,18,19]

| EBM BOX 44.2 | Characteristics of Severe Aortic Stenosis (All patients have Aortic Murmur)* | | | | |

Finding (Reference)[†]	Sensitivity (%)	Specificity (%)	Likelihood Ratio[‡] if Finding Is	
			Present	Absent
Arterial pulse				
Delayed carotid artery upstroke[5,9–13]	31–91	68–93	**3.5**	0.4
Reduced carotid artery volume[5,10,11]	44–80	65–81	2.3	0.4
Brachioradial delay[14]	97	62	2.5	**0.04**
Apical impulse				
Sustained apical impulse[10]	78	81	**4.1**	0.3
Apical-carotid delay[15]	97	63	2.6	**0.05**
Heart tones				
Absent or diminished S_2[5,9,11–13,16]	44–90	63–98	**3.8**	0.4
S_4 gallop[12,17]	29–50	57–63	NS	NS
Murmur				
Grade ≥3/6[5,18]	31–89	23–77	NS	NS
Early systolic timing[5]	4	61	**0.1**	1.6
Prolonged duration[5,9,12]	83–94	49–84	**3.0**	0.2
Late peaking[9,10,12,13]	83–91	70–88	**3.7**	0.2
Loudest over aortic area[11,12]	58–75	41–73	1.8	0.6
Radiation to neck[5,11–13]	90–98	11–51	1.4	**0.1**
Radiation to both sides of neck[5]	50	74	1.9	NS
Blowing quality[5]	4	67	**0.1**	1.4
Humming quality[5]	62	71	2.1	0.5

*Diagnostic standard: for *severe aortic stenosis*, aortic valve area <0.6 cm²/m², [13] <0.75 cm², [14,16] <0.8 cm², [11,15] <0.9 cm² [10]; peak gradient >50 mm Hg, [11,12] or aortic flow peak velocity >3.6 m/sec[9] or ≥4 m/sec.[5]

[†]Definition of findings: for *late peaking murmur*, murmur peaks at midsystole or beyond; for *aortic area*, second right intercostal space.

[‡]Likelihood ratio (LR) if finding present = positive LR; LR if finding absent = negative LR.

NS, Not significant.

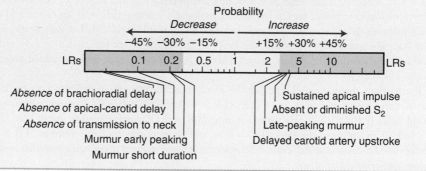

SEVERE AORTIC STENOSIS

The following findings are not helpful in identifying patients with severe aortic stenosis: narrow pulse pressure,[20] fourth heart sound, third heart sound,[16] reversed splitting of the second heart sound,[12] aortic ejection click,[12] and intensity of the murmur (see EBM Box 44.2).

2. Why Positive LRs Are So Low

The highest positive LR for the findings listed in EBM Box 44.2 is 4.1 (i.e., sustained apical impulse). In general, positive LRs are low when patients *without* disease also demonstrate the physical finding (i.e., specificity is low and there are many *false-positive* results). The cause of false-positive results in the studies of aortic stenosis is principally *moderate* aortic stenosis (defined as aortic valve area of 0.8 to 1.2 cm^2 or peak gradient of 25 to 50 mm Hg)*.

Therefore, if "disease" is instead defined as "combined moderate-to-severe aortic stenosis," the positive likelihood ratios improve dramatically, especially for delayed carotid upstroke (positive LR = 7.6, negative LR = 0.5), absent or diminished S$_2$ (positive LR = 7.4, negative LR = 0.5), prolonged duration of murmur (positive LR = 11.4, negative LR = 0.3), and late peaking murmur (positive LR = 13.7, negative LR = 0.3).[5,9,12,13,21]

This implies that clinicians examining patients with aortic flow murmurs can easily distinguish patients with moderate-to-severe aortic stenosis from those with milder stenosis or no obstruction, but they have greater difficulty distinguishing severe stenosis from those with moderate stenosis.

3. Combined Findings

One study has validated the use of combined findings in the diagnosis of aortic stenosis.[11] According to this diagnostic scheme, the clinician evaluates five bedside findings and assigns the following points: delayed carotid upstroke (3 points), diminished carotid volume (2 points), murmur loudest at right upper sternal border (2 points), single/absent second heart sound (3 points), and calcification of the aortic valve on chest radiography (4 points).

This diagnostic scheme distinguishes moderate-to-severe aortic stenosis from other causes of aortic flow murmurs. The probability of moderate-to-severe aortic stenosis is low with 0 to 6 points (LR = 0.2) and high with 10 to 14 points (LR = 10.6). Scores from 7 to 9 points are unhelpful (LR not significant).

References may be accessed online at *Elsevier eBooks for Practicing Clinicians*.

---

*This also explains why the LR for the characteristic systolic murmur in detecting *severe* aortic stenosis (LR = 3.5, EBM Box 44.1) is lower than that for *mild or worse* aortic stenosis (LR = 10.5, EBM Box 44.1).

Aortic Regurgitation

I. Introduction

The principal problem in aortic regurgitation is defective closure of the aortic valve, which allows blood to return from the aorta to the left ventricle during diastole. In patients with significant chronic regurgitation, the traditional physical findings are a diastolic murmur, dilated apical impulse, and abnormally forceful and collapsing arterial pulses (pulsus celer).

In the 1700s, clinicians associated the postmortem finding of damaged aortic valves with hearts "larger than that of an ordinary ox" (the origin of the phrase *cor bovinum*) and the finding during life of "violently throbbing" carotid arteries. In 1832, Sir Dominic John Corrigan, a Dublin surgeon, taught clinicians how to diagnose the disease during life, by emphasizing the importance of these dramatic arterial pulsations and the associated diastolic murmur.[1,2]

II. The Findings

A. THE MURMUR(S)

Severe aortic regurgitation may cause three distinct murmurs: (1) the early diastolic murmur of aortic regurgitation, (2) a systolic aortic flow murmur, and (3) the apical diastolic rumble of the Austin Flint murmur.

1. Early Diastolic Murmur of Regurgitation

The most important physical sign of aortic regurgitation is the early diastolic murmur, which is blowing, high-frequency, and decrescendo in shape (see Chapter 43)

Lub   PEWWWWWWW

The murmur may occupy all of diastole or just its early part.[3] Pressing firmly against the chest wall with the diaphragm of the stethoscope brings out the murmur, which is usually loudest in the left parasternal area at the third or fourth intercostal space. In some patients, the murmur is only audible when the patient sits up, leans forward, and holds his or her breath in exhalation.

2. Systolic Aortic Flow Murmur

Severe aortic regurgitation also produces a short systolic aortic flow murmur, which results from ejection over the aortic valve of the large stroke volume characteristic of the disease. The combination of this murmur and the early diastolic one causes a characteristic "to-fro" sound near the sternum (see Chapter 43)

Lub SHSHSH PEWWWWWWW

This murmur may superficially resemble that of aortic stenosis, although the flow murmur of pure regurgitation is shorter and associated with the peripheral pulse findings of severe regurgitation (see later).

3. Apical Diastolic Rumble: Austin Flint Murmur

a. Definition

The Austin Flint murmur is a diastolic rumbling murmur heard at the apex in patients with severe aortic regurgitation, which resembles mitral stenosis even though the mitral valve is completely normal. It was first described by the American physician Austin Flint in 1862.[4]

The Austin Flint murmur is found in up to 60% of patients with moderate or severe aortic regurgitation but is rarely heard in mild aortic regurgitation.[5,6] Austin Flint called his murmur *presystolic*, but by this he meant it was loudest before S_1 and thus different from the murmur of aortic regurgitation, which began immediately after S_2 and tapered off during diastole. About half of Austin Flint murmurs have two diastolic components (mid-diastolic and presystolic), whereas the other half have just a presystolic component.[6,7]

b. Pathogenesis

The cause of the Austin Flint murmur is still debated. Although all hypotheses assume the murmur depends on a strong regurgitant stream of blood being directed back toward the left ventricle during diastole, these hypotheses differ in how this regurgitant stream causes an apical rumbling sound. Proposed mechanisms include fluttering of the anterior leaflet of the mitral valve, premature closure of the mitral valve from elevated left ventricular end-diastolic pressure, collision of the regurgitant stream with the anterior mitral leaflet, ventricular vibrations caused by the regurgitant stream itself, and harmonic distortion of the aortic regurgitant murmur.[6,8–10] Many of these mechanisms may operate together to create the sound.[11] An instructive video showing the blood flow responsible for the Austin Flint murmur is available in the reference by Weir.[12]

B. WATER HAMMER PULSE AND INCREASED PULSE PRESSURE

Because of the large stroke volume and diastolic emptying of aortic blood into the left ventricle (i.e., aortic runoff), the arterial pulse wave of aortic regurgitation rises suddenly and collapses abruptly. This abnormality has many names, although the most common ones are **collapsing pulse**, **Corrigan pulse**, or the **water hammer pulse**.* In most patients with aortic regurgitation, the collapsing pulse becomes more prominent as the examiner elevates the patient's wrist.[13,14] This occurs because elevation of the arm with respect to the heart reduces the diastolic pressure in that arm, causing the vessel to collapse more completely with each beat. (The pounding sensation of the water-hammer pulse is identical to the sensation felt by the examiner when palpating a person's blood pressure, with the cuff pressure just above the person's diastolic pressure; see Chapter 17.)

C. ABNORMAL PULSATIONS OF OTHER STRUCTURES: THE AORTIC REGURGITATION EPONYMS

The large stroke volume and aortic runoff of aortic regurgitation may induce pulsations in other parts of the body, which has generated many eponyms of what is fundamentally a single physical finding (the number of eponyms for aortic regurgitation rivals those of some neurologic reflexes).[1,15–18] These various bobbings include the following: (1) an abnormally conspicuous capillary pulsation, best elicited by blanching a portion of the nail and then observing the pulsating border between the white and red color (**Quincke capillary pulsations**, described in 1868, although Heinrich Quincke should be known instead for inventing the lumbar puncture); (2) an anterior-posterior bobbing of the head, synchronous with the arterial pulsations (**de Musset sign**, named after the French poet Alfred de Musset, who was afflicted with aortic regurgitation)[19]; (3) alternate blanching and flushing of the forehead and face (**lighthouse sign**); (4) pulsations of organs or their parts, including the uvula (**Müller sign**, 1899), retinal arteries (**Becker sign**), larynx (**Oliver-Cardavelli sign**), spleen (**Sailer** sign, 1928),[20] and cervix (**Dennisons sign**).[21,†]

In many of the original descriptions of these eponymous findings, the sign was presented simply as an interesting observation, not one of particular diagnostic value. Excellent videos of patients with bounding carotids,[22] Quincke pulse,[23,24] and Müller sign[25] are available.

D. HILL TEST

In 1909, Leonard Hill of Britain observed that patients with severe aortic regurgitation often have a systolic pressure in the foot that is much greater than a simultaneously measured systolic pressure in the arm.[26,27] The **Hill test** specifically refers to the systolic pressure of the foot minus that of the arm (in the supine patient). The correct technique for measuring the pressure in the foot is to wrap the arm cuff around the patient's calf and to measure the systolic pressure in the dorsalis pedis and posterior tibial arteries by palpation. The higher of these two pressures is the "foot pressure."

---

*Corrigan actually emphasized the exaggerated *visible* pulsations of aortic regurgitation, not the palpable ones. The term *water hammer pulse* was coined in 1836 by Sir Thomas Watson, who likened the pulse to a Victorian toy called a water-hammer, which imparted to a child's hands the same sensation of a collapsing pulse of aortic regurgitation.[2]

†The eponym does not necessarily indicate priority: Sailor gave credit for the pulsating spleen to Tulp of the 1600s,[20] and Dennison gave credit for the pulsating cervix to Shelly, one of his house officers.[21]

E. AUSCULTATION OVER ARTERIES

Two auscultatory findings may appear over the peripheral arteries of patients with aortic regurgitation: **pistol shot sounds** and **Duroziez murmur** (or **Duroziez sign**).

1. Pistol Shot Sound

a. Definition

Pistol shot sounds are short, loud, snapping sounds with each pulse, heard over the femoral, brachial, or radial arteries. They are identical in quality to the Korotkoff sounds heard when measuring blood pressure. Pistol shot sounds are heard with only *light* pressure of the stethoscope and, like the water hammer pulse, may first appear only after elevation of the patient's arm.[14]

Pistol shot sounds were first described by Traube in 1872.[28,29]

b. Pathogenesis

Pistol shot sounds occur because of sudden expansion and tensing of the walls of the vessels during systole. Consequently, they are not only associated with the collapsing pulses of aortic regurgitation but also are inducible in normal individuals by administering intravenous vasodilator medications.[30] The sounds are analogous to the loud, snapping notes heard when a sail or parachute suddenly fills with wind.[31] The quicker the vessel dilates, the louder the note, and in patients with aortic regurgitation, the intensity of the pistol-shot sound correlates with the height of the pulse pressure[32] and the change in pressure over time (dP/dt) of the pulse.[30]

2. Duroziez Murmur or Sign[15,28,33–36]

a. Definition

The Duroziez sign is a *double* to-fro murmur heard over the brachial or femoral artery. It is heard only with *firm* pressure from the stethoscope. For the Duroziez sign to be positive, both a systolic and diastolic murmur must be present (many normal persons develop systolic murmurs with pressure on the stethoscope). The diastolic component often becomes louder with pressure applied distal to the stethoscope.

Although some claim the Duroziez murmur also may occur in normal individuals who have increased flow because of fever, anemia, or peripheral vasodilatation,[33] the vascular sound produced in these conditions does not have the characteristic to-fro sound of the Duroziez murmur, but instead resemble the continuous murmur of an arteriovenous fistula.[35]

PuSHSHSHSHPuSHSHSHSHSHSHSH

Duroziez described his "double intermittent murmur" in 1861.[28,37]

b. Pathogenesis

The diastolic component of Duroziez sign results from the blood actually reversing directions in the artery during diastole.[34,35]

III. Clinical Significance

A. DETECTING AORTIC INSUFFICIENCY

The presence of the characteristic early diastolic murmur of aortic insufficiency greatly increases the probability that an aortic leak is actually present (likelihood ratio [LR] = 10.1, EBM Box 45.1). Although some patients with mild regurgitation have no murmur, the *absence* of the characteristic murmur greatly *decreases* the probability of moderate-to-severe aortic regurgitation (LR = 0.1, EBM Box 45.1).

EBM BOX 45.1	Aortic Regurgitation*				
				Likelihood Ratio[†] if Finding Is	
Finding (Reference)	Sensitivity (%)	Specificity (%)		Present	Absent
Characteristic diastolic murmur					
Detecting mild aortic regurgitation or worse[38-46]	38–87	75–98		**10.1**	0.3
Detecting moderate-to-severe aortic regurgitation[42-45]	88–98	52–88		**4.3**	0.1
Early diastolic murmur loudest on right side of sternum					
Detecting dilated aortic root or endocarditis[3]	29	96		**8.2**	0.7
Early diastolic murmur softer with amyl nitrite inhalation					
Detecting aortic regurgitation (vs. Graham Steell murmur)[47]	95	83		NS	0.1

*Diagnostic standard: for *moderate-to-severe aortic regurgitation*, see EBM Box 45.2.
[†]Likelihood ratio (LR) if finding present = positive LR; LR if finding absent = negative LR.
NS, Not significant.

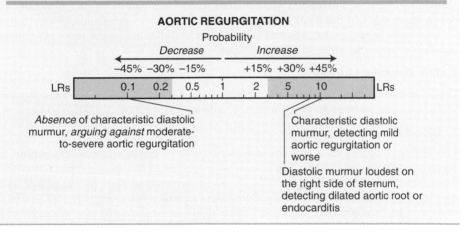

AORTIC REGURGITATION

Probability

Decrease   *Increase*

−45% −30% −15%   +15% +30% +45%

LRs   0.1   0.2   0.5   1   2   5   10   LRs

Absence of characteristic diastolic murmur, *arguing against* moderate-to-severe aortic regurgitation

Characteristic diastolic murmur, detecting mild aortic regurgitation or worse

Diastolic murmur loudest on the right side of sternum, detecting dilated aortic root or endocarditis

B. DISTINGUISHING AORTIC VALVE DISEASE FROM AORTIC ROOT DISEASE

The early diastolic murmur of aortic regurgitation is usually loudest in the left parasternal area. In some patients, the murmur may be loudest to the right of the sternum, which suggests an eccentric regurgitant stream from dilation of the aortic root (e.g., Marfan syndrome, aortic dissection, syphilitic aortitis) or damage to a single aortic cusp (e.g., endocarditis). This sign, introduced by Harvey in 1963,[48] increases the probability of a dilated root or endocarditis (LR = 8.2, EBM Box 45.1); its absence is diagnostically unhelpful (LR = 0.7).[‡]

[‡]The diagnostic accuracy of the "Harvey sign" is based on patients from the 1960s, when most patients with aortic insufficiency had either rheumatic valvular disease or syphilitic root disease. Whether it is as accurate today is unknown.

C. DISTINGUISHING AORTIC REGURGITATION FROM PULMONARY REGURGITATION

Distinguishing aortic from pulmonary regurgitation was particularly relevant in patients with rheumatic mitral stenosis, who often had associated aortic valve disease but who also could develop pulmonary hypertension and the early diastolic murmur of pulmonary insufficiency (i.e., the **Graham Steell murmur**).

In patients with mitral stenosis who also have an early diastolic murmur of regurgitation heard next to the sternum, the additional lesion is aortic regurgitation at least 80% of the time. Aortic regurgitation is the most common correct diagnosis even when there are no peripheral pulse findings of aortic regurgitation and the patient shows signs of severe pulmonary hypertension.[38,49,50] In the past, reducing afterload with amyl nitrite inhalation was used to distinguish aortic from pulmonary regurgitation, since amyl nitrite should diminish the intensity of the aortic regurgitation murmur (i.e., less regurgitant flow) but not affect the pulmonary regurgitation murmur. The finding of an early diastolic murmur that instead becomes louder or does not change after amyl nitrite inhalation *decreases* the probability of aortic regurgitation (LR = 0.1, see EBM Box 45.1).

D. SEVERITY OF AORTIC REGURGITATION

This section applies only to patients with the characteristic early diastolic murmur of chronic aortic regurgitation (EBM Box 45.2). It does not apply to acute aortic regurgitation. (See the section on acute aortic regurgitation.) Many of the patients enrolled in the studies also had additional murmurs of aortic stenosis or mitral regurgitation.

1. The Diastolic Murmur

The louder the murmur, the more severe the aortic regurgitation (r = 0.67).[51] Murmurs of grade 3 or more indicate moderate-to-severe aortic regurgitation (LR = 8.2, see EBM Box 45.2).

2. Blood Pressure

Two findings *increasing* the probability of moderate-to-severe regurgitation in these patients are diastolic blood pressure of 50 mm Hg or less (LR = 19.3, EBM Box 45.2) and pulse pressure of 80 mm Hg or more (LR = 10.9, see EBM Box 45.2). Two findings *decreasing* the probability of significant regurgitation are diastolic blood pressure of more than 70 mm Hg (LR = 0.2) and pulse pressure of less than 60 mm Hg (LR = 0.3). These signs have no diagnostic value when applied to other patients lacking the characteristic murmur of aortic regurgitation.[41]

3. Hill Test

If the abnormal response in the Hill test is defined as a foot-arm blood pressure difference of 40 mm Hg or more, the positive test increases the probability of significant regurgitation (LR = 6, see EBM Box 45.2).

Some doubt that the Hill test is accurate, citing experiments showing the intraarterial pressure in the *femoral arteries* of patients with aortic regurgitation to be identical to that of the brachial arteries.[55,56] The Hill test, however, measures the pressure of the pedal arteries, not the femoral arteries. It is possible that the systolic pressure is augmented in the foot, which is near the point of reflection of the abnormal pulse waveform.

4. Other Signs

The *absence* of an enlarged or sustained apical impulse *decreases* the probability of moderate-to-severe regurgitation (LR = 0.1; see EBM Box 45.2).

EBM BOX 45.2	Characteristics of Moderate-to-Severe Aortic Regurgitation*

Finding (Reference)[†]	Sensitivity (%)	Specificity (%)	Likelihood Ratio[‡] if Finding Is	
			Present	Absent
Diastolic murmur				
Murmur grade 3 or louder[41,51]	30–61	86–98	**8.2**	0.6
Blood pressure				
Diastolic blood pressure[38,52]				
>70 mm Hg	8–21	32–55	0.2	...
51–70 mm Hg	42–50	...	NS	...
≤50 mm Hg	30–50	98	**19.3**	...
Pulse pressure[52]				
<60 mm Hg	21	32	0.3	...
60–79 mm Hg	21	...	NS	...
≥80 mm Hg	57	95	**10.9**	...
Hill test				
Foot-arm systolic blood pressure difference > 40 mm Hg[52,53]	45–70	88–94	**6.0**	0.5
Other signs				
Enlarged or sustained apical impulse[52]	97	60	2.4	**0.1**
S_3 gallop[54]	20	97	**5.9**	0.8
Duroziez sign, femoral pistol shot, water hammer pulse[35,52]	37–55	63–98	NS	0.7

*Diagnostic standard: for *moderate-to-severe regurgitation*, regurgitation was either 3+ (moderate) or 4+ (severe) on a 0 to 4+ scale, using angiography,[35,38–40,44,45,52] doppler echocardiography,[42,43,46,51,53,54] or surgery.[41] Trivial regurgitation on echocardiography was classified as "absent regurgitation."
[†]Definition of findings: See text.
[‡]Likelihood ratio (LR) if finding present = positive LR; LR if finding absent = negative LR.
NS, Not significant.

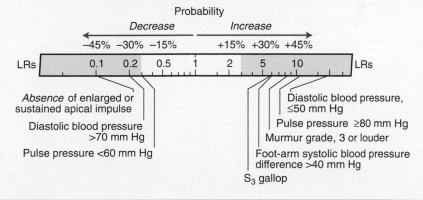

MODERATE-TO-SEVERE AORTIC REGURGITATION

In one study of patients with pure aortic regurgitation, the finding of a third heart sound increased the probability of severe regurgitation (LR = 5.9). Even so, the S_3 does not reliably indicate elevated left atrial pressure in these patients, because regurgitation alone may accelerate early diastolic filling sufficiently to produce the sound (see Chapter 41).[57,58] The Duroziez sign, femoral pistol shots, and the water hammer pulse are all unreliable indicators of severity of regurgitation.

E. ACUTE AORTIC REGURGITATION

Compared with chronic aortic regurgitation, acute aortic regurgitation (e.g., from endocarditis or acute aortic dissection) causes a shorter murmur, faster pulse rate (108 beats/min vs. 71 beats/min, mean values), smaller pulse pressure (55 mm Hg vs. 105 mm Hg), and lower systolic blood pressures (110 mm Hg vs. 155 mm Hg).[59] The murmur of acute aortic regurgitation is shorter because the combination of low arterial pressure and very high ventricular filling pressure eliminates the pressure gradient causing regurgitation by mid-diastole.[59] The first heart sound is faint or absent in acute aortic regurgitation, because of premature closure of the mitral valve (see Chapter 40).[60] In patients with aortic regurgitation from endocarditis, an associated pericardial rub often indicates extravalvular extension of the infection.[59]

F. DISTINGUISHING THE AUSTIN FLINT MURMUR FROM MITRAL STENOSIS

Based on an older analysis of 400 patients with severe aortic regurgitation, many of whom also had apical diastolic rumbles, the following findings increase the probability of associated mitral stenosis: atrial fibrillation, loud S_1, absent S_3, and presence of an opening snap. Findings suggesting that the apical rumble more likely is an Austin Flint murmur are sinus rhythm, faint S_1, S_3 gallop, and absent opening snap.[61] In addition, inhalation of amyl nitrite, which reduces systemic vascular resistance, makes the Austin Flint murmur (and the aortic regurgitation murmur) softer but the apical rumble of true mitral stenosis louder.[62]

References may be accessed online at *Elsevier eBooks for Practicing Clinicians*.

Miscellaneous Heart Murmurs

HYPERTROPHIC CARDIOMYOPATHY

I. The Murmur

The murmur of hypertrophic cardiomyopathy is usually midsystolic, harsh in quality, and loudest at the lower left sternal border or between the lower left sternal border and apex.[1] The murmur may obliterate the second heart sound and become late systolic, especially if there is associated mitral regurgitation. The intensity of the murmur behaves in distinctive ways during maneuvers altering venous return to the heart (see Chapter 43).

II. Associated Findings

The palpable apex beat may be sustained and the arterial pulse hyperkinetic (see Chapters 15 and 38). Although pulsus bisferiens has been described in hypertrophic cardiomyopathy,[2] this refers to a finding seen on intra-arterial pressure tracings, not a palpable one at the bedside.[3] The second heart sound is usually single or physiologically split, though in 10% splitting is paradoxic or reversed.[1] Over half of patients have audible fourth heart sounds.[1]

MITRAL REGURGITATION

I. The Finding

A. THE MURMUR

The murmur of chronic mitral regurgitation is usually holosystolic, high in frequency, and loudest at the apex.[4] It radiates to the axilla and inferior angle of the left scapula, although in some patients with isolated incompetence of the medial portion of the posterior leaflet, the murmur radiates instead to the right base and even into the neck, thus mimicking aortic stenosis.[4,5]

In 1832, James Hope was the first to describe the apical systolic murmur of mitral regurgitation.[4,6]

B. ASSOCIATED FINDINGS

In one study of 33 patients with chronic mitral regurgitation (mostly rheumatic in origin), the intensity of S_1 was normal 75% of the time and soft 12% of the time.[4] In contrast, a loud S_1 in mitral regurgitation is a clue to the diagnosis of mitral valve prolapse (see Chapter 40).[4,7] In 50% of patients with mitral regurgitation, S_2 splitting is wide and physiologic.[4] An associated S_3 is common, appearing in 89% with severe regurgitation. S_4 is rare.

Associated cardiac findings are an enlarged, laterally displaced palpable apical movement,[8] a palpable lower parasternal movement from an enlarged left atrium or associated tricuspid regurgitation (see Chapter 38)[9] and, in younger patients, a hyperkinetic arterial pulse (see Chapter 15).[10] Neck veins are normal unless the patient has decompensated heart failure.

II. Clinical Significance

A. DETECTING MITRAL REGURGITATION

The presence of the characteristic murmur of mitral regurgitation increases the probability that regurgitation is present, at least to a mild degree (likelihood ratio [LR] = 5.5, see Chapter 43). Although 25% to 49% of patients with *mild* regurgitation lack a murmur, the absence of the characteristic murmur decreases the probability of *moderate-to-severe* mitral regurgitation (LR = 0.4, see Chapter 43).

B. SEVERITY OF MITRAL REGURGITATION

1. The Murmur

In a very general way, the intensity of the murmur of mitral regurgitation correlates with the severity of regurgitation, especially for rheumatic mitral regurgitation (r = 0.67), but less so for ischemic or functional* mitral regurgitation (r = 0.45).[11-13] A mitral regurgitation murmur of grade 3 intensity or louder increases the probability of moderate-to-severe regurgitation (LR = 4.4, EBM Box 46.1).

2. Other Findings

Patients with severe mitral regurgitation may have a late systolic sustained left lower parasternal impulse from a dilated left atrium (Chapter 38 discusses how to distinguish this impulse from a right ventricular impulse or atrial impulse). The degree of this movement correlates well with

---

*Functional mitral regurgitation (or secondary mitral regurgitation) implies that the primary problem is cardiomyopathy, which dilates the atrioventricular ring and renders the valve incompetent. Initial therapy in these patients focuses on improving ventricular function, not replacing or repairing the valve.

EBM BOX 46.1	Severity of Mitral and Tricuspid Regurgitation*

Finding (Reference)[†]	Sensitivity (%)	Specificity (%)	Likelihood Ratio[‡] if Finding Is Present	Absent
Detecting moderate-to-severe mitral regurgitation (in patients with the characteristic murmur)				
Murmur grade 3 or louder[13]	85	81	**4.4**	0.2
S₃ gallop[14,15]	24–41	77–98	NS	0.8
Detecting moderate-to-severe tricuspid regurgitation				
Inspection of neck veins				
Early systolic outward movement (CV wave)[16]	37	97	**10.9**	0.7
Precordial and hepatic pulsations				
Lower sternal precordial pulsations[16]	17	99	**12.5**	0.8
Right ventricular (RV) rock[16]	5	100	**31.4**	NS
Pulsatile liver[16,17]	12–30	92–99	**6.5**	NS

*Diagnostic standard: for *moderate-to-severe mitral regurgitation*, regurgitant fraction >40% by Doppler echocardiography[13,15] or angiography[14]; for *moderate-to-severe tricuspid regurgitation*, 3+ or 4+ by angiography[17] or as assessed visually from echocardiography.[16]
[†]Definition of findings: for *RV rock*, see text and Chapter 38.
[‡]Likelihood ratio (LR) if finding present = positive LR; LR if finding absent = negative LR.
NS, Not significant.

MODERATE-TO-SEVERE MITRAL REGURGITATION (MR)

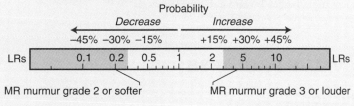

MODERATE-TO-SEVERE TRICUSPID REGURGITATION

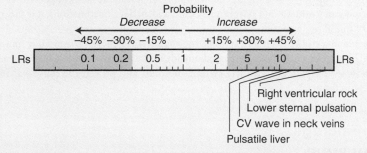

severity of regurgitation (r = 0.93, p < 0.01), as long as the patient does not have associated mitral stenosis (the presence of mitral stenosis confounds analyzing the parasternal impulse of patients with mitral regurgitation because the impulse could represent either a large left atrium from severe regurgitation or a hypertensive right ventricle from mitral stenosis).[9,18]

Some studies correlate the third heart sound with severity of mitral regurgitation,[15] whereas others do not.[14] Overall, the pooled LR is not significant (see EBM Box 46.1).

C. DISTINGUISHING ACUTE FROM CHRONIC MITRAL REGURGITATION

The physical signs of acute and chronic mitral regurgitation differ in several ways. In acute lesions, patients are acutely ill with elevated neck veins and signs of pulmonary edema; in chronic lesions, these signs may be absent. In acute lesions, the pulse is rapid and regular; in chronic lesions, it is often slow and irregular (from atrial fibrillation).[19] In acute lesions, the murmur may be short and confined to early systole (40% of patients in one series), because the left atrial pressure is so high it equilibrates with left ventricular pressures by mid-to-late systole and thus eliminates the regurgitation gradient[20,21]; in chronic lesions, the timing varies, although holosystolic and late systolic murmurs are most common. In acute lesions, the fourth heart sound is common (80% in one series); in chronic lesions, the fourth heart sound is rare, either because the atrial contraction is absent (i.e., atrial fibrillation) or the atrium is so dilated it cannot contract strongly.[11,19,22]

D. PAPILLARY MUSCLE DYSFUNCTION

Papillary muscle dysfunction refers to a murmur of mitral regurgitation that develops in the setting of myocardial ischemia. The murmur, which is usually transient, may be holosystolic, midsystolic, or late systolic. It appears in up to 20% of patients with myocardial infarction,[23] in whom it is associated with a higher incidence of persistent chest pain in the intensive care unit (45% vs. 26% without murmur) and a higher 1-year mortality (18% vs. 10%).[23]

MITRAL VALVE PROLAPSE

I. Introduction

Mitral valve prolapse describes an abnormal posterosuperior movement of the mitral valve leaflets into the left atrium after they close at the beginning of systole. It is an important cause of late systolic murmurs and mid-to-late systolic clicks,[24-26] and, in developed nations, it is the most common cause of mitral regurgitation.[27]

At the beginning of the twentieth century, most clinicians believed late systolic murmurs were benign and late systolic clicks were generated outside of the heart.[24,25] In 1963, Barlow performed angiograms in several patients with late systolic murmurs and proved the cause was mitral prolapse and regurgitation.[28]

II. The Findings

A. THE MURMUR

The murmur of mitral valve prolapse is loudest at the apex and is sometimes musical (see Chapter 43). It is characteristically late systolic because the mitral leaflets are well supported by chordae tendineae and competent during early systole, but lose this support as the ventricle becomes smaller during late systole, allowing the leaflets to buckle backwards toward the left atrium and create a regurgitant leak.[24-26]

B. THE CLICKS

The clicks of mitral valve prolapse occur during mid-to-late systole and are loudest at the apex or left lower sternal border.[24] They are sometimes multiple. In patients with both a click and a murmur, the click introduces the murmur 65% of the time and occurs just after the beginning of the murmur 35% of the time.[24] Sudden deceleration of the billowing mitral leaflet, as it prolapses into the left atrial cavity, causes the sound, which thus resembles the sound produced by a parachute or sail that suddenly tenses as it fills with wind.[29]

C. RESPONSE OF MURMURS AND CLICKS TO MANEUVERS

Bedside maneuvers that alter venous return or afterload (i.e., systemic vascular resistance) change both the timing of the clicks and murmurs and the intensity of the murmur, although they affect timing and intensity independently.

The *timing* of clicks and murmur depends on the venous return to the heart (Fig. 46.1). Reductions in venous return—by straining during the Valsalva maneuver or moving from squatting-to-standing—causes the ventricular chamber to become smaller and the mitral leaflets to prolapse earlier during systole, thus moving the click closer to S_1 and making the murmur longer.[24,26]

In contrast, the *intensity* of the murmur depends more on afterload, and in this way the response resembles that of chronic mitral regurgitation (see Chapter 43). As afterload is reduced with amyl nitrite inhalation, the murmur of mitral valve prolapse becomes fainter.[24] The Valsalva strain also often makes the murmur *softer*. Squatting-to-standing, however, makes the murmur *louder*, perhaps because the standing position invokes sufficient sympathetic tone to preserve afterload while at the same time making ventricular contractions more vigorous, thus intensifying the sound.[24,†]

III. Clinical Significance. Detection of Mitral Valve Prolapse

The presence of the characteristic click and murmur of mitral valve prolapse increases greatly the probability of prolapse, as detected by echocardiography (LR = 12.1, see Chapter 43). Indeed, some have argued that the auscultatory criteria alone are sufficient for diagnosis.[30,31] The criteria for diagnosing mitral valve prolapse are the reproducible finding in a young patient of a mid-to-late systolic click or late systolic murmur at or near the apex. These sounds should shift their timing with respect to S_1 and S_2 in response to the Valsalva and squatting-to-standing maneuvers (see the section on response of murmurs and clicks to maneuvers and Fig. 46.1). These criteria require the patient to be young to avoid confusion with papillary muscle dysfunction, a common cause of late systolic murmurs in older patients.[30] The click should be mobile and occur in mid-to-late systole to eliminate confusion with other short systolic sounds, such as the split S_1 and aortic ejection sound (Chapters 41 and 42 further differentiate these sounds).[30,31]

TRICUSPID REGURGITATION

I. The Findings

The physical findings of tricuspid regurgitation depend on the patient's pulmonary pressure, which may be high (high-pressure tricuspid regurgitation) or normal (low-pressure tricuspid

---

†Mitral valve prolapse is therefore an important cause of the false-positive result when using the squatting-to-standing maneuver to diagnose obstructive cardiomyopathy (see Chapter 43).

INCREASED VENTRICULAR VOLUME

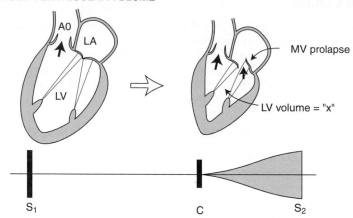

DECREASED VENTRICULAR VOLUME

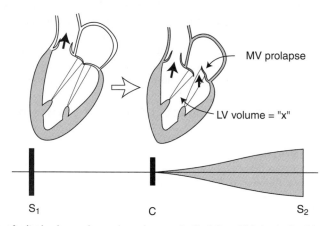

Fig. 46.1   Timing of mitral valve prolapse. In each example, the left ventricle is ejecting blood during systole and prolapse of the mitral valve occurs at the moment ventricular volume = "x." If ventricular systole begins with a relatively large ventricular volume (*top row*), the ventricular volume of "x" is delayed until late systole. If ventricular systole instead begins with a smaller ventricular volume (e.g., by straining during the Valsalva maneuver or moving from squatting-to-standing, *bottom row*), the ventricular volume of "x" is reached earlier during systole, causing the click and murmur to move towards S_1. *Ao*, Aorta; *C*, click; *LA*, left atrium; *LV*, left ventricle; *MV*, mitral valve.

regurgitation). **High-pressure tricuspid regurgitation** is commonly due to left-sided heart disease; **low-pressure tricuspid regurgitation** commonly results from endocarditis of the tricuspid valve.

A. THE MURMUR

Whether pulmonary pressures are high or low, the murmur of tricuspid regurgitation is typically loudest at the lower left sternal border, becomes louder during inspiration, and may radiate below the xiphoid process.[32]

1. High-Pressure Tricuspid Regurgitation

The murmur of high-pressure tricuspid regurgitation is holosystolic because the elevated right ventricular pressures exceed right atrial pressures throughout systole. The murmur becomes louder during inspiration (**Carvallo sign**) in 75% of patients and during manual pressure over the liver in 60% of patients.[17,33-37]

In some patients with high-pressure tricuspid regurgitation, the murmur is loudest at the apex because the enlarged right ventricle has replaced the normal position of the left ventricle. At this location, the resulting holosystolic apical murmur resembles mitral regurgitation, which, in the 1950s, led to the significant bedside error of misdiagnosing mitral regurgitation in some patients with mitral stenosis, thus inappropriately denying them valvuloplasty (a procedure contraindicated with severe mitral regurgitation).[38] Clues that help the clinician correctly recognize the apical holosystolic murmur as tricuspid regurgitation are the associated findings of an identical murmur at the lower sternal border, inspiratory augmentation of the murmur, elevated neck veins, and pulsatile liver.[38]

2. Low-Pressure Tricuspid Regurgitation

If pulmonary and right ventricular pressures are normal, the murmur of tricuspid regurgitation is confined to early systole, because right atrial and right ventricular pressures equilibrate by mid systole, thus eliminating the gradient causing the murmur.[39]

B. OTHER FINDINGS

1. High-Pressure Tricuspid Regurgitation

Other important cardiac findings are elevated neck veins (over 90% of patients), a systolic regurgitant wave in the neck veins (i.e., CV wave, 51% to 83% of patients), and systolic retraction of the apical impulse (22% of patients).[17,34,36] Thirty percent to 91% of patients have a pulsatile liver, and 90% have edema, ascites, or both.[17,32,34,36] In some patients there is an outward precordial pulsation of the lower sternum (from ejection of blood into the right atrium and liver). This sternal movement, when combined with simultaneous apical retraction (from right ventricular contraction), creates a distinctive rocking motion (i.e., apex moves in and lower sternum out at the same time), a motion called **right ventricular rock** (see Chapter 38).[16]

2. Low-Pressure Tricuspid Regurgitation

In these patients, the neck veins and apical impulse are normal, and there is no edema, pulsatile liver, or ascites.

C. ESTIMATING VENOUS PRESSURE IN TRICUSPID REGURGITATION

Estimates of venous pressure are useful because they indicate right ventricular *diastolic* pressures (or filling pressures), which provides important clues to the etiology of ascites and edema (see Chapter 36). In tricuspid regurgitation, however, the neck veins characteristically reveal a large *systolic* wave, raising the question of whether bedside estimates of venous pressure reliably indicate the right heart filling pressures.

In patients with tricuspid regurgitation (and no tricuspid stenosis), catheter measurements of the *mean* pressure in the right atrium correlate closely with right ventricular end diastolic pressure ($r = 0.94$, $p < 0.001$, slope = 1).[34] Mean atrial pressure is estimated at the bedside by identifying which patient position brings out the regurgitant waves. If the regurgitant waves are visible when the patient is supine, then venous diastolic pressure must be low (i.e., the waves collapse and become visible because the diastolic venous pressure is below the level of the sternum, or low). The mean atrial pressure (i.e., central venous pressure) in these patients is probably normal. On the other hand, if the regurgitant waves are only visible in the upright position, the diastolic pressure in the veins must be high (otherwise the neck veins would collapse and be visible in lower positions). The mean atrial and central venous pressure of these patients is probably high.

II. Clinical Significance

A. DETECTING TRICUSPID REGURGITATION

The presence of the characteristic systolic murmur of tricuspid regurgitation increases the probability of tricuspid regurgitation (LR = 10.1, see Chapter 43). Even so, many patients with tricuspid regurgitation lack a murmur, which means that the *absence* of a murmur has less diagnostic significance (i.e., negative LRs are either not significant or close to the value of 1; see Chapter 43).

B. SEVERITY OF TRICUSPID REGURGITATION

From palpation of the precordium or inspection of neck veins alone, the diagnosis of moderate-to-severe tricuspid regurgitation may be obvious (EBM Box 46.1). Diagnostic findings include the RV rock (LR = 31.4), lower sternal pulsations (LR = 12.5), early systolic outward venous pulsation (i.e., the CV wave, LR = 10.9; see Chapter 36), and hepatic pulsations (LR = 6.5). The absence of any of these findings, however, is diagnostically unhelpful.

PULMONIC REGURGITATION

I. The Finding

The murmur of pulmonic regurgitation is a diastolic murmur heard best at the second left intercostal space. Its timing and frequency depend on pulmonary pressures.

A. HIGH-PRESSURE PULMONIC REGURGITATION

Sustained pulmonary hypertension may cause the pulmonic valve to become incompetent, producing an early diastolic, high-frequency murmur at the second left intercostal space. The murmur begins immediately after a loud S_2, and most patients have elevated neck veins and other auscultatory findings of pulmonary hypertension, such as the pulmonary ejection sound, abnormal S_2 splitting, and right ventricular gallops (see Chapters 40 to 42).[40] Chapter 45 discusses how to distinguish this murmur from that of aortic regurgitation.

The high-pressure pulmonic regurgitation murmur was first described by the British clinician Graham Steell in 1888[41] and is often called the **Graham Steell murmur**.

B. LOW-PRESSURE PULMONIC REGURGITATION

When pulmonary pressures are normal, pulmonic regurgitation represents primary valvular disease (e.g., endocarditis). This murmur is mid-diastolic and contains a mixture of low and high frequency sound. It begins with a short delay after S_2.[39]

II. Clinical Significance

A. DETECTING PULMONIC REGURGITATION

Although the presence of the characteristic murmur is diagnostic (LR = 17.4, see Chapter 43), the absence of the murmur is unhelpful (LR not significant, see Chapter 43).

B. DETECTING PULMONARY HYPERTENSION

In patients with mitral stenosis, the presence of the high-pressure pulmonary regurgitation murmur (i.e., Graham Steell murmur) increases probability of pulmonary hypertension (mean pulmonary artery pressure ≥50 mm Hg; LR = 4.2, EBM Box 46.2).

EBM BOX 46.2	**Other Cardiac Findings in Mitral Stenosis***			
Finding (Reference)[†]	Sensitivity (%)	Specificity (%)	Likelihood Ratio[‡] if Finding Is	
			Present	Absent
Graham Steell murmur Detecting pulmonary hypertension[42]	69	83	**4.2**	0.4
Hyperkinetic apical movement Detecting associated mitral regurgitation or aortic valve disease[10]	74	93	**11.2**	0.3
Hyperkinetic arterial pulse Detecting associated mitral regurgitation[10]	71	95	**14.2**	0.3

*Diagnostic standard: for *pulmonary hypertension*, mean pulmonary pressure ≥50 mm Hg.[42]
[†]Definition of findings: for *Graham Steell murmur*, early diastolic decrescendo murmur of high pressure pulmonic regurgitation at second left intercostal space; for *hyperkinetic apical movement*, apical "thrust"[10] (see Chapter 38); for *hyperkinetic pulse*, arterial pulse strikes fingers abruptly and strongly (see Chapter 15).
[‡]Likelihood ratio (LR) if finding present = positive LR; LR if finding absent = negative LR.
NS, Not significant.

OTHER CARDIAC FINDINGS IN MITRAL STENOSIS

Probability

Decrease ← | → Increase

−45% −30% −15%   +15% +30% +45%

LRs   0.1   0.2   0.5   1   2   5   10   LRs

Absence of hyperkinetic arterial pulse, *arguing against* associated MR

Absence of hyperkinetic apical movement, *arguing against* associated MR or aortic valve disease

Hyperkinetic arterial pulse, detecting associated MR

Hyperkinetic apical movement, detecting MR or aortic valve disease

Graham Steell murmur, detecting pulmonary hypertension

C. HEMODIALYSIS PATIENTS

A common cause of an early diastolic murmur at the sternal border in patients with end-stage renal disease is pulmonic regurgitation.[43] This murmur presumably occurs from volume overload, because it is loudest immediately before dialysis and often disappears just after dialysis.

MITRAL STENOSIS

I. The Findings

A. THE MURMUR

Mitral stenosis causes a low-frequency, rumbling mid-diastolic murmur, which is usually heard with the bell lightly applied to the apex, often only after the patient has turned to the left lateral decubitus position. The murmur peaks during mid-diastole and again immediately before the first heart sound (**presystolic accentuation**). The mid-diastolic peak occurs because the mitral leaflets move backward toward the left atrium at this time, narrowing the mitral orifice and causing more turbulence (an analogy is the difficulty whistling with the mouth open).[44,45] The importance of these movements to the sound may explain why some patients with severe calcific mitral stenosis and inflexible leaflets lack murmurs.[45]

The traditional explanation for presystolic accentuation is atrial systole, but this is probably incorrect because presystolic accentuation also occurs in patients with atrial fibrillation.[46] Instead, there is some evidence that presystolic accentuation is actually caused by *ventricular* contraction: The crescendo sound occurs because the closing movement of the mitral leaflets, induced by ventricular systole, occurs when a pressure gradient is still maintaining forward flow across the valve. The sound continues and crescendos up until the moment the valves completely close at the first heart sound (therefore, the "presystolic" accentuation is not presystolic at all, but instead is systolic).[44-46]

Because the sound vibrations of mitral stenosis border on the threshold of human hearing, this murmur is indistinct and the most difficult to detect, as reflected in similes and metaphors used to describe the sound: "the faint sound of distant thunder," "the rumbling sound of a ball rolling down a bowling alley," and "the absence of silence."[47]

B. OTHER CARDIAC FINDINGS

Other cardiac findings in mitral stenosis include an irregular pulse (atrial fibrillation), loud first heart sound, opening snap (early diastolic sound), and associated findings of pulmonary hypertension, including elevated neck veins, right ventricular parasternal impulse, and a palpable P_2 (see Chapters 36, 38, and 40).[10] The palpable apical impulse is small or absent, because of obstruction of blood flow into the left ventricle.[10]

II. Clinical Significance

A. THE MURMUR

In countries where rheumatic heart disease is still prevalent, the apical diastolic rumble of mitral stenosis is diagnostic (LR = 31.2, see Chapter 43). Nonetheless, mitral stenosis has become a rare diagnosis in developed countries, where the characteristic apical diastolic rumble instead may reflect another disorder, such as mitral annular calcification, Austin-Flint murmur, atrial myxoma, or flow rumbles (i.e., increased flow over a nonobstructed mitral valve from mitral regurgitation, ventricular septal defect, or high output states; see Chapter 41). In one study of 529 elderly patients living in the United States, an apical diastolic rumble detected *mitral annular calcification* on echocardiography with a sensitivity of 10%, specificity of 99%, and positive LR = 7.5 (90% of patients with this murmur had *no* mitral stenosis).[48]

B. OTHER CARDIAC FINDINGS

In patients with mitral stenosis, the apical impulse should be absent or small and the arterial pulse should be normal or reduced. Consequently, the finding of a hyperkinetic apical movement in patients with mitral stenosis suggests additional mitral or aortic regurgitation (LR = 11.2, see EBM Box 46.2), and the finding of a hyperkinetic arterial pulse strongly suggests additional mitral regurgitation (LR = 14.2, see EBM Box 46.2)

ARTERIOVENOUS FISTULAE: THE HEMODIALYSIS FISTULA

The hemodialysis fistula provides a good example of the continuous murmur typical of arterio-venous fistulae: it is a high-frequency murmur, persisting throughout systole and diastole and peaking during late systole:

PuSHSHSHSHPuSHSHSHSHSHSHSH

Moving the stethoscope progressively away from the fistula and toward the heart makes the diastolic component of the murmur fainter until only a systolic murmur remains.[49]

The importance of this murmur is that its systolic remnants are transmitted to the upper sternal border, where than can be mistaken for cardiac murmurs unless the clinician traces them to the fistula (see "isolated base" murmur pattern in Fig. 43.1).[16,49]

In contrast to murmurs from arteriovenous fistulas, continuous murmurs generated from abnormal flow in veins (e.g., venous hums, mammary souffle) peak during diastole (see Chapter 43).

References may be accessed online at *Elsevier eBooks for Practicing Clinicians.*

Disorders of the Pericardium

PERICARDITIS AND THE PERICARDIAL RUB

I. Introduction

The pericardial rub is a physical sign of pericarditis, or inflammation of the pericardium, which is caused by a wide variety of disorders, including infections, connective tissue diseases, radiation injury, myocardial infarction, neoplasia, uremia, and trauma.

In the 1820s, shortly after the introduction of the stethoscope, Collin first described the pericardial rub, as a sound "similar to that of the crackling of new leather."[1]

II. The Finding

Pericardial rubs are grating, scratching, or creaking sounds that are loudest near the left sternal border and are most apparent when the patient is sitting upright, leaning forward, and holding his or her breath in deep exhalation.[2,3] They resemble the sound of two pieces of sandpaper being rubbed together. Compared with heart murmurs, the pericardial rub has more high-frequency energy and sounds closer to the ear,[2] it may completely disappear during inspiration or expiration, and up to one-fourth are palpable.[3,4]

In approximately 50% of patients, the rub has three components per cardiac cycle—one during ventricular systole and two during diastole (mid-diastole and atrial systole).* In approximately one-third of patients, only two components are heard (usually the atrial and ventricular systolic rub), and in the remaining 15%, only a single-component ventricular systolic rub is heard.[3]

---

*These three components represent the three moments in the cardiac cycle when the ventricle is moving the most.

III. Clinical Significance

A. THE RUB AND PERICARDITIS

Clinical studies of pericarditis require at least two of the following four criteria: (1) pericardial rub, (2) characteristic pericardial chest pain (precordial pleuritic pain radiating to the trapezius ridge which is relieved when sitting up), (3) characteristic electrocardiographic changes (diffuse concave ST elevation, PR segment depression, absence of Q waves), and (4) new or worsening pericardial effusion. Echocardiography alone cannot be used to diagnose pericarditis, because only 50% to 66% of patients have detectable pericardial effusions on echocardiography (and most of these effusions are mild).[5–9]

Therefore, because the pericardial friction rub is one of the bedside criteria for the diagnosis of pericarditis, the diagnostic accuracy of the rub cannot be assessed (see Chapter 1).

B. PERICARDITIS AND FEVER

In Western Europe and the United States, the specific cause of pericarditis is never discovered in 80% to 90% of cases.[8] Such idiopathic cases are often attributed to viral infection. In contrast, evaluation reveals a *specific* diagnosis (such as neoplasia, connective tissue disease, tuberculosis, or bacterial infection) in only 10% to 20% of cases. In one study of 453 patients with acute pericarditis, the presence of fever (temperature >38°C) increased the probability that one of these specific diagnoses would be found (likelihood ratio [LR] = 4.3) and decreased the probability of an idiopathic/viral diagnosis (LR = 0.2).[10]

C. THE RUB AND PERICARDIAL EFFUSION

Although the pericardial rub suggests the rubbing together of contiguous pericardial surfaces, the sound often persists after the accumulation of significant pericardial effusions.[3,11] The rub is heard, for example, in up to one-fourth of patients with cardiac tamponade (see later). Therefore, the *presence* of the rub cannot be used to argue *against* the development of pericardial effusion.

D. THE RUB AND NEOPLASTIC DISEASE

Pericardial rubs are less frequent in neoplastic pericarditis than in other etiologies. For example, in patients with known cancer who subsequently develop pericardial disease, the presence of a rub increases the probability that the pericarditis is idiopathic or radiation-induced, not neoplastic (positive LR = 5.5, negative LR = 0.4).[12] In another study of 322 patients presenting with undiagnosed moderate or severe pericardial effusion, the presence of a pericardial rub (among other inflammatory signs[†]) increased the probability of a non-neoplastic etiology (LR = 2.3).[13]

E. THE RUB AND MYOCARDIAL INFARCTION

A pericardial rub is found in 5% to 20% of patients with acute myocardial infarction, usually appearing from hospital days 1 to 3.[14–18] The incidence is lowest (i.e., 5% to 7%) in patients receiving immediate thrombolytic medications or angioplasty[16,18.] Compared with patients who do not develop rubs, patients with rubs have significantly larger myocardial infarctions, lower ejection fractions, more extensive coronary artery disease, and more complications, including congestive heart failure and atrial arrhythmias.[14,16,17] Nonetheless, in these patients tamponade is rare, even if they receive thrombolytic medications.[16]

[†]In this study, "inflammatory signs" were defined as two or more of the following: pericardial rub, characteristic pericarditis chest pain, fever, or characteristic Electrocardiographic changes.

CARDIAC TAMPONADE

I. Introduction

Cardiac tamponade occurs when a pericardial effusion has become so large and tense that intrapericardial pressures exceed the normal filling (i.e., diastolic) pressures of the heart, thus impairing the diastolic filling of the heart and reducing the cardiac output.

The history of diagnosing tamponade illustrates well the tension that sometimes exists between older diagnostic standards based on physical signs and newer ones based on clinical imaging. For example, early descriptions of tamponade, which were based on catastrophic acute intrapericardial hemorrhage, emphasized hypotension, elevated neck veins, and the small, quiet heart as diagnostic findings (**Beck triad**).[19,20] Later, after it became obvious that many medical patients with tamponade had normal blood pressure and loud heart tones, the definition of tamponade shifted to emphasize large pericardial effusions, elevated neck veins, pulsus paradoxus, and relief of symptoms and signs after pericardiocentesis.[21] Finally, in the 1980s, several echocardiographic criteria for tamponade were introduced,[20,22] although studies have subsequently shown that relying solely on echocardiographic criteria sometimes identifies patients who fail to improve symptomatically or physiologically after pericardiocentesis.[23–25]

Therefore, the diagnosis of tamponade should not rely solely on the echocardiographic report but requires synthesis of all the findings, emphasizing especially the ones from physical diagnosis—elevated neck veins, tachycardia, and pulsus paradoxus.[26]

II. The Findings

Table 47.1 presents the physical signs observed in several studies of patients with proven cardiac tamponade. Most of these patients presented with shortness of breath.[21,27] The definition and pathogenesis of pulsus paradoxus and elevated neck veins are discussed in Chapters 15 and 36.

TABLE 47.1 ■ Cardiac Tamponade*

Physical Finding†	Frequency (%)‡
Neck veins	
Elevated neck veins	100
Kussmaul sign	0
Arterial pulse	
Tachycardia (>100 bpm)	81–100
Blood pressure	
Systolic blood pressure greater than 100 mm Hg	58–100
Pulsus paradoxus >10 mm Hg	98
Pulsus paradoxus >20 mm Hg	78
Pulsus paradoxus >30 mm Hg	49
Pulsus paradoxus >40 mm Hg	38
Total paradox	23
Auscultation of heart	
Diminished heart tones	36–84
Pericardial rub	27
Other	
Hepatomegaly	58
Edema	27

Data from 128 patients from references 21,27,38–40.
*Diagnostic Standard: for *tamponade*, cardiac output that improved after drainage of pericardial effusion.
†Definition of finding: for *total paradox*, palpable pulse disappears completely during inspiration.
‡Results are overall mean frequency or, if statistically heterogeneous, the range of values.

The three key findings of tamponade are elevated neck veins (100% of patients), tachycardia (81% to 100% of patients), and pulsus paradoxus >10 mm Hg (98% of patients). In patients with pericardial effusions, the finding of pulsus paradoxus greater than 12 mm Hg detects tamponade with a sensitivity of 98%, specificity of 83%, positive LR = 5.9, and negative LR = 0.03 (see Chapter 15).[28] Furthermore, the *absence* of pulsus paradoxus on analysis of printed pulse oximetry tracings (see Chapter 15) greatly *decreases* the probability of tamponade (LR = 0.05).[29]

The complication of tamponade in patients with pericarditis greatly increases the probability that a specific diagnosis will be made (e.g., neoplasia, connective tissue disease, tuberculosis, or bacterial infection; LR = 21.5).[10]

Cardiac tamponade is one of the few causes of elevated neck veins with an absent *y* descent (see Chapter 36). This contrasts sharply with the exaggerated *y* descent of constrictive pericarditis (see later).

CONSTRICTIVE PERICARDITIS

I. Introduction

Constrictive pericarditis is present when calcification or fibrosis of the pericardium impairs diastolic filling, thus causing elevated venous pressure and reduced cardiac output.

II. The Findings

Table 47.2 presents the physical signs of patients with constrictive pericarditis; most patients present with edema, abdominal swelling, and dyspnea.[30–32] The key physical findings are elevated neck veins (94%), a prominent *y* descent in venous waveform (57% to 100%, median 94%), pericardial knock (20% to 94%), and hepatomegaly (53% to 100%).

TABLE 47.2 ■ Constrictive Pericarditis*

Physical Finding	Frequency (%)†
Neck veins	
Elevated neck veins	94
Prominent *y* descent (Friedreich sign)	57–100
Kussmaul sign	14–50
Arterial pulse	
Irregularly irregular (atrial fibrillation)	36–70
Blood pressure	
Pulsus paradoxus >10 mm Hg	13–64
Auscultation of heart	
Pericardial knock	20–94
Pericardial rub	3–16
Other	
Hepatomegaly	53–100
Edema	58–100
Ascites	37–89

Data from 780 patients from references 30,31,36,38,41–49.
*Diagnostic standard: For *constrictive pericarditis*, surgical and postmortem findings,[30,38,46–48] sometimes in combination with hemodynamic findings[31,36,41–45] and magnetic resonance imaging findings.[49]
†Results are the overall mean frequency or, if statistically heterogeneous, the range of values.

A. NECK VEINS

In addition to the elevated venous pressure, the venous waveform displays an unusually prominent *y* descent, which, combined with an exaggerated *x'* descent, creates two conspicuous dips per cardiac cycle, making the waveform appear to trace an M or W with each arterial pulse (**Friedreich sign**, see Chapter 36). Sometimes these movements are transmitted to the liver, causing it to pulsate inward twice with each cardiac cycle.[33]

The prominent *y* descent occurs because diastolic filling is only impaired during the last two-thirds of diastole. At the moment the tricuspid valve opens (beginning of diastole and beginning of *y* descent), the right atrium empties rapidly and without resistance (causing a prominent *y* descent), although eventually the relaxing ventricle meets the limits of the rigid pericardial shell and the pressures again increase.[34] This contrasts with tamponade, which impairs diastolic filling throughout diastole and thus eliminates the *y* descent.

B. KUSSMAUL SIGN

The Kussmaul sign is the paradoxical increase in venous pressure during inspiration. This sign, present in 14% to 50% of patients with constriction, is discussed fully in Chapter 36 (an excellent video of the Kussmaul sign is available in the reference by Mansoor).[35]

C. PERICARDIAL KNOCK

The pericardial knock is a loud, high-frequency early diastolic sound heard between the apex and left lower sternal border. It is discussed in Chapter 42.

D. OTHER FINDINGS

Up to 90% of patients with constrictive pericarditis have systolic retraction of the apical impulse (see Chapter 38).[36,37]

According to traditional teachings, pulsus paradoxus is a not a finding of constrictive pericarditis; however, the studies reviewed in Table 47.2 indicate that pulsus paradoxus does appear, occurring in 13% to 64% of patients with constrictive pericarditis (see Table 47.2). This seeming contradiction probably reflects the different definitions of pulsus paradoxus. When pulsus paradoxus is defined as an inspiratory fall in the systolic blood pressure of 10 mm Hg or more (i.e., the usual definition), 13% to 64% of patients with constriction have the finding; when it is instead defined as an inspiratory fall of 20 mm Hg or more, no patient has the finding.[38] In contrast, the usual pulsus paradoxus in patients with tamponade is 20 to 50 mm Hg (see Table 47.1).[21]

Therefore, mild degrees of pulsus paradoxus (10 to 20 mm Hg) are commonly observed in patients with constrictive pericarditis, but larger degrees (>20 mm Hg) are not and suggest tamponade or another cause of the finding (see Chapter 15).

References may be accessed online at *Elsevier eBooks for Practicing Clinicians*.

CHAPTER 48

Congestive Heart Failure

KEY TEACHING POINTS

- In patients with chest pain or dyspnea, the following physical signs *increase* probability of elevated left heart filling pressure and cardiac dyspnea: positive abdominojugular test, abnormal Valsalva response, displaced apical impulse, heart rate greater than 100 beats/min, the third heart sound, elevated neck veins, and a positive bendopnea test.
- A *normal* Valsalva response and *negative* abdominojugular test *decrease* probability of elevated left heart filling pressure.
- The following physical signs are accurate signs of low ejection fraction: Cheyne-Stokes respirations, displaced apical impulse, abnormal Valsalva response, elevated neck veins, and third heart sound.

I. Introduction

Heart failure is a clinical syndrome characterized by impaired ventricular performance, elevated diastolic filling pressure, and diminished exercise capacity. Patients with heart failure and ventricular disease may have a low ventricular ejection fraction (systolic dysfunction) or normal ejection fraction (diastolic dysfunction).

Clear descriptions of the signs of heart failure date to the Middle Ages.[1] In the 17th century, just after Harvey published his discovery of the circulation of blood, clinicians began to correlate the pathologic observation of large heart chambers and congested lungs with the clinical observations of dyspnea and edema.[2]

II. The Findings

Many of the findings of heart failure are discussed fully in other chapters of the book, including pulsus alternans and the dicrotic pulse (see Chapter 15), Cheyne-Stokes respirations (see Chapter 19), crackles (see Chapter 30), elevated neck veins (see Chapter 36), the abdominojugular test (see Chapter 36), displaced apical impulse (Chapter 38), and third heart sound (see Chapter 41).

This chapter reviews two findings not discussed extensively elsewhere, the bendopnea test and the abnormal Valsalva response, and then presents the diagnostic accuracy of all findings of congestive heart failure.

A. BENDOPNEA TEST

1. The Finding

Bendopnea describes shortness of breath that develops when a seated patient bends over. In 2013, clinicians began investigating this symptom in heart failure patients, most of whom had advanced disease with significant dyspnea on exertion.[3,4]

Researchers have developed a specific bedside test to determine whether or not bendopnea is present: The patient sits in a chair and is asked to bend forward at the waist "as if putting on their socks or shoes." The clinician then times the interval between bending over and the onset of shortness of breath (if it develops). If this interval is less than 30 seconds, bendopnea is present.[4] Alternative symptoms, such as lightheadedness and fullness in the head, chest, or abdomen do not constitute a positive test.[4] In clinical studies of patients with a positive test, dyspnea appears after a median interval of only 8 to 12 seconds.[4,5]

2. Pathogenesis of Bendopnea

The cause of bendopnea is elevated left heart filling pressure. Compared to those without bendopnea, patients with bendopnea have more orthopnea, more paroxysmal nocturnal dyspnea, and higher pulmonary capillary wedge pressure.[3,4] The action of bending over increases filling pressure even more, an increment sufficient to cause significant dyspnea in those with the positive bendopnea test.[4] Even so, the actual mechanism for increment in cardiac pressure with bending over is controversial. Some investigators believe it is due to an increase in intrathoracic pressure in the bended position,[4,6] whereas others believe it results from increased abdominal pressure (similar to the abdominojugular test).[7] The symptom is not explained by differences in cardiac output, ascites frequency, waist circumference, or body habitus.[4,5]

B. THE VALSALVA RESPONSE

1. Introduction

The **Valsalva maneuver** consists of forced expiration against a closed glottis after a full inspiration.[8] The **Valsalva response** refers to the changes in blood pressure and pulse that occur during both the strain phase of the maneuver and the recovery period after the strain is released.

Valsalva introduced his maneuver in 1704 as a technique to expel pus from the middle ear.[8–10] The maneuver was forgotten, however, until 1859, when Weber showed he could use it to interrupt his arterial pulse at will (an experiment he eventually abandoned after fainting and developing convulsions).[9] Beginning in the 1950s, many different investigators reported that the Valsalva response was distinctly abnormal in patients with congestive heart failure.[11–15]

2. Technique

To perform the maneuver, the patient should take a deep breath in and bear down, as if straining to have a bowel movement. The clinician measures the Valsalva response by using a blood pressure cuff, as described below. In clinical studies, the straining phase is standardized by having the patient's mouthpiece connected to a pressure transducer, which should demonstrate an increment of 30 to 40 mm Hg for at least 10 seconds.

The Valsalva maneuver is contraindicated in patients with recent eye or central nervous system surgery or hemorrhage. It is also unwise to perform the maneuver in patients with acute coronary ischemia, because it may induce arrhythmias, although in patients with chronic ischemic heart disease the maneuver is safe and was once even used to terminate episodes of angina.[16]

3. The Normal Valsalva Response

The normal Valsalva response is divided into four phases (Fig. 48.1).[8] In phase 1, the arterial systolic blood pressure rises briefly because increased intrathoracic pressure is transmitted directly to the aorta. In phase 2, blood pressure falls because of reduced venous return during continuing straining. In phase 3, just after release of straining, pressure falls further because of temporary pooling of blood in the pulmonary veins. In phase 4, the arterial pressure overshoots to levels above the control values, primarily because of reflex sympathetic activity induced by previous hypotension. The changes in heart rate are exactly out of phase with the blood pressure: the heart rate increases during phases 2 and 3 and decreases during phase 4.

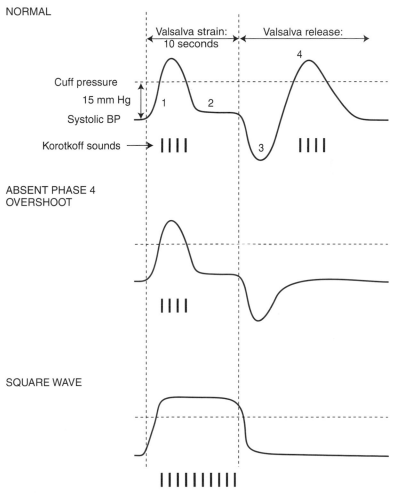

Fig. 48.1 **The Valsalva Response.** The *solid line* in each drawing depicts changes in systolic blood pressure over time during the Valsalva maneuver. The three types of Valsalva responses are normal (*top*), absent phase 4 overshoot (*middle*), and square wave (*bottom*). The clinician distinguishes these responses by inflating the blood pressure cuff 15 mm Hg above the patient's resting systolic blood pressure BP; (*horizontal dotted line*) and listening for Korotkoff sounds. Korotkoff sounds appear in phase 1 and 4 in the normal response, in phase 1 only in the absent phase 4 overshoot response, and in phases 1 and 2 only in the square wave response. See the text.

The clinician identifies these four phases by inflating a blood pressure cuff on the patient's arm 15 mm Hg higher than the patient's resting systolic blood pressure and maintaining this cuff pressure during the straining phase and for 30 seconds afterwards, at the same time listening for Korotkoff sounds just as if manually measuring blood pressure. Korotkoff sounds appear whenever the patient's systolic pressure exceeds the cuff pressure. Therefore, during the normal Valsalva response, Korotkoff sounds appear during phase 1 and phase 4 but are absent during phases 2 and 3.

4. The Abnormal Valsalva Response (Fig. 48.1)

In patients with congestive heart failure, there are two abnormal Valsalva responses: (1) **Absent phase 4 overshoot**, in which the arterial pressure fails to rise during phase 4 (Korotkoff sounds during phase 1 only), and (2) **Square wave response**, in which the arterial pressure rises in parallel with intrathoracic pressure (Korotkoff sounds during phases 1 and 2 only).

In all three interpretable responses—normal, absent phase 4 overshoot, and square wave response—Korotkoff sounds appear during phase 1. If sounds do not appear during this phase, the intrathoracic pressure did not increase to high enough levels during the maneuver, and the test is therefore *not* interpretable.

Beta-blocker medications may cause a false-positive response, primarily by eliminating the phase 4 overshoot.[17]

5. Pathogenesis of the Abnormal Valsalva Response

In patients with congestive heart failure, Korotkoff sounds fail to appear during phase 4 because the weakened heart cannot increase cardiac output in response to hypotension (there is a direct relationship between the degree of overshoot and patient's ejection fraction, r = 0.72).[17] Although the cause of the square wave response is still debated, it probably represents the combined effect of neurohormonal activation, peripheral venoconstriction, and increased central blood volume.[13,14,18,19] Phase 2 hypotension may not occur in these patients because increased central venous blood volume maintains the venous return to the right heart despite the Valsalva strain, and the congested lungs have an ample supply of blood for the left heart.*

III. Clinical Significance

EBM Box 48.1 and 48.2 present the diagnostic accuracy of physical signs for congestive heart failure. EBM Box 48.1 refers to the diagnosis of elevated left heart filling pressure and therefore applies to the diagnosis of systolic or diastolic dysfunction. The ability to accurately detect elevated left heart filling pressure is especially important in patients with dyspnea, because elevated pressure implicates the heart as the cause of the patient's symptoms. EBM Box 48.2 refers to the diagnosis of depressed left ventricular ejection fraction and therefore applies only to the diagnosis of systolic dysfunction.

This information should only be applied to patients similar to those enrolled in the studies cited in EBM Boxes 48.1 and 48.2. These patients were all adults presenting to clinicians primarily for evaluation of chest pain or dyspnea. Most had no prior history of congestive heart failure, and many had alternative explanations for dyspnea, such as lung disease.

A. DETECTING ELEVATED LEFT HEART FILLING PRESSURE

In descending order of their likelihood ratios (LRs), the findings *increasing* the probability of elevated filling pressure the most are a positive abdominojugular test (LR = 8, EBM Box 48.1), abnormal Valsalva response (i.e., either absent phase 4 overshoot or square wave response,

---

*The same pathophysiology probably explains the finding of reversed pulsus paradoxus in some patients with congestive heart failure receiving positive pressure ventilation (see Chapter 15).

EBM BOX 48.1	Congestive Heart Failure – Elevated Left Heart Filling Pressure*

Finding (Reference)[†]	Sensitivity (%)	Specificity (%)	Likelihood Ratio[‡] if Finding Is	
			Present	Absent
Vital signs				
Heart rate >100/min at rest[20]	6	99	**5.5**	NS
Abnormal Valsalva response[21]	95	88	**7.6**	0.1
Pulse increase of ≥10% during Valsalva strain[22]	11	54	**0.2**	1.7
Lung examination				
Crackles[17,20,23,24]	12–23	88–96	NS	NS
Heart examination				
Elevated jugular venous pressure[17,20,24]	10–58	96–97	**3.9**	NS
Positive abdominojugular test[24-26]	55–84	83–98	**8.0**	0.3
Supine apical impulse lateral to MCL[23]	42	93	**5.8**	NS
S_3 gallop[17,20,23,27]	12–37	85–96	**3.9**	0.8
S_4 gallop[17,28]	35–71	50–70	NS	NS
Other findings				
Edema[17,20]	10	93–96	NS	NS
Bendopnea test[4]	47	88	**3.2**	0.6

*Diagnostic standard: for *elevated left heart filling pressure*, pulmonary capillary wedge pressure >12 mm Hg,[23] >15 mm Hg,[21,24-26] or ≥ 22 mm Hg[4]; or left ventricular end diastolic pressure >15 mm Hg[17,20,27,28] or >18 mm Hg.[22]

[†]Definition of findings: for *abnormal Valsalva response*, absent phase 4 overshoot or square wave response (see text); for *positive abdominojugular test*, sustained rise in jugular venous pressure during 10–15 seconds of midabdominal pressure (see text); for *bendopnea test*, shortness of breath within 30 seconds of bending over (see text).

[‡]Likelihood ratio (LR) if finding present = positive LR; LR if finding absent = negative LR.

MCL, Midclavicular line; *NS*, not significant.

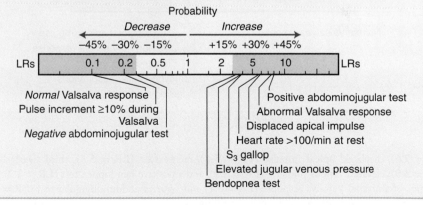

ELEVATED LEFT HEART FILLING PRESSURE

Probability

Decrease   *Increase*

−45% −30% −15%   +15% +30% +45%

LRs   0.1   0.2   0.5   1   2   5   10   LRs

Normal Valsalva response
Pulse increment ≥10% during Valsalva
Negative abdominojugular test

Positive abdominojugular test
Abnormal Valsalva response
Displaced apical impulse
Heart rate >100/min at rest
S_3 gallop
Elevated jugular venous pressure
Bendopnea test

| EBM BOX 48.2 | Congestive Heart Failure - Low Ejection Fraction* |

Finding (Reference)[†]	Sensitivity (%)	Specificity (%)	Likelihood Ratio[‡] if Finding Is	
			Present	Absent
Vital signs				
Heart rate >100 beats/min at rest[29]	22	92	2.8	NS
Cheyne-Stokes respirations[30]	33	94	**5.4**	0.7
Abnormal Valsalva response[31,32]	69–88	90–91	**7.6**	**0.3**
Lung examination				
Crackles[29,33-35]	10–29	77–98	NS	NS
Heart examination				
Elevated neck veins[29,33,35]	7–25	96–98	**6.3**	NS
Supine apical impulse lateral to MCL[29,33-35]	5–66	93–99	**10.3**	0.7
S₃ gallop[27,33,34,36,37]	11–51	85–98	**3.4**	0.7
S₄ gallop[28,38]	31–67	55–68	NS	NS
Murmur of mitral regurgitation[34]	25	89	NS	NS
Other				
Hepatomegaly[33]	3	97	NS	NS
Edema[29,33,35]	8–33	70–98	NS	NS

*Diagnostic standard: for *low ejection fraction*, radionuclide left ventricular ejection fraction <0.50[31,32,34,36] or <0.53,[33] echocardiographic ejection fraction <0.50[27,28,35,37,38] or <0.40,[30] or left ventricular fractional shortening <25% by echocardiography.[29]
[†]Definition of findings: for *abnormal Valsalva response*, absent phase 4 overshoot or square wave response (see text).
[‡]Likelihood ratio (LR) if finding present = positive LR; LR if finding absent = negative LR.
MCL, Midclavicular line; *NS*, not significant.

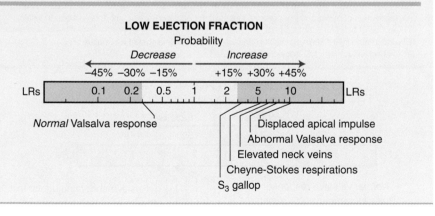

LOW EJECTION FRACTION
Probability

LR = 7.6), displaced apical impulse (LR = 5.8), tachycardia (LR = 5.5), third heart sound (LR = 3.9), elevated venous pressure (LR = 3.9), and a positive bendopnea test (LR = 3.2). The findings of a normal Valsalva response (LR = 0.1) and *negative* abdominojugular test (LR = 0.3) *decrease* the probability of elevated left heart filling pressure. The *absence* of tachycardia, elevated venous pressure, displaced apical impulse, or S₃ gallop are all diagnostically unhelpful (LRs not significant).

Because the pulse rate during the Valsalva maneuver is exactly out of phase of with the blood pressure changes, the pulse rate should accelerate during phases 2 and 3 of the normal response (i.e., when the systolic blood pressure is falling, see Fig. 48.1). In one study, the finding of pulse acceleration during Valsalva strain (i.e., an increase in rate of 10%, as detected by rhythm strips) *decreased* the probability of an elevated filling pressure (LR = 0.2, EBM Box 48.2).

The presence of crackles, fourth heart sound, or edema does not indicate elevated left heart filling pressure in these patients. Crackles are unhelpful because they are infrequent in chronic heart failure (sensitivity of only 12% to 23%) and because many other disorders causing dyspnea also produce crackles. Even so, if the finding of crackles is instead applied just to patients with known cardiomyopathy (e.g., those awaiting cardiac transplantation), they become a more accurate sign of elevated filling pressure, detecting a pulmonary capillary wedge pressure of 20 mm Hg or higher with a sensitivity of 15% to 64%, specificity of 82% to 94%, and positive LR = 2.1. The finding is more accurate in this setting probably because other diagnoses causing crackles have already been excluded.[24,39–41]

A small instrument similar to a digital pulse oximeter has been designed that measures and records the pulse pressure during the Valsalva maneuver.[42] This instrument calculates the **pulse-amplitude ratio**, which is the ratio of the pulse pressure at the end of phase 2 divided by that at the beginning of phase 1. Patients with a normal Valsalva response have a low pulse-amplitude ratio (because pulse pressure at the end of phase 2 is much less than that at the beginning of phase 1), whereas those with the square wave response have a higher ratio (near the value of 1). Several studies have shown a direct relationship between the pulse-amplitude ratio and the pulmonary capillary wedge pressure (r = 0.81 to 0.92).[19,42–45] In 3 studies, a pulse amplitude ratio of more than 0.7 detected a measured pulmonary capillary wedge pressure of more than 15 mm Hg with a sensitivity of 31% to 91%, specificity of 85% to 95%, and positive LR = 5.2 (negative LR not significant).[44,46,47]

B. DETECTING DEPRESSED LEFT VENTRICULAR EJECTION FRACTION

Some of the same signs that detect elevated filling pressure also indicate a depressed ejection fraction: displaced apical impulse (LR = 10.3, see EBM Box 48.2), abnormal Valsalva response (either absent phase 4 overshoot or square wave response, LR = 7.6), elevated neck veins (LR = 6.3), Cheyne-Stokes respirations (LR = 5.4), and third heart sound (LR = 3.4). Cheyne-Stokes respirations are a more accurate sign of depressed ejection fraction in patients 80 years old or younger (LR = 8.1) than they are in older patients (LR = 2.7) (see Chapter 19).

The *absence* of any of these findings (excepting Valsalva response) is diagnostically unhelpful (i.e., many patients with ejection fractions less than 50% lack these findings). Nonetheless, the absence of the third heart sounds does decrease the probability of an ejection fraction less than 30% (LR = 0.3, see Chapter 41).[34,36]

Some investigators believe that the abnormal Valsalva response is primarily a sign of elevated filling pressure, not low ejection fraction, citing data correlating the degree of Valsalva abnormality with left atrial pressure (r = 0.77, p = 0.005) but not ejection fraction.[21,42,48] This apparent contradiction may reflect varying prevalence of diastolic dysfunction in different investigators' practices. Assuming that the sign is primarily one of elevated filling pressure, it will therefore also be a good sign of depressed ejection fraction if most patients with heart failure in the clinician's practice have systolic dysfunction (EBM Box 48.2),[31,32] but it will not predict ejection fraction if there is a mixture of patients with systolic and diastolic dysfunction.[21,42,48]

Several findings provide no useful diagnostic information when assessing the patient's ejection fraction: crackles, murmur of mitral regurgitation, hepatomegaly, or edema (all LRs not significant; see EBM Box 48.2).

C. PROPORTIONAL PULSE PRESSURE

In patients with known dilated cardiomyopathy and severe left ventricular dysfunction, a proportional pulse pressure (i.e., arterial pulse pressure divided by the systolic blood pressure) less than 0.25 detects a low cardiac index (i.e., $\leq 2.2\,L/min/m^2$) with a sensitivity of 70% to 91%, specificity of 83% to 93%, positive LR = 6.9, and negative LR = 0.2.[40,49]

D. PHYSICAL SIGNS AND CONSENSUS DIAGNOSIS OF CONGESTIVE HEART FAILURE

Recent investigations[50-64] into the diagnostic accuracy of B-type natriuretic peptide (BNP) in patients with acute dyspnea have further addressed the value of physical examination. In contrast to the studies in EBM Boxes 48.1 and 48.2, these studies used expert judgment as the diagnostic standard for heart failure, based on the retrospective review of patient's presenting findings, laboratory tests, and response to treatment. These studies confirmed the value of the third heart sound (LR = 7.7), displaced apical impulse (LR = 6.7), and elevated neck veins (LR = 4); these findings actually increased probability of heart failure more than a BNP level $\geq 100\,pg/mL$ (LR = 2.7). Nonetheless, in these same studies a BNP level $<100\,pg/mL$ decreased the probability of the consensus diagnosis of heart failure (LR = 0.1) far more than the *absence* of third heart sound, displaced apical impulse, or elevated neck veins (LRs 0.7–0.9).

Because it is possible that judgments about final diagnosis in these studies were influenced by the physical findings themselves, they are excluded from the EBM Boxes.

E. PROGNOSIS IN HEART FAILURE

In patients with clinically suspected ischemic heart disease, the physical signs of heart failure are independent predictors of mortality, adding prognostic information to that already provided by the patient's age, exercise capacity, and measured ejection fraction.[65,66] Six-month to one-year cardiac mortality is significantly higher for those with a displaced apical impulse (39% vs. 12% without the finding, p = 0.005),[23] jugular vein distention (33% vs 28% without the finding, p < 0.001),[67] the third heart sound (57% vs. 14% without the finding, p = 0.002),[23] Kussmaul sign (41% vs. 12% without the finding, p = 0.001; see Chapter 36),[68] positive abdominojugular test (27% v 14% without the finding, p = 0.004),[69] and a positive bendopnea test (30% vs 17% without the finding, p = 0.02).[5]

In 1976, Forrester[70] showed that patients with acute myocardial infarction could be classified into four hemodynamic profiles, based on measurements of pulmonary capillary wedge pressure (elevated or not, i.e., *wet* or *dry*) and cardiac output (low or normal, i.e., *cold* or *warm*). Subsequently, clinicians have used physical examination to classify hospitalized patients with heart failure into the same 4 profiles (i.e., *dry-warm*, *wet-warm*, *wet-cold*, or *dry-cold*). In general, *cold* patients have signs of compromised perfusion, such as cool extremities, narrow proportional pulse pressure (<25%, see Chapter 17), pulsus alternans (see Chapter 15), symptomatic hypotension, and impaired mentation. In 4 studies of 8700 heart failure patients, the *cold* profile (either *wet-cold* or *dry-cold*) was associated with increased early mortality (sensitivity 24% to 55%, specificity 81% to 96%, positive LR = 3).[71-74]

References may be accessed online at *Elsevier eBooks for Practicing Clinicians*.

Coronary Artery Disease

I. Introduction

Coronary disease is the leading cause of heart disease and death in the United States,[1] and chest pain accounts for 8% to 10% of complaints of patients presenting to clinics or emergency departments.[2-4] The bedside diagnosis of chest pain is difficult and at times humbling, as illustrated by the fact that up to 1% to 6% of patients with myocardial infarction (confirmed by cardiac biomarkers) are misdiagnosed and discharged home from emergency departments.[5-10] The focus of this chapter is to identify all aspects of the initial patient encounter—patient interview, physical examination, and the electrocardiogram—that help distinguish patients with angina and myocardial infarction from those with mimicking disorders.

The first clear description of **angina pectoris** was given in 1768 by William Heberden, who coined the term* and provided a clinical description that has been unsurpassed. Just eight years later, Edward Jenner linked angina to "ossification" of the coronary arteries and insufficient coronary blood flow,[11] and in 1878 (more than 50 years before the introduction of electrocardiography), Adam Hammer correctly diagnosed the first case of myocardial infarction during life in a young man with sudden collapse, bradycardia, and enfeebled heart tones.[12,13] Coronary disease was once considered to be an

---

*Heberden based the term *angina* on the Greek *agkhone*, which means "strangling." This Greek root also forms the basis for the English words *anxiety* and *anguish*. Heberden's selection of *angina* was unfortunate, because the term had already been applied to other conditions of the throat, such as Vincent's angina and Ludwig's angina.

uncommon disorder—the great 19th century American cardiologist Austin Flint found only seven cases of angina in his clinical records,[14] and Osler personally observed only 40 cases during his career.[11]

II. The Findings

A. INTRODUCTION

Unlike other clinical problems in cardiology such as valvular disease and heart failure, patients with coronary artery disease have few or no physical findings. For over 100 years, the most important aspect of diagnosing coronary disease has been the patient's description of chest pain, whereas the most important element in diagnosing myocardial infarction (at least since 1918) has been the electrocardiogram.

B. DESCRIPTION OF CHEST PAIN

Heberden wrote that **angina** is a "most disagreeable sensation in the breast" that seizes patients "while they are walking" yet vanishes "the moment they stand still."[15] Modern definitions of **typical angina** retain most of Heberden's essential features, by defining it as substernal discomfort with three characteristics: (1) it is precipitated by exertion, (2) it is improved by rest or nitroglycerin (or both), and (3) it lasts less than 10 minutes. Many patients also describe radiation of the pain to the shoulders, jaw, or inner aspect of the arm. In contrast, **atypical angina** is substernal discomfort with atypical features (e.g., it is not always relieved by nitroglycerin, it is not always brought on by exertion, or it is relieved after 15 to 20 minutes of rest), and **nonanginal chest pain** lacks all features of typical angina (i.e., it is unrelated to activity, unrelieved by nitroglycerin, or otherwise not suggestive of angina).

C. HAND GESTURES DURING DESCRIPTION OF CHEST PAIN

According to traditional teachings, patients provide diagnostic clues to the physician by the hand gestures they spontaneously make when describing their chest pain. Four of these gestures are (1) **Levine sign** – placing clenched fist against the sternum, (2) **palm** sign – placing the extended palm against the sternum, (3) **arm** sign – gripping the left arm, and (4) **pointing** sign – pointing to a single point on the chest with one or two fingers.[16] According to traditional teachings, gestures suggesting deep, poorly localized visceral pain (Levine and palm signs) or pain radiating to the left arm (arm sign) increase the probability of coronary disease whereas gestures indicating well-localized somatic pain (pointing sign) decrease the probability of disease.

D. PHYSICAL FINDINGS

Some of the findings that appear in EBM Boxes 49.1 and 49.2 are discussed in other chapters: crackles (Chapter 30), displaced precordial pulsation (Chapter 38), and the third heart sound (Chapter 41).

1. Earlobe Crease

The earlobe crease is a diagonal crease across the earlobe, connecting the lowest point on the tragus to the outside of the earlobe (see Fig. 49.1). Some investigators define the finding as a crease traversing at least one-third the distance from tragus to posterior pinna,[36,37] whereas others require the crease to extend the total distance.[27,30,38] In a letter to the editor written in 1973,[77] Frank first presented the "positive earlobe sign" as a sign tightly associated with other cardiovascular risk factors. Although its association with coronary disease remains controversial and its pathogenesis a mystery, many investigators have shown that the earlobe crease is a modest risk factor for coronary

EBM BOX 49.1	Coronary Artery Disease*			
			Likelihood Ratio‡ if Finding Is	
Finding (Reference)†	Sensitivity (%)	Specificity (%)	Present	Absent
Patient interview				
Description of chest pain				
Classification of chest pain[17–24]				
Typical angina	50–91	78–94	**5.8**	...
Atypical angina	8–44	...	1.2	...
Nonanginal chest pain	4–22	14–50	**0.1**	...
Pain duration >30 minutes[25]	1	86	**0.1**	NS
Associated dysphagia[25]	5	80	**0.2**	NS
Other				
Male sex[22,23,26–32]	72–86	36–58	1.6	0.4
Age[23,26–28,31,33]				
<30 years	0–1	97–98	NS	...
30–49 years	16–38	...	0.6	...
50–70 years	62–73	...	1.3	...
>70 years	2–52	67–99	2.6	...
Prior myocardial infarction[22,24,28,29,31,34,35]	42–69	66–99	**3.8**	0.6
Physical examination				
Ear lobe crease[27,30,36–43]	26–80	32–96	2.1	0.5
Arcus senilis[44]	40	86	**3.0**	0.7
Chest wall tenderness[25,45–47]	1–69	16–97	0.8	NS
Ankle-to-arm pressure index <0.9[48–50]	9–26	93–97	**3.6**	NS
Laterally displaced apical impulse[51]	5	100	NS	NS
Electrocardiogram				
Normal[24,51,52]	15–33	50–69	NS	NS
ST/T wave abnormalities[17,24,35]	14–44	73–93	NS	NS

*Diagnostic standard: for *coronary artery disease*, positive myocardial perfusion scan[47] or coronary angiography reveals >50% to 75% stenosis of any epicardial vessel (all other studies).
†Definition of findings: for *classification of chest pain, earlobe crease*, and *arcus senilis*, see text.
‡Likelihood ratio (LR) if finding present = positive LR; LR if finding absent = negative LR.
NS, Not significant.

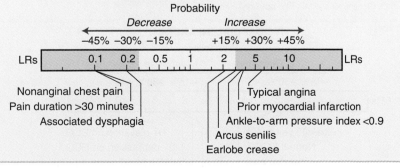

CORONARY ARTERY DISEASE
Probability
Decrease — Increase
−45% −30% −15%   +15% +30% +45%
LRs 0.1 0.2 0.5 1 2 5 10 LRs

Nonanginal chest pain
Pain duration >30 minutes
Associated dysphagia
Typical angina
Prior myocardial infarction
Ankle-to-arm pressure index <0.9
Arcus senilis
Earlobe crease

EBM BOX 49.2	**Myocardial Infarction***

Finding (Reference)[†]	Sensitivity (%)	Specificity (%)	Likelihood Ratio[‡] if Finding Is Present	Absent
Patient interview				
Male sex[53–62]	59–72	24–61	1.3	0.7
Age[53,58,59]				
<40 years	4	81	**0.2**	...
40–59 years	34	...	NS	...
≥60 years	47–74	54–68	1.5	...
Sharp or stabbing pain[58,63–66]	8–21	43–91	0.5	1.2
Pleuritic pain[58,59,63–66]	3–19	69–82	**0.3**	1.2
Positional pain[58,59,64–66]	3–43	75–87	NS	1.1
Relief of pain with nitroglycerin[67–70]	35–92	12–59	NS	NS
Physical examination				
Hand gestures[16]				
Levine sign	7	87	NS	NS
Palm sign	32	63	NS	NS
Arm sign	18	83	NS	NS
Pointing sign	2	95	NS	NS
Chest wall tenderness[58,59,63,64,66]	3–15	51–83	**0.3**	1.2
Diaphoretic appearance[59,62,63]	28–56	71–94	2.2	0.7
Pallor[62]	70	49	1.4	0.6
Systolic blood pressure <100 mm Hg[55]	6	98	**3.6**	NS
Jugular venous distension[54]	10	96	2.4	NS
Pulmonary crackles[54,63]	20–38	82–91	2.1	NS
Third heart sound[63]	16	95	**3.2**	NS
Electrocardiogram[53,55,58,62,63,65,71–76]				
Normal	1–13	48–77	**0.2**	...
Nonspecific ST changes	5–8	...	**0.2**	...
T wave inversion	9–39	...	2.0	...
ST depression	20–62	...	**3.8**	...
ST elevation	9–56	96–100	**18.4**	...

*Diagnostic standard: for *myocardial infarction*, development of new electrocardiographic Q waves, elevations of cardiac biomarkers (CK-MB or troponin), or both; except for the studies of nitroglycerin effect, which used a broader definition of "active coronary disease" that combined myocardial infarction, positive stress test, or abnormal coronary arteriogram.[67–69]

[†]Definition of findings: for *relief of pain with nitroglycerin*, nitroglycerin provided moderate or complete relief within. All electrocardiographic abnormalities refer to findings that are new or of unknown duration.

[‡]Likelihood ratio (LR) if finding present = positive LR; LR if finding absent = negative LR.

CK-MB, Creatine kinase MB; *NS,* not significant.

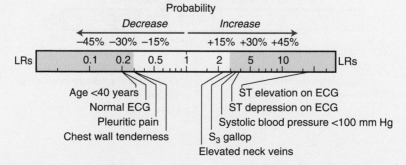

MYOCARDIAL INFARCTION
Probability

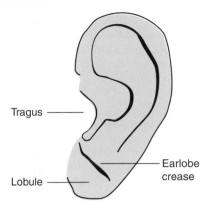

Fig. 49.1   Earlobe crease. The earlobe crease is a diagonal crease extending from the lowest point on the tragus to the outside of the earlobe. See the text.

artery disease, independent of other traditional risk factors such as hypertension, age, diabetes mellitus, family history, hyperlipidemia, obesity, and cigarette smoking.[30,36,38,78,79]

2. Arcus Senilis

Arcus senilis is a white or grayish opaque ring about the circumference of the cornea. Since the 1830s, this sign has been associated with both older age (hence, "senilis") and vascular disease (Virchow considered it a definite sign of heart disease).[80] Modern investigators[81,82] continue to suggest arcus senilis is linked to coronary disease, independent of its association with hyperlipidemia, although others challenge this view.[80]

3. Ankle-to-Arm Pressure Index

After positioning the patient supine, the clinician uses a handheld doppler stethoscope to measure the highest systolic blood pressure in the posterior tibial or dorsalis pedis artery (i.e., the "ankle" pressure). The **ankle-to-arm pressure index** represents this ankle pressure divided by the systolic pressure in the brachial artery (see Chapter 54).

E. GI COCKTAIL

For many years, clinicians working in emergency departments have mixed liquid antacids with other substances (most commonly viscous lidocaine, a topical anesthetic, and an elixir with the trade name of Donnatol, an antispasmotic) to create GI **cocktails**, which are administered orally to patients presenting with chest or upper abdominal discomfort. Because GI cocktail should act topically only on gastrointestinal mucosa, prompt relief of a patient's discomfort is said to support a gastrointestinal cause of pain (and, by inference, argue against a cardiac cause of the pain). Although antacid, lidocaine, and Donnatol are the standard ingredients of GI cocktail, some investigators have shown that antacid alone (without lidocaine or Donnatol) may relieve pain just as well.[83]

III. Clinical Significance

A. DIAGNOSING CORONARY ARTERY DISEASE

EBM Box 49.1 summarizes the accuracy of bedside findings in diagnosing coronary artery disease (based on study of more than 10,000 patients).[84] Almost all of the patients in these studies presented to outpatient clinics with intermittent chest pain, and the diagnosis of coronary artery disease was based on subsequent cardiac catheterization revealing a significant stenosis (>50 to 70% luminal narrowing) in any major epicardial vessel (i.e., single-vessel disease or worse).

According to the likelihood ratios (LRs) in EBM Box 49.1, the findings *increasing* the probability of coronary disease the most in patients with intermittent chest pain are typical angina (LR = 5.8), previous myocardial infarction (LR = 3.8), ankle-to-arm pressure index of less than 0.9 (LR = 3.6), arcus senilis (LR = 3), age older than 70 years (LR = 2.6), and a positive ear lobe crease (LR = 2.1).

These studies confirm Heberden's original impression that the key diagnostic finding in patients with chest pain is the patient's actual description of pain. Many investigators have attempted to improve on Heberden's definition of typical angina by dissecting apart the individual components of the patient's description (e.g., response to nitroglycerin or the pain's quality) or by creating complicated angina scoring schemes, but each of these attempts to improve diagnosis is less accurate than the clinician's global perception of whether the patient's pain is typical angina or not.[84]

The findings that *decrease* the probability of coronary artery disease in these studies are chest pain that is nonanginal (i.e., pain unrelated to activity, unrelieved by nitroglycerin, or otherwise not suggestive of angina, LR = 0.1), pain duration longer than 30 minutes (LR = 0.1), and associated dysphagia (LR = 0.2).

Unhelpful findings include atypical angina, chest wall tenderness, and a displaced apical impulse. Additional descriptors of the pain, such as burning pain, pain made worse by food or emotion, and radiation of the pain to the arms, are also unhelpful (i.e., they appear just as often in patients with coronary disease as in patients with noncardiac chest pain, and the LRs are not different from the value of 1).[84] Neither the Levine sign nor the palm sign affects the probability of coronary disease.[85] Interestingly, electrocardiographic findings (i.e., normal vs. abnormal, presence or absence of nonspecific ST changes) also are diagnostically unhelpful in these studies (LR not significant, EBM Box 49.1).

Assessment of the patient's traditional risk factors—hypertension, diabetes mellitus, cigarette smoking, family history, or combinations of these—carry much less diagnostic weight than the patient's description of pain. Each of these risk factors—except for cholesterol level higher than 300 mg/dL (LR = 4) and cholesterol level lower than 200 mg/dL (LR = 0.3)—has an LR between the values of 1.2 and 2.3, thus changing probability of disease little if at all.[84,86,87] Even combinations of three or more risk factors change probability of coronary disease relatively little (LR = 2.2, a value similar to the LR for the earlobe crease).[84]

B. DIAGNOSING MYOCARDIAL INFARCTION

EBM Box 49.2 summarizes the findings in thousands of patients presenting to emergency departments with sustained acute chest pain unrelated to trauma and unexplained by the chest radiograph. The diagnosis of myocardial infarction was confirmed by the development of new Q waves on the electrocardiogram, elevations of cardiac biomarkers (CK-MB or troponin), or both.

According to the LRs in Table 45.2, the finding *increasing* the probability of myocardial infarction the most are new electrocardiographic ST elevation (LR = 18.4) or ST depression (LR = 3.8). Several additional physical findings have modest value in diagnosing myocardial infarction: systolic blood pressure lower than 100 mm Hg (LR = 3.6), a third heart sound (LR = 3.2), jugular venous distention (LR = 2.4), diaphoretic appearance (LR = 2.2), and pulmonary crackles (LR = 2.1). Radiation of pain to the right arm (LR = 2.7) increases probability of myocardial infarction more than radiation to the left arm (LR = 1.5).[53,54,63-66,84,88,89] The only findings *decreasing* the probability of myocardial infarction in these studies are pain that is pleuritic (LR = 0.3), a normal electrocardiogram (LR = 0.2), chest wall tenderness (LR = 0.3), and age younger than 40 years (LR = 0.2).

In another study of 1635 patients presenting with sustained chest pain, the finding of chest wall tenderness (reproducing the patient's pain) *decreased* significantly the probability of acute coronary syndrome (i.e., myocardial infarction or unstable angina) during the next 30 days (LR = 0.1).[90]

The response to nitroglycerin fails to discriminate between cardiac and noncardiac causes of chest pain (LR not significant, EBM Box 49.2). This may reflect the temporary nature of most chest pain or perhaps the noncardiac effects of nitroglycerin. Nonetheless, even though the response to nitroglycerin lacks diagnostic value in patients with sustained chest pain, it remains a key element in the definition of typical angina. (See the previous discussion in the section on description of chest pain.)

The different hand signs also lack diagnostic value in studies of patients admitted with chest discomfort (EBM Box 49.2).

One interesting contrast between the diagnosis of coronary disease (EBM Box 49.1) and myocardial infarction (EBM Box 49.2) is that chest wall tenderness decreases the probability of myocardial infarction (LR = 0.3, EBM Box 49.2) but lacks diagnostic value when considering coronary artery disease (LR = 0.8, EBM Box 49.1). This difference may reflect a higher prevalence of chest wall disorders in patients without disease in the acute chest pain studies.

C. RISK FACTORS AND CORONARY DISEASE

In patients with sustained chest pain, the presence or absence of traditional cardiovascular risk factors again carries little or no diagnostic weight (positive LRs = 1.2 to 1.7).[84] There are two important reasons why risk factors fail to discriminate well in diagnostic studies. One, traditional cardiovascular risk factors are mostly derived from study of middle-aged white residents of Framingham, Massachusetts.[91] They may thus overestimate the risk in other populations, something that has been demonstrated in British men,[92] elderly Americans,[93] and Japanese-American, Native American, and Hispanic populations.[94] A second reason is the fundamental difference between risk factors and diagnostic signs. Risk factors precede disease, presumably play a role in causing the disease, and become apparent only after study of large groups of *asymptomatic* individuals for long periods of time. Diagnostic signs, in contrast, usually first appear after the onset of disease, are *caused by* the disease, and become evident after study of a relatively smaller group of *symptomatic* individuals. It is possible, for example, that certain risk factors associated with coronary disease are also associated with noncardiac causes of pain, which would neutralize any diagnostic value (e.g., cigarette smoking may also increase the risk of chest wall pain, making it appear just as often in patients with noncardiac pain as those with cardiac pain. The resulting LR would therefore have a value near 1).

D. GI COCKTAIL

The existing literature suggests that the GI cocktail has questionable diagnostic value. One problem is that clinicians usually administer the GI cocktail just minutes away from other active medications, such as narcotics, nitroglycerin, antiemetics, histamine blockers, or ketorolac, thus clouding interpretation of the test's results.[95] Another problem is that the viscous lidocaine is absorbed, and even though most patients have levels below 1 ug/mL (usual therapeutic levels are 2 to 5 ug/mL), instances of toxicity and seizures have occurred.[95–97] A final and most troubling problem is the many documented examples of the GI cocktail relieving the discomfort of disorders distant from the gastroesophageal mucosa, such as myocardial infarction,[96,98] hepatitis, pancreatitis, or cholecystitis.[99]

References may be accessed online at *Elsevier eBooks for Practicing Clinicians*.

Abdomen

Inspection of the Abdomen

This chapter reviews two physical signs, ecchymosis of the abdominal wall and Sister Mary Joseph nodule. Other chapters discuss jaundice (Chapter 8), dilated abdominal veins (Chapter 8), signs of malnutrition (Chapter 12), and abnormal respiratory movements of the abdominal wall (Chapter 19).

ECCHYMOSIS OF THE ABDOMINAL WALL

I. The Findings

Ecchymosis of the abdominal wall is an important sign of retroperitoneal or intraperitoneal hemorrhage. Periumbilical ecchymosis is called the **Cullen sign**, after the American pathologist and clinician who first described the finding in a patient with ectopic pregnancy in 1918.* Flank ecchymosis is often called **Grey Turner sign** or **Turner sign**, after the British surgeon Gilbert Grey Turner who described the sign in a patient with hemorrhagic pancreatitis in 1920.[1] Nonetheless, the Cullen and Turner signs are rare, occurring in less than 1% of patients with ruptured ectopic pregnancy[2] and less than 3% of patients with pancreatitis.[3] Both signs have since been described in a wide variety of other disorders, including intrahepatic hemorrhage from tumor,[4] amebic liver abscess,[5] ischemic bowel,[6] splenic rupture,[7,8] rectus sheath hematoma,[9] perforated duodenal ulcer,[10] ruptured abdominal aortic aneurysm,[11] and as complications of percutaneous liver biopsy[12] and coronary angiography.[13] Sometimes, the same patient will have both Cullen and Grey Turner signs.[14–16]

II. Pathogenesis

The discoloration of the skin is actually due to the collection of blood in the subcutaneous fascial planes, not to the dispersion of red cells within lymphatics as has been sometimes surmised.[17] In patients with pancreatitis, computed tomography often reveals collections of retroperitoneal blood

---

*Cullen was well versed in the anatomy of the umbilicus, having just 2 years earlier published his book *Embryology, Anatomy, and Diseases of the Umbilicus, Together with the Urachus*, which contained 27 chapters on the umbilicus.[32,33]

within the fascial planes behind the kidney, which may then pass to the subcutaneous tissues of the lateral abdominal wall via the lateral border of the quadratus lumborum muscle.[18] Presumably, the mechanism of the Grey Turner sign in other disorders is the same. In most patients with the Cullen sign, blood travels to the periumbilical area through the falciform ligament, which connects to the retroperitoneum via the lesser omentum and transverse mesocolon (the falciform ligament and lesser omentum are the embryologic remnants of the ventral mesentery, into which the liver has grown).

Even so, in patients with ectopic pregnancy the falciform ligament is probably not responsible for the Cullen sign, because the ecchymosis of these patients is often located on the abdominal wall below the umbilicus, yet the falciform ligament attaches to the abdominal wall above the umbilicus. Some investigators have hypothesized that fascial planes connecting the broad ligament and the lower abdominal wall are responsible for the Cullen sign in ectopic pregnancy,[18] although this does not explain why the sign sometimes appears in patients with free rupture into the peritoneal cavity outside of the broad ligament.[2]

SISTER MARY JOSEPH NODULE

I. The Finding

Sister Mary Joseph nodule is metastatic carcinoma of the umbilicus. It usually presents as a hard dermal or subcutaneous nodule and, in about 20% of patients with the lesion, it represents the initial sign of malignancy.[19] Most patients have metastatic adenocarcinoma, usually from the stomach, large bowel, ovary, or pancreas (usually the tail of the pancreas, not the head).[19–25] It is an ominous sign, with the average survival after discovery being only 10 to 11 months.[19,22]

The finding is named after Sister Mary Joseph, who, as first surgical assistant to William J. Mayo, noted the association between umbilical nodules and intraabdominal malignancy (Sister Mary Joseph was born Julia Dempsey in 1856; before Vatican II in 1965, all Franciscan nuns took the name of Mary as a prefix to an additional name).[26,27] Dr. Mayo discussed the sign as early as 1928, calling it the **pants-button umbilicus**.[28] It was not until Sir Hamilton Bailey's 1949 edition of *Physical Signs in Clinical Surgery* (10 years after Sister Mary Joseph's death) that the term **Sister Joseph nodule** was used.[29] A mimic of the Sister Mary Joseph nodule is an omphalith, which is the hardened concretion of keratin and sebum in the umbilicus from inadequate hygiene.[30] Careful examination of these patients, however, manages to extract the debris.

II. Pathogenesis

There are many potential avenues of spread to the umbilicus: vascular and lymphatic connections to the retroperitoneum, axilla, and inguinal regions, and embryologic remnants that connect the umbilicus to the bladder and retroperitoneum.[31] Nonetheless, the umbilicus and periumbilical tissues represent the thinnest part of the abdominal wall, and in one series of patients, direct spread from peritoneal tumor implants through the abdominal wall was the most common cause of the umbilical nodule.[19]

References may be accessed online at *Elsevier eBooks for Practicing Clinicians.*

Palpation and Percussion
of the Abdomen

I. Introductory Comments on Technique

Palpation of the abdomen may reveal abnormal tenderness, tumors, hernias, aneurysms, or organomegaly (i.e., of the liver, spleen, or gallbladder). To help the patient relax and to minimize pain during palpation, experienced clinicians recommend that the clinician's hands should be warm, the technique soft and gentle, and the expected tender areas palpated last. Other maneuvers designed to help the patient relax include drawing up the patient's knees, encouraging deep breathing, and engaging the patient in conversation.

In the days before clinical imaging, palpation of a relaxed abdomen was so essential that patients with tense abdominal muscles were often reexamined after immersion in a hot bath or after anesthesia had been induced with ether or chloroform, to determine whether an abnormality was present or not.[1]

II. Liver

A. LIVER SPAN

1. The Finding

The liver span is the distance in centimeters between the upper border of the liver in the right midclavicular line (as determined by percussion, i.e., where lung resonance changes to liver dullness) and the lower border (as determined by either percussion or palpation). Clinicians have been measuring the liver span ever since Piorry introduced topographic percussion in 1828,[2] although after introduction of the x-ray it became apparent that the estimated span often differed from the actual span, leading most clinicians to adopt the view that the percussed liver span was just an index of liver size, not a precise measurement.[3]

2. Clinical Significance

The clinician's assessment of liver span almost always underestimates the actual value. Clinicians place the upper border too low (2 to 5 cm)[4,5] and lower border too high (more than 2 cm in about half of patients),[4,6] except in patients with chronic obstructive lung disease, in whom the error with the top border is less.[4] The liver span is the same whether the patient is percussed during quiet respirations or full held expiration.[7]

Nonetheless, most studies of liver percussion make two points: (1) The estimated span does correlate modestly with actual span, as determined by ultrasonography or scintigraphy (r = 0.6 to 0.7).[3,5,6,8,9] This correlation is much better in patients with diseased livers than in those with healthy livers.[5,8] (2) The percussed liver span is very dependent on the clinician's technique, and consequently, one clinician's "normal liver span" is not the same as another's. The heavier the clinician's percussion stroke, the smaller the measured span and the greater the error in underestimating the actual liver size (see also Chapter 29).[4,7] This explains why published estimates of the "normal liver span" range from as low as 6 cm to as high as 15 cm* [6,9,11–13] and why experienced clinicians, each examining the same patient, differ in their estimate of the patient's span, *on average*, by 8 cm.[14]

These comments imply that each clinician could determine his or her own "normal liver span," based on examination of hundreds of healthy persons, and then use this span as a benchmark to indicate whether a patient's span is abnormally large or not. Nonetheless, two studies applying a standardized percussion technique failed to accurately detect hepatomegaly (likelihood ratio [LR] not significant, see EBM Box 51.1).

B. PALPABLE LIVER EDGE

1. The Finding

To palpate the liver edge, the clinician begins by gently palpating the patient's right lower quadrant. As the patient breathes in and out, the clinician moves the palpating hand upward 1 to 2 cm at a time, at each location searching for a liver edge that moves down during inspiration and strikes the clinician's fingers. Once the edge is located, the clinician should note its consistency (a cirrhotic liver is firmer than a healthy one)[8] and whether the edge has any irregularities or masses.[30]

Anatomically, the normal liver extends on average 4 to 5 cm below the right costal margin at the midclavicular line.[5,31]

2. Clinical Significance

a. Detection of Hepatomegaly

If clinicians palpate what they believe is the patient's liver edge extending below the costal margin, they are virtually always correct (LR = 233.7, EBM Box 51.1). Nonetheless, the distance between the liver edge and costal margin correlates poorly with overall liver size, and the finding of a palpable liver edge is an unreliable sign of hepatomegaly (LR only 1.9; EBM Box 51.1). Moreover, approximately half of livers that extend below the costal margin are not palpable.[8,16] The *consistency* of the liver parenchyma probably determines in part whether a liver is palpable, because in patients with cirrhosis, whose livers are smaller but firmer than normal, the liver's edge is palpable 95% of the time.[8]

---

*The normal upper limit for the cephalocaudad dimension of the liver on ultrasonography, from its lower border in the midclavicular line to its upper margin with the lung, is 13 cm.[10]

EBM BOX 51.1	Detection of Enlarged Liver and Spleen*				
				Likelihood Ratio‡ if Finding Is	
Finding (Reference)†	Sensitivity (%)	Specificity (%)		Present	Absent
Liver					
Percussion span ≥10 cm in MCL					
Detecting enlarged liver[6,15]	61–92	30–43		NS	NS
Palpable liver					
Detecting liver edge below costal margin[16]	48	100		**233.7**	0.5
Detecting enlarged liver[15,17–19]	39–71	56–85		1.9	0.6
Spleen					
Palpable spleen					
Detecting enlarged spleen[17,18,20–28]	18–78	89–99		**8.5**	0.6
Splenic percussion signs					
Detecting enlarged spleen[21,22,26–29]					
Spleen percussion sign	25–85	32–94		1.7	0.7
Nixon method	25–66	68–95		2.0	0.7
Traube's space dullness	11–76	63–95		2.1	0.8

*Diagnostic standard: for *enlarged liver*, liver enlarged by scintigraphy,[17,19] craniocaudal span >13 cm by ultrasonography,[6,15] or postmortem weight of liver >2000 g[18]; for *enlarged spleen*, spleen enlarged by ultrasonography,[22,25–29] scintigraphy,[17,20,21,23] or postmortem weight >200 g[18] or >250 g.[24]

†Definition of findings: for *percussed liver span*, using light percussion technique; for *splenic percussion signs*, see text.

‡Likelihood ratio (LR) if finding present = positive LR; LR if finding absent = negative LR.

MCL, Midclavicular line; *NS*, not significant.

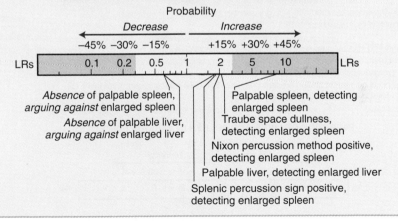

DETECTION OF ENLARGED LIVER AND SPLEEN

Probability

Decrease | *Increase*

−45% −30% −15%   +15% +30% +45%

LRs | 0.1   0.2   0.5   1   2   5   10 | LRs

Absence of palpable spleen, *arguing against* enlarged spleen

Absence of palpable liver, *arguing against* enlarged liver

Palpable spleen, detecting enlarged spleen

Traube space dullness, detecting enlarged spleen

Nixon percussion method positive, detecting enlarged spleen

Palpable liver, detecting enlarged liver

Splenic percussion sign positive, detecting enlarged spleen

b. Palpable Liver and Other Disorders

In patients with chronic liver disease, a few findings modestly increase the probability of cirrhosis: enlarged palpable liver edge (LR = 2.3, EBM Box 51.2), palpable liver in the epigastrium (LR = 2.7), and a liver edge that is unusually firm (LR = 3.3). In patients with jaundice, the

| EBM BOX 51.2 | Palpation of Liver and Spleen in Various Disorders* |

Finding (Reference)	Sensitivity (%)	Specificity (%)	Likelihood Ratio)† if Finding Is Present	Absent
Liver				
Enlarged palpable liver in patients with chronic liver disease, detecting cirrhosis[32–39]	31–96	20–96	2.3	0.6
Palpable liver in epigastrium in patients with chronic liver disease, detecting cirrhosis[37,39]	50–86	68–88	2.7	**0.3**
Liver edge firm to palpation in patients with chronic liver disease, detecting cirrhosis[33,36,40]	71–78	71–90	**3.3**	0.4
Palpable liver in patients with jaundice, detecting hepatocellular disease (nonobstructive jaundice)[41,42]	71–83	15–17	NS	NS
Liver tenderness in patients with jaundice, detecting hepatocellular disease (nonobstructive jaundice)[41,42]	37–38	70–78	NS	NS
Palpable liver in patients with lymphadenopathy, detecting serious disease[43,44]	14–16	86–89	NS	NS
Spleen				
Palpable spleen in returning travelers with fever, detecting malaria[45–47]	19–25	95–98	**6.5**	0.8
Palpable spleen in patients with jaundice, detecting hepatocellular disease (nonobstructive jaundice)[41,42]	29–47	83–90	2.9	0.7
Palpable spleen in patients with chronic liver disease, detecting cirrhosis[33–39,48–51]	5–85	35–100	2.5	0.8
Palpable spleen in patients with lymphadenopathy, detecting serious disease[43,44,52]	5–10	92–96	NS	NS
Palpable spleen in patients with fever of unknown origin, predicting diagnostic bone marrow examination.[53–55]	35–53	82–89	2.9	0.7

*Diagnostic standard: for *nonobstructive (vs. obstructive) jaundice*, needle biopsy of liver, surgical exploration, or autopsy; for *cirrhosis*, needle biopsy of liver (see Chapter 8); for *serious disease* (in patients with lymphadenopathy), see Chapter 27.
†Likelihood ratio (LR) if finding present = positive LR; LR if finding absent = negative LR.
MCL, Midclavicular line; *NS*, not significant.

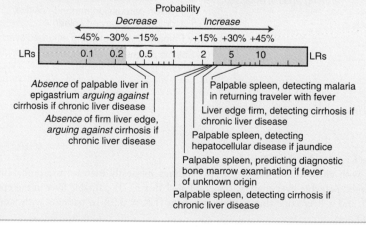

PALPATION OF LIVER AND SPLEEN IN VARIOUS DISORDERS

findings of a palpable liver and liver tenderness are unhelpful, both appearing equally often in patients with hepatocellular disease (i.e., nonobstructive jaundice) as in those with obstructive jaundice (LR not significant, see Chapter 8). In patients with lymphadenopathy, the finding of palpable liver fails to distinguish those with serious infections and malignancies from those with benign self-limited disorders (LR not significant, see Chapter 27).

The clinician's assessment of stiffness or firmness of the liver, determined by palpation, correlates well with noninvasive measures of liver fibrosis, such as ultrasound-based elastography.[56]

C. AUSCULTATORY PERCUSSION – SCRATCH TEST

1. The Finding

Auscultatory percussion (see also Chapter 29) is frequently used to locate the lower border of the liver. According to traditional teachings, the moment the clinician's percussing digit crosses the border of the liver and begins to strike abdominal wall over the liver, the sound heard through the stethoscope becomes louder.

Nonetheless, the lack of consensus on the proper technique of locating the liver will quickly discourage the serious student of auscultatory percussion. Various experts recommend placing the stethoscope on the xiphoid,[4,57] near the umbilicus,[58] superior to[59] or at the costal margin,[60] at four separate positions over the liver,[61] or above the suspected center.[62] According to various authorities, the clinician should percuss with a finger and pleximeter,[62] a finger alone,[59] a bristle brush,[61] or a corrugated rod.[61] The direction of the stroke should be circular,[1] centripetal,[62] centrifugal,[61] left to right,[60] or always in a longitudinal axis and toward the liver.[4,59]

2. Clinical Significance

The evidence supporting auscultatory percussion of the liver is mixed and meager. Two studies support the technique's accuracy, showing that 78% to 82% of estimates of the lower border are within 2 cm of the actual border (by ultrasonography),[31,59] whereas a third study demonstrated only 37% of estimates from the scratch test within 2 cm from actual edge.[63] Another study showed that palpation of the liver was more accurate than auscultatory percussion.[4] A final study showed that there was no correlation whatsoever between the distance of the liver edge below the costal margin, located by auscultatory percussion, and the actual distance (by ultrasonography) for any of 11 different examiners.[57]

D. PULSATILE LIVER

The finding of a pulsatile liver has been described in tricuspid regurgitation with high pulmonary pressures (see Chapter 46) and constrictive pericarditis.[64,65] In patients with the holosystolic murmur of tricuspid regurgitation, the finding of a pulsatile liver increases the probability that the regurgitation is moderate-to-severe (LR = 6.5, see EBM Box 46.1).

III. The Spleen

A. PALPABLE SPLEEN

1. The Finding

Experts recommend many different ways to palpate the spleen: some palpate from the patient's right side, and others from the patient's left side (curling the fingers over the costal margin to "hook" the spleen edge); some position the patient supine, others position the patient supine with the patient's left fist under his or her left posterior chest, and still others position the patient in the right lateral decubitus position. One study comparing the different positions found all three to be equivalent[22]; the approach clinicians use probably depends most on personal preference.

2. Clinical Significance

a. Detection of Splenomegaly

EBM Box 51.1 indicates that the finding of a palpable spleen increases greatly the probability of splenomegaly (LR = 8.5, EBM Box 51.1). Although many enlarged spleens are not palpable (median sensitivity is only 51%; range, 18% to 78%), virtually all massively enlarged spleens (i.e., weight >1 kg or scintigraphic span >22 cm) are detectable by palpation.[24,66]

b. Etiology of Splenomegaly

The common causes of splenomegaly are hepatic disease (i.e., portal hypertension), hematologic disorders (e.g., leukemias, lymphomas, myelofibrosis), infectious disease (e.g., HIV infection), and primary splenic disorders (e.g., splenic infarction or hematoma).[67,68] The presence of left upper quadrant tenderness and pain increases the probability of a primary splenic disorder or hematologic disorder.[68] Associated lymphadenopathy practically excludes hepatic disease and points to one of the other disorders (LR = 0.1).[68,69] The finding of massive splenomegaly (i.e., spleen extends to level of umbilicus) increases the probability of underlying hematologic disease (LR = 2.8).[68–71]

c. Palpable Spleen and Other Disorders

In returning travelers from tropical countries who are febrile, the finding of a palpable spleen significantly increases the probability of malaria (LR = 6.5, EBM Box 51.2). In patients with jaundice, the palpable spleen modestly increases probability of hepatocellular disease (i.e., nonobstructive jaundice, LR = 2.9, see Chapter 8), and in patients with chronic liver disease a palpable spleen increases probability of cirrhosis (LR = 2.5). In patients with lymphadenopathy, a palpable spleen is found just as often in patients with serious infections and malignancies as in those with benign, self-limited disorders (LR not significant, see Chapter 27). In patients with fever of unknown origin (i.e., unexplained fever lasting more than 3 weeks), the finding of a palpable spleen increases probability that a bone marrow biopsy will be diagnostic (LR = 2.9).

B. SPLENIC PERCUSSION SIGNS

1. The Findings

There are three commonly used splenic percussion signs:

a. Spleen Percussion Sign

Castell described this sign in 1967,[12] finding it a useful way to measure splenic size in patients with infectious mononucleosis. The clinician percusses the lowest left intercostal space in the anterior axillary line (usually the eighth or ninth); if the percussion note in this location, usually resonant, becomes dull with a full inspiration, the test is positive. Since Castell's original description, other investigators have regarded any dullness at this location as a positive response (i.e., whether during inspiration or expiration).

b. Nixon Method

Nixon described this sign in 1954,[72] finding it accurate in his experience of 60 splenic aspiration biopsies. The patient is positioned in the right lateral decubitus position, and the clinician percusses from the lower level of pulmonary resonance in the posterior axillary line downwards obliquely to the lower midanterior costal margin. The test is positive if the border of dullness on this line lies more than 8 cm from the costal margin.

c. Traube Space Dullness

Traube's space is the triangular space, normally tympanic, that is over the left lower anterior part of the chest. Its upper border is marked by the limits of cardiac dullness (usually the sixth rib), its lower border is the costal margin, and its lateral border is the anterior axillary line. Although Traube suggested that dullness in this space was a sign of pleural effusion,[73] Parrino in 1987 suggested that it could be a sign of splenic enlargement.[74]

2. Clinical Significance

Positive percussion signs are less convincing (positive LRs = 1.7 to 2.1; see EBM Box 51.1) than the technique of palpation. Traube's space dullness becomes even less accurate in overweight patients or those who have recently eaten.[75]

IV. Gallbladder: Courvoisier Sign

A. THE FINDING

The Courvoisier sign is a *palpable nontender* gallbladder in a patient with *jaundice*, a finding that has been traditionally associated with malignant obstruction of the biliary system. Many textbooks call the sign **Courvoisier law**, as if the positive result were pathognomonic of malignancy, although the Swiss surgeon Courvoisier originally presented the finding in 1890 as only an interesting observation.[76] Writing in a monograph on biliary tract disorders, he stated that, among 187 patients with jaundice and common duct obstruction, a dilated gallbladder was found in only 20% of patients with stones, compared with 92% of patients having other disorders, mostly malignancy.[77]

B. CLINICAL SIGNIFICANCE

Summarizing the information about Courvoisier sign is difficult because various authors define the sign differently. Some apply it to patients without jaundice (clearly not what Courvoisier intended)[78]; others define the positive sign as any palpable gallbladder, whether tender or nontender (some patients with cholecystitis have tender enlarged gallbladders)[79-81]; and still others expand the positive sign to include a dilated gallbladder discovered during surgery, clinical imaging, or even autopsy.[82]

Restricting analysis to those studies defining the positive sign as a palpable gallbladder in a jaundice patient, EBM Box 51.3 indicates that Courvoisier sign is pathognomonic for extrahepatic obstruction of the biliary system (i.e., stones or malignancy, LR = 26; i.e., *not* hepatocellular jaundice). Among patients with biliary obstruction, however, the sign increases probability only modestly for malignancy and against stones (LR = 2.6). In another series of 86 hospitalized patients with distended gallbladders (as detected by computed tomography or at laparotomy), only 46 (53%) were palpable at the bedside: 83% had a malignant cause of the obstruction, 17% a benign one.[94]

Consequently, if there is a "law" to the Courvoisier sign, it is that the palpable gallbladder in a jaundiced patient indicates extrahepatic obstruction, not that the obstruction is necessarily caused by malignancy.

C. PATHOGENESIS

Courvoisier's original hypothesis—that the gallbladder of choledocholithiasis resists dilation because its walls are fibrotic from chronic cholecystitis—is probably incorrect, because experiments with gallbladders of jaundiced patients show that both dilated and nondilated gallbladders have similar wall stiffness.[95] Instead, patients with dilated gallbladders differ from patients without

| EBM BOX 51.3 | **Palpation of Gallbladder, Bladder, and Aorta*** |

Finding (Reference)	Sensitivity (%)	Specificity (%)	Likelihood Ratio[†] if Finding Is	
			Present	Absent
Gallbladder				
Palpable gallbladder				
Detecting obstructed bile ducts in patients with jaundice[41]	31	99	**26.0**	0.7
Detecting malignant obstruction in patients with obstructive jaundice[41,78,80,83]	26–55	83–90	2.6	0.7
Bladder				
Palpable bladder				
Detecting ≥400 mL urine in bladder[84]	82	56	1.9	**0.3**
Aorta				
Expansile pulsating epigastric mass				
Detecting AAA[85-93]	22–69	75–99	**8.4**	0.6

*Diagnostic standard: for *obstructive jaundice* and *malignant obstruction*, needle biopsy of liver, surgical exploration, or autopsy; for *≥400 mL urine in bladder*, bladder ultrasound[84]; for *abdominal aortic aneurysm*, ultrasonography revealing focal dilation of infrarenal aorta >3 cm in diameter,[86,87,89-93] >4 cm in diameter,[88] or >1.5 cm larger than proximal aorta.[85]
[†]Likelihood ratio (LR) if finding present = positive LR; LR if finding absent = negative LR.
AAA, Abdominal aortic aneurysm; *NS*, not significant.

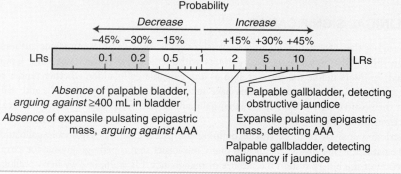

PALPATION OF GALLBLADDER, BLADDER, AND AORTA

dilated gallbladders in two important ways: Dilated gallbladders are associated with much higher operative intraductal pressures and longer duration of jaundice.

The relationship between duration of jaundice and dilation of gallbladder explains why Courvoisier's original findings are different from the studies in EBM Box 51.3. When analysis is restricted to just those patients with extrahepatic obstruction, the sensitivity of the dilated gallbladder in malignant obstruction today (25% to 55%) is lower than it was for Courvoisier (i.e., 92%) (although the specificity is similar at 80% to 90%). The reduced sensitivity may simply reflect the fact that patients with malignant obstruction today, compared with those from a century ago, are diagnosed more quickly using clinical imaging, before pressures increase enough to enlarge the gallbladder greatly.

V. Bladder Volume

For over a century, clinicians have investigated percussing the suprapubic area to detect bladder volume, most studies revealing that the bladder volume must be approximately 400 to 600 mL before dullness reliably appears.[96] Although the extent of dullness above the symphysis pubis does correlate with bladder volume,[96,97] the sign is overall unreliable because the results vary tremendously among individual patients and because many patients have inexplicable dullness of the lower abdomen, even without bladder distention.[2,96]

There are few studies of palpation of the bladder. One study has demonstrated that the *absence* of a palpable bladder in the suprapubic area *decreases* the probability of bladder volumes ≥400 mL (LR = 0.3, EBM Box 51.3).[84]

VI. Ascites

A. THE FINDINGS

In supine patients with ascites, peritoneal fluid gravitates to the flanks and air-filled intestines float to occupy the periumbilical space. This distribution of fluid and air causes four characteristic signs of ascites: (1) **Bulging flanks**; (2) **Flank dullness**. Flank dullness is positive if there is a *horizontal* border between dullness in the flank area and resonance (or tympany) in the periumbilical area. (3) **Shifting dullness**. Shifting dullness describes flank dullness whose position shifts as the patient changes position, usually by rolling on to one side. The sign is based on the principle that air-filled loops of intestine, floating on peritoneal fluid, move to the uppermost position in the abdomen. In a patient with a positive response, the border between resonance and dullness shifts away from the side that is most dependent. To be positive, the shifting border should remain horizontal. (4) **Fluid wave**. To elicit the fluid wave, the clinician places one hand against the lateral wall of the abdomen and uses the other hand to tap firmly on the opposite lateral wall. In the positive response, the tap generates a wave that is transmitted through the abdomen and felt as a sudden shock by the other hand. Since a false-positive response may result from waves travelling through the subcutaneous tissue of the anterior abdominal wall, the clinician should always use the patient's hand or that of an assistant to apply firm pressure against the anterior abdominal wall.

In addition to these four signs, most patients with ascites also have edema, from hypoalbuminemia and the weight of the peritoneal fluid compressing the veins to the legs.[98]

B. PATHOGENESIS

In experiments with cadavers performed over a century ago, Müller showed that 1000 mL of fluid injected into the peritoneal space was undetectable by physical examination (i.e., flank or shifting dullness), 1500 mL resulted in some flank dullness, and 2000 mL was the smallest volume to cause shifting dullness.[96] The living abdominal wall is probably more elastic than the cadaver's, and it is likely that the careful clinician can detect smaller amounts of ascites in patients, but one small study of healthy volunteers still showed that injection of 500 to 1100 mL of fluid was necessary before shifting dullness appeared.[99] A significant cause of false-positive flank dullness or shifting dullness is accumulation of fluid within loops of the colon.[99,100] This condition, called *pseudoascites* in the days before clinical imaging,[100] typically occurred in patients with diarrheal illnesses.

C. CLINICAL SIGNIFICANCE

In patients with abdominal distention, the findings *increasing* probability of ascites the most are the positive fluid wave (LR = 5, EBM Box 51.4) and presence of edema (LR = 3.8). The findings *decreasing* probability of ascites the most are *absence* of edema (LR = 0.2) and *absence* of flank dullness (LR = 0.3). Shifting dullness shifts probability of ascites modestly upward when present (LR = 2.3) and modestly downward when absent (LR = 0.4). Findings having relatively little diagnostic value are positive flank dullness, positive bulging flanks, and negative fluid wave. The finding of a flat or everted umbilicus was also diagnostically unhelpful in one study.[102]

Auscultatory percussion also has been recommended to detect ascites,[104-106] although only the puddle sign (auscultatory percussion of the prone patient) has been formally tested,[101,102] proving to be diagnostically unhelpful.

EBM BOX 51.4	Ascites*			

Finding (Reference)[†]	Sensitivity (%)	Specificity (%)	Likelihood Ratio[‡] if Finding Is Present	Absent
Inspection				
Bulging flanks[101-103]	73–93	44–70	1.9	0.4
Edema[102]	87	77	**3.8**	**0.2**
Palpation and percussion				
Flank dullness[101,102]	80–94	29–69	NS	**0.3**
Shifting dullness[101-103]	60–87	56–90	2.3	0.4
Fluid wave[101-103]	50–80	82–92	**5.0**	0.5

*Diagnostic standard: for *ascites*, peritoneal fluid by ultrasonography.
[†]Definition of findings: for *shifting dullness*, border between resonance and dullness "shifts" when patient rolls from supine to left lateral decubitus position or right lateral decubitus position; Cattau required a shift in both positions,[101] Simel in only 1 of 2 positions,[102] and Cummings used only the right lateral decubitus position at 45 degrees and required a shift >1 cm.[103]
[‡]Likelihood ratio (LR) if finding present = positive LR; LR if finding absent = negative LR.
NS, Not significant.

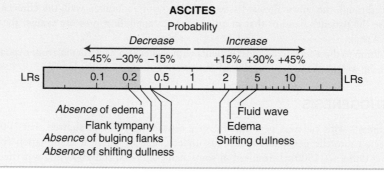

ASCITES
Probability

VII. Abdominal Aortic Aneurysm

A. INTRODUCTION

Abdominal aortic aneurysm is a focal ballooning of the infrarenal abdominal aorta, traditionally defined as a diameter greater than 3 to 4 cm. It is a disorder of elderly patients, affecting 1% to 2% of patients over the age of 50.[107,108] Abdominal aortic aneurysms tend to enlarge slowly, but some rupture catastrophically with an overall mortality of up to 90%.[109]

B. THE FINDING

Because the normal aorta bifurcates at the level of the umbilicus, palpable aortic aneurysms are found usually in the epigastrium or left upper quadrant. The clinician should place one hand on each side of the aorta and measure its diameter, subtracting the estimated thickness of two layers of skin and subcutaneous tissue. Most studies do not specifically define the positive finding (instead stating simply the positive finding is "aortic aneurysm present by palpation"), although others define it as an estimated diameter greater than 3 cm using the previously described method.[86]

Importantly, an aortic aneurysm pushes the two hands *apart*, a finding called *expansile* pulsation.[110] Other prominent epigastric pulsations sometimes occur in patients with thin abdomens or in those with epigastric masses overlying the normal aorta, but unless these pulsations are expansile, they do not indicate an aneurysm.

C. CLINICAL SIGNIFICANCE

According to EBM Box 51.3, the finding of a palpable epigastric pulsation suggestive of aneurysm increases probability that one is present (LR = 8.4; see EBM Box 51.3). In contrast, the absence of this finding is much less helpful (LR is only 0.6), simply because the sensitivity for the finding is as low as 22% (i.e., up to 78% of patients with aneurysms lack a prominent pulsation).

The two most important variables governing whether an aneurysm is palpable are the size of the aneurysm and the patient's abdominal girth. Aneurysms between 3 and 5 cm in diameter are difficult to detect, and if *aneurysm* is instead defined as a focal bulging more than 5 cm in diameter—a diameter approaching the threshold for surgical repair—the sensitivity of bedside examination increases to over 80% in almost all series.[86,108,111] Aneurysms are also more difficult to detect in patients with larger abdominal girths.[85,86,111,112] After restricting the analysis to just patients with abdominal girth of less than 100 cm (measured at the umbilicus)[85,86] or to patients in whom the clinician can palpate the aorta,[86,112,113] the sensitivity of the examination exceeds 88% in all studies. These results indicate that the negative examination decreases probability of an aneurysm of more than 5 cm in diameter, especially if the patient has a girth of less than 100 cm or has a palpable aorta.

The most common cause for a false-positive examination is an abnormally tortuous aorta.[114,115] Rare causes are a horseshoe kidney, intraabdominal tumor, or paraaortic adenopathy.[114,115]

References may be accessed online at *Elsevier eBooks for Practicing Clinicians.*

Abdominal Pain and Tenderness

- In patients with acute abdominal pain, the findings of rigidity, guarding, and percussion tenderness increase the probability of peritonitis. All three of these findings are more accurate than is rebound tenderness.
- In patients with right lower abdominal pain, McBurney point tenderness, and an Alvarado score of 7 or more *increases* the probability of appendicitis; an Alvarado score of 4 or less *decreases* the probability of appendicitis.
- In patients with acute abdominal pain, the administration of analgesics does not diminish the accuracy of bedside signs for appendicitis.
- In patients with acute abdominal pain, visible peristalsis, a distended abdomen, and hyperactive bowel sounds all increase the probability of bowel obstruction.
- In patients with acute or chronic abdominal pain, the positive abdominal wall tenderness test *decreases* the probability of intraabdominal pathology.

ACUTE ABDOMINAL PAIN

I. Introduction

Among patients presenting with acute abdominal pain and tenderness (i.e., pain lasting less than 7 days), the most common diagnoses are nonspecific abdominal pain (31% to 43% of patients), acute appendicitis (4% to 20%), acute cholecystitis (3% to 11%), small bowel obstruction (4% to 7%), and ureterolithiasis (3% to 4%).[1-5] The term *acute abdomen* usually refers to those conditions causing abrupt abdominal pain and tenderness and requiring urgent diagnosis and surgical intervention, such as appendicitis, bowel obstruction, and perforated intraabdominal organs.

Although many patients with the acute abdomen undergo computed tomography (to distinguish perforation, abscess, and appendicitis from alternative disorders), bedside diagnosis remains a fundamental diagnostic tool in all patients with the acute abdomen.[6] Based just on the bedside findings, some patients can be safely discharged home without further imaging because the probability of peritonitis is so low, whereas others should proceed directly to the operating room because the probability of peritonitis is so high.[7] Those patients whose bedside findings are equivocal or suggest abscess formation benefit the most from further imaging.[8]

II. The Findings

The two most common causes of the acute abdomen are (1) **peritonitis** from inflammation (appendicitis, cholecystitis) or perforation of a viscus (appendix, peptic ulcer of stomach or duodenum, diverticulum) and (2) **bowel obstruction**. Both peritonitis and obstruction cause abdominal tenderness. Additional findings are discussed below.

A. PERITONITIS

The additional findings of peritonitis are guarding and rigidity, rebound tenderness, percussion tenderness, a positive cough test, and a *negative* abdominal wall tenderness test.

1. Guarding and Rigidity

Guarding refers to the *voluntary contraction* of the abdominal wall musculature, usually the result of fear, anxiety, or the laying on of cold hands.[9] Rigidity refers to the *involuntary contraction* of the abdominal musculature in response to peritoneal inflammation, a reflex that the patient cannot control.[9] Experienced surgeons distinguish these two findings by (1) distracting the patient during examination (e.g., engaging the patient in conversation or using the stethoscope to palpate the abdomen gently)[10,11] and (2) examining the patient repeatedly over time. Guarding, but not rigidity, diminishes with distraction and fluctuates in intensity or even disappears over time.

The first clinician to clearly describe rigidity was the Roman physician Celsus, writing in 30 AD.[12]

2. Rebound Tenderness

To elicit rebound tenderness, the clinician maintains pressure over an area of tenderness and then withdraws the hand abruptly. If the patient winces with pain upon withdrawal of the hand, the test is positive. Many expert surgeons discourage using the rebound tenderness test, regarding it "unnecessary,"[9,13] "cruel,"[6] or a "popular and somewhat unkind way of emphasizing what is already obvious."[14]

Rebound tenderness was originally described by J. Moritz Blumberg (1873–1955), a German surgeon and gynecologist, who believed that pain in the lower abdomen after abrupt withdrawal of the hand from the *left* lower abdominal quadrant was a sign of appendicitis (i.e., Blumberg sign).[15]

3. Percussion Tenderness

In patients with peritonitis, sudden movements of the abdominal wall cause pain, such as those produced during abdominal percussion. Percussion tenderness is present if light percussion causes pain.

4. Cough Test

The cough test is based on the same principle as percussion tenderness (i.e., jarring movements of the abdominal wall cause pain in patients with peritonitis). The cough test is positive if the patient, in response to a cough, shows signs of pain, such as flinching, grimacing, or moving hands toward the abdomen.[16]

5. Abdominal Wall Tenderness Test

In 1926 Carnett introduced the abdominal wall tenderness test[17] as a way to diagnose lesions in the abdominal wall that cause abdominal pain and tenderness and sometimes mimic peritonitis. In this test, the clinician locates the area of maximal tenderness by gentle palpation and then applies enough pressure to elicit moderate tenderness. The patient is then asked to fold the arms on the chest and lift the head and shoulders, as if performing a partial sit-up. If this maneuver causes increased tenderness at the site of palpation, the test is positive,[18] suggesting the origin of pain is the abdominal wall, not the peritoneal cavity. In patients with peritonitis or serious intra-abdominal pathology, this maneuver should decrease the tenderness because tense abdominal wall muscles are protecting the peritoneum from the clinician's hands.

One well-recognized cause of acute abdominal wall tenderness is diabetic neuropathy (i.e., thoracoabdominal neuropathy involving nerve roots T7-T11; lesions of T1-T6 cause chest pain).[19–21] In addition to a positive abdominal wall tenderness test, characteristic signs of this disorder are cutaneous hypersensitivity, often of contiguous dermatomes, and weakness of the abdominal muscles causing ipsilateral bulging of the abdominal wall that resembles a hernia.[20–22]

B. APPENDICITIS

1. McBurney Point Tenderness

In a paper read before the New York Surgical Society in 1889, citing the advantages of early operation in appendicitis, Charles McBurney stated that all patients with appendicitis have maximal pain and tenderness "determined by the pressure of the finger (at a point) very exactly between an inch and a half and two inches from the anterior superior spinous process of the ilium on a straight line drawn from that process to the umbilicus."[23–25]

2. Rovsing Sign (Indirect Tenderness)

Rovsing sign (Neils T. Rovsing, 1862–1927, Danish surgeon) is positive when pressure over the patient's *left* lower quadrant causes pain in the right lower quadrant.[9] Rovsing believed that firm pressure in the left abdomen would force gas backward to the splenic flexure and through the transverse colon to the cecum, where the extra distension would produce pain in the right lower quadrant if the appendix is inflamed.[26]

3. Rectal Tenderness

In patients with appendicitis and inflammation confined to the pelvis, rectal examination may reveal tenderness, especially on the right side; additionally, some patients with perforation may have a rectal mass (i.e., pelvic abscess).

4. Psoas Sign

The inflamed appendix may lie against the right psoas muscle, causing the patient to shorten that muscle by drawing up the right knee. To elicit the psoas sign, the patient lies down on the left side and the clinician hyperextends the right hip. Painful hip extension is the positive response.[9,13]

5. Obturator Sign

The obturator sign is based on the same principle as the psoas sign, that stretching a pelvic muscle irritated by an inflamed appendix causes pain. To stretch the right obturator internus muscle and elicit the sign, the clinician flexes the patient's right hip and knee and then internally rotates the right hip.[9,13]

C. CHOLECYSTITIS AND MURPHY SIGN

Patients with acute cholecystitis present with continuous epigastric or right upper quadrant pain, nausea, and vomiting. The traditional physical signs are fever, right upper quadrant tenderness, and a positive **Murphy sign**. In 1903, the American surgeon Charles Murphy stated that the hypersensitive gallbladder of cholecystitis prevents the patient from taking in a "full, deep inspiration when the clinician's fingers are hooked up beneath the right costal arch below the hepatic margin. The diaphragm forces the liver down until the sensitive gallbladder reaches the examining fingers, when the inspiration suddenly ceases as though it had been shut off."[27]

Most clinicians elicit the Murphy sign by palpating the right upper quadrant of the supine patient. In his original description, Murphy proposed other methods, such as the **deep-grip**

palpation technique, in which the clinician examines the seated patient from behind and curls the fingertips of his or her right hand under the right costal margin, and the **hammer stroke percussion technique,** in which the clinician strikes a finger pointed into the right upper quadrant with the ulnar aspect of the other hand.[27]

D. SMALL BOWEL OBSTRUCTION

Small bowel obstruction presents with abdominal pain and vomiting. The traditional physical signs are abdominal distention and tenderness, visible peristalsis, and abnormal bowel sounds (initially, high-pitched tickling sounds followed by diminished or absent bowel sounds).[9,13] Signs of peritonitis (e.g., rigidity, rebound) may appear if portions of the bowel become ischemic.

III. Clinical Significance

EBM Boxes 52.1 through 52.4 present the physical findings of the acute abdomen. Two of the EBM Boxes (52.1 and 52.4) apply to *all* patients with acute abdominal pain, addressing diagnosis of peritonitis (EBM Box 52.1) or small bowel obstruction (EBM Box 52.4) (many of these pooled likelihood ratio [LR] estimates are based on more than 6000 patients). EBM Box 52.2 addresses bedside findings specific for appendicitis (i.e., focusing on patients with right lower quadrant pain), whereas EBM Box 52.3 applies to patients with right upper quadrant pain and suspected cholecystitis.

A. PERITONITIS

In the studies reviewed in EBM Box 52.1, the principal cause of peritonitis was appendicitis, although some patients had perforated ulcers, perforated diverticuli, or cholecystitis. According to these studies, the findings increasing the probability of peritonitis the most are rigidity (LR = 3.6), percussion tenderness (LR = 2.4), and guarding (LR = 2.3). The finding that *decreases* the probability of peritonitis is a *positive* abdominal wall tenderness test (LR = 0.1). The presence or absence of rebound tenderness (positive LR = 2, negative LR = 0.4) shifts probability relatively little, confirming the long-held opinion of expert surgeons that rebound tenderness adds little to what clinicians already know from gentle palpation.

Unhelpful findings in these studies are fever, character of the bowel sounds, and rectal tenderness.

B. SPECIAL TESTS FOR APPENDICITIS

In patients with acute abdominal pain, the *absence* of right lower quadrant tenderness decreases the probability of appendicitis (LR = 0.3, EBM Box 52.2).

1. Individual Findings

All of the findings in EBM Box 52.1 apply to patients with suspected appendicitis (in fact, the most common cause of peritonitis in these studies was appendicitis). Additional special tests that further increase the probability of appendicitis are McBurney point tenderness (LR = 3.4), positive Rovsing sign (LR = 2.1), and positive psoas sign (LR = 1.7). The only special finding decreasing the probability of appendicitis (other than absence of right lower quadrant tenderness) is the absence of McBurney point tenderness (LR = 0.4).

McBurney point tenderness may have even greater accuracy if every patient's appendix were precisely at the McBurney point, but radiologic investigation reveals that the normal appendix sometimes lies a short distance away.[89] In one study of patients with acute abdominal pain, clinicians

EBM BOX 52.1	Acute Abdominal Pain, Signs Detecting Peritonitis*

Finding (Reference)[†]	Sensitivity (%)	Specificity (%)	Likelihood Ratio[‡] if Finding Is Present	Absent
Vital signs				
Fever[28–40]	20–96	11–86	1.4	0.7
Abdominal examination				
Guarding[2,29,34,36,38,39,41–48]	13–90	40–97	2.3	0.6
Rigidity[2,30,32,41,42,44,46,48–50]	6–66	76–100	**3.6**	0.7
Rebound tenderness[2,28–30,32–34,36–41,43–48,51–57]	37–95	13–91	2.0	0.4
Percussion tenderness[32,45,53]	57–65	61–86	2.4	0.5
Abnormal bowel sounds[2,42]	25–61	44–95	NS	0.8
Rectal examination				
Rectal tenderness[28–30,34,35,37,39,41–43,45,46,48,54,58]	22–82	41–95	NS	NS
Other tests				
Positive abdominal wall tenderness test[18,59]	1–5	32–72	**0.1**	NS
Positive cough test[16,32,35,48,49,53,56]	44–85	38–85	1.9	0.5

*Diagnostic standard: for *peritonitis*, surgical exploration and follow-up of patients not operated on; causes of peritonitis included appendicitis (most common), cholecystitis, and perforated ulcer. One study also included patients with pancreatitis.[42]

[†]Definition of findings: for *fever*, most studies used >37.3°C; for *abnormal bowel sounds*, absent, diminished, or hyperactive; for *abdominal wall tenderness test*, see text; for *positive cough test*, the patient is asked to cough, and during the cough shows signs of pain or clearly reduces the intensity of the cough to avoid pain.[32]

[‡]Likelihood ratio (LR) if finding present = positive LR; LR if finding absent = negative LR.

NS, Not significant.

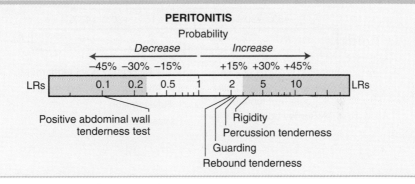

first located the patient's appendix using handheld ultrasound equipment. Maximal pinpoint tenderness over this "sonographic McBurney point" had superior diagnostic accuracy for detecting appendicitis (sensitivity of 87%, specificity of 90%, positive LR = 8.4, negative LR = 0.1).[101]

In contrast to a long-held traditional teaching, administering analgesics to patients with acute abdominal pain does not change the accuracy of individual signs nor reduce the clinician's overall diagnostic accuracy.[91]

Rectal tenderness (EBM Box 52.1) and the obturator sign (EBM Box 52.2) were diagnostically unhelpful in these studies. Nonetheless, a rectal examination should still be performed to detect the rare patient (2% or less) with a pelvic abscess and rectal mass.[41,42]

EBM BOX 52.2	Acute Abdominal Pain: Findings of Appendicitis*

Finding (Reference)[†]	Sensitivity (%)	Specificity (%)	Likelihood Ratio[‡] if Finding Is Present	Absent
Abdominal examination				
Right lower quadrant tenderness[28–30,32–34,38,39,41–43,46,48,53,56,60]	65–100	1–92	1.9	**0.3**
McBurney point tenderness[29,32,61]	50–94	75–86	**3.4**	0.4
Rovsing sign[29,34,35,44,57]	7–68	58–96	2.1	0.8
Other signs				
Psoas sign[34,43,45,57]	13–42	79–97	1.7	NS
Obturator sign[43,57]	8–28	81–94	NS	NS
Combination of findings - Alvarado score[4,28,33,57,62–79]				
7 or more	24–95	46–99	**3.0**	...
5–6 points	4–43	...	NS	...
4 or less	0–28	6–95	**0.1**	...

*Diagnostic standard: for *appendicitis*, surgical findings, histology, and follow-up of patients not operated on.
[†]Definition of findings: for *Rovsing sign*, see the text; for *Alvarado Score*, see Table 52.1.
[‡]Likelihood ratio (LR) if finding present = positive LR; LR if finding absent = negative LR.
NS, Not significant.

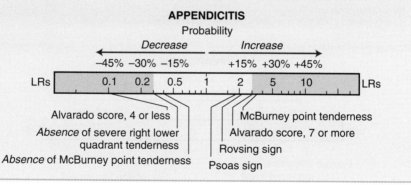

Many scoring systems have been developed to improve diagnostic accuracy and reduce the negative appendectomy rate in patients with acute right lower quadrant tenderness. One of the earliest and most widely used ones is the **Alvarado score** (see Table 52.1), which is also called the MANTRELS **score**, based on the mnemonic **M**igration to the right iliac fossa, **A**norexia, **N**ausea/Vomiting, **T**enderness in the right iliac fossa, **R**ebound pain, **E**levated temperature (fever), **L**eukocytosis, and **S**hift of leukocytes to the left.[28] In 19 studies of more than 4700 patients with acute abdominal pain, an Alvarado score of 7 or more increased the probability of appendicitis (LR = 3, EBM Box 52.2) and a score of 4 or less significantly decreased the probability of appendicitis (LR = 0.1).

2. Combination of Findings: The Alvarado Score

| EBM BOX 52.3 | **Acute Right Upper Quadrant Tenderness; Signs Detecting Cholecystitis*** |

Finding (Reference)[†]	Sensitivity (%)	Specificity (%)	Likelihood Ratio[‡] if Finding Is Present	Likelihood Ratio[‡] if Finding Is Absent
Fever[80-83]	29–44	37–83	NS	NS
Right upper quadrant (RUQ) tenderness[42,60,80,82,84-86]	60–98	1–97	2.4	0.4
Murphy sign[60,84,86-88]	48–97	48–98	**3.9**	0.5
Right upper quadrant mass[80,82,83,85]	2–23	70–99	NS	NS

*Diagnostic standard: for *cholecystitis*, positive hepatobiliary scintiscan[84] or surgical findings and histology.[42,60,80,82,83,85-88]

[†]Definition of findings: for *fever*, temperature >37.5°C[83]; >37.7°C,[81] >38°C,[82] or undefined.[80]

[‡]Likelihood ratio (LR) if finding present = positive LR; LR if finding absent = negative LR.

NS, Not significant.

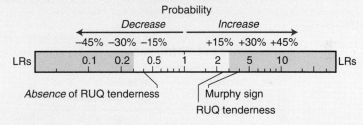

CHOLECYSTITIS

Probability

C. CHOLECYSTITIS

In patients with right upper quadrant pain and suspected cholecystitis (see EBM Box 52.3), the findings that increase the probability of cholecystitis are a positive Murphy sign (LR = 3.9) and right upper quadrant tenderness (LR = 2.4). The absence of right upper quadrant tenderness decreases the probability (LR = 0.4). The presence or absence of a right upper quadrant mass is unhelpful, probably because a palpable tender gallbladder is uncommon in cholecystitis (sensitivity less than 25%) and because the sensation of a right upper quadrant mass may occur in other diagnoses, such as liver disease or localized rigidity of the abdominal wall from other disorders.

There is also a *sonographic Murphy sign*, elicited during ultrasonography of the right upper quadrant, which is simply the finding of maximal tenderness over the gallbladder. Studies of this sign in patients with right upper quadrant pain reveal much better diagnostic accuracy than that of conventional palpation: sensitivity of 42% to 63%, specificity of 94% to 99%, positive LR = 15.7, and negative LR = 0.5.[92] The superior accuracy of this sign, which also relies on palpation of the abdominal wall, suggests that the poorer accuracy of conventional palpation is due to the difficulty in precisely locating the position of the gallbladder.

The Murphy sign may be less accurate in elderly patients, because up to 25% of patients over 60 years of age with cholecystitis lack any abdominal tenderness whatsoever.[93] Although most

EBM BOX 52.4 | Acute Abdominal Pain; Signs Detecting Bowel Obstruction*

Finding (Reference)†	Sensitivity (%)	Specificity (%)	Likelihood Ratio‡ if Finding Is	
			Present	Absent
Inspection of abdomen				
Visible peristalsis[3]	6	100	**18.8**	NS
Distended abdomen[1,3,42]	58–67	89–96	**9.6**	0.4
Palpation of abdomen				
Guarding[1,2,42]	20–63	47–78	NS	NS
Rigidity[1–3,42]	6–18	75–99	NS	NS
Rebound tenderness[1,2,42]	22–40	52–82	NS	NS
Auscultation of abdomen				
Hyperactive bowel sounds[3,42]	40–42	89–94	**5.0**	0.6
Abnormal bowel sounds[1–3,42]	63–93	43–88	**3.2**	0.4
Rectal examination				
Rectal tenderness[1,2,42]	4–26	72–94	NS	NS

*Diagnostic standard: for *small bowel obstruction*, surgical findings, abdominal radiographs, and clinical follow-up.
†Definition of findings: for *abnormal bowel sounds*, hyperactive, absent, or diminished bowel sounds.
‡Likelihood ratio (LR) if finding present = positive LR; LR if finding absent = negative LR.
NS, Not significant.

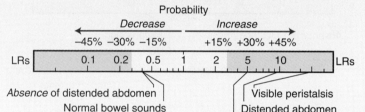

BOWEL OBSTRUCTION
Probability

TABLE 52.1 ■ The Alvarado Score*

Finding†	Points
Symptoms	
Migration	1
Anorexia	1
Nausea and vomiting	1
Signs	
Tenderness, right lower quadrant	2
Rebound tenderness	1
Elevation of temperature	1
Laboratory	
Leucocytosis (white blood cell count >10,000/μL)	2
Shift to the left (>75% neutrophils)	1
Total Possible Points	10

*"*MANTRELS*" is an acronym for the Alvarado score (i.e., each letter represents the initial letters of items in the score; see the text).
†*Definition of findings*: for *migration*, classic migration of pain from periumbilical or epigastric area to right lower quadrant; for *anorexia*, may substitute acetone in urine; for *elevation of temperature*, oral temperature ≥37.3°C.

of these patients have abdominal pain, some lack this symptom as well, likely because of altered mental status.

In patients with a pyogenic liver abscess, the presence of the Murphy sign increases the probability of associated biliary tract sepsis (sensitivity of 32%, specificity of 88%, positive LR = 2.8, negative LR not significant).[94]

D. SMALL BOWEL OBSTRUCTION

In patients with acute abdominal pain (See EBM Box 52.4), the findings of visible peristalsis (LR = 18.8), abdominal distention (LR = 9.6), and hyperactive bowel sounds (LR = 5) increase the probability of bowel obstruction (although visible peristalsis is rare, occurring in only 6% of affected patients). Diminished or absent bowel sounds also occur in obstruction, being found in one of four patients.[3,42]

The findings that decrease the probability of obstruction slightly are normal bowel sounds (i.e., not hyperactive, absent, or diminished) and absence of a distended abdomen (both LRs = 0.4). Nonetheless, 33% to 42% of patients with obstruction lack abdominal distention, especially early in the course or if the obstruction is high in the intestines. The findings of peritoneal irritation—rigidity and rebound tenderness—do not change the probability of obstruction.

E. DIVERTICULITIS

Two studies have investigated the accuracy of **left lower quadrant tenderness** in patients with suspected diverticulitis. In an older study of 600 patients with acute abdominal pain (using the operative findings as the diagnostic standard), left lower quadrant tenderness was specific (98%) but not sensitive (22%; positive LR = 13.8, negative LR = 0.8).[42] Sensitivity was low in this study because most patients with diverticulitis had more generalized abdominal tenderness. In another study of 163 patients with acute lower abdominal pain (using CT scan as the diagnostic standard), left lower quadrant tenderness was more sensitive (76%) but less specific (65%; positive LR = 2.2, negative LR = 0.4).[95] Specificity was lower in this study because many more patients with mimicking disorders were enrolled (compared to the previously mentioned study), disorders such as enteritis, colon cancer, gynecologic abnormalities, and ischemic colitis. In one study of 172 patients with diverticulitis (confirmed by CT scan), the presence of guarding greatly increased the probability of abscess or generalized peritonitis (sensitivity of 9%; specificity of 99%, positive LR = 8.4).[96]

F. RENAL COLIC

In a study of 1333 patients presenting with acute abdominal pain, two findings were accurate signs of ureterolithiasis (as diagnosed by imaging or follow-up): loin tenderness (sensitivity of 15%, specificity of 99%, positive LR = 27.7, negative LR = 0.9) and renal tenderness (sensitivity of 86%, specificity of 76%, positive LR = 3.6, negative LR = 0.2). As compelling as these findings are, they are less accurate than the finding of microscopic hematuria, which has a sensitivity of 75%, specificity of 99%, positive LR = 73.1, and negative LR = 0.3.[90]

CHRONIC ABDOMINAL PAIN

In two studies of patients with chronic abdominal pain, the abdominal wall tenderness test (see the section on abdominal wall tenderness test) significantly *decreased* the probability of a visceral cause of the pain (LR = 0.1, see EBM Box 52.5). Furthermore, a positive abdominal wall

| EBM BOX 52.5 | Chronic Upper Abdominal Pain* | | | |

Finding (Reference)†	Sensitivity (%)	Specificity (%)	Likelihood Ratio‡ if Finding Is	
			Present	Absent
Positive abdominal wall tenderness test, detecting visceral pain[97,98]	11–13	15–21	0.1	4.9
Right upper quadrant tenderness, detecting cholelithiasis[99]	53	51	NS	NS
Lower abdominal tenderness, detecting cholelithiasis[99]	21	57	0.5	1.4
Epigastric tenderness, detecting positive upper endoscopy[100]	63	31	NS	NS

*Diagnostic standard: for *visceral pain*, pain originating from an intraabdominal organ or structure (i.e., not abdominal wall); for *cholelithiasis*, ultrasonography or oral cholecystogram[99]; for *positive upper endoscopy*, findings on upper gastrointestinal endoscopy, most of which were peptic ulcers.
†Definition of findings: for *abdominal wall tenderness test*, see the text.
‡Likelihood ratio (LR) if finding present = positive LR; LR if finding absent = negative LR.
NS, Not significant.

CHRONIC ABDOMINAL PAIN
Probability

Decrease   *Increase*

−45% −30% −15%   +15% +30% +45%

LRs | 0.1   0.2   0.5   1   2   5   10 | LRs

Positive abdominal wall tenderness
test, *arguing against* visceral pain

tenderness test increased the probability that the patient's pain would respond to an injection of combined anesthetic/corticosteroid into the tender spot and that *no* serious pathology would be discovered during 3 or more months of follow-up (LR = 7).[97]

Beyond this finding, there is relatively little information on the accuracy of examination in diagnosing chronic abdominal pain. Most studies show that the finding of abdominal tenderness is common in many nonorganic disorders and has little diagnostic value. In patients with suspected biliary colic, right upper quadrant tenderness does not distinguish patients with cholelithiasis from those without, although lower abdominal tenderness modestly decreases the probability of cholelithiasis (LR = 0.5, EBM Box 52.5). In patients with dyspepsia, epigastric tenderness does not help predict whether upper endoscopy will reveal an ulcer, some other abnormality, or normal findings.

Even if the finding of tenderness has little diagnostic value in patients with chronic abdominal pain, abdominal examination is still important to detect masses, organomegaly, and signs of a surgical abdomen.

References may be accessed online at *Elsevier eBooks for Practicing Clinicians*.

Auscultation of the Abdomen

ABDOMINAL BRUITS

I. The Finding

Abdominal bruits are murmurs heard during auscultation of the abdomen. Like any murmur generated outside the four heart chambers, abdominal bruits may extend beyond the confines of the first and second heart sounds, from systole into diastole (i.e., they may be *continuous* murmurs; see Chapter 43). Most bruits are detected in the epigastrium or upper abdominal quadrants.

II. Clinical Significance

A. BRUITS IN HEALTHY PERSONS

Bruits occur in 4% to 20% of healthy persons.[1-3] Abdominal bruits are more common in those younger than 40 years of age than in older persons.[1-4]

Characteristically, the abdominal bruit of a healthy individual is systolic, medium-pitched to low-pitched, and audible between the xiphoid process and umbilicus.[1] Only rarely does it spread to the patient's sides, in contrast to abnormal bruits, which are often loudest away from the epigastrium (see following sections). Arteriograms reveal that the most common source for the normal abdominal bruit is the patient's celiac artery.[4]

B. BRUITS IN RENOVASCULAR HYPERTENSION

In patients with renal artery stenosis and renovascular hypertension, an abdominal bruit may be heard in the epigastrium, although the sound sometimes radiates to one side.[1] In one study of patients referred because of severe hypertension that was difficult to control—a setting suggesting renovascular hypertension—the finding of a *systolic/diastolic* abdominal bruit (i.e., continuous bruit) was virtually diagnostic for renovascular hypertension (likelihood ratio [LR] = 38.9, EBM Box 53.1). In contrast, the finding in similar patients of *any* abdominal bruit (i.e., one not necessarily extending into diastole) is less compelling (LR = 5.6), probably because they also occur in persons without renovascular hypertension (see the section on bruits in healthy persons).

The abdominal bruit of renovascular hypertension, however, does not always originate in the renal artery. In one study of patients undergoing surgery for renal artery stenosis, intraoperative auscultation localized the bruit to the renal arteries as the sole source only about half the time.[1] In the remaining patients, other vessels generated or contributed to the sound. Bruits in these patients are possibly general markers of vascular disease, just as the finding of a carotid bruit has been associated with disease in other distant vascular beds, such as the coronary vasculature.[11]

C. OTHER DISORDERS

Harsh epigastric or right upper quadrant bruits (systolic and continuous) have been repeatedly described in patients with hepatic malignancies[12,13] and hepatic cirrhosis.[12,14] In these patients, the sound may represent extrinsic compression of vessels by tumor or regenerating nodules, the hypervascular tumor, or portosystemic collateral vessels. Left upper quadrant bruits occur in patients with carcinoma of the body of the pancreas (8 of 21 patients in one study).[15] Other rare causes of abdominal bruits are renal artery aneurysms,[16] aortocaval fistulae,[17,18] ischemic bowel disease,[19] hepatic arteriovenous fistula of hereditary hemorrhagic telangiectasia,[20,21] and celiac compression

---

EBM BOX 53.1   Auscultation of the Abdomen*

Finding (Reference)	Sensitivity (%)	Specificity (%)	Likelihood Ratio[†] if Finding Is Present	Likelihood Ratio[†] if Finding Is Absent
Abdominal bruit—any				
Detecting renovascular hypertension[5-8]	27–56	89–96	**5.6**	0.6
Detecting abdominal aortic aneurysm[9]	11	95	NS	NS
Abdominal bruit—systolic/diastolic				
Detecting renovascular hypertension[10]	39	99	**38.9**	0.6

*Diagnostic standard: for *renovascular hypertension*, renal angiography,[5-8] sometimes combined with renal vein renin ratio >1.5[10] or cure of hypertension after surgery;[7] for *abdominal aortic aneurysm*, ultrasonography revealing focal dilation of infrarenal >1.5 cm larger than proximal aorta.[9]

†Likelihood ratio (LR) if finding present = positive LR; LR if finding absent = negative LR.

NS, Not significant.

RENOVASCULAR HYPERTENSION
Probability

Systolic/diastolic abdominal bruit
Any abdominal bruit

syndrome.[22,23] Although an abdominal bruit is traditionally associated with abdominal aortic aneurysm, the finding lacked diagnostic value in one study (LR not significant, EBM Box 53.1).[9]

HEPATIC RUB

In the absence of recent liver biopsy, the finding of a hepatic friction rub has been repeatedly associated with intrahepatic malignancy, either hepatoma or metastatic disease.[13,24] In one study of tumors metastatic to the liver, 10% of patients had a hepatic friction rub.[25]

BOWEL SOUNDS

I. The Finding

Most clinicians have great difficulty making any sense out of a patient's bowel sounds, for two reasons: (1) Normal bowel sounds, from moment to moment, vary greatly in pitch, intensity, and frequency. One healthy person may have no bowel sounds for up to 4 minutes, but when examined later may have more than 30 discrete sounds per minute.[26] The activity of normal bowel sounds may cycle with peak-to-peak periods as long as 50 to 60 minutes,[27] meaning that any analysis based on even several minutes of bedside auscultation is incomplete. (2) Bowel sounds generated at one point of the intestinal tract radiate widely over the entire abdominal wall.[26,28] The sounds heard in the right lower quadrant, for example, may actually originate in the stomach. This dissemination of bowel sounds makes the practice of listening to them in all four quadrants fundamentally unsound, because, as an example, the left lower quadrant may be quieter than the left upper quadrant not because the descending colon is making less noise than the stomach but instead because the entire abdomen has become quieter, at least for the moment the clinician is listening to the lower quadrant.

Most bowel sounds are generated in the stomach, followed by the large intestine and then the small bowel.[29] The overall frequency of bowel sounds increases after a meal.[30] The actual cause of bowel sounds is still debated; experiments with exteriorized loops of bowel in dogs show many intestinal contractions to be silent, although sound often appears when contractions propel contents through a bowel segment that is not relaxed.[26]

II. Clinical Significance

Analysis of the bowel sounds has modest value in diagnosing small bowel obstruction. After experimental complete bowel obstruction in animals, bowel sounds are hyperactive for about 30 minutes before becoming diminished or absent.[27] In patients with small bowel obstruction, clinical observation shows that about 40% have hyperactive bowel sounds and about 25% have diminished or absent bowel sounds.[31,32] Consequently, since most patients with small bowel obstruction have abnormal bowel sounds, the finding of *normal* bowel sounds in a patient with acute abdominal pain modestly *decreases* the probability of bowel obstruction (LR = 0.4, see EBM Box 52.4 in Chapter 52).

A traditional finding of peritonitis is diminished or absent bowel sounds, although studies of patients with acute abdominal pain show this finding to be inaccurate (see Chapter 52).

Clinicians have traditionally listened postoperatively to the patient's bowel tones to gauge return of peristaltic activity after postoperative ileus. Nonetheless, in one study of 124 patients who had undergone major abdominal surgery, there was no correlation between presence of bowel tones during any of the first 10 postoperative days and whether the patient had passed flatus, had a bowel movement, or tolerated oral intake.[33]

References may be accessed online at *Elsevier eBooks for Practicing Clinicians*.

Extremities

Peripheral Vascular Disease

- By analysis of the patient's symptoms, examination of the patient's pulses, and knowledge of the anatomy of peripheral vascular disease, clinicians can accurately diagnose the distribution and severity of a patient's vascular disease.
- Peripheral vascular disease affects three distinct anatomic segments: aortoiliac, femoropopliteal, and peroneotibial. Significant disease of a single segment causes claudication; disease of multiple segments causes rest pain and limb-threatening ischemia. Disease in the peroneotibial segment is uncommon unless the patient has diabetes or thromboangiitis obliterans.
- In patients with claudication, the following signs increase probability of peripheral vascular disease: absence of both pedal pulses, presence of foot wounds or sores, absence of femoral pulses, asymmetric coolness, and presence of a limb bruit.
- In critically ill patients, three signs of reduced peripheral perfusion—cool limbs, capillary refill time of more than 5 seconds, and mottling of the skin—increase probability of poor perfusion and adverse outcome.

I. Introduction

Chronic arterial disease usually affects the lower limbs in three distinct segments: (1) the aortoiliac segment (especially the infrarenal abdominal aorta and common iliac arteries), (2) the femoropopliteal segment (especially the superficial femoral artery in the adductor canal), and (3) the peroneotibial segment (below the knee).[1] Disease in each segment produces distinct patterns of claudication (Table 54.1). Most patients have aortoiliac disease, femoropopliteal disease, or both.[2] Disease below the knee is uncommon unless the patient has diabetes or thromboangiitis obliterans.

The diagnostic standard for chronic lower-extremity ischemia is the ankle-brachial blood pressure index (ABI), which is obtained by positioning the patient supine and measuring the highest systolic blood pressure at the ankle (dorsalis pedis and posterior tibial arteries), using a handheld doppler flowmeter, and dividing it by the blood pressure in the brachial artery.[3]* Values less than 0.97 are abnormal (i.e., the lower 2.5% of measurements from large numbers of young, nonsmoking, asymptomatic persons),[4-6] although most investigators define chronic leg ischemia as an ABI less than 0.9.[3] Most patients with claudication have ABIs between 0.5 and 0.8 and significant disease in only a single segment; those with limb-threatening ischemia (i.e., rest pain, gangrene) have ABIs less than 0.5 and disease in at least two segments.[5,6†]

---

*The blood pressure cuff should be placed just above the ankle, wrapping the cuff's edges parallel to each other (*spiral* wrapping increases interobserver disagreement).
†Oscillometric blood pressure cuffs (i.e., automated blood pressure cuffs) are increasingly being used, though they are not yet generally recommended for measuring the ABI.[7] In one meta-analysis of 20 studies, the diagnostic accuracy of the oscillometric ABI (vs. doppler ABI) was sensitivity of 65%, specificity of 96%, positive LR = 15.3, and negative LR = 0.3.[8]

TABLE 54.1 ■ Diagnosis of Peripheral Arterial Disease: Traditional Approach

Anatomic segment	Location of claudication	Pulse examination		
		Femoral*	Popliteal	Pedal
Aortoiliac	Buttock, thigh, calf†	Absent	Absent	Absent
Femoropopliteal*	Calf	Present	Absent	Absent
Peroneotibial	None or foot‡	Present	Present	Absent

Adapted from reference 1.
*The *femoro* of femoropopliteal indicates the superficial femoral artery; the *femoral* of femoral pulse indicates the common femoral artery.
†May cause erectile dysfunction if internal iliac arteries are involved.
‡Disease in this segment usually causes no claudication in patients with diabetes but causes foot pain in those with thromboangiitis obliterans (Buerger disease).

II. The Findings

A. APPEARANCE OF THE FOOT

The earliest clinicians writing about peripheral vascular disease emphasized the physical sign of gangrene, but in 1924, the American surgeon Leo Buerger described in his book *The Circulatory Disturbances Of The Extremities*[9] various prodromal signs of vascular disease, including toe and foot ulcers, poor capillary refill, impaired nail growth, atrophic skin, foot pallor with elevation, and dependent foot rubor (i.e., redness of the foot first appearing after dangling it in a dependent position, i.e., over the edge of a bed).[10] Clinicians have since regarded these findings as characteristic of chronic lower limb ischemia, although some of them—especially poor capillary refill and dependent rubor—were controversial even in Buerger's time.[11,12]

B. PULSES

In studies of large numbers of healthy individuals, the dorsalis pedis pulse is not palpable 3% to 14% of the time and the posterior tibial pulse is not palpable 0% to 10% of the time.[13-18] Nonetheless, when one of these arteries is congenitally small or absent, the other enlarges to make up the difference, explaining why only 0% to 2% of healthy persons lack *both* pedal pulses.[13,14,17]

The absence of both pedal pulses is common to vascular disease in each of the three vascular segments and thus represents the best screening test for peripheral vascular disease (see Table 54.1).

C. BRUITS

A traditional finding of vessel stenosis is the limb bruit, either iliac (above the inguinal crease), femoral (in the thigh), or popliteal. Complete occlusion of a vessel should make bruits disappear.

In patients who have undergone femoral artery puncture for cardiac catheterization, the presence of a continuous femoral bruit (i.e., one extending beyond the second heart sound and thus having both systolic and diastolic components) suggests an abnormal communication between an artery and vein (i.e., arteriovenous fistula, see Chapter 43).

D. ANCILLARY TESTS

1. Venous Filling Time

In patients with peripheral vascular disease, the veins of the feet fill abnormally slowly once they are emptied. After positioning the patient supine and identifying a prominent vein on the top of the foot, the clinician empties this vein by elevating the patient's leg to 45° above the table surface for 1 minute. The patient then sits up and dangles the foot over the edge of the examining table, the clinician then recording how long it takes for the vein to rise above the level of the skin surface. Measurements of more than 20 seconds are abnormal.[19]

2. Capillary Refill Time

Normal values of capillary refill time, based on observation of thousands of persons, average about 2 seconds.[20,21] Women have slightly longer times compared to men, and capillary refill times normally increase in elderly patients and in cooler ambient temperatures.

In the studies of capillary refill of patients with suspected peripheral vascular disease, investigators applied firm pressure for 5 seconds to the plantar skin of the great toe and then timed how long it took for normal skin color to return after releasing the pressure. Measurements of 5 seconds or more were regarded abnormal.[19] In studies of capillary refill of critically ill patients, investigators tested the patient's finger (usually index finger) by applying firm pressure for 15 seconds and regarded times of 5 seconds or more as abnormal.[22-24]

3. Buerger Test

In the Buerger test, the clinician observes the color of the patient's leg when it is elevated and again when it is lowered. Abnormal pallor with elevation and a deep rubor in the lowered position are features of vascular disease.[1,9] In Buerger's version of the test, the clinician elevated the leg to produce pallor and then simply recorded the angle at which the reddish hue returned as the limb was lowered (his *angle of circulatory sufficiency*).[9] In the only investigated version of this test (see section on distribution of vascular disease), the clinician elevated the patient's leg 90 degrees from the table surface for 2 minutes and then dangled it perpendicular to the table edge for another 2 minutes. The positive response was abnormal pallor with elevation and the appearance of a dusky red flush spreading proximally from the toes in the dependent position.[25]

III. Clinical Significance

A. DIAGNOSIS OF PERIPHERAL VASCULAR DISEASE

EBM Box 54.1 shows that the following physical signs *increase* probability of peripheral vascular disease (i.e., ABI <0.9) if found in a symptomatic leg: absence of both pedal pulses (likelihood ratio [LR] = 9.9), presence of wounds or sores on the foot (LR = 7), absence of femoral pulse (LR = 6.1), presence of asymmetric coolness of the foot (LR = 6.1), and presence of any limb bruit (LR = 5.4). In another study,[19] the presence of foot coolness was diagnostically unhelpful, although this study defined the abnormal finding as "foot cooler than ipsilateral calf," which actually is a normal finding (i.e., the skin surface temperature of healthy persons normally diminishes toward the feet, paralleling progressively reduced cutaneous blood flow to conserve body heat).[1]

The presence of one or both pedal pulses decreases probability only modestly (LR = 0.4). Studies show that approximately one of three patients with disease have this finding. In these patients, however, the pulses often diminish or disappear during exercise (e.g., running in place, walking, toe-stands, or ankle flexion repeatedly against resistance), just as normal resting coronary blood flow in a patient with coronary artery disease may become abnormal after exercise.[3,32]

| EBM BOX 54.1 | Peripheral Vascular Disease* |

Finding (Reference)[†]	Sensitivity (%)	Specificity (%)	Likelihood Ratio[‡] if Finding Is Present	Absent
Inspection				
Wounds or sores on foot[26]	2	100	**7.0**	NS
Foot color abnormally pale, red, or blue[26]	35	87	2.8	0.7
Atrophic skin[19]	50	70	1.7	NS
Absent lower limb hair[19]	48	71	1.7	NS
Palpation				
Foot asymmetrically cooler[26]	10	98	**6.1**	0.9
Absent femoral pulse[26]	7	99	**6.1**	NS
Absent posterior tibial and dorsalis pedis pulses[26-29]	50–73	91–99	**9.9**	0.4
Auscultation				
Limb bruit present[26,28-31]	11–50	92–99	**5.4**	0.7
Ancillary tests				
Capillary refill time ≥5 seconds[19]	28	85	1.9	NS
Venous filling time >20 seconds[19]	22	94	**3.6**	NS

*Diagnostic standard: for *peripheral vascular disease*, ankle-brachial index <0.8–0.97 except for the study by Boyko[19] (i.e., atrophic skin, absent lower limb hair, capillary refill time, and venous filling time), which recruited only diabetic patients and defined disease as ABI <0.5.
[†]Definition of findings: for *limb bruit present*, femoral artery bruit[26,28,29,31] or iliac, femoral, or popliteal bruit.[30]
[‡]Likelihood ratio (LR) if finding present = positive LR; LR if finding absent = negative LR.
NS, Not significant.

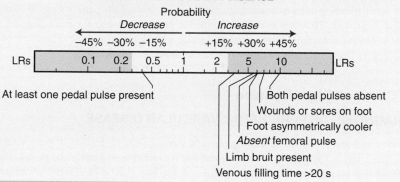

Findings that are unhelpful diagnostically are atrophic skin, hairless lower limbs,[33,34] and prolonged capillary refill time. Writing soon after Buerger introduced the capillary refill time as a test of peripheral vascular disease (his *expression test*), Lewis[12] and Pickering[11] showed it was an unreliable sign, because prompt refill could occur from the veins of a limb rendered completely ischemic experimentally. In critically ill patients, however, a prolonged capillary refill time in the patient's finger does have proven diagnostic value (see section on detecting hypoperfusion in intensive care unit).

Some investigators have wondered whether clinicians could accurately measure the ABI by palpating the pedal pulses distal to the blood pressure cuff instead of using a Doppler flowmeter.

In 2 studies,[35,36] such an ABI <0.9 *by palpation* detected an ABI <0.9 *by Doppler testing* with a sensitivity of 88%, specificity of 72% to 82%, positive LR = 4, and negative LR = 0.2. Another innovative way to detect peripheral vascular disease (without Doppler) places a bedside pulse oximeter sequentially on the patient's fingers and great toes: a positive result is either a supine toe measurement 2% lower than the finger measurement *or* a toe measurement that decreases 2% after 12 inches of foot elevation. This test detects vascular disease with a sensitivity of 77%, specificity of 97%, positive LR = 30.5, and negative LR = 0.2.[37] Nonetheless, studies of ABI by palpation and toe pulse oximetry have enrolled mostly asymptomatic patients, and it is unlikely these tests would be easy to apply in patients with more serious vascular disease, who may lack pedal pulses or have undetectable toe arterial waveforms.

B. DISTRIBUTION OF PERIPHERAL VASCULAR DISEASE

One study showed that vascular surgeons using traditional methods accurately localized the distribution of disease in 96% of 102 symptomatic patients, although the study omitted information about the relative value of specific findings.[38] Of the few studies available, one confirms the traditional teaching (Table 54.1) that an absent or severely diminished femoral pulse in a symptomatic limb increases probability of aortoiliac disease (sensitivity of 39%, specificity of 99%, positive LR = 31, negative LR = 0.6).[39] Also, in symptomatic limbs with preserved popliteal pulses (i.e., a finding arguing against *occlusion* of the aortoiliac or femoropopliteal segments), the presence of a limb bruit argues *for* the presence of stenoses on angiography, a finding of therapeutic importance because these patients may be candidates for angioplasty (sensitivity of 80%, specificity of 75%, positive LR = 3.2, negative LR = 0.3).[40] Finally, patients who have a positive Buerger test have more extensive disease than those who are test negative, including more rest pain (60% vs. 8%) and gangrene (23% vs. 0%) and lower ABIs (mean ± SD, 0.37 ± 0.29 vs. 0.62 ± 0.23).[25]

C. COMPLICATIONS OF ARTERIAL PUNCTURE

Femoral artery puncture for cardiac catheterization may rarely be complicated by the formation of false aneurysms or arteriovenous fistulae. In one study of patients with significant groin hematomas or new limb bruits after cardiac catheterization, two findings were diagnostic.[41] A **continuous femoral bruit** (i.e., one having both systolic and diastolic components) was diagnostic for arteriovenous fistula (sensitivity of 96%, specificity of 99%, positive LR = 80.8, negative LR = 0.04), and an **expansile femoral pulsation** (i.e., a dilated arterial pulsation whose walls expanded laterally with each beat) was diagnostic for false aneurysm formation (sensitivity of 92%, specificity of 93%, positive LR = 13.8, negative LR = 0.1). In this study, the diagnostic standard was duplex scanning, surgery, or both.

D. DETECTING HYPOPERFUSION IN INTENSIVE CARE UNIT (ICU)

The body normally responds to decreased cardiac output by reducing cutaneous blood flow to the skin, which may produce cool limbs, longer capillary refill times, and mottling of the limbs (mottling is a blotchy or lacelike pattern of dusky erythema).[42] In patients with critical illness, each of these signs, alone or in combination, identifies patients with reduced cardiac output, worse prognosis, or both. For example, the finding of cool legs in ICU patients increases the probability of low cardiac output (LR = 3.7, EBM Box 54.2), even in the subset of patients with sepsis (LR = 5.2). A capillary refill time of 5 seconds or more predicts major postoperative complications after intraabdominal surgery (LR = 12.1) and predicts 14 day mortality in patients with sepsis (LR = 4.6). In patients with sepsis, testing capillary refill time *after* initial fluid resuscitation is more accurate than testing before it (LRs 10.5 vs. NS, predicting mortality).[49] Mottling of the skin

| EBM BOX 54.2 | **Peripheral Perfusion of ICU Patients*** |

Finding (Reference)†	Sensitivity (%)	Specificity (%)	Likelihood Ratio‡ if Finding Is Present	Absent
Detecting low cardiac output				
Both legs cool (all patients)[43]	23	94	**3.7**	0.8
Both legs cool (patients with sepsis)[43]	30	94	**5.2**	0.7
Combinations of hypoperfusion findings[44]				
0 of 3 findings present	36	24	0.5	...
1 of 3 findings present	52	...	2.3	...
3 or 3 findings present	12	98	**7.5**	...
Capillary refill time ≥5 s[45]	25	85	1.6	NS
Detecting elevated arterial lactate level				
Limb is cool *or* capillary refill time ≥5 s[22]	67	69	2.2	0.5
Predicting multiorgan dysfunction				
Limb is cool *or* capillary refill time ≥5 s[22]	77	70	2.6	**0.3**
Predicting major postoperative complications after intraabdominal surgery				
Capillary refill time ≥5 s[23]	79	93	**12.1**	**0.2**
Predicting mortality if septic shock				
Capillary refill time ≥5 s[24]	50	89	**4.6**	0.6
Mottling of skin extending to upper thigh[46-48]	9–41	96–97	**10.2**	NS

*Diagnostic standard: for *low cardiac output, cardiac index* < 2.2 L/min/M^2,[45] < 2.5 L/min/M^2,[44] or < 3 L/min/M^2;[43] for *elevated lactate level*, blood lactate >2 mmol/L; for *multiorgan dysfunction*, SOFA score that increases during the first 48 hours of hospitalization (SOFA score is the Sequential Organ Failure Assessment, a score tabulating the following variables: P$_a$O$_2$/F$_i$O$_2$, number of vasoactive pressors being administered, bilirubin, platelet count, Glasgow coma scale, and creatinine or urine output); for *major postoperative complication*, one requiring endoscopy, repeat surgery, general anesthesia, or ICU transfer[23]; for *mortality*, 14 day[46] or 28 day[47,48] mortality.

†Definition of findings: for *both legs cool*, either all 4 limbs have cool temperature or legs cool despite warm arms (patients with known peripheral vascular disease were excluded)[43]; for *combinations of hypoperfusion findings*, there are 3: (1) capillary refill time >2 S, (2) skin mottling over the knees, and (3) cool limbs[44]; for all *capillary refill times*, testing performed on the patient's finger or nailbeds; and for *mottling of skin over knees*, mottling extending at least to the level of mid-thigh (only light-skinned patients were tested).[46]

‡Likelihood ratio (LR) if finding present = positive LR; LR if finding absent = negative LR.
ICU, Intensive care unit; *NS*, not significant.

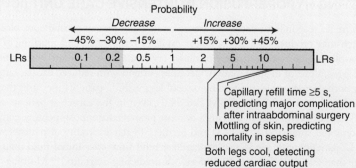

HYPOPERFUSION IN THE ICU

Probability

Decrease ← → Increase

−45% −30% −15%   +15% +30% +45%

LRs 0.1 0.2 0.5 1 2 5 10 LRs

Capillary refill time ≥5 s, predicting major complication after intraabdominal surgery
Mottling of skin, predicting mortality in sepsis
Both legs cool, detecting reduced cardiac output

over the knees and extending to the upper thigh also predicts mortality in patients with sepsis (LR = 10.2), independent of the use of vasopressor medications,[48] and its course over time heralds the patient's outcome (i.e., patients whose mottling diminishes over time have better survival than those whose mottling persists).[46] Studies of mottling excluded patients with dark skin.

Other investigators have focused on combinations of findings. For example, in one study of intubated patients with acute lung injury, the simultaneous presence of capillary refill time more than 2 seconds,[‡] mottling over the knees, and cool limbs increased the probability of low cardiac output (LR = 7.5; EBM Box 54.2). In another series of ICU patients, the findings of *either* cool limbs or capillary refill time of 5 seconds or more increased probability of an elevated lactate levels (LR = 2.2) and predicted future progressive multiorgan dysfunction (LR = 2.6).

References may be accessed online at *Elsevier eBooks for Practicing Clinicians.*

[‡]This study contrasts with other studies of capillary refill by applying only *mild* pressure on the patient's fingertip to elicit the finding, not firm pressure, and by defining the abnormal test as just 2 seconds or more.

The Diabetic Foot

I. Introduction

The term *diabetic foot* refers to those complications occurring in a foot rendered hypesthetic from diabetic polyneuropathy. These include ulceration, Charcot arthropathy, and infection. Each year, 2% to 6% of diabetics develop a foot ulcer,[1] and the diabetic foot is the leading cause of hospitalization among diabetics and the overall leading cause of amputation in the United States.[2]

II. The Findings

A. FOOT ULCERATION

Most diabetic foot ulcers involve the forefoot, especially the toes or plantar surface of the metatarsal heads. Less often, they develop over the heel, plantar midfoot, or previous amputation sites. The term *ulcer area* refers to the product of the maximum ulcer width and maximum ulcer length.

B. DIABETIC NEUROPATHY AND SEMMES-WEINSTEIN MONOFILAMENTS

Although neuropathy, ischemia, and infection all contribute to ulceration, the most important is probably neuropathy. Conventional examination often fails to detect diabetic polyneuropathy, and about half of patients with diabetic ulceration lack complaints of numbness or pain[3] and can still detect the touch of a cotton wisp or pinprick.[4,5] Consequently, most diabetologists use a simple and more sensitive bedside tool, the Semmes-Weinstein monofilament, to identify which patients have sufficient neuropathy placing them at risk for ulceration.

According to traditional teachings, a foot that is able to sense the 5.07 monofilament* is protected from ulceration, whereas one that fails to perceive the 5.07 monofilament is predisposed

---

*The nominal value of a monofilament represents the common logarithm of 10 times the force in milligrams required to bow it (e.g., the 5.07 monofilament will buckle with 11.8 g of pressure, $\log_{10}[10 \times 11,800] = 5.07$).[6] Therefore, monofilaments with higher numbers are stiffer and more easily perceived than those with lower numbers.

to ulceration. To use the monofilament, the patient should be lying supine with eyes closed, and the monofilament should be applied perpendicular to the skin with enough force to buckle it for approximately one second. The patient responds "yes" each time he or she senses the monofilament, as the clinician randomly tests each site on the foot multiple times. In clinical studies, anywhere from 1 to 10 different sites on the foot are tested, but each study defines the abnormal result as inability to consistently sense the monofilament at *any* site. Testing the plantar surface of the first and fifth metatarsal heads may be the most efficient and overall accurate bedside maneuver.[7]

Monofilaments were first developed in 1898 by von Frey who glued thorns to hairs of various stiffness and calibrated them with a chemical balance (**von Frey hairs**).[6] Nylon monofilaments were introduced in 1960 by Josephine Semmes and Sidney Weinstein, who used filaments of 20 different diameters (from 0.06 to 1.14 mm) to study sensation in patients with penetrating brain injuries.[8,9] Although the 5.07 monofilament is firmly entrenched as the standard for testing diabetic feet, this is based on an older study of patients with neuropathic foot ulcers from diabetes or leprosy, which used just three of the twenty monofilaments available.[10] The monofilaments studied were the 4.17 monofilament, which was selected because virtually all normal persons are able to sense it, and the stiffer 5.07 and 6.10 monofilaments. In the study, none of the patients with ulcers could sense the 4.17 or 5.07 monofilaments, although some could sense the 6.10 monofilament. These findings led the investigators to conclude that the ability to sense the 5.07 monofilament was protective (i.e., 6.10 was not protective and 4.17 was normal sensation). It is also possible, however, that a better indicator of protective sensation is one of the other seven monofilaments between 6.10 and 4.17 not used in the study, and in support of this hypothesis, one study has suggested that the 4.21 monofilament may be a better discriminatory threshold.[4]

C. CHARCOT JOINT

Charcot joint (neuro-arthropathy) refers to accelerated degenerative changes and ultimate joint destruction that follows repetitive trauma to insensitive, neuropathic joints. Although historically the most common causes were syphilis (affecting the larger joints of the lower extremity) and syringomyelia (affecting the larger joints of the upper extremity), the most common cause currently is diabetes. In diabetic patients, Charcot joint characteristically affects the foot, including ankle, tarso-metatarsal, and metatarso-phalangeal (MTP) joints.[11,12]

Most patients present with a limp, difficulty putting on shoes, or soft tissue swelling suggesting fracture, acute arthritis, or sprain.[12,13] The characteristic physical findings are anesthetic or hypesthetic feet (100% of patients), bony deformities (69% of patients), and soft tissue swelling (17% of patients). Many patients also have ulceration and abnormal callus formation. The most common bony deformities are abnormal projections on the plantar arch (rocker sole) or other unusual prominence of the dorsal or medial arches of the midfoot or the MTP joint. In the acute phase, soft tissue swelling typically appears at the ankle and midfoot, sometimes with marked rubor and warmth mimicking arthritis or cellulitis (in one study, the affected foot was about 5°C [9.2°F] warmer than the unaffected side).[13]

Jean-Martin Charcot described Charcot neuro-arthropathy in 1868 in patients with tabes dorsalis,[14] although he credited the American Mitchell (1831) with the original description.[15]

D. OSTEOMYELITIS

In diabetic patients with foot ulceration and underlying radiographic abnormalities of the bone, it is very difficult to distinguish Charcot foot from osteomyelitis. One proposed test is the **probe test**, in which the clinician gently probes the ulcer base with a sterile blunt, 14.0 cm 5 Fr, stainless-steel eye probe. The test is positive, suggesting osteomyelitis, if the clinician detects a rock-hard, often gritty structure at the ulcer base without any intervening soft tissue.[16]

III. Clinical Significance

A. THE SEMMES-WEINSTEIN MONOFILAMENT

According to the information presented in EBM Box 55.1, the *inability* to feel the 5.07 monofilament is a modest predictor of ulceration during 1 to 4 years of follow-up (likelihood ratio [LR]

EBM BOX 55.1   The Diabetic Foot*

Finding (Reference)†	Sensitivity (%)	Specificity (%)	Likelihood Ratio‡ if Finding Is Present	Absent
Predictors of subsequent foot ulceration				
Insensate to 5.07 monofilament[17–25]	50–90	34–86	2.7	0.5
Predictors of osteomyelitis, in patients with foot ulcers				
Ulcer area[26–28]				
>2 cm²	44–88	20–92	NS	NS
>3 cm²	79	77	3.5	0.3
>4 cm²	67	91	7.3	0.4
>5 cm²	50	95	11.0	0.5
Positive probe test[16,27,29–33]	38–98	78–93	6.0	0.2
Ulcer depth >3 mm or bone exposed[27,28]	65–82	77–85	3.9	0.3
Erythema, swelling, purulence[27,28]	36–41	77–80	NS	NS
Predictors of nonhealing wound at 20 weeks, in patients with foot ulcers[34]				
0 findings	14	70	0.5	…
1 finding	37	…	0.8	…
2 findings	35	…	1.8	…
3 findings	13	96	3.5	…

*Diagnostic standard: for *foot ulceration*, the appearance of an ulcer during 1.2 to 4 years of follow-up; for *osteomyelitis*, biopsy of the bone (histology or microbiology); a small number of patients in two studies[26,31] underwent MRI magnetic resonance imaging to confirm osteomyelitis.
†Definition of findings: for *positive probe test, ulcer area*, and *predictors of nonhealing wound*, see text.
‡Likelihood ratio (LR) if finding present = positive LR; LR if finding absent = negative LR.
NS, Not significant

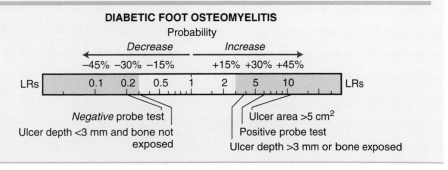

DIABETIC FOOT OSTEOMYELITIS
Probability
Decrease   *Increase*
−45% −30% −15%   +15% +30% +45%

LRs   0.1   0.2   0.5   1   2   5   10   LRs

Negative probe test
Ulcer depth <3 mm and bone not exposed

Ulcer area >5 cm²
Positive probe test
Ulcer depth >3 mm or bone exposed

= 2.7). Abnormal monofilament sensation also weakly predicts future amputation during 1 to 4 years of follow-up (positive LR = 2.6, negative LR = 0.4).[17,25,35] Monofilament sensation predicts complications better than do other quantitative measures of sensation, including the 128 Hz tuning fork[36] and graded vibratory or thermal stimuli.[4,37]

The "Ipswich Touch Test" was developed as an alternative way to test for protective foot sensation, particularly when non-professionals are examining diabetics and lack access to monofilaments.[38] In this test, the clinician (or caregiver) uses his or her index finger to lightly touch the tips of the patient's first, third, and fifth toes on both feet. Lack of sensation at 2 or more of the 6 sites is a positive test (the patient closes his or her eyes and indicates sensation by saying "yes"). In two studies of 596 diabetics undergoing evaluation of their feet, a positive Ipswich Touch test detected abnormal monofilament sensation with sensitivity of 76% to 78%, specificity of 90% to 94%, positive LR = 9.9, and negative LR = 0.3.[38,39]

B. OSTEOMYELITIS

In diabetic patients with foot ulceration, three findings *increase* the probability of underlying osteomyelitis (defined by bone biopsy): ulcer size (>3 cm², LR = 3.5; >4 cm², LR = 7.3; >5 cm², LR = 11), positive probe test (LR = 6), and ulcer depth >3 mm or exposed bone (LR = 3.9). The findings of erythema, swelling, or purulence are unhelpful in diagnosing osteomyelitis.[28] The negative probe-to-bone test decreases probability of osteomyelitis (LR = 0.2).

C. PREDICTORS OF NONHEALING WOUNDS

In one study of over 27,000 diabetic foot ulcers treated with debridement, moist wound dressings, and measures to reduce pressure on the foot (e.g., special footwear, crutches, or wheelchairs), 53% failed to heal after 20 weeks.[34] This study identified three independent predictors of nonhealing ulcers: (1) wound age of more than 2 months, (2) wound size of more than 2 cm², and (3) full-thickness wound associated with either exposed tendons, exposed joint, abscess, osteomyelitis, necrotic tissue, or limb gangrene.[34] The presence of all three of these predictors increases the likelihood that a diabetic foot ulcer will not heal by 20 weeks (LR = 3.5).

References may be accessed online at *Elsevier eBooks for Practicing Clinicians*.

Edema and Deep Vein Thrombosis

EDEMA

I. Introduction

Edema of a limb may occur because of increased venous pressure (e.g., venous insufficiency, congestive heart failure), increased vascular permeability (e.g., inflammation), decreased oncotic pressure (e.g., hypoalbuminemia), lymphatic obstruction (i.e., lymphedema), and deposition of additional tissue (e.g., lipedema). The most common causes of bilateral edema are congestive heart failure, chronic venous insufficiency, pulmonary hypertension, and drug-induced edema (e.g., nifedipine, amlodipine, or nonsteroidal anti-inflammatory medications).[1] The most common causes of unilateral swelling of the leg are deep vein thrombosis, Baker cyst, and cellulitis (see later section).[2–4]

II. The Findings

The pitting characteristics of edema reflect the viscosity of the edema fluid, which in turn depends largely on its protein concentration.[5–8] Edema fluid with low protein levels (e.g., hypoalbuminemia, congestive heart failure) pits easily and recovers relatively quickly compared with edema fluid that has higher protein levels (lymphedema, inflammatory edema).[6,7] A clue to low-protein edema (i.e., edema associated with a serum albumin level less than $3.5\,g/dL$) is edema that pits easily with just 1 to 2 seconds of thumb pressure over the tibia, and then, after removal of the thumb, begins to recover within 2 to 3 seconds.[8]

Lymphedema is painless, firm edema that characteristically causes squaring of the toes and a dorsal hump on the foot. In contrast to venous edema, lymphedema varies little during the day and ulceration is uncommon unless there is secondary infection. Even though lymphedema has high protein levels, clinical experience reveals that lymphedema does pit early in its course although it eventually becomes nonpitting, hard, and "woody" as secondary fibrosis ensues.[5,9,10]

Lipedema consists of bilateral deposition of excess subcutaneous fatty tissue in the legs that does not pit with pressure and whose most characteristic feature is sparing of the feet.[11,12] Lipedema occurs exclusively in obese women.

III. Clinical Significance

A. PITTING EDEMA

In patients with bilateral pitting edema of the legs, the most important diagnostic finding is the patient's venous pressure, estimated from examination of the neck veins. If the neck veins are abnormally distended, cardiac disease or pulmonary hypertension is at least partly responsible for the patient's edema; if they are normal, another cause is responsible, such as liver disease, nephrosis, chronic venous insufficiency, or one of the patient's medications. Clinicians' estimates of venous pressure are accurate, with studies showing that the finding of elevated neck veins predicts an abnormally increased central venous pressure (i.e., >8 cm H_2O) with a positive likelihood ratio [LR] of 8.9 (see Chapter 36).

In contrast, the finding of pitting edema by itself and without knowledge of the patient's venous pressure is an unreliable sign of cardiac disease. For example, in patients undergoing cardiac catheterization because of chest pain or dyspnea, the finding of edema (without knowledge of venous pressure) lacked any significant relationship with the patient's left heart pressures (see Chapter 48).

B. LYMPHEDEMA

Lymphedema is classified as *primary* (i.e., a congenital abnormality of the lymphatic systems) or *secondary* (damage to the lymphatics from previous radiation or surgery, malignant obstruction, or recurrent episodes of cellulitis).[10] Primary lymphedema begins before the age of 40 years, may be bilateral (50% of cases), and affects women ten times more often than men.[13] Secondary lymphedema from infection, radiation, or surgery affects men and women of all ages, is usually unilateral, and is preceded by the characteristic history. Malignant obstruction affects patients older than 40 years and is almost always unilateral (>95% of cases).[13] The most common cause of malignant lymphedema in the leg is metastatic prostate carcinoma in men and lymphoma in women.[13] Lymphedema of the arm is almost always due to breast cancer, either from the tumor itself or combined treatment with surgery and radiation.[14]

DEEP VEIN THROMBOSIS

I. Introduction

Deep vein thrombosis of the leg is conventionally divided into *proximal* thrombosis (popliteal vein and above) and *distal* thrombosis (calf veins). In patients with acutely painful and swollen calves, accurate diagnosis is essential, not only because untreated proximal thrombi may cause fatal pulmonary emboli, but also because inappropriate administration of anticoagulants to persons without proximal thrombi unnecessarily risks life-threatening hemorrhage.

II. The Findings

A. INSPECTION AND PALPATION

The most important signs of vein thrombosis are tenderness and swelling. Calf asymmetry of more than 1.5 cm is abnormal, indicating significant edema of the larger limb or atrophy of the smaller one.[15]

Other traditional signs associated with deep vein thrombosis are a palpable cord, dilated superficial veins, Homans sign, skin erythema, and altered skin temperature (both coolness and warmth have been proposed by different authorities). The basis for these signs, however, seems dubious. Since large muscles and dense fascial tissues encompass the deep veins of the legs, concealing them from the examiner's eyes and hands, it is difficult to conceive how a clinician could ever palpate the cord of a thrombosed deep vein. The increased collateral flow around an obstruction could make the superficial veins more conspicuous, but skin surface temperature and color reflect blood flow and vessel size of the minute vessels *of the dermis*,[16] which would not necessarily be different after venous obstruction.

B. HOMANS SIGN

In his extensive writings about venous thrombosis, the American surgeon John Homans contrasted two forms of the disease: bland thrombosis of the calf veins, which caused few symptoms other than mild swelling and pain, and iliofemoral thrombophlebitis (phlegmasia alba dolens), which caused generalized leg edema and cyanosis.[17-19] Homans believed that most pulmonary emboli originated in the bland calf thrombi, and that, once diagnosed, the disorder should be treated by femoral vein ligation to prevent pulmonary emboli (anticoagulation was not yet being used). In 1941, Homans proposed that the **dorsiflexion sign**, defined as "discomfort behind the knee on forced dorsiflexion of the foot," was a sign of these difficult-to-diagnose calf thrombi.[18] Although contemporaries called the sign **Homans sign**,[20] Homans never did and instead later credited another clinician for making the original description.[21]

Surgeons soon learned that there were many examples of a false-positive Homans sign (i.e., positive dorsiflexion sign but no clot found at surgery),[20,22] and in 1944, Homans redefined the positive response, stating that "discomfort need have no part in the reaction." Eventually, Homans became unenthusiastic about the sign[23,24] and has been quoted as saying "if you wanted to name a sign after me, why didn't you pick a good one?"[25]

C. PSEUDOTHROMBOPHLEBITIS

In a large series of patients presenting with suspected deep vein thrombosis, only one out of every four or five patients actually has the diagnosis.[26-30] An important mimic of deep vein thrombosis (i.e., **pseudothrombophlebitis**) is Baker cyst, which is a distended gastrocnemius-semimembranosus bursa that has dissected or ruptured into the calf or is compressing the popliteal vein.[31,32] A telltale sign of this disorder (and any other cause of calf hematoma) is crescent-shaped ecchymosis near either malleolus.[33,34]

III. Clinical Significance

A. INDIVIDUAL FINDINGS

EBM Box 56.1 presents the diagnostic accuracy of physical signs for deep vein thrombosis of the lower extremity, as applied to thousands of patients with acute calf pain, swelling, or both. Although some studies recruited outpatients[26,35-48] and others both inpatients and outpatients,[28,29,49] the accuracy

EBM BOX 56.1   Lower Extremity Deep Vein Thrombosis*

Finding (Reference)†	Sensitivity (%)	Specificity (%)	Likelihood Ratio‡ if Finding Is	
			Present	Absent
Inspection				
Any calf or ankle swelling[23,24,29,35-37,50,51]	41–90	8–74	1.2	0.7
Asymmetric calf swelling, ≥2 cm difference[28,38]	61–67	69–71	2.1	0.5
Swelling of entire leg[29,36,37,39]	34–57	58–80	1.5	0.8
Superficial venous dilation[24,36,37,39,49]	28–33	79–85	1.6	0.9
Erythema[35,49,50]	16–48	61–87	NS	NS
Superficial thrombophlebitis[51]	5	95	NS	NS
Palpation				
Tenderness[23,24,35-37,39,49-51]	19–85	10–80	NS	NS
Asymmetric skin coolness[24]	42	63	NS	NS
Asymmetric skin warmth[49,50]	29–71	51–77	1.4	NS
Palpable cord[29,49]	15–30	73–85	NS	NS
Other tests				
Homans sign[23,24,29,35,49-51]	10–54	39–89	NS	NS

*Diagnostic standard: for *deep venous thrombosis*, positive contrast venography[23,24,29,35-51] or compression ultrasonography.[28,36-39]

†Definition of findings: All findings refer to the symptomatic leg.

‡Likelihood ratio (LR) if finding present = positive LR; LR if finding absent = negative LR.

NS, Not significant.

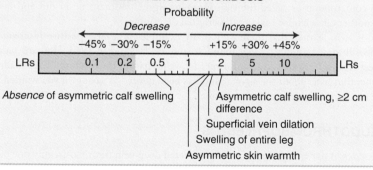

DEEP VENOUS THROMBOSIS

of individual signs is the same whether or not inpatients are included in the analysis. In almost all studies, "deep vein thrombosis" refers only to proximal thrombosis (popliteal vein or higher),[29,35-47,50] although a few studies included patients with proximal vein or isolated calf vein thrombosis.[28,48,49,51] Most studies excluded patients with symptoms suggesting pulmonary embolism.

According to these studies, only the findings of asymmetric calf swelling (≥2 cm difference, LR = 2.1), superficial vein dilation (LR = 1.6), swelling of the entire leg (LR = 1.5), and asymmetric skin warmth (LR = 1.4) increase the probability of thrombosis, although the discriminatory value of all these signs is slight. The presence or absence of erythema, tenderness, skin coolness, palpable cord, and Homans sign lack diagnostic value. As expected, the finding of superficial thrombophlebitis (i.e., visibly inflamed and tender subcutaneous veins) also lacks any relationship to pathology in the deep veins. No individual finding convincingly *decreases* the probability of thrombosis (i.e., no LR <0.5).

TABLE 56.1 ■ **Wells Scoring Scheme for Pretest Probability of Deep-Vein Thrombosis[26]***

Clinical feature	Points
Risk factors	
Active cancer	1
Paralysis, paresis, or recent plaster immobilization of the lower extremities	1
Recently bedridden >3 days or major surgery, within 4 weeks	1
Signs	
Localized tenderness along the distribution of the deep venous system	1
Entire leg swollen	1
Asymmetric calf swelling (>3 cm difference, 10 cm below tibial tuberosity)	1
Asymmetric pitting edema	1
Collateral superficial veins (non-varicose)	1
Alternative diagnosis	
Alternative diagnosis as likely or more likely than deep venous thrombosis	−2

*Interpretation of score: high probability if 3 points or more, moderate probability if 1 or 2 points, and low probability if 0 points or less.

These same studies show that certain risk factors assist diagnosis, most importantly the presence of active cancer (sensitivity of 7% to 39%, specificity of 90% to 97%, positive LR = 2.9).[26,28,29,36–40,52] The findings of "recent immobilization" or "recent surgery" both increase the probability of deep venous thrombosis a smaller amount (positive LR for each finding is 1.6).

B. COMBINED FINDINGS

Given the meager accuracy of individual findings, Wells and others developed a simple scoring scheme (Table 56.1) that combines findings, stratifying patients into groups of low, moderate, or high probability for deep vein thrombosis of the leg.[26] The findings entering his model were all proven to be independent predictors in an earlier analysis.[27,53] This model has now been validated in many studies enrolling more than 6800 patients with suspected deep venous thrombosis: a low pretest probability (0 or fewer points by this model) decreases probability of deep vein thrombosis (LR = 0.2, EBM Box 56.2), and a high pretest probability (3 or more points) significantly increases the probability of deep vein thrombosis (LR = 6.3). The finding of a moderate pretest probability is diagnostically unhelpful.

The Wells score has been tested mostly in outpatients and may be less accurate in inpatients.[54] Also, Wells's original rule was later modified by adding one extra variable ("previous documented deep vein thrombosis") to the original rule (earning 1 additional point if present). This *modified Wells rule* is also accurate, whether it is trichotomized as the original rule (i.e., low probability [0 or fewer points], LR = 0.3; intermediate probability [1 or 2 points], LR not significant; and high probability [3 or more points], LR = 3.9)[40,55,56] or is dichotomized into DVT "likely" (2 or more points, LR = 1.8) or "unlikely" (<2 points, LR = 0.3).[57]

If the clinical probability is low using any of these Wells rules and a quantitative D-dimer measurement is normal, the probability of deep vein thrombosis is so low that anticoagulants and further testing may safely be withheld. Randomized studies show that this approach is as accurate and safe as performing compression ultrasonography in all patients.[57]

C. DIAGNOSING UPPER EXTREMITY DEEP VEIN THROMBOSIS

Constans and others have derived and validated a bedside rule to diagnose deep venous thrombosis of the upper extremity.[58] According to this rule, the clinician adds one point for each of three

EBM BOX 56.2	Lower Extremity Deep Vein Thrombosis (Wells Score)*

Pretest probability[26,30,41,43–48,55,59–61]†	Sensitivity (%)	Specificity (%)	Positive LR‡
Low pretest probability	2–29	24–77	0.2
Moderate pretest probability	13–46	…	NS
High pretest probability	35–87	71–99	6.3

*Diagnostic standard: for *deep vein thrombosis*, proximal vein clot by compression ultrasonography,[26,30,43–48,55,59–61] sometimes with contrast venography.[26,60] In some studies,[44,46,55,60,61] deep venous thrombosis was excluded without compression ultrasonography in patients with low clinical risk, normal D-dimer assay, and absence of venous thromboembolism during 3 months of follow-up.
†Definition of findings: for *pretest probability*, see Table 56.1.
‡Likelihood ratio (LR) if finding present = positive LR; LR if finding absent = negative LR.
NS, Not significant.

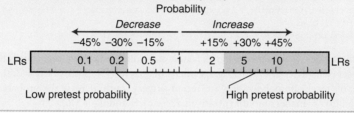

DEEP VENOUS THROMBOSIS (LEG) - WELLS SCORE

EBM BOX 56.3	Upper Extremity Deep Vein Thrombosis[58,62]*

Finding†	Sensitivity (%)	Specificity (%)	Positive LR
Constans score 1 or less, detecting arm DVT	12–42	…	0.3
Constans score 2 or 3, detecting arm DVT	58–88	…	3.0

*Diagnostic standard: for *arm deep vein thrombosis*, compression ultrasonography.
†Definition of findings: for *Constans score*, see text.
DVT, Deep vein thrombosis; *LR*, likelihood ratio.

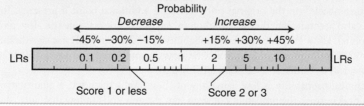

DEEP VENOUS THROMBOSIS (ARM) - CONSTANS SCORE

clinical findings—(1) venous material (i.e., catheter, pacemaker, or access device in a subclavian or jugular vein), (2) pitting edema of arm, (3) localized pain of the arm—and then *subtracts* one point if another diagnosis is at least as plausible as arm deep venous thrombosis (possible scores thus range from −1 to 3). A Constans score of 1 or less decreases probability of arm thrombosis (LR = 0.3, EBM Box 56.3), and a score of 2 or 3 increases probability of thrombosis (LR = 3).

References may be accessed online at *Elsevier eBooks for Practicing Clinicians*.

CHAPTER 57

Examination of the Musculoskeletal System

KEY TEACHING POINTS

- In patients with shoulder pain, the presence of a painful arc increases probability of rotator cuff tendinitis, and a positive dropped arm test, infraspinatus weakness, and age ≥60 years increase probability of rotator cuff tear.
- In patients with hip pain, the following findings increase probability of hip osteoarthritis: limitation of internal rotation (<15 degrees), posterior hip pain during a squat, and groin pain during hip abduction or adduction.
- In patients with knee pain, the following findings increase probability of knee osteoarthritis: palpable osteophytes, genu varum, and stiffness lasting less than 30 minutes.
- In patients with trauma to the knee, all of the traditional signs of ligament injuries (drawer signs, Lachman sign, collateral ligament laxity tests) are accurate when positive.
- In patients with blunt trauma to the knee, ankle, or midfoot, Ottawa rules specific to each area accurately exclude clinically important fractures.
- Three signs accurately diagnose Achilles tendon rupture: the calf squeeze test, the knee flexion test, and palpation of a gap in the tendon itself.

Examination of the musculoskeletal system includes *inspection* (for joint swelling, redness, and deformity), *palpation* (for joint warmth, tenderness, and crepitus*), and investigation of the joint's *range of motion*. Of these tests, range of motion is the most sensitive indicator of joint disease. The normal range of motion of joints is presented in Table 57.1.

Joint pain may originate in the joint itself (i.e., articular disease) or in extra-articular structures such as tendons, ligaments, bursae, or nerves. Articular disease characteristically causes swelling and tenderness that surrounds the entire joint. Articular disease also limits the joint's entire repertoire of motion during both active and passive movements. Extra-articular disease, in contrast, causes swelling and tenderness localized to particular regions of the joint; it affects some aspects of the joint's range of motion while sparing others. Extra-articular disease also tends to limit active joint movements (i.e., voluntary movements) more than it does passive ones (i.e., movements with the muscles relaxed).

In joints lacking normal alignment, **dislocation** implies complete lack of contact between the two articular surfaces whereas **subluxation** implies residual contact but abnormal alignment. In a **valgus deformity**, the distal part of the limb is directed *away* from the body midline (e.g., **genu valgum** of knock-knees; or **hallux valgus** of bunions). In a **varus deformity**, the distal part is directed *toward* the body midline (e.g., **genu varum** of bowlegs). A **recurvatum deformity**

---

*Crepitus is a vibratory sensation felt over joints during movement.

TABLE 57.1 ▦ Normal Range of Motion of Joints*

Joint	Flexion/extension	Abduction/adduction	Rotation
Shoulder	180 degrees	180 degrees (abduction)	90 degrees (internal rotation)
		45 degrees (adduction, across body)	90 degrees (external rotation)
Elbow	150 degrees (humero-ulnar)		180 degrees (radio-humeral)
Wrist and carpal joints	70 degrees (wrist extension)	50 degrees (ulnar deviation)	
	80–90 degrees (palmar flexion)	20–30 degrees (radial deviation)	
Fingers (MCP, PIP, and DIP joints)	90 degrees (MCP)	30–40 degrees (MCP combined abduction/adduction)	
	120 degrees (PIP)		
	80 degrees (DIP)		
Hip	10–20 degrees (extension)	40 degrees (abduction)	40 degrees (internal rotation)
	120 degrees (flexion, knee flexed)	25 degrees (adduction)	45 degrees (external rotation)†
Knee	130 degrees		
Ankle and feet	45 degrees (plantar flexion)		30 degrees (inversion)
	20 degrees (dorsiflexion)		20 degrees (eversion)

*From reference 82.
†Internal and external rotation if hip and knee flexed; less if hip and knee extended.
DIP, Distal interphalangeal; *MCP*, metacarpophalangeal; *PIP*, proximal interphalangeal.

describes abnormal hyperextension of a joint (e.g., **genu recurvatum** of back-kneed individuals, common in patients with chronic quadriceps weakness, see Chapter 7).

An attentive physical examination is fundamental to musculoskeletal diagnosis because, in contrast to other organ systems, the diagnostic standard for many musculoskeletal disorders *is* the bedside findings (Table 57.2 and Chapter 1). For example, in patients with symmetric arthritis of the wrists and hands, ulnar deviation of the metacarpophalangeal joints, and swan-neck deformities of the fingers, the diagnosis of rheumatoid arthritis is likely whether or not serologic biomarkers are present (i.e., if rheumatoid factor and anti-citrullinated peptide antibodies are absent, the patient has **seronegative rheumatoid arthritis**). Instead of focusing on such syndrome-defining findings (for which calculating likelihood ratios [LRs] is impossible), this chapter will focus on those disorders of the shoulder, hip, knee, and ankle for which diagnosis relies on clinical imaging or surgical findings (e.g., osteoarthritis and orthopedic injuries). Other chapters of this book review stance and gait (see Chapter 7), back pain (see Chapter 64), and hand pain (see Chapter 64).

THE SHOULDER

I. Introduction

Shoulder pain is the third most common musculoskeletal complaint (the first two are back pain and knee pain).[1] The shoulder is vulnerable to pain because it is the only location in the human body where tendons (i.e., the rotator cuff tendons†) pass between moving bones (i.e., the acromion

---

†The tendons of the supraspinatus, infraspinatus, subscapularis, and teres minor muscles make up the rotator cuff.

TABLE 57.2 ▪ Abnormal Articular Findings and Implied Diagnosis*

Finding	Diagnosis
Shoulder	
Inspection:	
Flattening of rounded lateral aspect of shoulder	Anterior dislocation
Swelling over anterior aspect	Glenohumeral synovitis; synovial cyst
Elbow	
Inspection:	
Localized cystic swelling over olecranon	Olecranon bursitis
Swelling obscuring para-olecranon grooves	Elbow synovitis
Nodules over extensor surface of ulna	Gouty tophi; rheumatoid nodules
Palpation:	
Elbow pain and tenderness over lateral epicondyle	Lateral epicondylitis (tennis elbow)
Elbow pain and tenderness over medial epicondyle	Medial epicondylitis (golfer's elbow)
Wrists and carpal joints	
Inspection:	
Firm, painless cystic swelling, often located over volar or dorsal wrist	Ganglion (synovial cyst)
Thickening of palmar aponeurosis, causing flexion deformity of MCP joints (4th finger > 5th finger > 3rd finger)	Dupuytren contracture
Abnormal prominence of distal ulna	Subluxation of ulna (from chronic inflammatory arthritis, especially rheumatoid arthritis)
Nonpitting swelling proximal to wrist joint, sparing joint itself; associated clubbing of digits	Hypertrophic osteoarthropathy
Special tests:	
Flexion and extension of digits causes snapping or catching sensation in palm	Trigger finger (flexor tenosynovitis)
Finkelstein test: pain when patient makes fist with fingers over thumb and bends the wrist in an ulnar direction	Tenosynovitis of long abductor and short extensor of thumb (de Quervain stenosing tenosynovitis)
Fingers	
Inspection:	
Loss of normal knuckle wrinkles	PIP or DIP synovitis
Loss of "hills and valleys" appearance of metacarpal heads	MCP synovitis
Ulnar deviation at metacarpophalangeal joints	Chronic inflammatory arthritis
Swan-neck deformity (flexion at MCP joint, hyperextension of PIP joint, flexion of DIP joint)	Chronic inflammatory arthritis, especially rheumatoid arthritis
Boutonniere deformity (flexion of PIP, hyperextension of DIP)	Detachment of central slip of extensor tendon to PIP, common in rheumatoid arthritis
Osteophytes: Heberden nodes at DIP, Bouchard nodes at PIP	Osteoarthritis
Mallet finger: flexion deformity of DIP	Detachment of extensor tendon from base of distal phalanx or fracture
"Telescoping" or "opera glass hand": shortening of digits and destruction of IP joints	Arthritis mutilans, in rheumatoid or psoriatic arthritis
Hip	
Inspection:	
Trauma, hip externally rotated	Femoral neck fracture; anterior dislocation
Trauma, hip internally rotated	Posterior dislocation

continued

TABLE 57.2 ■ Abnormal Articular Findings and Implied Diagnosis*—Cont'd

Finding	Diagnosis
Pelvic tilt (imaginary line through the anterior iliac spines is not horizontal)	Scoliosis; anatomic leg-length discrepancy; hip disease
Palpation:	
Hip pain, tenderness localized over greater trochanter	Trochanteric bursitis
Hip pain, tenderness localized over middle third of inguinal ligament, lateral to femoral pulse	Iliopsoas bursitis
Hip pain and tenderness localized over ischial tuberosity	Ischiogluteal bursitis (weaver's bottom)
Knee	
Inspection:	
Localized tenderness and swelling over patella	Prepatellar bursitis (housemaid's knees)
Generalized swelling of popliteal space	Baker cyst (enlarged semimembranosus bursa, which communicates with knee joint)
Genu varum and genu valgum	See text
Palpation:	
Knee pain and tenderness localized over medial aspect of upper tibia	Anserine bursitis
Distressed reaction if patella moved laterally (apprehension test)	Recurrent patellar dislocation
Ankle and feet	
Inspection:	
Flattening of longitudinal arch	Pes planus
Abnormal elevation of medial longitudinal arch	Pes cavus
Outward angulation of great toe with prominence over medial 1st MTP joint (bunion)	Hallux valgus
Hyperextension of MTP joints and flexion of PIP joints	Hammer toes
Palpation:	
Nodules within Achilles tendon	Tendon xanthoma
Foot pain, localized tenderness over calcaneal origin of plantar fascia	Plantar fascitis
Foot pain, localized tenderness over plantar surface of MT heads	Metatarsalgia
Forefoot pain, tenderness between 2nd or 3rd toes or between 3rd and 4th toes	Morton interdigital neuroma
Ankle pain, dysesthesias of sole, aggravated by forced dorsiflexion and eversion of foot	Tarsal tunnel syndrome

*Special tests of the shoulder, hip, knee, and ankle are discussed in the text.
DIP, Distal interphalangeal; *MCP*, metacarpophalangeal; *MT*, metatarsal; *MTP*, metatarsophalangeal; *PIP*, proximal interphalangeal.

and humerus). This anatomy grants the shoulder great flexibility but also renders the rotator cuff tendons and accompanying bursa susceptible to inflammation, degeneration, and tears.

One popular method of classifying shoulder pain (see Table 57.3), based on the work of the British orthopedic surgeon James Cyriax,[2,3] distinguishes the causes of shoulder pain by location of pain, range of passive motion, strength of rotator cuff muscles, and **painful arc** (i.e., pain during arm elevation between the angles of 70 and 100 degrees, angles that compress the subacromial tissues the most). Using this classification, 5% to 12% of patients with shoulder pain have capsular syndromes, 17% acute bursitis, 5% to 11% acromioclavicular syndromes, 47% to 65% subacromial syndromes, and 5% to 10% referred shoulder pain (e.g., cervical disc disease or myofascial pain).[4–7]

TABLE 57.3 ■ Shoulder Syndromes

Syndrome	Location of pain	Range of passive motion	Other findings
Capsular syndromes Adhesive capsulitis Glenohumeral arthritis	Outer arm	Limited* (all motions limited; especially external rotation and abduction)	
Acute bursitis†	Outer arm	Limited* (abduction especially limited)	
Acromioclavicular pain	Point of shoulder	Normal	Tenderness of acromioclavicular joint Pain worse during adduction of arm across body
Subacromial syndromes Rotator cuff tendonitis Rotator cuff tear	Outer arm	Normal	Painful arc Rotator cuff muscle strength: Normal in tendonitis Weak in rotator cuff tears

Adapted from references 2–4.
*One way to test for limitation of passive motion is to ask the patient to bend over and try to touch his or her toes. In those with normal shoulder passive motion, the arms dangle toward the floor.
†*Acute bursitis* and *subacromial disorders* both represent disorders of the subacromial space, but bursitis causes inflammation and swelling that is more acute and severe, thus limiting motion.

Nonetheless, some clinicians have questioned the utility and accuracy of this classification, for several reasons: (1) most shoulder syndromes are treated similarly with anti-inflammatory medications, injections, and physical therapy, no matter what the diagnosis is[4]; (2) different shoulder syndromes are indistinguishable from the patient's perspective, causing similar pain and disability over time[4,5]; (3) if patients are examined a second time, the specific diagnosis often changes[5]; and (4) legions of bedside tests have been proposed to diagnose shoulder disorders (one website lists 129 tests[8]), and new ones continue to appear[9-11] suggesting that a comprehensive understanding of shoulder pain is still lacking.

Nonetheless, the bedside examination continues to play an important role in patients with shoulder pain, especially in distinguishing intrinsic shoulder syndromes from disorders causing referred pain, and in identifying rotator cuff tears, a condition sometimes requiring surgical repair. These subjects are the focus of this section.

II. The Findings

A. IMPINGEMENT SIGNS

Impingement signs reproduce subacromial pain by compressing the rotator cuff tendons between the head of the humerus and acromion. Of the many different impingement signs, the most popular are the **Neer impingement sign** and **Hawkins impingement sign** (Figs. 57.1 and 57.2). Both of these maneuvers were originally introduced to select patients for specific surgical procedures. The Neer maneuver forces the humerus (and the overlying rotator cuff tendons) against the *anterior* acromion, which Neer proposed resecting (i.e., anterior acromioplasty) in patients with persistent pain.[12] The Hawkins maneuver forces the greater tuberosity of the humerus against the coracoacromial ligament (the ligament forming the anterior roof over the rotator cuff). If patients develop pain during this maneuver and surgery is contemplated, Hawkins believed the coracoacromial ligament should be resected.[13]

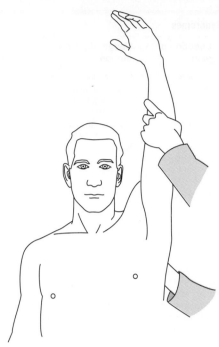

Fig. 57.1 Neer impingement sign.[12] The clinician prevents scapular motion with one hand and uses the other hand to raise the patient's arm in forward flexion, a position that presses the greater tuberosity of the humerus against the acromion.[12,117] Neer believed his sign was nonspecific (i.e., shoulder pains of all types worsened with this maneuver), but he taught that subacromial pain was the only shoulder syndrome whose positive impingement sign disappeared after injection of lidocaine into the subacromial space.

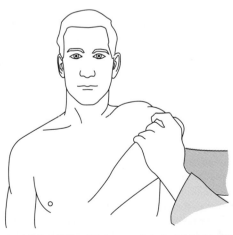

Fig. 57.2 Hawkins impingement sign.[13] The clinician stands in front of the patient, flexes both the patient's shoulder and elbow to 90 degrees, and then internally rotates the patient's arm, a position that presses the greater tuberosity against the coracoacromial ligament.[117]

B. YERGASON SIGN

The **Yergason sign** (Fig. 57.3) has traditionally been associated with bicipital tendonitis, as if that were an isolated entity, but in fact most patients with inflammation of the biceps tendon also have disease of the rotator cuff. This occurs because progressive subacromial impingement causes wearing away of the supraspinatus tendon and underlying capsule, which then exposes the long head of the biceps tendon and subjects it to the same injurious forces. Indeed, most tears of the biceps tendon are associated with advanced rotator cuff disease.[12,14,15]

C. SPEED TEST

Like the Yergason sign, the **Speed test** (Fig. 57.4) was originally developed to identify pain originating in the biceps tendon,[16] but studies apply the test now to the diagnosis of subacromial impingement syndromes in general.

D. MUSCLE ATROPHY

The clinician detects atrophy of the supraspinatus or infraspinatus muscles by inspecting the posterior scapula on the symptomatic side and noting any increased prominence of the scapular spine when compared with the contralateral side. Atrophy of these muscles may appear as soon as 2 to 3 weeks after a rotator cuff tear.

E. MUSCLE TESTING

The most important muscles to test in suspected tears of the rotator cuff are the supraspinatus muscle (involved in most rotator cuff tears) and the infraspinatus muscle (involved in 11% to

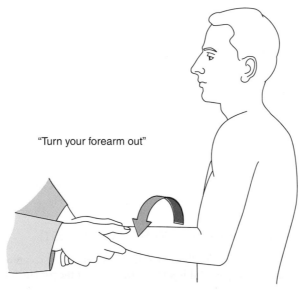

"Turn your forearm out"

Fig. 57.3 Yergason sign.[118] The clinician stands in front of the patient, flexes the patient's forearm 90 degrees at the elbow, and pronates the patient's wrist. The clinician then asks the patient to supinate the forearm against resistance (i.e., turn forearm in the direction of the arrow). Pain in the shoulder indicates a positive test, implying inflammation of the long head of the biceps tendon (the main supinator of the forearm).

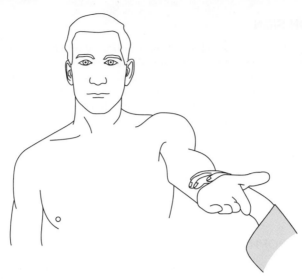

Fig. 57.4 Speed test. The patient flexes the shoulder forward to 60 to 90 degrees, with his or her elbow extended and arm fully supinated (i.e., palm up), as the clinician applies a downward force. Pain in the shoulder (in the bicipital groove) is the positive response.

45% of tears).[15,17] The supraspinatus muscle abducts the shoulder, and the infraspinatus externally rotates it. Figs. 57.5 and 57.6 describe testing the strength of these muscles.

F. DROPPED ARM TEST

The examiner abducts the patient's arm as far as possible and releases it, asking the patient to lower the arm slowly back down to the side. In patients with a positive test, indicating a rotator cuff tear, the patient lowers the arm smoothly until about 100 degrees, after which the smooth movements become irregular and the arm may fall suddenly to the side.[18]

The dropped arm test becomes positive below angles of 100 degrees, not because the supraspinatus is the most powerful abductor at this angle,‡ but because the rotator cuff muscles must be intact to pull the humeral head tightly against the glenoid fossa, creating a fulcrum that allows the deltoid to smoothly lower the arm.

G. PALPATING ROTATOR CUFF TEARS

Early descriptions of rotator cuff tears emphasized the importance of actually palpating the tear, just anterior to the acromial edge and through the deltoid muscle (Fig. 57.7).[19]

H. CROSSED BODY ADDUCTION TEST (SCARF TEST)

Crossing the arm horizontally maximally across the chest (Fig. 57.8) compresses the ipsilateral acromioclavicular joint, causing pain if this joint is the source of the patient's symptoms.

---

‡The supraspinatus muscle is responsible for only the initial 30 degrees of abduction, whereas the deltoid muscle (uninvolved in rotator cuff disease) accounts for abduction between 30 degrees and 180 degrees.

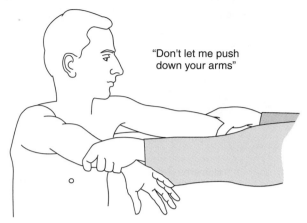

Fig. 57.5 **Supraspinatus test (empty can test, Jobe test).**[119] The clinician stands in front of the patient and elevates the patient's arms to 90 degrees in the plane of the scapula (i.e., *scaption*, midway between forward flexion and sideways abduction). The patient's arms are internally rotated with thumbs pointing down (as if emptying a can). The patient is asked to hold this position and resist attempts to lower the arms to the side. Some investigators propose testing the supraspinatus muscle in a slightly different way, with the arms externally rotated and thumbs pointing up (i.e., **full can test**), because this position causes less pain than the empty can test. In clinical studies, both versions have similar diagnostic accuracy.[17,89]

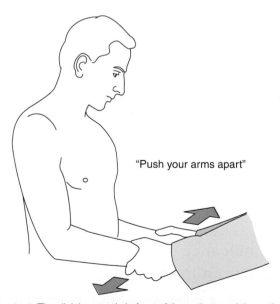

Fig. 57.6 **Infraspinatus test.** The clinician stands in front of the patient, and the patient's arms are at his or her side with elbows flexed 90 degrees and thumbs up. The examiner places his or her hands outside those of the patient's and directs the patient to move his arms out (i.e., direction of arrow), resisting the clinician's opposing inward pressure.[87]

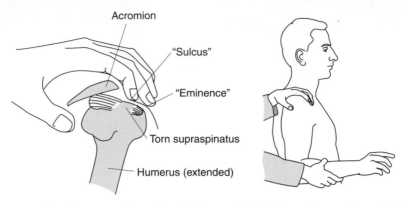

Fig. 57.7 Palpation of rotator cuff tears. The clinician stands behind the patient, and the patient's arm is relaxed at the side with elbow flexed 90 degrees. The clinician palpates just below the patient's acromion with one hand and holds the patient's forearm with the other. The clinician then gently extends the patient's arm as far as possible and rotates the shoulder internally and externally to fully reveal the greater tuberosity and attached tissues. In patients with tears of the supraspinatus tendon (which inserts on the greater tuberosity), the clinician detects both an abnormal eminence and an abnormal sulcus posterior to this eminence. The abnormal eminence is the greater tuberosity with attached remnant of tendon, and the sulcus just behind it is the actual rent in the supraspinatus tendon. Comparison with the contralateral shoulder helps determine whether the suspected tear is real or not.

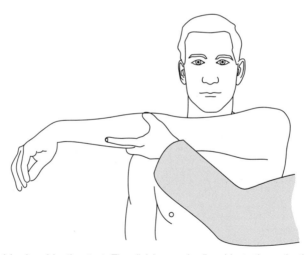

Fig. 57.8 Crossed body adduction test. The clinician maximally adducts the patient's arm (ipsilateral to the symptomatic shoulder) across the patient's chest. Pain in the symptomatic acromioclavicular joint is the positive response.

III. Clinical Significance

A. ACROMIOCLAVICULAR JOINT PAIN

In patients with shoulder pain, a positive crossed body adduction test increases probability of acromioclavicular joint pain (LR = 3.7, EBM Box 57.1) and its absence decreases it (LR = 0.3). Acromioclavicular joint tenderness and compression tenderness are diagnostically unhelpful (LRs not significant).

B. ROTATOR CUFF TENDONITIS

According to the LRs in EBM Box 57.1, the findings that increase probability of rotator cuff tendonitis the most are positive painful arc (LR = 2.9), Yergason sign (LR = 2.8), and positive Speed test (LR = 1.9). The diagnostic accuracy of Yergason sign and Speed test emphasizes again the association between biceps tendon pain and rotator cuff disease (see the section on Yergason sign).

The presence of Neer or Hawkins impingement signs fails to change the probability of rotator cuff tendonitis much (LRs = 1.6 to 1.7), simply because shoulder pain of all types worsens during these maneuvers (i.e., specificity is low and there are many false positives. Nonetheless, these studies did not repeat the impingement signs after lidocaine injection as Neer originally proposed, a maneuver that might improve specificity). The *absence* of Hawkins sign (LR = 0.3) and the *absence* of both impingement signs (LR = 0.1) significantly *decreases* probability of rotator cuff tendinitis.

EBM BOX 57.1   **Shoulder Pain-Individual Findings***

Finding (Reference)[†]	Sensitivity (%)	Specificity (%)	Likelihood Ratio[‡] if Finding Is Present	Absent
Detecting acromioclavicular joint pain				
Acromioclavicular joint tenderness[7]	96	10	NS	NS
Tenderness with compression of acromioclavicular joint[7]	79	50	NS	NS
Crossed body adduction test[83]	77	79	**3.7**	0.3
Detecting rotator cuff tendinitis				
Neer impingement sign[22,84–86]	68–89	32–69	1.6	0.5
Hawkins impingement sign[22,84–86]	72–93	26–66	1.7	**0.3**
Hawkins or Neer impingement sign[85]	96	41	1.6	**0.1**
Yergason sign[84]	37	87	2.8	0.7
Speed test[22,84]	38–69	55–83	1.9	0.7
Painful arc[22,84,86]	32–74	80–82	2.9	NS
Detecting rotator cuff tear - individual findings				
Age[18]				
≤39 years	5	58	**0.1**	...
40–59 years	34	...	NS	...
≥60 years	62	81	**3.2**	...
Supraspinatus atrophy[87]	55	73	2.0	0.6
Infraspinatus atrophy[87]	55	73	2.0	0.6
Painful arc[22,87,88]	39–97	10–84	NS	0.5
Neer impingement sign[11,22,85,88]	59–88	43–89	2.1	0.5
Hawkins impingement sign[11,22,85,88]	36–83	48–77	1.7	0.7
Supraspinatus testing causes pain[15,17,89–91]	54–90	11–62	1.5	0.5
Supraspinatus weakness[11,17,22,87–93]	32–90	46–89	2.1	0.4
Infraspinatus weakness[22,87,88]	16–76	57–84	2.6	0.6
Dropped arm test[18,22,88]	6–35	87–98	2.9	NS
Palpable tear[20,21]	91–96	75–97	**10.2**	**0.1**

continued

EBM BOX 57.1	Shoulder Pain-Individual Findings*—Cont'd

*Diagnostic standard: for *acromioclavicular joint pain*, reduction of pain after injecting lidocaine into the acromioclavicular joint; for *rotator cuff tendonitis*, reduction of pain after injection of the subacromial space with lidocaine[84] or subacromial bursitis at arthroscopy[22,85,86]; for *rotator cuff tear*, arthrography,[22,87] MRI,[17,88,89] ultrasonography,[90,93] or surgery (arthroscopy or open repair).[11,15,18,20,21,85,91,92]

†Definition of findings: for *tenderness with compression of the acromioclavicular joint*, the clinician stands behind the patient and compresses the joint by placing his or her thumb over the patient's posterolateral acromion and index/middle fingers on the patient's midclavicle.[7]

‡Likelihood ratio (LR) if finding present = positive LR; LR if finding absent = negative LR.
MRI, Magnetic resonance imaging; *NS*, not significant.

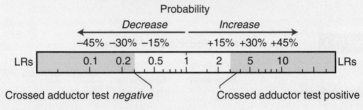

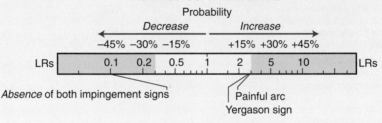

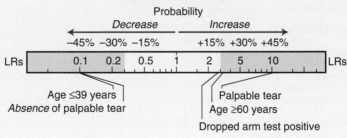

C. ROTATOR CUFF TEARS

1. Individual Findings

In patients with shoulder pain, the bedside findings increasing the probability of rotator cuff tear the most are age of 60 years or older (LR = 3.2), positive dropped arm test (LR = 2.9), and infraspinatus weakness (LR = 2.6). The positive supraspinatus test increases probability slightly, and diagnostic accuracy is similar whether the clinician regards the positive response to be weakness (LR = 2.1) or pain (LR = 1.5). Age of 39 years or younger (LR = 0.1) decreases probability of rotator cuff tear.

Although the reported diagnostic accuracy of palpating actual rents in the supraspinatus tendon is impressive (positive LR = 10.2, negative LR = 0.1, EBM Box 57.1), these LRs have been derived from examinations by orthopedic surgeons who have comprehensive understanding of the anatomy of the shoulder and considerable experience treating shoulder pain.[20,21] Whether other practitioners will duplicate this accuracy is unknown.

2. Combined Findings

Two investigations of rotator cuff tears that combined clinical findings demonstrated superior diagnostic accuracy. Each focused on three clinical findings. Murrell[18] combined (1) impingement signs, (2) supraspinatus weakness, and (3) infraspinatus weakness, and Park[22] combined (1) Hawkins sign, (2) painful arc, and (3) infraspinatus weakness. When all three signs are present, the probability of rotator cuff tear is greatly increased (LR = 48 for the Murrell findings; LR = 15.9 for the Park findings, EBM Box 57.2), whereas when all three signs are absent, probability is greatly diminished (LR = 0.02 for the Murrell findings; LR = 0.2 for the Park findings).

EBM BOX 57.2	Shoulder Pain - Combined Findings*			
			Likelihood Ratio[†] if Finding Is	
Finding (Reference)	**Sensitivity (%)**	**Specificity (%)**	**Present**	**Absent**
Detecting rotator cuff tear				
Number of findings present (Murrell): (1) impingement signs, (2) supraspinatus weakness, (3) infraspinatus weakness[18]				
3 findings	24	100	**48.0**	...
2 findings	37	...	**4.9**	...
1 finding	39	...	NS	...
0 findings	1	52	**0.02**	
Number of findings present (Park): (1) Hawkins sign, (2) painful arc, (3) infraspinatus weakness[22]				
3 findings	33	98	**15.9**	...
2 findings	35	...	**3.6**	...
1 finding	24	...	NS	...
0 findings	9	42	**0.2**	

*Diagnostic standard: for *rotator cuff tear*, arthroscopy.[18,22]
[†]Likelihood ratio (LR) if finding present = positive LR; LR if finding absent = negative LR.
NS, Not significant.

ROTATOR CUFF TEAR (COMBINED FINDINGS)

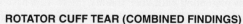
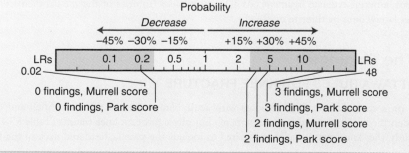

Probability

Decrease | Increase

−45% −30% −15% | +15% +30% +45%

LRs 0.02 — 0.1 0.2 0.5 1 2 5 10 — LRs 48

0 findings, Murrell score
0 findings, Park score

3 findings, Murrell score
3 findings, Park score
2 findings, Murrell score
2 findings, Park score

THE HIP

I. Introduction

Hip pain may result from a variety of disorders including hip arthritis, sacroiliac disease, extra-articular disease (e.g., trochanteric bursitis, iliopsoas bursitis), neurogenic causes (e.g., meralgia paresthetica, sciatica), and rarely, miscellaneous distant disorders (e.g., hernia).

II. The Findings

The hip joint lies deep in the lower pelvis, surrounded by large muscles that protect it from direct contact with the external world, thus limiting the development of well-localized somatic sensations. Consequently, some patients with hip arthritis develop groin pain, but many experience pain at distant sites in the cutaneous distribution of nerves innervating the hip joint capsule, such as the thigh and knee (obturator and femoral nerves) or buttock (sciatic nerve). Unlike extraarticular causes of hip pain (e.g., trochanteric bursitis), hip disease affects the entire repertoire of hip motion, including flexion, extension, abduction, adduction, and internal and external rotation.

Many patients with hip disease develop a characteristic limp, the **coxalgic gait** (see Chapter 7).

III. Clinical Significance

In a study of 78 patients presenting with unilateral hip pain (38),[23] pain localized to the ipsilateral buttock (LR = 6.7) or groin (LR = 3.6) increased the probability of hip osteoarthritis. Additional findings increasing the probability of hip disease were posterior hip pain with squatting (LR = 6.1, EBM Box 57.3), groin pain with abduction or adduction (LR = 5.7), and hip pain with active flexion (LR = 3.6) or extension (LR = 2.7). In another study of 598 elderly patients with joint pain, limitation of hip internal rotation to less than 15 degrees was a compelling argument for hip osteoarthritis (LR = 9.9).[24]

THE KNEE

I. Introduction

Knee pain affects up to 13% of the adult population and is second only to back pain among musculoskeletal complaints.[25] Common causes include arthritis (osteoarthritis, rheumatoid arthritis, gout, and pseudogout), bursitis (prepatellar and anserine bursitis), and injuries to ligaments or menisci. Among patients presenting with knee trauma, 6% to 12% have significant fractures on knee radiographs,[26–34] and the most frequently injured internal structures are the medial collateral ligament, anterior cruciate ligament (ACL), and menisci (injuries of the medial meniscus outnumber lateral ones by three to one).[35–40]

II. The Findings

A. OTTAWA RULES FOR KNEE FRACTURE

Based on a study of over 1000 patients with acute blunt injury to the knee, Stiell and others have identified five independent predictors of clinically significant knee trauma (Table 57.4).[27] In this study, the "knee" was broadly considered to include the patella, head and neck of the fibula,

EBM BOX 57.3	Diagnosis of Osteoarthritis, in Patients With Hip Pain*

Finding (Reference)	Sensitivity (%)	Specificity (%)	Likelihood Ratio† if Finding Is Present	Likelihood Ratio† if Finding Is Absent
Squat causes pain in posterior hip[23]	24	96	**6.1**	NS
Abduction or adduction causes groin pain[23]	33	94	**5.7**	NS
Active hip flexion causes lateral hip pain[23]	43	88	**3.6**	NS
Active hip extension causes hip pain[23]	52	80	2.7	0.6
Passive internal rotation				
≤25 degrees[23]	76	61	1.9	0.4
<15 degrees[24]	39	96	**9.9**	0.6

*Diagnostic standard: for *diagnosis of osteoarthritis*, Kellgren-Lawrence score on plain radiographs[23] ≥2 or presence of radiographic osteophytes and joint space narrowing.[24]
†Likelihood ratio (LR) if finding present = positive LR; LR if finding absent = negative LR.
NS, Not significant.

HIP OSTEOARTHRITIS
Probability

Decrease ← → Increase

−45% −30% −15%   +15% +30% +45%

LRs   0.1   0.2   0.5   1   2   5   10   LRs

Internal rotation >25°

Internal rotation <15°
Squat causes posterior hip pain
Abduction or adduction causes groin pain
Active hip flexion causes lateral hip pain

proximal 8 cm of the tibia, and distal 8 cm of the femur; *significant trauma* implied an injury requiring orthopedic consultation, splinting, or surgery.

B. TESTS OF LIGAMENT INJURIES

The stability of the knee depends on the joint capsule and two pairs of ligaments: the medial and lateral collateral ligaments, and the anterior and posterior cruciate ligaments (ACL and (PCL).§ The clinician tests each of these four ligaments by stressing the knee in a direction that the intact ligament would normally resist (specific tests appear below). If no movement occurs during stress testing or if small movements occur but abruptly end with a firm stop (i.e., a "hard" end point),

§The crossed cruciate ligaments are named for their attachment to the *tibial* surface, i.e., the anterior cruciate liga-ment (ACL) crosses from the posterior femur to the *anterior* tibia; the *posterior* cruciate ligament (PCL) crosses from the anterior femur to the *posterior* tibia. "Cruciate" derives from Latin *cruciatus*, meaning "cross-shaped."

TABLE 57.4 ■ **Ottawa Rule for Knee Fracture[26,27]**

A knee radiograph is indicated (and the rule is positive) if *any* of the following are present:
  Aged ≥55 years
  Tenderness at head of fibula
  Isolated tenderness of patella*
  Inability to flex to 90 degrees
  Inability to bear weight both immediately and in the emergency department (four steps)†

*No bone tenderness of knee other than patella.
†Unable to transfer weight twice onto each lower limb regardless of limping.

the ligament is intact. If there is excessive laxity of movement or a "soft" or "mushy" end point, the ligament is damaged.

Blunt trauma to the outside of the knee is associated with injury of the medial collateral ligament; trauma to the inside of the knee suggests injury of the lateral collateral ligament. Twisting of the knee after planting the foot is the characteristic mechanism of ACL injury, whereas deceleration of the flexed knee on a hard surface (e.g., striking the knee against the dashboard in an automobile accident) often precedes PCL injury. The mechanism of meniscal injuries, resembles that of ACL injuries—twisting the knee after planting the foot—but unlike ACL injuries, which are associated with immediate knee swelling, meniscal injuries cause swelling that appears only after a delay of several hours (because the menisci are relatively avascular).[41,42]

1. Anterior Cruciate Ligament

The ACL prevents anterior subluxation of the tibia on the femoral head. There are three common tests for this ligament: the anterior drawer sign, Lachman sign, and the pivot shift sign (Figs. 57.9 to 57.11).

The **pivot shift sign** refers to the tendency of the tibia to sublux anteriorly in ACL-deficient knees when the knee is between 0 and 30 degrees of flexion, and the *spontaneous reduction* of the subluxed tibia as the knee is flexed past 40 degrees.[43,44] Patients with ACL injuries notice the pivot-shift phenomenon themselves when they plant their foot with extended knee in front of them (e.g., stopping suddenly from a run causes the tibia to shift forward, producing the sensation of the knee "giving away"). Fig. 57.12 explains the mechanism of the pivot shift phenomenon. What specifically is responsible for the sudden reduction at 40 to 50 degrees is controversial, but most experts believe it is the pull of the iliotibial tract (whose action abruptly changes from a knee extensor to knee flexor beyond 40 degrees of flexion)[43,45,46] and the geometric peculiarities of the convex tibial surface.[44,47]

Descriptions of the **anterior drawer sign** have been found in writings from the 1870s.[48] The **Lachman test** was attributed to the American orthopedic surgeon John Lachman by one of his students in 1976,[49] although the same sign was described a century earlier by European clinicians.[48] Photographs of patients demonstrating their own pivot shift phenomenon were published in 1920,[50] but the pivot shift test was formerly described in 1972.[51] The term itself is confusing, but according to Liorzou[45] it originated from an interview with a hockey player who stated "When I pivot, my knee shifts."

2. Posterior Cruciate Ligament

The PCL is the least likely internal structure of the knee to be injured.[36] Since this ligament resists posterior subluxation of the tibia on the femur, the conventional test is the **posterior drawer sign** (Fig. 57.13).

3. Collateral Ligaments

Injury to either collateral ligament is identified by applying a varus or valgus stress to the knee and noting abnormal movement when compared to the contralateral side. Testing is performed with

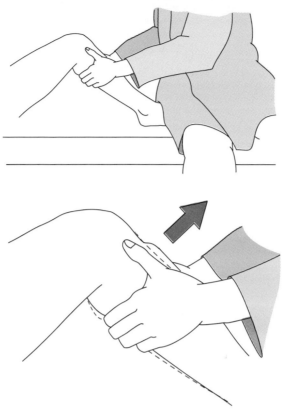

Fig. 57.9 Anterior drawer sign. The patient lies supine with hip flexed at 45 degrees, knee flexed at 90 degrees, and foot flat on the table. The clinician sits on top of the patient's foot to stabilize it and then stresses the ACL ligament by grasping the patient's upper calf and pulling forward. Abnormal anterior subluxation of the tibia (*arrow*) with a soft end point is a positive test.

the knee straight and at 20 degrees flexion. Excessive movement during valgus stress indicates injury to the medial collateral ligament; excessive movement during varus stress indicates injury to the lateral collateral ligament.

C. TESTS OF MENISCAL INJURIES: THE MCMURRAY TEST

Tears of the *anterior* meniscus or large bucket-handle tears often displace tissue between the articular surfaces of the anterior tibia and femur, thus preventing full extension of the knee (or **locking**), a characteristic sign of meniscal injury.

Because tears of the posterior half of the meniscus are unlikely to cause locking and are therefore more difficult to detect, the British orthopedic surgeon McMurray proposed in 1949 additional diagnostic tests, one of which is now called the McMurray test (Fig. 57.14).[40],¶

¶One way to help recall the correct positioning of the McMurray test: testing the medial (i.e., *inner*) meniscus is analogous to the patient squatting with both feet *externally* rotated; testing the lateral (*outer*) meniscus is analogous to the patient squatting with both feet *internally* rotated (i.e., pigeon-toed). One author has converted this squatting maneuver into a clinical test (the Ege test).[52]

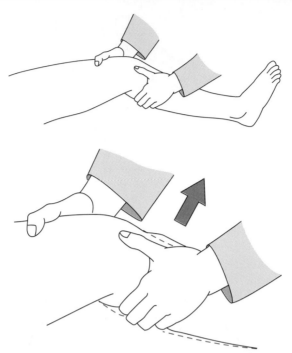

Fig. 57.10 Lachman sign. The Lachman sign differs from the anterior drawer sign (see Fig. 57.9) by the position of the knee during testing. In the Lachman test, the hip is extended and the knee flexed at only 20 degrees. The clinician grasps the lower thigh with one hand and the upper calf with the other, pulling forward on the tibia to stress the ligament and reveal the abnormal anterior subluxation of the tibia (*arrow*).

III. Clinical Significance

A. DETECTING OSTEOARTHRITIS

In a study of 237 patients with various forms of chronic knee pain (i.e., osteoarthritis, rheumatoid arthritis, meniscal or ligament injuries, osteonecrosis, gout, septic arthritis, and other assorted connective tissue disorders),[53] the following findings increased the probability of osteoarthritis in the knee: palpable bony enlargement (LR = 11.8, EBM Box 57.4), genu varum deformity (LR = 3.4), stiffness lasting for less than 30 minutes (LR = 3), and presence of at least three of six characteristic findings listed in EBM Box 57.4 (LR = 3.1). The findings that decreased probability of osteoarthritis in the knee are fewer than three characteristic findings (LR = 0.1), morning stiffness lasting for more than 30 minutes (LR = 0.2), and absence of crepitus (LR = 0.2). The presence of valgus deformity is diagnostically unhelpful (LR not significant), occurring just as often in patients with osteoarthritis as alternative diagnoses.

In another study of 598 elderly patients with painful, stiff joints, inability to flex the knee more than 120 degrees accurately detected radiographic changes of osteoarthritis (sensitivity of 13%, specificity of 96%, positive LR = 3.4).[24]

B. DETECTING KNEE FRACTURE

In patients presenting to emergency departments with knee trauma, the following findings increase probability of a clinically significant knee fracture: inability to flex the knee beyond 60

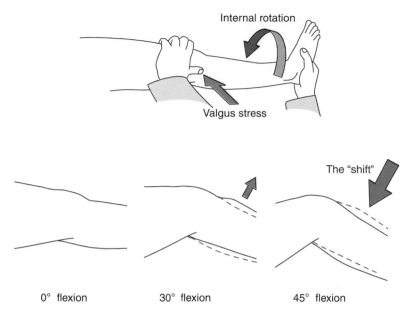

Fig. 57.11 **Pivot shift sign.** Many variations of this test have been published,[120] but the most common version begins with the patient supine, hip and knee extended. The clinician lifts the patient's leg, one hand over the fibula and the other at the ankle, pushing medially on the fibula (i.e., providing a valgus stress) and rotating internally the ankle and foot (and thus tibia). While maintaining these valgus and rotational stresses, the examiner slowly flexes the patient's knee. In the ACL-deficient knee, the tibia subluxes anteriorly, almost imperceptibly, during the initial 0 to 30 degrees flexion with these applied forces (*small arrow*). At 40 to 50 degrees, however, the tibia suddenly subluxes posteriorly (the shift), which constitutes a positive pivot shift test (and recalls for many patients the sensation of their "knee giving way").[121]

degrees (LR = 4.7, EBM Box 57.5), inability to bear weight immediately after the injury and in the emergency department (LR = 3.6), tenderness at the head of the fibula (LR = 3.4), and age of 55 years or older (LR = 3). A negative Ottawa knee rule (i.e., lacking all five predictors from Table 57.4) greatly decreases probability of knee fracture (LR = 0.1).

C. DETECTING LIGAMENT AND MENISCAL INJURIES

Most studies of soft tissue injuries of the knee are vulnerable to both *selection bias* (i.e., only patients scheduled for surgery are enrolled) and *verification bias* (i.e., the surgeons who operated on the patients are also the clinicians who examined the patients). Nonetheless, these biases may be less important than expected because other studies using independent diagnostic standards (e.g., magnetic resonance imaging [MRI][54,55] reveal similar diagnostic accuracy for these clinical signs.

1. Anterior Cruciate Ligament Injury

Any of the three physical tests of ACL injury, when positive, are increase probability of ACL injury: Lachman sign (LR = 20.5, EBM Box 57.6), anterior drawer sign (LR = 12.2), and pivot shift sign (LR = 8.2). Only the *absence* of Lachman sign, however, significantly decreases the probability of ACL injury (LR = 0.2).

The Lachman sign is more sensitive than the anterior drawer sign for three reasons[49]: (1) Hemarthrosis from acute ACL injury impairs knee flexion and thus prevents the testing of the anterior drawer test. (2) Tense hamstring muscles, irritated from pain, directly oppose forward subluxation of the tibia during the anterior drawer sign (knee at 90°) but not when the knee is at

INTERNAL ROTATION

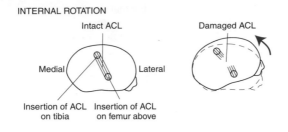

0–30° FLEXION → ANTERIOR DISPLACEMENT OF TIBIA

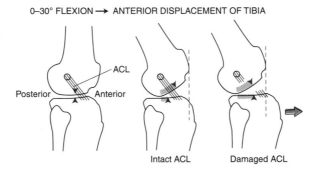

>40–50° FLEXION → SUDDEN POSTERIOR SHIFT

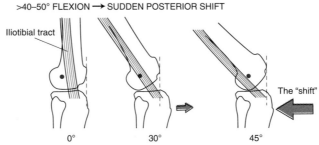

Fig. 57.12 Mechanism of the pivot shift. The pivot shift phenomenon (i.e., positive test) refers to anterior displacement of the tibia with respect to the distal femur during the first 30 degrees of flexion and the sudden backward return of the tibia to its normal position after about 40 to 50 degrees flexion (see Fig. 57.11). This figure depicts what happens during internal rotation (*top row*), 0 to 30 degrees flexion (*middle row*), and beyond 40 to 50 degrees flexion (*bottom row*) in the ACL-deficient knee. **(1) Top row** (view of the tibial plateau from above): Because of its oblique orientation (*left*), the ACL is the key ligament resisting internal rotation of the tibia (this also explains why many ACL injuries occur after the athlete plants the foot and then rotates the knee). If the ACL is torn (*right*), internal rotation causes excessive anterior movement of the tibia (with respect to the femur). **(2) Middle row** (0 to 30 degrees flexion): The *left* figure shows the orientation of the ACL, and the *purple arrowheads* mark contiguous points on the femur and tibia when the knee is fully extended. During flexion of the knee when the ACL is intact (*middle figure*), the femur glides on the tibia, which results in a large surface area of the femur (*blue shading*) contacting a relatively small area on the tibia. If the ACL is damaged (*right* figure), such gliding does not occur and instead the femur rolls back on the tibia, which displaces the tibia anteriorly (see *vertical dotted line*). A valgus stress is applied during the pivot shift test because it ensures contact between the lateral femoral condyle and lateral tibial plateau, as occurs during normal weight-bearing. **(3) Bottom row**: When the knee is extended (*left*), the iliotibial tract is relaxed and lies in front of the axis of flexion (solid purple circle). At 30 degrees flexion (*middle*), the iliotibial tract is still in front of the axis of flexion, but it becomes taut in the ACL-deficient knee as the tibia is displaced anteriorly. At 45 degrees flexion (*right*), the iliotibial tract suddenly falls behind the axis of flexion, thus shifting from an extensor to a flexor of the knee and pulling the tibia backward into its normal alignment (the shift).

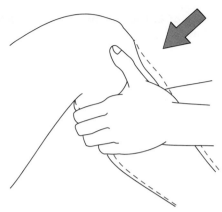

Fig. 57.13   Posterior drawer sign. With the patient positioned as for the anterior drawer sign (see Fig. 57.9), the clinician pushes posteriorly on the patient's upper calf. In the PCL-deficient knee, this force reveals an abnormal posterior tibial movement (*arrow*) with a soft end point.

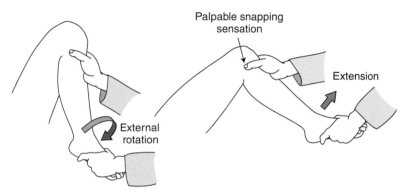

Fig. 57.14   The McMurray test. The clinician flexes the patient's knee fully against the buttock and rotates the tibia (by grasping the patient's foot and ankle). The purpose of rotation is to bring the torn meniscal fragment, located on the posterior half of the meniscus, *anterior* to the curved surface of the femoral condyle: external rotation brings forward the *medial* meniscus; internal rotation, the *lateral* meniscus. This figure, therefore, depicts testing of the medial meniscus: the clinician places a free hand over the medial joint line, fully flexes the patient's knee, and then rotates the tibia externally. The clinician slowly extends the knee while maintaining this rotational force, thereby forcing the medial femoral condyle to glide forward on the tibia and *over* any torn fragment of the meniscus. When the femur passes over the torn fragment, a palpable snapping sensation may be detected at the medial joint line (a positive test). To test the lateral meniscus, the clinician repeats the test while internally rotating the knee and palpating the lateral joint line. Popular orthopedic textbooks[122] and review articles[42,59,123] add varus and valgus stresses to their definitions of the McMurray test, although McMurray did not include this in his original description nor were they used in clinical studies testing the sign's accuracy (see EBM Box 57.6).

20 degrees (i.e., at this angle the hamstring's pull is almost perpendicular to anterior subluxation of the tibia). (3) The thick posterior edge of the medial meniscus acts as a wedge against the curved femoral condyles and prevents anterior subluxation of the tibia when the knee is at 90 degrees (i.e., anterior drawer sign) but not when it is at 20 degrees (i.e., Lachman sign). In support of this last hypothesis, the sensitivity of the anterior drawer sign in one study increased from 50% to 100% after medial meniscectomy.[49]

| EBM BOX 57.4 | **Diagnosis of Osteoarthritis, in Patients With Chronic Knee Pain*,53** |

| | Sensitivity (%) | Specificity (%) | Likelihood Ratio‡ if Finding Is | |
Finding (Reference)†			Present	Absent
Individual findings				
Stiffness <30 minutes	85	72	**3.0**	0.2
Crepitus, passive motion	89	58	2.1	0.2
Bony enlargement	55	95	**11.8**	0.5
Palpable increase in temperature	14	52	**0.3**	1.6
Valgus deformity	24	83	NS	NS
Varus deformity	22	93	**3.4**	0.8
Combined findings: (1) age >50 years; (2) stiffness <30 min; (3) crepitus; (4) bony tenderness along margins of joint; (5) bone enlargement; (6) no palpable warmth				
At least 3 out of 6:	95	69	**3.1**	0.1

*Diagnostic standard: for *diagnosis of osteoarthritis*, consensus of experts after review of patient's course, laboratory tests, and radiographs.
†Definition of findings: for *morning stiffness <30 minutes*, when applied only to patients complaining of morning stiffness and knee pain.
‡Likelihood ratio (LR) if finding present = positive LR; LR if finding absent = negative LR.
NS, Not significant.

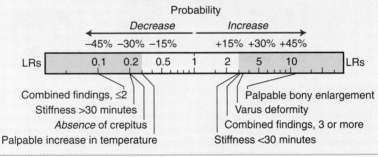

KNEE OSTEOARTHRITIS

In three clinical studies, expert clinicians combining the patient interview and clinical examination accurately diagnosed ACL tears (as detected by subsequent arthroscopy: sensitivity of 86% to 96%, specificity of 98% to 99%, positive LR = 49.6, negative LR = 0.1).[36,56,57]

2. Posterior Cruciate Tear

Two studies demonstrated the accuracy of bedside examination for posterior cruciate tears (positive LR = 97.8, negative LR = 0.1; EBM Box 57.6). Unfortunately, neither study specifically identified the technique used at the bedside, although it almost certainly included the posterior drawer sign.

3. Meniscal Injury

Both the positive McMurray sign (LR = 3.6) and block to full extension of the knee (LR = 3.2) increase probability of a meniscal tear. Nonetheless, no finding significantly the decreases probability of meniscal tear, except for absence of joint line tenderness (LR = 0.4), which decreases

EBM BOX 57.5	Clinically Significant Knee Fracture*			
			Likelihood Ratio‡ if Finding Is	
Finding (Reference)†	Sensitivity (%)	Specificity (%)	Present	Absent
Individual findings				
Age ≥55 years[26,28]	23–48	87–88	**3.0**	NS
Joint effusion[26-28,94]	54–79	71–81	2.5	0.5
Ecchymosis[28]	19	91	NS	NS
Limitation of knee flexion[26-28]				
Not able to flex beyond 90 degrees	42–65	78–80	2.9	0.5
Not able to flex beyond 60 degrees	46–49	90	**4.7**	0.6
Isolated tenderness of patella[26-28]	25–31	85–89	2.2	0.8
Tenderness at head of fibula [26-28]	12–32	92–95	**3.4**	NS
Inability to bear weight, immediately and in emergency department [26-28]	46–58	81–89	**3.6**	0.6
Combined findings				
Ottawa rule positive[26-34]	81–99	19–54	1.7	**0.1**

*Diagnostic standard: for *clinically significant knee fracture*, one requiring orthopedic consultation, splinting, or surgery (i.e., one >5mm in breadth or one associated with complete tendon or ligament disruption).

†Definition of findings: for *isolated tenderness of the patella*, no bony tenderness elsewhere on the knee[26]; for *inability to bear weight immediately and in emergency department*, unable to transfer weight twice onto each lower limb regardless of limping; for *Ottawa rule positive*, see Table 57.4.

‡Likelihood ratio (LR) if finding present = positive LR; LR if finding absent = negative LR.

NS, Not significant.

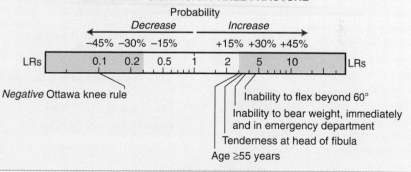

CLINICALLY SIGNIFICANT KNEE FRACTURE

Probability

Decrease — Increase

−45% −30% −15%   +15% +30% +45%

LRs | 0.1 0.2 0.5 1 2 5 10 | LRs

Negative Ottawa knee rule

Inability to flex beyond 60°
Inability to bear weight, immediately and in emergency department
Tenderness at head of fibula
Age ≥55 years

probability slightly. It is possible that the presence of joint line tenderness reflects accompanying injury of the joint capsule or collateral ligaments, rather than injury to the meniscus per se.

The above studies address diagnosis of *any* meniscus injury. Four studies have addressed whether expert clinicians combining the patient interview with clinical examination can accurately diagnose *and localize* the injured meniscus. In these studies, clinicians were slightly more

EBM BOX 57.6   Ligament and Meniscal Injuries*

Finding[†] (Reference)	Sensitivity (%)	Specificity (%)	Likelihood Ratio[‡] if Finding Is	
			Present	Absent
Detecting anterior cruciate ligament tear				
Anterior drawer sign[37,49,54,55,95-98]	27–94	91–99	**12.2**	0.4
Lachman sign[37,49,54,55,95,97,98]	48–96	90–99	**20.5**	**0.2**
Pivot shift sign[37,54,95,97,98]	6–61	94–99	8.2	0.7
Detecting posterior cruciate ligament tear				
Posterior drawer sign[36,99]	90–95	99	**97.8**	**0.1**
Detecting meniscal injury				
McMurray sign[38,39,52,100-105]	17–80	70–98	**3.6**	0.6
Joint line tenderness[39,52,100-102,106,107]	55–92	30–83	1.9	0.4
Block to full extension[39]	44	86	**3.2**	0.7
Pain on forced extension[39,100]	47–51	67–70	1.6	0.7
Detecting medial collateral ligament injury				
Valgus stress laxity[37,108,109]	79–89	49–99	**7.7**	**0.2**
Detecting lateral collateral ligament injury				
Varus stress laxity[109]	25	98	**16.2**	NS

*Diagnostic standard: for ACL *tear*, MRI,[54,55,98] arthroscopy[37,95,97] or surgery[49,96]; for *posterior cruciate tear*, arthroscopy; for *meniscal tear*, arthroscopy; for *collateral ligament tears*, arthroscopy[37,109] or MRI.[108]
[†]Definition of findings: all examination performed in awake patients (i.e., *not* examinations under anesthesia).
[‡]Likelihood ratio (LR) if finding present = positive LR; LR if finding absent = negative LR.
ACL, Anterior cruciate ligament; *LCL,* lateral collateral ligament; *MCL,* medial collateral ligament; *MRI,* magnetic resonance imaging; *NS,* not significant; *PCL,* posterior cruciate ligament.

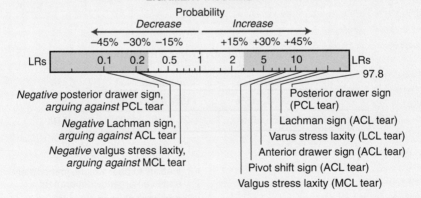

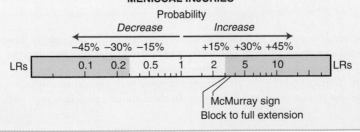

accurate *ruling out* medial meniscus injury (sensitivity of 88% to 95%, specificity of 56% to 87%, positive LR = 3.6, negative LR = 0.1) and *ruling in* lateral meniscus injury (sensitivity of 51% to 86%, specificity of 90% to 96%, positive LR = 8.6, negative LR = 0.5).[36,56–58]

4. Collateral Ligaments

The presence of valgus stress laxity accurately indicates a tear of the medial collateral ligament (positive LR = 7.7, EBM Box 57.6) and the presence of a varus stress laxity indicates a tear of the lateral collateral ligament (LR = 16.2). The *absence* of a valgus stress laxity *decreases* probability of a medial collateral ligament tear (LR = 0.2).

5. Variables Affecting Sensitivity of Signs

Signs of ligament injury are more likely to be positive if (1) the ligament tear is complete, not partial,[59] (2) the injury is chronic, not acute,[60,61] and (3) multiple ligaments are injured (e.g., in ACL-deficient knees, the anterior drawer sign is more likely to be positive if the medial collateral ligament is also injured).[62] In addition, the degree to which the patient is relaxed influences the sensitivity of these signs, as illustrated by the observation that the sensitivity of most tests increases when patients are examined under anesthesia.[37,59,60,62]

6. Predicting the Need for Knee Surgery

If all knee injuries were managed conservatively (e.g., by rest, bracing, and physical therapy), the detailed bedside examination described above would have limited clinical utility. One study, however, enrolled patients with knee pain and demonstrated that many of these physical signs—limited knee flexion (<120 degrees) or extension, medial or lateral joint line tenderness, a positive McMurray test, a positive Lachman test, and a positive anterior drawer sign—independently predicted whether an experienced orthopedic surgeon would recommend nonarthroplasty knee surgery to the patient.[63]

THE ANKLE

I. Introduction

In patients presenting to emergency departments with ankle or foot injuries to emergency departments, 8% to 14% are found to have a clinically significant fractures.[64–70] Achilles tendon rupture typically occurs during sports activities when the athlete forcibly plantarflexes the ankle ("pushes off" during running or jumping) or dorsiflexes it forcibly.[71]

II. The Finding

A. OTTAWA ANKLE AND MIDFOOT RULES

Stiell and others have developed a prediction rule for clinical significant injuries, called the Ottawa ankle rule.[72,73] This rule focuses on the presence of tenderness at four locations and whether the patient is able to bear weight both immediately after the accident and later in the emergency department (Fig. 57.15). Importantly, it applies only to patients with injury of the ankle (i.e., distal 6 cm of tibia and fibula and talus) and midfoot (i.e., navicular bone, cuboid, cuneiforms, anterior process of the calcaneus, and base of the 5th metatarsal) and *not* to injury of the body and tuberosities of the calcaneus or injury more than 10 days old.

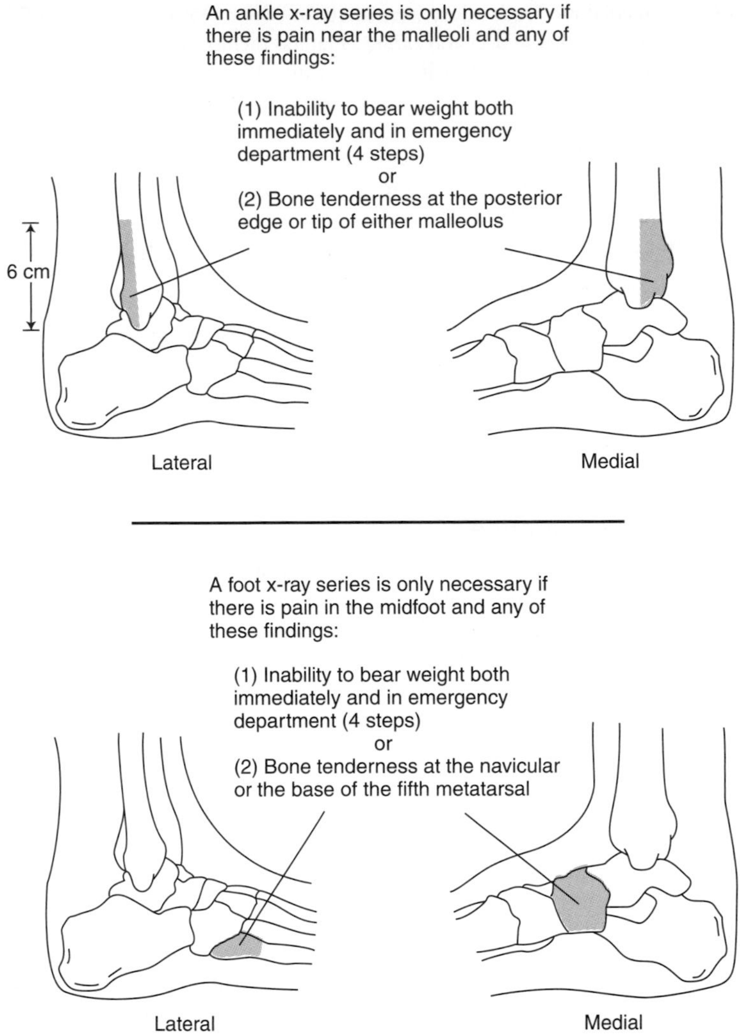

An ankle x-ray series is only necessary if there is pain near the malleoli and any of these findings:

(1) Inability to bear weight both immediately and in emergency department (4 steps)
or
(2) Bone tenderness at the posterior edge or tip of either malleolus

6 cm

Lateral   Medial

A foot x-ray series is only necessary if there is pain in the midfoot and any of these findings:

(1) Inability to bear weight both immediately and in emergency department (4 steps)
or
(2) Bone tenderness at the navicular or the base of the fifth metatarsal

Lateral   Medial

Fig. 57.15   Ottawa rule for ankle or midfoot fracture. The rule for ankle pain is the *top figure*; the rule for midfoot pain is the *bottom figure*. The rule is positive if any indication for radiography is met. "Inability to take 4 steps" means the patient is unable to transfer weight twice onto each lower limb regardless of limping. Importantly, these rules apply *only* to patients with injury of the ankle or midfoot, and they exclude patients with injury to the body or tuberosities of the calcaneus. Adapted from reference 72 with permission.

B. ACHILLES TENDON RUPTURE

Many patients with ruptured Achilles tendons can still plantarflex the ankle, thus potentially misleading clinicians into thinking the Achilles tendon is intact (i.e., the tibialis posterior and peroneus muscles, which attach to the midfoot bones, plantar flex the foot). Consequently, special tests for Achilles tendon rupture have been developed. These tests, illustrated in Fig. 57.16, rely on palpation of the injured tendon (**palpable gap**) or demonstration of absent tendon function (**calf squeeze test** and **knee flexion test**).

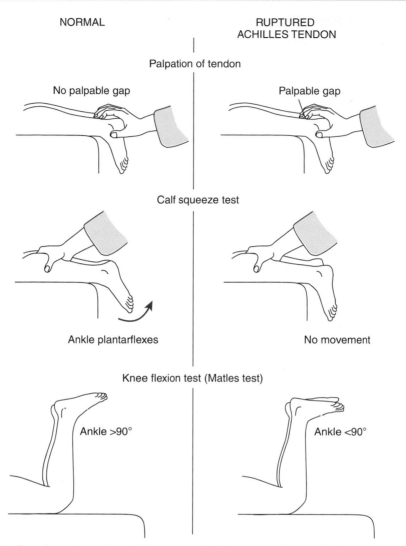

NORMAL

RUPTURED
ACHILLES TENDON

Palpation of tendon

No palpable gap

Palpable gap

Calf squeeze test

Ankle plantarflexes

No movement

Knee flexion test (Matles test)

Ankle >90°

Ankle <90°

Fig. 57.16 Tests for rupture of the Achilles tendon.[116] All tests are performed with the patient lying prone and his or her feet extending over the end of the examination table. The patient's asymptomatic side serves as a control (for each test, a patient with an intact Achilles tendon is depicted on the *left*, compared with a patient with a ruptured Achilles tendon on the *right*). **(1) Palpable gap in tendon** (*top*): The clinician gently palpates the course of the tendon, searching for gaps, which if present usually lie between 2 to 6 cm from the calcaneus.[71] **(2) Calf squeeze test (Simmonds-Thompson test,** *middle*)[124]: The clinician gently squeezes the patient's calf in its middle third and just below the place of widest girth, observing the ankle for movement. If the tendon is intact, the ankle should plantarflex. Absence of movement or minimal movement is a positive response. The normal plantar flexion of the ankle results from compression of the soleus muscle, which bows the Achilles tendon away from the tibia resulting in plantar flexion.[125] **(3) Knee flexion test (Matles test,** *bottom*). The clinician observes the position of the patient's ankles as the patient flexes both knees to 90 degrees (the knees may be flexed individually or simultaneously). The ankle remains slightly plantar flexed if the tendon is intact; slight dorsiflexion or a neutral position of the ankle is the positive response. Thompson described the calf squeeze test in 1962,[71] pointing out that the test could be performed with the patient prone or kneeling on a chair. Simmonds described the identical test in 1957.[126] Matles described the knee flexion test in 1975.[127]

III. Clinical Significance

A. ANKLE AND MIDFOOT FRACTURES

In patients with ankle injury, the finding of tenderness of the posterior medial malleolus increases probability of fracture (LR = 4.8, EBM Box 57.7), and a negative Ottawa ankle rule (LR = 0.1) and ability to bear weight 4 steps in the emergency room (LR = 0.3) decrease probability. Specificity of the Ottawa ankle rule may improve by substituting *tuning-fork tenderness* for *tenderness with palpation.*[74]

EBM BOX 57.7	Ankle and Midfoot Fracture*			
			Likelihood Ratio‡ if Finding Is	
Finding (Reference)†	Sensitivity (%)	Specificity (%)	Present	Absent
Detecting ankle fracture				
Tenderness over posterior lateral malleolus[72,73]	69–76	65–74	2.4	0.4
Tenderness over posterior medial malleolus[72,73]	34–47	87–95	**4.8**	0.6
Inability to bear weight immediately after injury[72,73]	61–68	72–79	2.6	0.5
Inability to bear weight 4 steps in the emergency room[72,73]	80–85	64–70	2.5	**0.3**
Ottawa ankle rule[65,67,72,77,110–114]	94–100	16–46	1.5	**0.1**
Detecting midfoot fracture				
Tenderness at the base of the 5th metatarsal[72,73]	92–94	66–69	2.9	**0.1**
Tenderness of navicular bone[72,73]	3–12	74–90	0.4	NS
Inability to bear weight immediately [72,73]	18–28	74–82	NS	NS
Inability to bear weight 4 steps in the emergency room[72,73]	38–45	58–67	NS	NS
Ottawa foot rule[67,72,77,110,111,115]	88–99	21–79	2.1	**0.1**

*Diagnostic standard: for *clinically significant ankle or midfoot fracture*, bone fragments >3 mm in breadth (i.e., a size that might require plaster immobilization).
†Definition of findings: for *Ottawa ankle and foot rules*, see Fig. 57.15.
‡Likelihood ratio (LR) if finding present = positive LR; LR if finding absent = negative LR.
NS, Not significant.

ANKLE AND MIDFOOT FRACTURE

Probability

Decrease   *Increase*

←————————————   ————————————→
−45% −30% −15%   +15% +30% +45%

LRs | 0.1   0.2   0.5   1   2   5   10 | LRs

Negative Ottawa ankle rule,   Tender posterior medial malleolus,
arguing against ankle fracture   detecting ankle fracture

Negative Ottawa foot rule,   Tender base of 5th metatarsal,
arguing against midfoot fracture   detecting midfoot fracture

In patients with midfoot pain, tenderness at the base of the fifth metatarsal bone increases the probability of fracture a small amount (LR = 2.9). A negative Ottawa foot rule greatly decreases probability midfoot fracture (LR = 0.1), though much of this argument rests on the absence of tenderness at the base of the fifth metatarsal (LR = 0.1).

Other studies combining the ankle and foot rules have confirmed their accuracy[64–70,75,76] and shown they reduce the need for radiographs by 14% to 34% and decrease medical costs and patient waiting times.[65,67–69,72,77–81]

B. ACHILLES TENDON RUPTURE

All three signs of Achilles tendon rupture accurately increase probability of a torn tendon if present (LRs = 6.2 to 13.5, EBM Box 57.8) and decrease probability if absent (LRs 0.05 to 0.3).

EBM BOX 57.8   **Achilles Tendon Tear[116,*]**

Finding (Reference)	Sensitivity (%)	Specificity (%)	Likelihood Ratio[†] if Finding Is Present	Absent
Palpable gap in Achilles tendon	73	89	6.8	0.3
Calf squeeze test	96	93	13.5	0.05
Knee flexion test	88	86	6.2	0.1

*Diagnostic standard: for *Achilles tendon tear*, surgical findings or (in patients without surgery) ultrasonography or magnetic resonance imaging.
†Likelihood ratio (LR) if finding present = positive LR; LR if finding absent = negative LR.

ACHILLES TENDON TEAR

Probability

Decrease   Increase

−45% −30% −15%   +15% +30% +45%

LRs   0.1   0.2   0.5   1   2   5   10   LRs

Calf squeeze test *negative*   Calf squeeze test positive
Knee flexion test *negative*   Palpable gap
Absence of palpable gap   Knee flexion test positive

References may be accessed online at *Elsevier eBooks for Practicing Clinicians.*

Neurologic Examination

Visual Field Testing

I. Introduction

Abnormalities of peripheral vision are called **visual field defects**. These defects, many of which can be detected at the bedside, provide important clues to the diagnosis of lesions throughout the visual pathways—retina, optic nerve, optic chiasm, optic tracts, optic radiations (parietal and temporal lobes), and occipital cortex (Fig. 58.1).

II. Definitions

The term **hemianopia** describes visual defects that occupy about one-half of an eye's visual space. **Quadrantanopia** describes defects confined mostly to about one-fourth of an eye's visual space. **Homonymous** describes defects that affect the same side of the vertical meridian (i.e., right or left side) of both eyes. For example, a right homonymous hemianopia affects the right visual space of both eyes (i.e., the temporal field of the right eye and the nasal field of the left eye). The term *homonymous* implies the defect does not cross the vertical meridian.

III. The Anatomy of the Visual Pathways

The key anatomic points in Fig. 58.1 are the following: (1) Images from the visual fields are inverted throughout the retina and all neural pathways. Images from the temporal visual field fall on the nasal retina, and those from the nasal field on the temporal retina. Images from the *superior* visual fields are transmitted throughout the *inferior* visual pathways (inferior retina, inferior optic

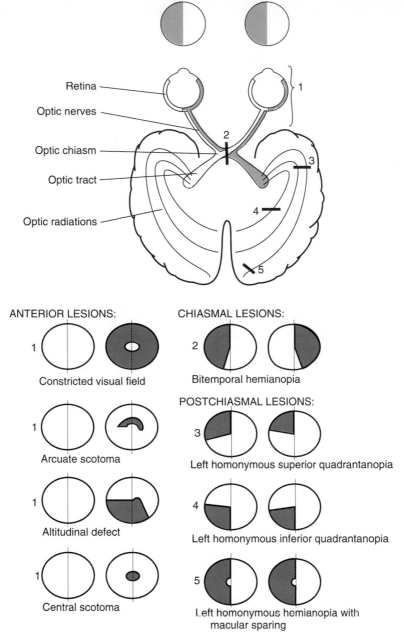

Fig. 58.1   Anatomy of the visual pathways. The anatomy of the visual pathways appears at the top of the figure, the *light blue shading* indicating how visual information from the left visual space eventually courses to the right brain. Visual field defects are at the bottom of the figure. Anterior defects (labeled "1," from disease of the optic nerve or retina) characteristically affect one eye and cause defects (the *blue shading*) that may cross the vertical meridian (i.e., the vertical meridian is the *vertical line* bisecting each visual field). Chiasmal defects (labeled "2") and postchiasmal defects (labeled "3" for a lesion in the anterior temporal lobe, "4" for the parietal lobe, and "5" for the occipital cortex) characteristically affect both eyes and respect the vertical meridian.

nerve and chiasm, and temporal lobe), and those from the *inferior* visual fields throughout the *superior* visual pathways (superior retina, superior optic nerve and chiasm, parietal lobe). (2) The nasal retinal fibers cross in the optic chiasm; therefore, disease of the optic chiasm causes defects in both temporal visual fields (**bitemporal hemianopia**). (3) The visual pathways posterior to the optic chiasm contain information from the same visual space of each eye: lesions in the *right* postchiasmal pathways cause defects in the *left* visual space of each eye (i.e., temporal field of left eye and nasal field of right eye), and those of the *left* postchiasmal pathways cause defects in the *right* visual space. Such defects, respecting the vertical meridian in each eye, are called *homonymous*. (4) The visual pathways in the occipital cortex that contain information from the macula (point of fixation) are distant from those connected to the more peripheral fields.[1] Therefore, lesions of the occipital cortex may cause either homonymous defects sparing the macula or visual defects confined to central vision.

IV. Technique

There are many ways to test visual fields at the bedside,[2] but the two traditional techniques are static confrontational testing and kinetic confrontational testing. In all techniques, the patient sits about 70 to 100 cm from the clinician and fixes on the clinician's own eye. Only one eye of the patient is tested at a time; the other is occluded with a card or the patient's hand.

A. STATIC TECHNIQUE

Using this technique, the clinician presents objects at a fixed point in the visual field, usually about 20 to 30 degrees from fixation. The clinician presents one, two, or five fingers to each visual quadrant and asks the patient to count the number of fingers. Testing two quadrants simultaneously (e.g., by asking the patient to count the total number of fingers) has the advantage of detecting some parietal lobe lesions, which may allow patients to see an object in the contralateral field if it appears alone, but not if another object is presented simultaneously to the healthy visual field (i.e., visual extinction).

Throughout the examination, the clinician focuses on whether a defect respects the vertical or horizontal meridians of the visual field (see later). Defects crossing the vertical meridian are due to anterior disease (see later), whereas those respecting the vertical meridian are due to chiasmal disease (if the defect is bitemporal) or postchiasmal disease (if it is homonymous).

B. KINETIC TECHNIQUE

In this technique, the clinician tests one quadrant at a time by slowly moving an object (e.g., wiggling finger, <5 degrees of oscillation) from an extreme peripheral field toward fixation, the patient then indicating the moment he or she sees the object. The trajectory of the moving object is an imaginary line bisecting the horizontal and vertical meridians (e.g., 45, 135, 225, and 315 degrees from the vertical meridian), and the direction of movement is from periphery to central fixation.

V. The Findings

Visual field defects are classified as *prechiasmal* defects (from disease in retina or optic nerves, often called *anterior* defects), *chiasmal* defects, and *postchiasmal* defects (optic tracts, optic radiations, and occipital cortex).

A. ANTERIOR OR PRECHIASMAL DEFECTS

The characteristic features are the following:
1. **One Eye is Affected** (unless the retinal or optic nerve disorder is bilateral).
2. **Visual Acuity is Poor**. Most patients have diminished acuity or, if acuity is normal, other signs of anterior disease, such as an afferent pupillary defect (see Chapter 21), red color desaturation, abnormal retina examination, or an abnormal optic disc (drusen, cupping, or atrophy).
3. **The Defects May Cross the Vertical Meridian**. This occurs because retinal nerve fibers from the temporal retina arch across the vertical meridian to reach the optic disc and nerve (which lie on the nasal side of the retina). Damage to these fibers thus may cause a defect that crosses the vertical meridian. Small nerve fiber defects may cause an *arcuate defect* (see Fig. 58.1), larger ones an *altitudinal defect* (having a sharp horizontal border in the nasal field). Damage to fibers from the macula may cause *central scotomas* and, to those preferentially affecting the most peripheral vision, *constricted visual fields*.[3]

B. CHIASMAL DEFECTS

These defects are bitemporal hemianopias (see Fig. 58.1).

C. POSTCHIASMAL DEFECTS

The characteristics of these defects are the following:
1. **Both Eyes are Affected**, causing homonymous hemianopias or quadrantanopias.
2. **Visual Acuity is Normal**. This is true in greater than 90% of cases. If visual acuity is abnormal, it is because of bilateral disease and thus the acuity in both eyes is the same.[4]
3. **Pupil and Retinal Examination are Normal**. One important exception is the occasional finding of papilledema, caused by brain tumors affecting the optic radiations.

VI. Clinical Significance

A. ETIOLOGY

Most anterior defects are caused by severe glaucoma, age-related macular degeneration, retinal emboli, and optic nerve disorders.[2,5] Chiasmal defects are usually from a pituitary tumor just below the optic chiasm. Over 95% of postchiasmal defects are due to lesions of the temporal, parietal, and occipital lobes, most frequently stroke, traumatic brain injury, and tumors.[5] Lesions of the optic tracts are uncommon.[4,6]

Although parietal and temporal lobe disease may cause inferior and superior quadrantanopias, respectively (Fig. 58.1), lesions in these areas more often cause dense hemianopias or hemianopias that are denser inferiorly or superiorly, respectively.[4,7]

B. DIAGNOSTIC ACCURACY

EBM Box 58.1 summarizes the diagnostic accuracy of the confrontational technique for diagnosing visual field defects. According to these likelihood ratios (LR)s, the finding of a visual field defect by confrontation significantly increases the probability that one is actually present (i.e.,

EBM BOX 58.1	Visual Field Defects*				

Finding (Reference)†	Sensitivity (%)	Specificity (%)	Likelihood Ratio‡ if Finding Is	
			Present	Absent
Confrontation technique, detecting the following visual field defects[2,8–15]				
Anterior defects (retina and optic nerve)	11–58	93–99	**5.7**	0.7
Patchy defects	6			
Constriction of visual fields	58			
Arcuate defects	20–51			
Altitudinal defects	88			
Posterior defects (optic chiasm to occipital cortex)	43–90	81–98	**9.5**	0.4
Bitemporal hemianopia	45			
Homonymous hemianopia	80			
Patients with homonymous hemianopias, detecting parietal lobe disease				
Asymmetric optokinetic nystagmus[4]	93	84	**5.7**	**0.1**
Associated hemiparesis or aphasia.[16]	90	95	**18.3**	**0.1**

*Diagnostic standard: for *visual field defects*, conventional perimetry.
†Definition of findings: abnormal static finger counting, static kinetic finger testing, kinetic finger boundary testing, or combinations of these tests.
‡Likelihood ratio (LR) if finding present = positive LR; LR if finding absent = negative LR.

VISUAL FIELD DEFECTS

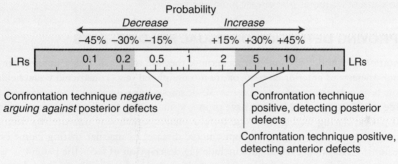

Confrontation technique *negative, arguing against* posterior defects

Confrontation technique positive, detecting posterior defects

Confrontation technique positive, detecting anterior defects

PARIETAL LOBE DISEASE (IF HOMONYMOUS HEMIANOPIA)

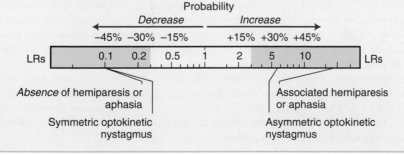

Absence of hemiparesis or aphasia

Symmetric optokinetic nystagmus

Associated hemiparesis or aphasia

Asymmetric optokinetic nystagmus

by perimetry, LRs = 5.7 to 9.5). Nonetheless, the absence of a defect on bedside testing only modestly decreases the probability of an actual defect (especially for anterior defects, LR = 0.7). Sensitivity is lower for anterior defects because anterior defects are much less dense than posterior ones (see the section on improving detection of visual defects).[2]

C. DIFFERENTIAL DIAGNOSIS OF POSTCHIASMAL DEFECTS

Homonymous hemianopias may be either an isolated finding or associated with other neurologic findings. The most common cause of an *isolated* homonymous hemianopia is an ischemic infarct of the occipital cortex.[16,17] In patients with associated hemiparesis, aphasia, or asymmetric optokinetic nystagmus, the most common diagnosis is parietal lobe disease.[4,16,18,19] Optokinetic nystagmus is a normal horizontal nystagmus that occurs when patients look at a vertically-striped tape moving in front of them. The clinician moves the tape first to one side and then the other, comparing the amplitude of horizontal nystagmus produced, which should be equal in each direction. Parietal lobe lesions reduce or eliminate optokinetic nystagmus when the tape is moved *toward* the side with the lesion (Barany first made this observation in 1921).

In patients undergoing computed tomography of the head (because of stroke, headache, seizures), the finding of a homonymous hemianopia increases probability of contralateral focal cerebral disease (sensitivity of 22% to 30%, specificity of 93% to 98%, positive LR 4.3; see Chapter 61).[20,21] In those patients with homonymous defects, the presence of asymmetric optokinetic nystagmus, associated aphasia or hemiparesis, increases probability of a parietal lobe lesion (LR = 5.7 for optokinetic nystagmus and LR = 18.3 for hemiparesis or aphasia), whereas the absence of these findings decreases probability of a parietal lobe lesion (both LRs = 0.1) and thus makes occipital or temporal lobe disease more likely.

D. IMPROVING DETECTION OF VISUAL FIELD DEFECTS

Confrontation fails to detect some defects because they are too small, lack a sharp linear border (e.g., patchy defects of anterior disease), or are too peripheral (e.g., constricted visual fields; confrontation tests only the most central 20 to 30 degrees of visual space). To increase sensitivity of bedside examination, some experts have proposed increasing the distance between the clinician and patient during testing from one to four meters, which may improve the detection of subtle arcuate scotomata (glaucoma or optic nerve disease) or macular sparing (some occipital cortex lesions).[22] Additional techniques include (1) **description of face**: The patient is asked to report if any part of the examiner's face is distorted or missing; (2) **kinetic red boundary** testing: The patient is asked to report when a moving red target (5- to 20- mm diameter) first appears the color red as it is moved inward from the periphery; (3) **red target comparison**: The examiner presents two 20-mm red targets (often the caps of mydriatic solutions) to two quadrants simultaneously and asks the patient if the bottle tops appear equally red; and (4) **laser target testing**: The clinician uses a conventional red laser pointer and projects it in front of the patient on a screen 1 m away.[11,23]

According to studies comparing these various techniques (EBM Box 58.2), static finger counting, kinetic finger boundary testing, and description of the clinician's face have similar diagnostic accuracy (LR 13.3 to 54.4). Kinetic testing with a red target and laser pointer testing improves sensitivity but at the cost of diminished specificity. In these studies, the red target comparison test was diagnostically unhelpful (LRs not significant).

| EBM BOX 58.2 | Visual Field Testing: Comparison of Techniques* |

Finding (Reference)[†]	Sensitivity (%)	Specificity (%)	Likelihood Ratio[‡] if Finding Is	
			Present	Absent
Finger counting[2,12]	25–35	99–100	**54.4**	0.7
Kinetic finger boundary testing[2,12]	39–41	97–99	**13.3**	0.6
Description of face[2,12]	36–44	99	**26.4**	0.6
Kinetic red boundary testing[2,12]	56–74	93–99	**13.6**	0.4
Laser target testing[11]	71	89	**6.3**	**0.3**
Red target comparison[2,12]	59–77	27–99	NS	NS

*Diagnostic standard: for *visual field defect*, conventional perimetry testing (most patients in these studies had anterior visual field defects).
[†]Definition of findings: for *kinetic red boundary testing*, the moving target was either 5 mm^2 or 20 mm[12] in diameter and the patient was asked to report when it first appeared red. For all other findings, see text.
[‡]Likelihood ratio (LR) if finding present = positive LR; LR if finding absent = negative LR.

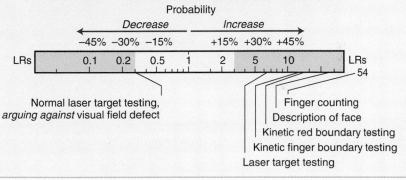

References may be accessed online at *Elsevier eBooks for Practicing Clinicians*.

CHAPTER 59

Nerves of the Eye Muscles (III, IV, and VI): Approach to Diplopia

KEY TEACHING POINTS

- In patients with diplopia, the clinician should distinguish monocular diplopia (which persists after closing one eye) from binocular diplopia (which resolves after closing one eye). Monocular diplopia is usually due to problems with the optics of the affected eye (spectacles, contact lenses, cataracts, corneal disease).
- In patients with binocular diplopia, the clinician should first inquire whether there is associated variability of symptoms (myasthenia), ptosis (cranial nerve III palsy, myasthenia), orbital disease or injury (thyroid eye disease, orbital wall fracture), or associated neurologic signs (posterior fossa disease).
- Only after these questions are addressed should the clinician identify which of the 12 eye muscles is weak in the patient with binocular diplopia. First, by moving the eyes through the 6 cardinal directions of gaze and observing which direction the diplopia is worse, the clinician narrows the diagnostic possibilities to 2 eye muscles, one in each eye. Then, by using inspection, the red glass test, or the cover/uncover test, the clinician determines which of these 2 muscles is abnormal.
- Weakness of each specific eye muscle has a unique differential diagnosis (discussed in the text). Almost all of these syndromes can be diagnosed at the bedside.

DIPLOPIA

I. Introduction

Patients with lesions of cranial nerves III, IV, and VI have paralysis of one or more ocular muscles, which prevents the eyes from aligning properly and causes double vision, or **diplopia**. The most common mistake in analyzing diplopia, however, is to prematurely conclude that affected patient must have neuropathy of one of these three nerves. Because only 39% to 68% of patients with diplopia actually have a cranial neuropathy, this chapter first emphasizes the general approach to *all* causes of diplopia.

II. Definitions

Diplopia may be monocular or binocular. **Monocular diplopia** persists after occluding one eye. **Binocular diplopia** depends on the visual axes of each eye being out of alignment and therefore disappears when one eye is occluded.

Several other terms are used to describe the findings of patients with binocular diplopia. **Heterotropia** is a general term for the finding of visual axes that are not parallel. (Synonyms are **squint** or **strabismus**.) **Esotropia** means that one eye is converging or is deviated toward the nose (e.g., a left esotropia means that the left eye is deviated toward the nose). **Exotropia** means that one eye is diverging or is deviated toward the temple (e.g., a right exotropia means that the right eye is deviated out). **Hypertropia** means that one eye is deviated upwards (e.g., a left hypertropia means that the left eye is elevated with respect to the right eye). Diplopia may be **horizontal**, with the two images side by side, or **vertical**, with one image higher than the other (the term **vertical diplopia** also encompasses diplopia with images separated both vertically and horizontally).

III. Technique

A. GENERAL APPROACH

Fig. 59.1 outlines the general approach to diplopia. The most important initial question is whether the diplopia is monocular or binocular, which can easily be addressed by covering one of the patient's eyes. Overall, 12% to 25% of all diplopia is monocular and 75% to 88% is binocular.[4,5]

In patients with binocular diplopia, the clinician can avoid misdiagnosing cranial neuropathy by first addressing the five questions listed in Fig. 59.1. Only after asking these questions should the clinician attempt to identify which eye muscle is weak.

B. IDENTIFYING THE WEAK MUSCLE

When examining the eye muscles, the clinician holds up his or her index finger or penlight and asks the patient to track it toward each of the six cardinal directions of gaze (i.e., left, left and up, left and down, right, right and up, right and down). These directions parallel the principal action of the six eye muscles, as described in Fig. 59.2.

There are two steps in identifying which eye muscle is weak. Step 1 reduces the number of possible weak eye muscles from 12 to 2. Step 2 then identifies which of these 2 muscles is causing the diplopia.

1. Step #1: **The Worst Diplopia (and Heterotropia) Occurs When the Patient Looks in the Direction of the Weak Muscle**. The clinician asks the patient which of the six cardinal directions aggravates the diplopia the most. According to this rule, the weak muscle is one of the two muscles responsible for this movement, one of which moves the right eye and the other the left eye. For example, diplopia that is worse on far right lateral gaze indicates weakness of the right lateral rectus or the left medial rectus. Diplopia that is worse when the patient looks to the left and down indicates a problem of the left inferior rectus or the right superior oblique.*

2. Step #2: **The Clinician Identifies Which of the Two Identified Muscles Is Weak**. There are three techniques (a, b, and c following):

a. Simple Inspection of the Eyes

In patients with diplopia on far right lateral gaze, the weak muscle is the right lateral rectus if there is an esotropia, but it is the left medial rectus if there is an exotropia. In patients with diplopia that is worse when looking up and to the right, the weak muscle is the right superior rectus if there is a left hypertropia but the left inferior oblique if there is a right hypertropia.

---

*Because the actions of the four vertical muscles are sometimes difficult to recall, a mnemonic by Maddox (1907) may be helpful: the affected muscle is "either the same-named rectus muscle or the most crossed-named oblique muscle." For example, if diplopia is worse when the patient looks to the *left* in a *superior* direction, the affected muscles are either the *left superior* rectus or *right inferior* oblique.

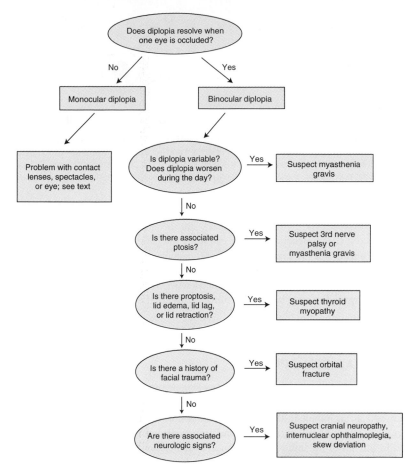

Fig. 59.1 General approach to diplopia. The clinician should first distinguish monocular from binocular diplopia and, in patients with binocular diplopia, address the five questions on the middle of the figure. Only then should the clinician identify which muscle is weak, although this is unnecessary if the clinician already suspects myasthenia (from fatigability) or full third nerve palsy (from weakness of the medial rectus, superior rectus, inferior rectus, and inferior oblique muscles, with or without a dilated pupil). Uncommon causes of diplopia and associated *ptosis*, not presented in the figure, are botulism, the Fisher variant of Guillain-Barre syndrome, and aberrant regeneration of the third nerve.[1,2] Uncommon causes of diplopia and associated *orbital findings* (e.g., proptosis) are carotid-cavernous fistula (which may produce an orbital bruit),[3] orbital tumor, and pseudotumor.

Often, however, the heterotropia is not obvious, either because the visual axes are out of line only by a degree or two (too small to observe) or because the patient can compensate and temporarily pull the visual axes back into line. In these patients, the following techniques are helpful.

b. The Affected Eye is the One with the Most Peripheral Image

By placing a red glass over one eye (usually the right eye), the patient is less likely to fuse the images, and, when looking at a penlight in the direction of maximal diplopia, sees two images, one red and one white. The most peripheral image belongs to the weak eye (Fig. 59.3).

For example, in a patient whose maximal diplopia is to the left and down (and who has the red glass over the right eye), the weak muscle is the right superior oblique if the red image is most peripheral but the left inferior rectus if the white image is most peripheral.

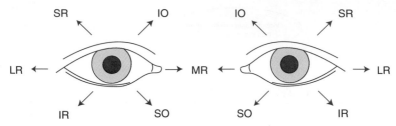

Fig. 59.2 Principal Actions of Ocular Muscles. There are 12 ocular muscles, 6 in each eye. The actions of the medial rectus (*MR*) and lateral rectus (*LR*) are simple right and left lateral movements. Although the actions of the four vertical eye muscles—the superior rectus (*SR*), inferior rectus (*IR*), superior oblique (*SO*), and inferior oblique (*IO*)—are more complex, there is one direction of gaze, indicated in the figure, in which weakness is most apparent.

c. The Cover/Uncover Test

To perform this test the clinician covers one eye while the patient looks in the direction of maximal diplopia. Covering one eye prevents fusion of the images, and any heterotropia that exists will return, although it is now obscured by occlusion of the eye. The clinician then observes which way that eye moves to pick up the image after it is uncovered. If it moves out, there was an esotropia; if it moves in, there was an exotropia, and if it moves down, that eye had a hypertropia.

IV. Clinical Significance

A. MONOCULAR DIPLOPIA

Almost all patients with monocular diplopia have extraocular or ocular causes.[4,6] Common extraocular causes are the patient's spectacles (e.g., reflections off one or both surfaces of the lenses) or contact lenses (e.g., air bubble in the pupillary area, abnormal curves, or uneven thicknesses). This diplopia resolves after removal of the lenses and, in patients with spectacles, varies as the spectacles are moved in and out or up and down. Common ocular causes include problems in the lens (e.g., fluid clefts, early cataracts), cornea (e.g., astigmatism, keratitis), and eyelids (e.g., chalazion, or prolonged reading, which may allow drooping lids to temporarily deform the cornea). The diplopia of these patients resolves when patients look through a pinhole or when a card is held over half of the pupillary aperture (it resolves because the diplopia depends on irregularities of the optic media acting as tiny prisms that divert some rays off the fovea; the pinhole or card blocks these wayward rays and thus eliminates the problem).

Rare patients with monocular diplopia have cerebral disease.[7] Despite traditional teachings, hysteria is a rare cause of monocular diplopia.

B. BINOCULAR DIPLOPIA

1. Etiology

Among patients with binocular diplopia, common final diagnoses are cranial neuropathy (III, IV, or VI; 39% to 68% of patients), eye muscle disease (thyroid ophthalmopathy, myasthenia gravis; 12% of patients), trauma (11%), supranuclear causes (internuclear ophthalmoplegia, skew deviation, 3% to 12%), other causes (4% to 16%), and unknown (4% to 11%).[4,5,8]

2. Weak Muscles and Their Clinical Significance

Incomplete palsies of the third cranial nerve are rare (in one study of 579 third nerve palsies, less than 1% were partial).[9,10] Therefore, if only one or two of the third nerve muscles (i.e., superior

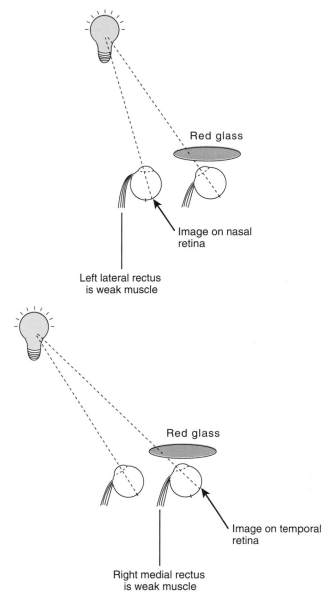

Fig. 59.3 The use of red glass to identify the weak muscle. In this example, the patient has horizontal binocular diplopia when looking to the left, indicating that the possible weak muscles are the either the left lateral rectus or right medial rectus (see Fig. 59.2). A red glass is placed in front of the right eye, causing the image seen by the right eye to be red and that from the left eye to be white. Importantly, images projecting on the nasal side of the retina are perceived to belong to the temporal visual space (see Chapter 58); those on the temporal side retina, to the nasal visual space. If the left lateral rectus is the weak muscle (*top* figure), the image in the left eye falls on the nasal retina, whereas that of the right eye falls on the fovea; therefore, the white image is more *peripheral* than the red image (i.e., it is farther leftward in the patient's left visual field). If the right medial rectus is the weak muscle (*bottom* figure), the image in the left eye falls on the fovea and that of the right eye falls on the temporal retina; therefore, the red image is more *peripheral* than the white image (i.e., it is farther leftward in the patient's left visual space). In both cases, the most peripheral image belongs to the paralyzed eye. In both of these examples, it is the stronger eye that is fixing on the target (i.e., the image falls on the fovea of the stronger eye), but the results are the same if it is the weaker eye that fixates on the object (i.e., the more peripheral image belongs to the weaker eye). See the text.

rectus, inferior rectus, medial rectus, and inferior oblique) are weak, the diagnosis is almost certainly *not* a partial third nerve palsy but instead one of the diagnoses listed below.

a. Weak Superior Rectus Muscle

The clinician should consider **myasthenia gravis** (see Fig. 59.4). Most patients with myasthenia gravis present with ocular symptoms, usually diplopia and ptosis,[11] although the pupils are always normal. Symptoms often fluctuate, worsening at the end of the day or even alternating between the eyes. Ocular myasthenia may mimic any ocular misalignment, although the most commonly affected muscles are the superior or medial rectus muscles, whose weakness is provoked by having the patient sustain upward or far lateral gaze for 30 seconds or more.

One important bedside test for myasthenia is the ice pack test (see the section on ice pack test for myasthenia gravis).

b. Weak Inferior Rectus Muscle

The clinician should consider thyroid myopathy and orbital floor fracture.

(1) ***Thyroid Myopathy.*** Patients may have associated proptosis, lid lag, lid retraction, chemosis, and hyperemia at the insertions of the recti muscles (see Chapter 25). These findings are sometimes subtle, and because many patients are also clinically euthyroid, the only finding of thyroid myopathy may be heterotropia. The cause of diplopia is mechanical restriction of the eye muscles, which ophthalmologists can confirm using the forced duction test (i.e., after anesthetization of the conjunctiva, the ophthalmologist grasps the conjunctiva with toothed forceps and attempts to passively rotate the eye, detecting abnormal resistance in patients with thyroid myopathy).[9]

(2) ***Orbital Fracture.*** Diplopia is a complication of 40% to 82% of blowout fractures of the orbit and 20% of all midfacial fractures.[12-14] The heterotropia occurs because of swelling or entrapment of one of the eye muscles, most often the inferior rectus. In addition to the history of previous trauma, some patients have an additional clue, hypesthesia of the ipsilateral infraorbital area, which results from accompanying injury to the infraorbital branch of the trigeminal nerve. Diplopia may first become a problem for the patient days after the injury, when the swelling has had time to partially resolve.[9]

In one study of 912 patients presenting with orbital trauma, the following findings increased probability that an orbital fracture would be found on subsequent computed tomography: periorbital emphysema (subcutaneous crepitation on palpation, likelihood ratio [LR] = 4.9), infraorbital hypesthesia (LR = 3.5), and presence of diplopia during testing of eye movements (LR = 2.6). The *absence* of any of these findings, however, was diagnostically unhelpful (negative LRs 0.7–0.8).[14]

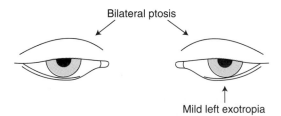

Bilateral ptosis

Mild left exotropia

Fig. 59.4 Myasthenia gravis. Myasthenia gravis may mimic any ocular disorder causing diplopia, although most often it mimics weakness of the superior rectus muscle or medial rectus muscle (i.e., difficulty with sustained elevation or adduction of the eye, respectively). Clues to the diagnosis of myasthenia gravis are associated ptosis, fluctuating course, and *normal* pupils.

c. Weak Medial Rectus

The clinician should consider internuclear ophthalmoplegia and myasthenia gravis.

    (1) ***Internuclear Ophthalmoplegia[15–17].*** Lesions in the medial longitudinal fasciculus (the peri-aqueductal pathway in the brainstem that links the nuclei of cranial nerves III, IV, and VI and coordinates conjugate eye movements) cause **internuclear ophthalmoplegia (INO)** (Fig. 59.5). The features of INO are the following: (1) incomplete adduction of one eye on lateral gaze (i.e., the "weak" medial rectus) and (2) jerk nystagmus of the contralateral abducting eye. Many patients also have vertical nystagmus on upward gaze. The finding is named according to the side with weak adduction. For example, in efforts to look to the far right, if the patient's left eye is unable to completely adduct and the right eye develops a jerk nystagmus, the patient has a left internuclear ophthalmoplegia (and a lesion in the left medial longitudinal fasciculus).

        Ninety-seven percent of patients with *bilateral* INOs have multiple sclerosis, whereas *unilateral* INO has many causes, although the most common one is vertebrobasilar cerebrovascular disease.[16]

    (2) ***Myasthenia Gravis.*** Myasthenia gravis (see the section on weak superior rectus muscle) sometimes causes medial rectus weakness. In contrast to the finding in patients with internuclear ophthalmoplegia, there is no jerk nystagmus of the abducting eye.

d. Weak Lateral Rectus

Weakness of this muscle almost always indicates damage to the **sixth cranial nerve** (see later), although mimics include myasthenia gravis and thyroid myopathy.[18]

e. Weak Superior Oblique

Weakness of this muscle indicates damage to the **fourth cranial nerve** (see later).

f. Weak Inferior Oblique

Weakness of the inferior oblique usually indicates **Brown syndrome**.[19,20] These patients appear to have a weak inferior oblique muscle, but the problem actually is in the superior oblique muscle and

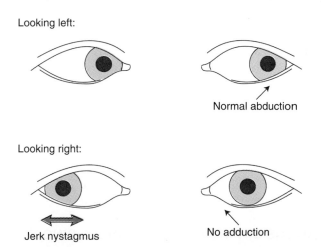

Looking left:

Normal abduction

Looking right:

Jerk nystagmus

No adduction

Fig. 59.5   **Internuclear ophthalmoplegia.** When the patient in the figure looks to the left (*top* row), both eyes move normally, but when the patient looks to the right (*bottom* row), the left eye fails to adduct ("weak" medial rectus) and the contralateral eye develops a jerk nystagmus. The finding is named for the side with weak adduction (i.e., in this example, a *left* internuclear ophthalmoplegia), and the lesion is in the *ipsilateral* medial longitudinal fasciculus (i.e., *left* medial longitudinal fasciculus in this example). See the text.

tendon, which are unable to move freely through their pulley (i.e., the trochlea). In some patients, Brown syndrome is congenital. Acquired Brown syndrome is a complication of orbital inflammation, surgery, and metastases.

3. Skew Deviation

Skew deviation has the following diagnostic features: (1) acquired hypertropia, (2) associated cerebellar or brainstem disease, and (3) lack of alternative etiology for hypertropia. Skew deviation mimics a weak inferior rectus 40% of the time, a weak inferior oblique 25% of the time, a weak superior rectus 17% of the time, and a weak superior oblique 17% of the time (although the head tilt test, described later, is negative).[9,21]

Skew deviation is believed to represent an abnormal **ocular tilt reaction** (see Fig. 59.6),[22] caused by an imbalance in neuronal signals to cranial nerves III, IV, and VI from the right and left otolith organs (utricles). These organs normally sense the position of the patient's head, especially when the patient is upright (i.e., otoliths allow normal persons to detect if they are tilting to the left or right when their eyes are closed). Damage to the cerebellum or brainstem may cause input from the utricles to the ocular motor nuclei to be asymmetric, thus producing an abnormal ocular tilt reaction and skew deviation.

Because the utricles are most active when the head is upright and less active when supine, Wong hypothesized that the hypertropia of skew deviation would be more pronounced when the patient is upright than supine.[23] In a study of 125 patients with diverse causes of vertical diplopia, *resolution* of hypertropia after the patient moves from the upright to supine position (i.e., a positive **upright-supine test**)[24] accurately diagnosed skew deviation (sensitivity of 37%, specificity of 100%, positive LR = 73.8, negative LR = 0.6).[25]

C. ICE PACK TEST FOR MYASTHENIA GRAVIS

Clinicians have observed that sunlight may aggravate the ptosis of myasthenic patients and that hot liquids (vs. cold liquids) may provoke myasthenic dysphagia.[26] Based on these observations and the fact that results of electromyography in myasthenia are temperature-dependent, Salvedra devised the ice pack test in 1979[27] as a test for ptosis. In this test, the clinician places a surgical glove filled with crushed ice for two minutes over the patient's closed eye and then compares the ptosis before application of the ice (by measuring the palpebral fissure, i.e., the vertical height of eye opening, to the nearest 0.5 mm) to that after application of the ice. Digital pressure is applied on the forehead just above the eyebrow to avoid contributions from the frontalis muscle in elevating the lid. Since cold temperature improves the weakness of myasthenia, the positive result is *diminished* ptosis after application of the ice (i.e., the palpebral fissure increases 2 mm or more).[28]

Several investigators have studied this test in patients presenting with ptosis, demonstrating that the positive ice test increases probability of myasthenia gravis (LR = 8.1, EBM Box 59.1) and the negative result decreases the probability (LR = 0.1). Also, in two investigations of patients with diplopia (with or without ptosis), the positive ice pack test accurately detected the ophthalmoplegia of myasthenia gravis and distinguished it from other causes of diplopia (positive LR = 30.6, negative LR = 0.1, EBM Box 59.1). (In these patients, the test was positive if the patient's ophthalmoplegia and diplopia improved after application of ice.)

D. COMBINATIONS OF FINDINGS TO DIAGNOSE BINOCULAR DIPLOPIA

In 2016, Butler published the "Edinburgh diplopia diagnostic algorithm," a simplified method of combining findings to diagnose binocular diplopia (i.e., diplopia that resolves after occlusion of one eye).[8] The initial question in this algorithm is to distinguish *horizontal* diplopia from *vertical*

NORMAL OCULAR TILT REACTION

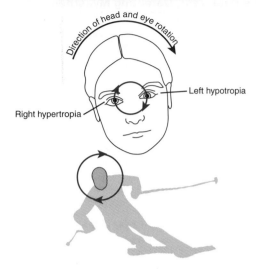

SKEW DEVIATION

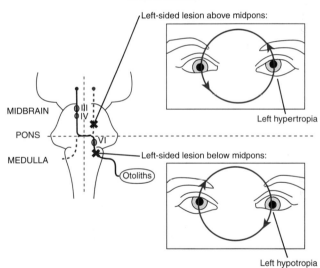

Fig. 59.6 Skew deviation and the ocular tilt reaction. When a person leans to one side, his or her head and eyes normally compensate by rotating the opposite direction. For example, in the skier in the top figure, whose body is leaning to the right, the natural compensatory movements are tilting the head to the left, eleva-tion of the right eye and depression of the left eye, and torsion of both eyes (the right eye *intorts* and the left eye *extorts*), all of which are movements that restore the normal vertical position of the head and eyes (*top* figure). All of these compensatory movements are part of the ocular tilt reaction, a normal reflex that stabilizes retinal images and is mediated by the otolith organs (especially the gravity-sensing utricle and its connections to the ocular motor nuclei and the vestibulospinal tract). Skew deviation (*bottom* figure) is an abnormal hetero-tropia that appears in disorders (especially cerebellar or brainstem lesions) that produce asymmetry in these pathways.[22] Unilateral lesions below the mid-pons, the point where these gravity-adjusting pathways cross in the brainstem, cause *ipsiversive* tilt reactions (i.e., the patient's *lowermost eye* indicates the side of the lesion; *right bottom*; see Wallenberg stroke in Chapter 62); lesions above the mid-pons cause *contraversive* tilt reac-tions (i.e. the *uppermost eye* indicates the side of the patient's lesion; *right top*). *III,* Oculomotor nucleus; *IV,* trochlear nucleus; *VI,* abducens nucleus.

EBM BOX 59.1	Ice Pack Test, Detecting Myasthenia*

Finding (Reference)[†]	Sensitivity (%)	Specificity (%)	Likelihood Ratio[‡] if Finding Is	
			Present	Absent
Improvement in ptosis after application of ice[26,27,29-38]	39–96	78–98	8.1	0.1
Improvement in diplopia and ophthalmoplegia after application of ice[26,35]	75–97	97–98	30.6	0.1

*Diagnostic standard: for *myasthenia gravis*, a positive edrophonium (Tensilon) test, positive anti-acetylcholine receptor antibody, electromyography, or combinations of these tests.
[†]Definition of findings: for *ice pack test*, see text. The ice was applied to the eye for 2 minutes[29-31,36-38] or 5 minutes[26,35] before determining the results of the test.
[‡]Likelihood ratio (LR) if finding present = positive LR; LR if finding absent = negative LR.

ICE-PACK TEST FOR MYASTHENIA
Probability

Decrease				Increase		
−45%	−30%	−15%		+15%	+30%	+45%

LRs   0.1   0.2   0.5   1   2   5   10   LRs

Negative test, *arguing against* myasthenia if diplopia
Negative test, *arguing against* myasthenia if ptosis

Positive test, detecting myasthenia if diplopia
Positive test, detecting myasthenia if ptosis

diplopia (see earlier section on definitions). In 41 patients with binocular diplopia, the combination of horizontal diplopia and eyes *converging* when looking to the side of worse diplopia (i.e., *esotropia*) increased probability of sixth nerve palsy (LR = 19.2); horizontal diplopia and eyes *diverging* when looking to the side of worse diplopia (i.e., *exotropia*) increased probability of internuclear ophthalmoplegia (LR = 68.4). Vertical diplopia with anisocoria or ptosis increased probability of third nerve palsy (LR = 7.4). Vertical diplopia with signs of orbitopathy (e.g., lid edema, proptosis, gritty eyes) and without anisocoria or ptosis increased probability of orbital disease (LR = 68.4). Finally, isolated vertical diplopia (without anisocoria, ptosis, or signs of orbitopathy) increased probability of fourth nerve palsy (LR = 11.3). The most common error using this algorithm was for the clinician to conclude there was a third nerve palsy (i.e., vertical diplopia with anisocoria or ptosis), but the correct diagnosis was instead a less common disorder, such as myasthenia, Miller Fisher variant, or multiple cranial neuropathies.[8]

DISORDERS OF CRANIAL NERVES III, IV, AND VI

I. Introduction

Table 59.1 reviews the causes of *isolated* palsies of these three cranial nerves, based on analysis of over 3500 patients reported in the literature. Major causes are ischemic infarcts (all three nerves),

TABLE 59.1 ■ Etiology of Isolated Palsies of Cranial Nerves III, IV, and VI

	Oculomotor Nerve	Trochlear Nerve	Abducens Nerve	Mixed*
Proportion (%)†	31	11	45	13
Etiology (%)				
Head trauma	13	34	11	18
Neoplasm	11	5	19	29
Ischemic	25	22	20	7
Aneurysm	17	1	3	11
Other	14	8	21	19
Idiopathic	20	30	26	16

Based upon references. 39–51
*"Mixed" refers to combinations of cranial nerves III, IV, and VI.
†*Proportion* is ratio of palsies affecting designated cranial nerve to total number of palsies affecting any of cranial nerves III, IV, and VI.

intracranial aneurysms (especially the third cranial nerve), head trauma (especially the fourth cranial nerve), and tumors (especially when more than one of these nerves are affected). At least one fourth of isolated cranial neuropathies affecting these nerves remain idiopathic, even in the modern era of advanced clinical imaging.[47]

II. Rules For Diagnosing Ischemic Infarcts

One of the most common causes of *isolated* palsies of cranial nerves III, IV, and VI is ischemic infarction, a diagnosis made at the bedside based on the following criteria: (1) The palsy is isolated (i.e., no other neurologic or ophthalmologic findings), (2) the onset is abrupt, (3) the patient has risk factors for cerebrovascular disease (i.e., age >50 years, hypertension, and diabetes), (4) no other cause is apparent, and (5) the palsy is self-limited (i.e., resolves over several months). Seventy-five percent of ischemic mononeuropathies resolve within 4 months; persistence beyond this should prompt evaluation for other causes.

III. Oculomotor Nerve (Cranial Nerve III)

A. THE FINDING

Complete weakness causes downward and outward deviation of the affected eye and ptosis (Fig. 59.7). The pupil may or may not be dilated, depending on the etiology of the patient's neuropathy.

B. CLINICAL SIGNIFICANCE

1. Pupil-Sparing Rule[52,53]

The most common identified causes of *isolated nontraumatic* third nerve paralysis are posterior communicating artery aneurysm (which must be managed aggressively) and ischemic infarction of the third nerve (which is managed conservatively). In over 95% of aneurysmal palsies, the pupil reacts sluggishly to light or is fixed and dilated, but in 73% of ischemic palsies, the pupil is spared.[41,42,44,51,54–65] These observations have led to the **pupil-sparing rule**, which states that patients with third nerve palsies sparing the pupil do not have aneurysms and can be safely managed expectantly.

Looking ahead

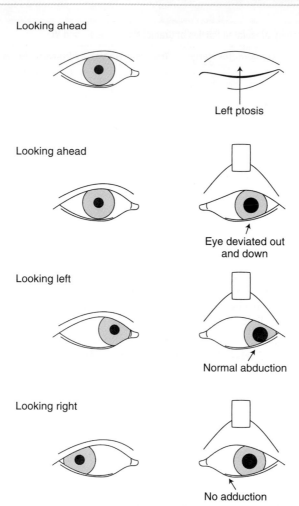

Left ptosis

Looking ahead

Eye deviated out
and down

Looking left

Normal abduction

Looking right

No adduction

Fig. 59.7 Third nerve palsy. Complete third nerve palsy (of the left eye in this example) causes ptosis that obscures the position of the eye (*first row*). When the lid is held open (by a piece of tape in this example), the eye appears deviated outward and slightly downward (*second row*), because of unopposed action of the lateral rectus muscle (abducting the eye) and superior oblique muscle (depressing the eye). In this example of third nerve palsy, the pupil is dilated because the cause is an intracranial aneurysm: many ischemic third nerve palsies spare the pupil. (See the section on the pupil-sparing rule in the text.) When the patient looks to the left (*third row*), the intact lateral rectus abducts the eye normally. When the patient looks to the right (*fourth row*), the left eye fails to adduct past the midline. Further tests would also demonstrate that the left eye cannot look up or down.

Before applying this rule, however, there are three important caveats: (1) The rule applies only to patients with *complete* paralysis of the ocular muscles of the cranial nerve III and *complete* sparing of the pupil. Up to 4% of patients with aneurysms do have sparing of the pupil although the third nerve muscles are only partially paralyzed; (2) The rule should be applied sparingly to patients aged 20 to 50 years, an age-group in which ischemic infarcts are uncommon; and (3) The rule only applies to patients with isolated third nerve palsies. Any other neurologic or ophthalmologic finding (e.g., hemiparesis, proptosis, other cranial neuropathy) invalidates the rule.

Nonetheless, the pupil-sparing rule had greater value in an earlier era when the only diagnostic test for intracranial aneurysms was catheter angiography (a test carrying a 2% risk of stroke). In this earlier era, clinicians sought ways to identify those patients who could safely avoid this potentially dangerous test, and the pupil-sparing rule was the result. Today, with the availability of safer noninvasive testing methods (computed tomographic angiography and magnetic resonance imaging), most experts recommend noninvasive vascular imaging of all patients with new-onset isolated nontraumatic third nerve palsies, whether or not the pupil is spared.[66-68]

2. Clinical Syndromes

Associated findings distinguish the different causes of third nerve palsy.[69]

a. Ipsilateral Brainstem Injury
Damage to the third nerve fascicle as it exits the ipsilateral brainstem causes accompanying ipsilateral cerebellar signs (**Nothnagel syndrome**, involving the superior cerebellar peduncle), contralateral hemitremor (**Benedikt syndrome**, involving the red nucleus), or contralateral hemiparesis (**Weber syndrome**, involving the cerebral peduncle).

b. Injury to the Nerve in the Subarachnoid Space
Important causes include uncal herniation (i.e., patient is comatose) and internal carotid posterior communicating artery aneurysm (i.e., the third nerve palsy is isolated; see Chapter 21).

c. Ipsilateral Cavernous Sinus or Orbit Injury
Lesions of the cavernous sinus or orbit cause simultaneous injury to cranial nerves III, IV, and VI (which causes total ophthalmoplegia), to the sympathetic nerves of the iris (contributing to a pupil that is small and unreactive), and to the ophthalmic distribution of the trigeminal nerve (causing hypesthesia of upper third of face). Orbital disease also causes early, prominent proptosis.

d. Ischemic Infarcts
Ischemic infarction causes isolated third nerve palsy. (See the sections on rules for diagnosing ischemic infarcts and pupil sparing rule.)

IV. Trochlear Nerve (Cranial Nerve IV)

A. THE FINDING

1. Isolated IV Palsy

Paralysis of cranial nerve IV causes vertical diplopia and hypertropia of the affected eye. Nonetheless, the hypertropia may not be evident on examination, and often the clinician will have to tilt the patient's head toward the affected side to bring out the finding (Fig. 59.8). Tilting the head aggravates the diplopia because it requires the ipsilateral eye to intort, which calls upon simultaneous contraction of the superior oblique and superior rectus muscles. These two muscles work together, and the tendency of the superior oblique to depress the eye is normally balanced by that of the superior rectus to elevate the eye. If the superior oblique is weak, however, attempts to intort the eye (e.g., during tilting of the head) instead bring about unopposed action of the superior rectus, which elevates the eye and aggravates the vertical diplopia and hypertropia.

2. Combined III and IV Palsy

In patients with third nerve palsy, testing cranial nerve IV is particular difficult because the eye is already deviated outward and down (Fig. 59.7). Nonetheless, if cranial nerve IV is intact in these patients, the eye will *intort* as the patient is asked to look down. Absence of intorsion (which is

Looking down and *left*

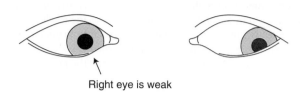

Right eye is weak

Head tilted *left*

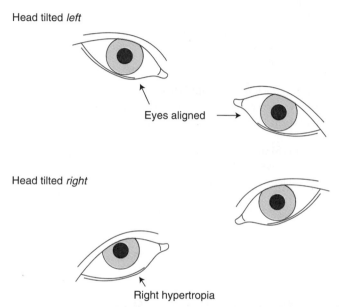

Eyes aligned ⟶

Head tilted *right*

Right hypertropia

Fig. 59.8 Fourth nerve palsy. The patient in this example has a right fourth nerve palsy. Diplopia is worst when looking down and to the left, indicating that the weak muscle is either the left inferior rectus muscle or right superior oblique muscle (see Fig. 59.2 for principal actions of eye muscles). Simple inspection (*first row*) reveals that the right eye lags behind the left eye, indicating that the weak muscle is indeed on the right side (i.e., right superior oblique). Tilting the head *away* from the affected side (i.e., to the *left* side, away from the weak *right* superior oblique, *second row*) aligns the eyes normally, but tilting the head *toward* the affected side (i.e., to the right side, *third row*) brings out a prominent right hypertropia (i.e., right eye is higher than the left eye). See the text.

apparent by observing the medial conjunctival vessels) indicates combined third and fourth nerve palsies. An instructive video of this finding appears in the reference by Reich.[70]

B. CLINICAL SIGNIFICANCE

1. Head Position

In studies of patients with isolated fourth nerve palsies, 45% actually habitually tilt their head away from the side of the lesion (to minimize any need for intorsion in the affected eye).[46,71,72] This habitual head tilting may be apparent in old photographs of patients with chronic fourth nerve palsies. As expected, when the head is tilted toward the affected side, the diplopia and hypertropia worsen in 92% to 96% of patients.[46,72,73]

2. Clinical Syndromes

The trochlear nerve has the longest intracranial course of any cranial nerve, in part explaining why trauma is the most common explanation for isolated lesions. Associated findings distinguish the different clinical syndromes.

a. Contralateral Midbrain Injury

Associated findings are contralateral Horner syndrome, contralateral dysmetria, and contralateral internuclear ophthalmoplegia. In all of these syndromes the associated findings are contralateral because the trochlear nerves cross on their way to the eyes (i.e., the fourth cranial nerve innervating the right eye originates in the left brainstem).[69]

b. Ipsilateral Cavernous Sinus or Orbit Injury

These lesions cause combinations of findings discussed previously in the section on ipsilateral cavernous sinus or orbit injury.

c. Ischemic Infarcts

Ischemic infarction causes isolated fourth nerve palsy. (See the section on rules for diagnosing ischemic infarcts.)

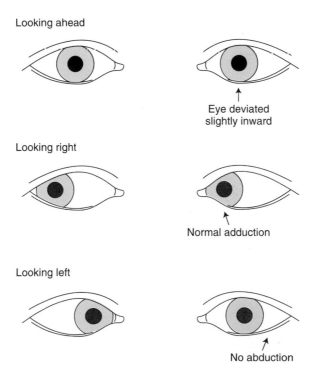

Fig. 59.9 **Sixth nerve palsy.** When the patient in this example (who has a *left* sixth nerve palsy) looks ahead, there is a mild left esotropia (i.e., left eye is deviated toward the nose, *first row*). When looking to the right, the affected eye adducts normally (*second row*). When looking to the left, the left eye fails to abduct (*third row*).

V. Abducens Nerve (Cranial Nerve VI)

A. THE FINDING

Paralysis of the sixth cranial nerve causes esotropia and an inability to fully abduct the affected eye (Fig. 59.9).

B. Clinical Significance

The various clinical syndromes are distinguished by their associated findings.

1. Ipsilateral Pons Injury

Associated findings are contralateral hemiparesis (**Raymond syndrome**), ipsilateral seventh nerve palsy and contralateral hemiparesis (**Millard-Gubler syndrome**), or ipsilateral Horner syndrome, ipsilateral horizontal gaze palsy, and ipsilateral involvement of cranial nerves V, VII, and VIII (**Foville syndrome**).

2. Injury to the Nerve in the Subarachnoid Space

Injury to the nerve in the subarachnoid space often causes isolated sixth nerve palsy. Examples are meningitis, recent lumbar puncture (with subsequent leak of cerebrospinal fluid that leads to stretching of the nerve), and pseudotumor cerebri (also from stretching of the nerve, brought on by elevated intracranial pressure; these patients may have associated papilledema).

3. Injury at the Petrous Apex

Examples are complicated otitis media (**Gradenigo syndrome**, which causes associated ipsilateral decreased hearing, facial pain from involvement of the fifth cranial nerve, and ipsilateral seventh nerve palsy), petrous bone fracture (associated with hemotympanum and **Battle sign**), and naso-pharyngeal carcinoma.

4. Ipsilateral Cavernous Sinus or Orbit Injury

These lesions cause combinations of findings discussed previously in the section on ipsilateral cavernous sinus or orbit injury.

5. Ischemic infarcts

Ischemic infarction causes an isolated sixth nerve palsy. (See the section on rules for diagnosing ischemic infarcts.)

References may be accessed online at *Elsevier eBooks for Practicing Clinicians*.

Miscellaneous Cranial Nerves

- Abnormalities of the cranial nerves may reflect local disorders of the nerve itself, injury to its nucleus in the brainstem, or cerebral hemispheric disease interrupting the supranuclear input to the cranial nerve nucleus. Cerebral hemispheric disease must be *bilateral* before there are *motor* abnormalities of cranial nerves V, IX, or X.
- Diagnosis of many well-defined syndromes depends entirely on the clinician's observation of cranial nerves: Foster Kennedy syndrome, herpes zoster ophthalmicus, Bell palsy, pseudobulbar palsy, and jugular foramen syndrome are examples.
- In patients with herpes zoster ophthalmicus (i.e., zoster infection of V1, the ophthalmic branch of cranial nerve V), Hutchison sign (i.e., involvement of the tip of the nose) increases probability of future ocular complications. Even so, all patients with this infection—whether or not Hutchinson sign is present—should receive antiviral medications and be examined by eye specialists.
- In patients who have had a stroke, several findings increase the patient's risk of aspiration, especially the findings of drowsiness, oxygen desaturation of 2% or more after swallowing a liquid, and the positive water swallow test. Normal pharyngeal sensation decreases probability of aspiration.

Table 60.1 reviews the physical examination of the 12 cranial nerves. Only cranial nerves I, V, VII and IX through XII are discussed in this chapter. Cranial nerve II is discussed in Chapters 21 and 58; cranial nerve VIII, in Chapter 24; and cranial nerves III, IV, and VI, in Chapter 59.

OLFACTORY NERVE (I)

I. Technique

The usual test for the sense of smell is placing a nonirritative substance, such as wintergreen or cloves, under one nostril at a time. One simple method uses the standard 70% isopropyl alcohol pad available in most clinics and wards.[1] Pungent substances like ammonia should be avoided because they stimulate trigeminal nerve endings (i.e., cranial nerve V).

II. Clinical Significance

A. ANOSMIA

Anosmia is the complete absence of smell. The most common causes are upper respiratory infection and sinus disease (which obstructs the nasal passages) and previous head trauma

TABLE 60.1 ■ The Twelve Cranial Nerves

Cranial Nerve	Motor Examination	Sensory Examination	Reflex Examination
Olfactory nerve (I)		Detection of nonirritating odors	
Optic nerve (II)		Visual acuity Retinal examination	Afferent pupillary defect (swinging flashlight test)
Nerves of the eye muscles: Oculomotor nerve (III) Trochlear nerve (IV) Abducens nerve (VI)	Extraocular movements (III, IV, and VI) Lid elevation (III only)		Pupillary constriction (III only)
Trigeminal nerve (V)	Masseter muscle Lateral pterygoid muscle	Pain, temperature, and touch sensation of the ipsilateral face	Corneal reflex (afferent limb) Jaw jerk (afferent and efferent limb) Glabellar reflex (afferent limb)
Facial nerve (VII)	All facial movements except lid elevation	Taste sensation to anterior two-thirds of the tongue	Corneal reflex (efferent limb) Glabellar reflex (efferent limb)
Vestibulocochlear nerve (VIII)		Tests of hearing (cochlear component)	Vestibulo-ocular reflex (vestibular component)
Glossopharyngeal nerve (IX)	Ipsilateral palate elevation (with X)	Sensation posterior pharynx Taste sensation to posterior two-thirds of tongue	Gag reflex (afferent limb and, with X, efferent limb)
Vagus nerve (X)	Ipsilateral palate elevation (with IX)		Gag reflex (efferent limb with IX)
Spinal accessory nerve (XI)	Trapezius muscle Sternocleidomastoid muscle		
Hypoglossal nerve (XII)	Genioglossus muscle		

(which damages the olfactory fibers).[2,3] Less common causes are **Kallman syndrome** (hypogonadotropic hypogonadism) and sphenoid ridge masses (e.g., meningioma, which causes the **Foster-Kennedy syndrome**, i.e., ipsilateral anosmia, ipsilateral optic atrophy, and contralateral papilledema).[2,4]

B. OLFACTORY DYSFUNCTION

Patients with olfactory dysfunction are able to detect odors but frequently misidentify them. Olfactory dysfunction is common in patients with Parkinson disease or after frontal or temporal lobectomies.[5,6] Patients with Parkinson disease are much more likely to have olfactory dysfunction than patients with other parkinsonian syndromes such as vascular parkinsonism or progressive supranuclear palsy (see Chapter 66).[6-11]

TRIGEMINAL NERVE (V)

I. Introduction

The trigeminal sensory and motor nuclei are located in the pons, although the sensory nucleus extends through the medulla into the cervical spinal cord. The sensory branches of the trigeminal nerve innervate the upper face (V1, ophthalmic division), mid-face (V2, maxillary division), and lower face (V3, mandibular division). The motor fibers to the masseter and lateral pterygoid muscles travel with the mandibular division (V3).

II. The Finding

A. MOTOR WEAKNESS

Lesions of the motor component of the trigeminal nerve affect the masseter muscle (causing difficulty clenching that side of the jaw, sometimes with atrophy that flattens the contour of the cheek) and lateral pterygoid muscle (causing difficulty deviating the jaw to the opposite side; at rest, the jaw may deviate toward the weak side).

B. SENSORY LOSS

Lesions of the sensory component cause diminished pain, temperature, and touch sensation in any or all of the three divisions on one side of the face. Sensation to most of the external ear (excluding the tragus) and the angle of the jaw is preserved in trigeminal lesions, because these areas are supplied by cervical sensory roots (see Fig. 62.1 in Chapter 62).

C. CORNEAL REFLEX

Unilateral gentle stimulation of the cornea normally causes bilateral blinking. The afferent limb of this reflex is the ipsilateral trigeminal nerve (only V1 and V2) and the efferent limb is both facial nerves (i.e., both eyes blink after stimulation of one cornea).

III. Clinical Significance

A. MOTOR WEAKNESS

Unilateral weakness of the trigeminal muscles indicates disease of the proximal mandibular division (e.g., skull metastases) or a lesion in the ipsilateral pons (patients with pontine lesions have other associated neurologic findings, such as abnormalities of cranial nerves VI or VII, or contralateral hemiparesis). Unilateral weakness of the trigeminal muscles does not occur with cerebral hemispheric lesions because each trigeminal nucleus receives bilateral cortical innervation.[12] *Bilateral* weakness, however, may occur in bilateral cerebral hemispheric disease and cause great difficulty chewing (see the section on pseudobulbar palsy).

B. SENSORY LOSS

Sensory loss of the face may be part of a broader neurologic syndrome affecting the sensation of the whole body and other neurologic functions (lesions of the cerebral hemisphere, thalamus, or brainstem) or may be isolated to the face (lesions of the peripheral nerve and its branches).

1. Sensory Loss of Face and Body

In thalamic and cerebral hemispheric lesions, sensation of the face and body is abnormal on the side of the body contralateral to the lesion. There is often associated hemiparesis, aphasia, or both. In brainstem lesions, the sensory abnormalities of the face and body are on *opposite* sides: sensation is diminished on the face *ipsilateral* to the lesion but on the body *contralateral* to the lesion (Fig. 62.2; Table 62.2). Pontine lesions affect intraoral more than facial sensation, whereas medullary lesions affect facial more than intraoral sensation.[13]

2. Sensory Loss Isolated to the Face

Sensory loss isolated to the face is part of syndromes affecting the apex of the temporal bone (see Chapter 59, section on cranial nerve VI), the cavernous sinus syndrome (V1 division only, see Chapter 59), and **numb chin syndrome**. The numb chin syndrome describes the loss of sensation on the lower lip and chin, an ominous finding in cancer patients because it suggests metastatic disease to the ipsilateral mandible, base of skull, or leptomeninges.[14,15] Some affected patients also have other cranial nerve abnormalities.

C. ABNORMAL CORNEAL REFLEX

The two limbs of the corneal reflex are cranial nerves V and VII. According to traditional teachings, unilateral trigeminal nerve dysfunction (i.e., in the ipsilateral brainstem, V1, or V2 divisions) prevents both eyes from blinking after stimulation of the ipsilateral cornea, whereas unilateral facial nerve dysfunction prevents the ipsilateral eye from blinking when its cornea is stimulated, although the contralateral eye blinks normally. The absent corneal reflex is felt to be particularly important in patients with unilateral sensorineural hearing loss, in whom it raises the possibility of cerebellopontine angle tumors such as acoustic neuroma.

Nonetheless, the clinical utility of the asymmetric corneal reflex is limited. The reflex is inexplicably absent unilaterally in 8% of healthy elderly patients,[16] and the sensitivity of the absent reflex for acoustic neuroma is only 33%, the finding usually indicating the tumor has already grown to a large size (more than 2 cm in diameter).[17]

D. HERPES ZOSTER INFECTION AND THE NASOCILIARY BRANCH OF THE TRIGEMINAL NERVE ("HUTCHINSON SIGN")

About half of patients with *herpes zoster* infection of the ophthalmic division of the trigeminal nerve (V1; "**herpes zoster ophthalmicus**") develop vision-threatening complications such as uveitis or keratitis within 1 to 4 weeks of the onset of the rash (mean onset of ocular complications is 11 to 13 days).[18–20] In 1865, Hutchinson noted that the tip of the nose, cornea, and iris all share the same branch of the trigeminal nerve (the nasociliary nerve) and that if patients with herpes zoster ophthalmicus develop vesicles on the tip of the nose (i.e., **Hutchinson sign**), they were at increased risk of ocular complications.[21] Nonetheless, the clinical utility of this sign is limited: its accuracy is only modest (sensitivity of 16% to 84%, specificity of 76% to 97%, positive likelihood ratio [LR] = 4, negative LR = 0.4),[18–20,22–24] and today all patients with herpes zoster ophthalmicus, whether or not the tip of the nose or the eye is involved, should receive antiviral medications and be examined by eye specialists.

FACIAL NERVE (VII)

I. The Finding

Lesions of the facial nerve may cause facial asymmetry (diminished ipsilateral nasolabial fold and widened ipsilateral palpebral fissure) and weakness of most ipsilateral facial muscles (muscles used during speaking, blinking, raising eyebrows, smiling, wrinkling the forehead, closing the eyes, showing teeth, and retracting the chin). There may be abnormalities of ipsilateral tearing (lacrimal gland), hearing (stapedius muscle), taste (anterior two thirds of the tongue), and the corneal and glabellar reflexes.

Facial nerve lesions do not cause ptosis, because the muscles elevating the lid are not innervated by the facial nerve but rather by sympathetic nerves and cranial nerve III.

II. Clinical Significance

A. CENTRAL VERSUS PERIPHERAL FACIAL WEAKNESS

Unilateral facial weakness may be *central* (i.e., in upper motor neurons, from lesions in the contralateral motor cortex or descending pyramidal tracts) or *peripheral* (i.e., in lower motor neurons, from lesions in the peripheral nerve or facial nucleus in the ipsilateral pons).* These lesions are distinguished by the following two features:

1. Distribution of Weakness

Peripheral lesions affect both upper and lower facial muscles, whereas central lesions affect predominately the lower facial muscles. Wrinkling of the forehead is relatively spared in central lesions because the facial nuclei innervating these muscles receive bilateral cortical innervation.

2. Movements Affected

Peripheral lesions paralyze all facial movements on the side affected, whereas central lesions affect the voluntary movements but spare emotional ones. The patient with central weakness (e.g., cerebral hemispheric stroke) may be unable to wrinkle one corner of the mouth volitionally yet is able to move it briskly when laughing or crying. This occurs because the emotional input to the facial nuclei does not come from the motor cortex.[†,25,26]

B. PERIPHERAL NERVE LESIONS

1. Etiology

The causes of isolated peripheral facial palsies are idiopathic (50% to 87%), surgical or accidental trauma (5% to 22%), herpes zoster infections (**Ramsey Hunt syndrome**, 7% to 13%), tumors (e.g., cholesteatoma, parotid tumors, 1% to 6%), and miscellaneous disorders (8% to 11%). (These figures originate from specialty referral centers and may overrepresent unusual etiologies.)[27–32] **Bell palsy** refers to the idiopathic disorders, although evidence suggests it may represent a viral infection.[33,34]

2. Associated Findings

In patients with Bell palsy, associated findings are diminished taste (52%), hyperacusis (8% to 30%), increased tearing (19% to 34%), and decreased tearing (2% to 17%).[28–31,35–37] Increased tear production occurs because the weak orbicularis oculi muscle cannot contain and direct the tears down the nasolacrimal duct; decreased tearing reflects lacrimal gland dysfunction. Although 23% of patients also have sensory complaints, the finding of hypesthesia of the face (i.e., cranial nerve V) is variable: Some investigators, arguing that Bell palsy is part of a multiple cranial neuropathy, have found hypesthesia in as many as 48% of patients[30,35] while other investigators have never found associated hypesthesia of the face.[28]

---

*Chapter 61 defines upper and lower motor neurons.
†The opposite clinical finding, emotional paralysis without volitional paralysis, occurs with lesions of the thalamus or frontal lobe.[25,26]

3. Topographic Diagnosis

The branches of the facial nerve diverge from the main trunk in predictable order: They are, proximally to distally, branches to the lacrimal gland, stapedius muscle, tongue (taste), and facial muscles.[30] Therefore, tests of tearing (Schirmer's tear test), stapedius function (stapedius reflex during audiometry), and taste should pinpoint the location of the lesion, although this is only accurate when the nerve is completely severed. In patients with patchy lesions (Bell palsy or partial injuries), topographic diagnosis is often nonsensical (e.g., tearing reduced but taste and stapedius function preserved) and has minimal clinical value.[30,35,38,39]

4. Complications of Bell Palsy[29,31,36,37]

Three complications occur after recovery from Bell palsy:

a. Associated Movements

Associated movements, or **synkinesis**, occur in 55% to 94% of patients. These are unexpected movements that probably result from aberrant regeneration. Examples of associated movements are narrowing of the palpebral fissure when the patient smiles, or motion of the corner of the mouth when the patient tightly closes his or her eyes.

b. Contracture

Contracture occurs in 3% to 36% of patients. Despite the name, this actually represents increased muscle tone, not fibrotic scar. Contracture often restores facial symmetry, even though some weakness persists.

c. Crocodile Tears

Crocodile tears are seen in 2% to 6% of patients, from aberrant regeneration of salivary gland fibers to the lacrimal gland. When affected patients eat, tears form and run down the cheek or collect in the nose.

GLOSSOPHARYNGEAL (IX) AND VAGUS (X) NERVES

I. Finding

These nerves are considered together because their function is difficult to separate at the bedside and because clinical disorders usually affect both nerves simultaneously. There are three abnormal findings: **(1) Absent pharyngeal sensation**. This is usually tested with a cotton applicator stick touching the posterior oropharynx, **(2) Diminished velar movement**. The posterior edge of the soft palate is called the **velum** and its elevation, **velar movement**. The soft palate should elevate as the patient vocalizes a prolonged "ah," **(3) Abnormal gag reflex**. During stimulation of the posterior tongue, pharynx, or soft palate, there is reflex elevation of the tongue and soft palate and constriction of the pharyngeal muscles. The gag reflex is labeled abnormal when it is diminished, absent, hyperactive, or asymmetrical.

II. Clinical Significance

Abnormalities of these nerves may occur because of *bilateral* cerebral hemispheric disease or because of disease in the *ipsilateral* medulla or peripheral nerves (i.e., cranial nerves IX and X). *Unilateral* cerebral hemispheric disease does not ordinarily cause palatal weakness because the nuclei of these nerves normally receive bilateral corticobulbar innervation.

A. BILATERAL CEREBRAL HEMISPHERIC LESIONS: PSEUDOBULBAR PALSY

Bilateral lesions above the level of the pons that disrupt the descending pyramidal tracts innervating brainstem motor nuclei may cause significant paralysis of the palate and pharynx, along with paralysis of the tongue, face, and muscles of chewing. This syndrome, **pseudobulbar palsy**, affects about 4% of patients with cerebrovascular disease, who mostly have lacunar infarcts in both internal capsules.[40,41] The main clinical features are dysarthria, dysphagia, and paralysis of voluntary movements of the face.[42] Other findings are hyperactive jaw jerk (70% of patients), absent gag reflex (70%), and hyperactive emotional reflexes that cause spasmodic and often inappropriate crying and laughing (24%).[40,41] The animated facial movements during laughter or uncontrollable crying contrast markedly with the lack of voluntary facial movement and the patient's inability to mimic gestures.

The term *pseudobulbar*, coined by Lepine in 1877,[41] is used because the lesion is supranuclear, to distinguish this syndrome from similar motor paralysis that may occur after damage to the brainstem nuclei themselves (i.e., **bulbar paralysis**). The term is a misnomer, however, because *bulbar* refers to the medulla and two of the motor nuclei prominently affected in pseudobulbar palsy—those of the facial muscles (VII) and of chewing (V)—reside in the pons.

B. BEDSIDE PREDICTORS OF RISK OF ASPIRATION AFTER STROKE

In patients who have suffered bilateral strokes, significant dysfunction of cranial nerves IX and X makes the airway vulnerable to aspiration during swallowing. EBM Box 60.1 presents the accuracy of several bedside signs predicting aspiration in patients after strokes. The findings that increase probability of aspiration risk the most are drowsiness (LR = 3.6), oxygen desaturation of 2% or more after the patient swallows a liquid (LR = 3.5), and abnormal water swallow test (LR = 2.6; see footnote to EBM Box 60.1 for definitions of findings). The findings *decreasing* the risk of aspiration the most are normal pharyngeal sensation (LR = 0.03), absence of oxygen desaturation following a swallow (LR = 0.4), and a normal water swallow test (LR = 0.4). The accuracy of other findings, including the abnormal gag reflex, presence of dysphonia, and abnormal cough, is only modest. Findings without predictive value are abnormal sensation of face and tongue, tongue weakness, bilateral cranial nerve findings, and abnormal chest radiograph.[43]

The poor predictive value of the gag reflex is not surprising because the pharyngeal muscles involved in this reflex are not necessarily the same ones activated during normal swallowing to protect the airway. Moreover, the gag reflex is often absent in normal individuals, especially elderly patients.[62,63] Pharyngeal sensation, on the other hand, is rarely absent in normal individuals.[62]

C. LESIONS OF IPSILATERAL BRAINSTEM OR PERIPHERAL NERVE

The lateral medullary syndrome causes ipsilateral absence of pharyngeal sensation and reduced velar elevation, associated with the Horner syndrome and other sensory and cerebellar signs (see Table 62.2 in Chapter 62). The jugular foramen syndrome (e.g., basilar skull fracture or glomus jugulare tumors) simultaneously disrupts cranial nerves IX, X, and XI, causing ipsilateral paralysis of the palate, vocal cords (hoarseness), and trapezius and sternocleidomastoid muscles.

| EBM BOX 60.1 | **Aspiration After Stroke*** | | | |

Finding (Reference)†	Sensitivity (%)	Specificity (%)	Likelihood Ratio‡ if Finding Is Present	Absent
Voice and cough				
Abnormal voluntary cough[43-53]	28–89	36–94	2.1	0.7
Dysphonia[43-48,50,52-54]	12–98	13–98	1.5	0.5
Dysarthria[46,50,53,55]	60–77	53–81	2.0	0.5
Neurologic examination				
Drowsiness[51,53,56]	3–76	65–100	**3.6**	NS
Abnormal sensation face and tongue[43]	22	52	NS	NS
Absent pharyngeal sensation[56]	98	60	2.4	**0.03**
Tongue weakness[51,52,54]	50–72	47–91	NS	0.6
Bilateral cranial nerve signs[43,48]	71–73	30–39	NS	NS
Abnormal gag reflex[43-48,50-52,54,55]	53–91	18–82	1.4	0.6
Other tests				
Water swallow test[49-51,53,54,56-59]	36–85	58–93	2.6	0.4
Oxygen desaturation 0–2 min after swallowing[49,58,60,61]	56–84	40–97	**3.5**	0.4

*Diagnostic standard: for *aspiration*, fiberoptic examination[49,58] or videofluoroscopy (all other studies).
†Definition of findings: for *abnormal voluntary cough*, the patient is asked to cough as hard as possible and the resulting cough is absent, weak, breathy, or sluggish; for *dysphonia*, the patient is asked to sing a prolonged "ah" and the voice is breathy, hoarse, wet, harsh, or strained; for *absent pharyngeal sensation*, the patient cannot sense an applicator stick applied to the posterior oropharynx, on one or both sides; for *abnormal gag reflex*, the gag reflex is diminished, absent, hyperactive, or asymmetric; for *water swallow test*, drinking 5 to 90 mL of water in 5 to 10 mL sips causes coughing, choking, or alteration of the voice; for *oxygen desaturation after swallowing*, oxygen saturation decreases ≥2% 0–2 min after swallowing 10 mL of water[49,] 50 mL of water[58,] or 20 mL[61] to 150 mL[60] of liquid barium.
‡Likelihood ratio (LR) if finding present = positive LR; LR if finding absent = negative LR.
NS, Not significant.

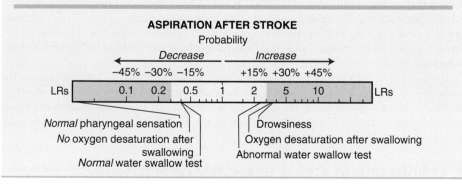

ASPIRATION AFTER STROKE

SPINAL ACCESSORY NERVE (XI)

I. Finding

The primary findings are a weakness or atrophy, or both, of the sternocleidomastoid muscle (which turns the head to the opposite side) and trapezius muscle (which elevates the ipsilateral shoulder).

II. Clinical Significance

Unilateral weakness of these muscles may represent disease of the cerebral hemispheres, brainstem, spinal cord, or peripheral nerve. Atrophy indicates that the lesion is in the nucleus (i.e., brainstem or high cervical spinal cord) or peripheral nerve (i.e., the lesion is not in the cerebral hemispheres).

A. CEREBRAL HEMISPHERE

Lesions of the cerebral hemispheres affect the trapezius and sternocleidomastoid muscles differently: Lesions in one cerebral hemisphere weaken the *contralateral* trapezius but the *ipsilateral* sternocleidomastoid muscle.[‡,64] Therefore, in a hemispheric stroke, the patient may demonstrate weakness turning the head toward the hemiparetic side.[65] In a focal seizure, the head often deviates toward the seizing limbs.

B. BRAINSTEM OR HIGH CERVICAL SPINAL CORD

Lesions of the accessory nucleus, located in the medulla and high cervical spinal cord (e.g., syringomyelia), may cause atrophy and weakness of the *ipsilateral* trapezius and sternocleidomastoid muscle.

C. PERIPHERAL NERVE

Injuries to the peripheral nerve, which occur from trauma to the posterior triangle of the neck (e.g., surgical excision of lymph nodes, blunt trauma), may paralyze the *ipsilateral* trapezius or sternocleidomastoid muscles, although the sternocleidomastoid muscle is often spared because its branches diverge proximally from the main trunk of the nerve.[66] The **jugular foramen syndrome**, discussed above under the glossopharyngeal nerve, also affects cranial nerve XI along with cranial nerves IX and X.

HYPOGLOSSAL NERVE (XII)

I. Finding

During protrusion of the tongue, each genioglossus muscle acts to push the tongue out and towards the opposite side. Normally these laterally directed forces balance each other, and the tongue remains in the midline. With unilateral hypoglossal weakness, however, the intact genioglossus muscle acts to deviate the tongue toward the opposite, or weak, side.

II. Clinical Significance

Weakness of the genioglossus may represent disease in the cerebral hemisphere, brainstem, or peripheral nerve. Atrophy or fasciculations of the tongue indicate the lesion is either in the hypoglossal nucleus (brainstem) or hypoglossal nerve (i.e., *not* cerebral hemispheres).

---

‡Descending corticobulbar fibers to the sternocleidomastoid muscle are believed to cross twice to innervate the ipsilateral side. This innervation makes teleologic sense, because the sternocleidmastoid muscle turns the head to the opposite side, and the cerebral hemisphere is interested in turning the head to same side for which it controls visual fields, eye movements, and motor function.[64]

A. CEREBRAL HEMISPHERE

Lesions of the cerebral hemisphere may cause weakness of the contralateral genioglossus. Therefore, the tongue deviates *toward* the side of the weak arm and leg.[67]

B. BRAINSTEM

The medial medullary syndrome causes ipsilateral hypoglossal paralysis, contralateral hemiparesis, and contralateral loss of proprioceptive and vibratory sensation (preserving pain and temperature sensation). Therefore, the tongue deviates *away* from the side of the weak arm and leg.

C. PERIPHERAL NERVE

The most common causes of lesions of the hypoglossal nerve are metastatic cancer (to base of skull, subarachnoid space, or neck) and trauma (e.g., gunshot wounds to the neck, radical neck surgery, carotid endarterectomy).[68]

Hypoglossal palsy in association with other cranial nerve findings occurs with both brainstem and peripheral nerve disorders, and therefore has little localizing value.[68]

References may be accessed online at *Elsevier eBooks for Practicing Clinicians*.

Examination of the Motor System: Approach to Weakness

- Neuromuscular weakness can have any of four causes: upper neuron disease (central weakness), lower motor neuron disease (peripheral weakness), neuromuscular junction disorders, or muscle disease. Each of these disorders is associated with distinct physical signs, neuroanatomy, and etiologies.
- The combination of both upper and lower motor neuron findings indicates disease of the spinal cord, the only anatomic location where both segments reside.
- Special tests such as pronator drift, forearm rolling test, and finger tapping test accurately detect contralateral cerebral hemispheric disease, even when muscle power is largely preserved.
- In patients with stroke, the presence of aphasia or conjugate eye deviation accurately localizes the stroke to the anterior circulation (i.e., distribution of the internal carotid arteries). In contrast, a posterior circulation stroke (i.e., distribution of the vertebral and basilar arteries) is more likely if there is Horner syndrome, crossed sensory or crossed motor findings, nystagmus, heterotropia, or ataxia.

THE MOTOR EXAMINATION

Examination of the muscles includes inspection (for atrophy, hypertrophy, fasciculations, and tremor), percussion (for myotonia), palpation (for abnormal tone), full flexion and extension of the elbows and knees (for abnormal tone and nonneurologic restrictions to movement, such as contractures or joint disease), and tests of muscle strength.

I. Muscle Strength

A. DEFINITIONS

Paralysis refers to loss of power of any degree, from mild weakness to complete loss. The suffixes **plegia** and **paresis** also indicate paralysis (e.g., hemiplegia), although the term paresis is usually used to indicate incomplete paralysis.[1] **Tetraparesis** indicates weakness of all four limbs (specialists in spinal cord disorders prefer this term over *quadriparesis*).[1] **Paraparesis** indicates weakness of both legs; **hemiparesis**, weakness of an arm and leg on one side of the body; and **monoparesis**, weakness of just one arm or leg.

B. THE FINDINGS

1. Technique

The clinician tests single muscles at a time by asking the patient to contract the muscle strongly while the clinician tries to resist any movement. Unilateral weakness is recognized by comparing the muscle to its companion on the opposite side; bilateral weakness, by comparing the strength to some standard recalled from clinical experience. The clinician grades the muscle's strength according to a 6-point system (0 through 5), as described later. (See the section on grading muscle strength.)

In patients with weakness, the clinician should systematically test all the muscles from head to foot, paying particular attention to which muscles are weak, whether proximal and distal muscles of a limb differ in strength, and whether the weakness of a monoparetic limb involves only muscles from a single spinal segment or peripheral nerve (see Chapter 64). An excellent, inexpensive handbook describes the proper technique for testing all of the important muscles of the arms and legs.[2]

Testing muscles by resisting their action, however, tends to overlook significant weakness at the hips and knees, where powerful antigravity muscles can easily overcome the physician's resistance even when significant weakness is present.[3] A better way to test these muscles is to use the patient's own body weight as the load the muscle must lift. For example, quadriceps weakness is more apparent by asking the patient to arise from a chair on the symptomatic leg than by manually resisting the patient's attempt to extend the knee.[4] Another method measures the time required by the patient to rise up from a chair and sit down 10 times. Patients without weakness accomplish this in 20 to 25 sec (<20 sec if 50 years old and <25 sec if 75 years old). If patients require more time, proximal weakness of the legs is present unless an alternative explanation is present, such as joint or bone disease.[5]

2. Grading Muscle Strength

Muscle strength is graded using a conventional scale developed by the British Medical Research Council (MRC) during World War II (Table 61.1).[6] This scale, which is universally used, has one important drawback: it assigns a disproportionate amount of a muscle's power to grade 4 strength. For example, the biceps muscle uses just 2% of its full power to overcome gravity (i.e., grade 3 strength), meaning almost 98% of the remaining range of power is grade 4.[7] Because of this drawback, many neurologists subdivide grade 4 into 3 more grades: 4 minus (i.e., barely moves against resistance), 4, and 4 plus (i.e., almost full power).

3. Special Tests for Unilateral Cerebral Lesions

In patients with cerebral lesions, measures of muscle power alone often underestimate the size of the lesion and the patient's functional disability. Special tests have been developed as more

TABLE 61.1 ■ Grading Muscle Strength

Grade	Finding
0	No contraction
1	Flicker or trace of contraction
2	Active movement with gravity eliminated
3	Active movement against gravity
4	Active movement against gravity and resistance
5	Normal power

From reference 2.

sensitive tests of motor function in these patients: upper limb drift (**pronator drift**), the **forearm rolling test** (and its variants—index finger test, little finger test, and thumb rolling test),[8,9] and the **rapid finger tapping** and **foot tapping** tests (Fig. 61.1).

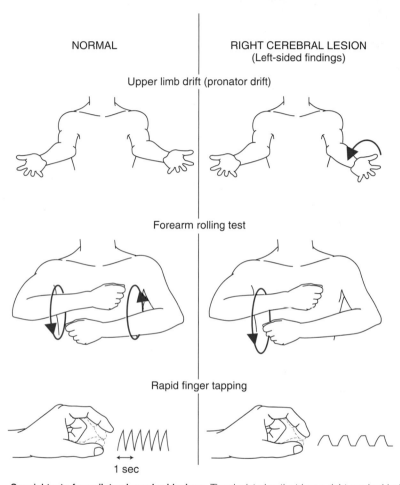

Fig. 61.1 Special tests for unilateral cerebral lesions. The depicted patient has a right cerebral lesion with left-sided findings during three different tests: **(1) Upper limb drift** (**pronator drift**, *top row*). The patient stretches out both arms directly in front of him or her with palms upright (i.e., forearms supinated) and closes his or her eyes. This position is held for 45 seconds.[10,11] The arm contralateral to the hemispheric lesion drifts downward and pronates. **(2) Forearm rolling test** (*middle row*).[8] The patient bends each elbow and places both forearms parallel to each other. He or she then rotates the forearms about each other in a rapid rolling motion for 5 to 10 seconds in each direction. In the abnormal response, the forearm contralateral to the lesion is held still while the other arm "orbits" around it. **(3) Rapid finger tapping** (*bottom row*). The patient rapidly taps the thumb and index finger repeatedly at a speed of about two taps per second. In normal persons the movement has an even rhythm and large amplitude. Hemispheric lesions cause the contralateral finger and thumb to tap more slowly and with diminished amplitude, as if the finger and thumb are sticking together.[10] The index finger rolling test and little finger rolling test are similar to the forearm rolling test (each index finger or little finger is rotated about the other for 5 seconds in both directions). In the foot tapping test, the seated patient taps one forefoot at a time for 10 seconds on the floor, as fast as possible, while the heel maintains contact with the floor. A discrepancy of more 5 taps between the left and right foot indicates cerebral disease contralateral to the slower foot.[12]

C. CLINICAL SIGNIFICANCE

See the section on approach to weakness, later.

II. Atrophy And Hypertrophy

A. ATROPHY

1. Definition

Atrophy describes muscles that are emaciated or wasted.

2. Technique

Atrophy is detected during inspection of the muscle. Examples are (1) an abnormally flat thenar eminence, when viewed from the side (e.g., cervical radiculopathy or carpal tunnel syndrome), (2) missing shadows on the anterior neck from atrophic sternocleidomastoid muscles (e.g., syringomyelia), or (3) metacarpal bones appearing unusually prominent on the back of the hand, from atrophic intrinsic muscles (e.g., polyneuropathy).

Significant asymmetry of the circumference of the arms or legs indicates atrophy of the smaller side (or edema of the other side). In normal persons, the difference in calf circumference between the right and left sides is less than 1 cm in 90% and less than 1.5 cm in 100% (measured 10 cm below the tibial tuberosity).[13]

3. Clinical Significance

Atrophy is a feature of lower motor neuron disease* and muscle disuse (especially from adjacent joint disease or trauma). In patients with sciatica, the finding of ipsilateral calf wasting (i.e., maximum circumference at least 1 cm less than contralateral side) accurately indicates lumbosacral nerve compression from disc herniation (likelihood ratio [LR] = 5.2, see Chapter 64).

B. HYPERTROPHY

Hypertrophy describes abnormal enlargement of a muscle. Bilateral calf hypertrophy is a typical feature of some muscular dystrophies, although it is found in a wide variety of neuromuscular diseases.[15]

III. Fasciculations

A. DEFINITION

Fasciculations are involuntary rapid muscle twitches that are too weak to move a limb but are easily felt by patients and seen or palpated by clinicians.[16] Most healthy people experience fasciculations at some time, especially in the eyelid muscles.

B. CLINICAL SIGNIFICANCE

Isolated fasciculations without other neurologic findings are benign.[17] When accompanied by weakness or atrophy, however, fasciculations indicate lower motor neuron disease, usually of

---

*In the evaluation of weakness, a fundamental distinction is the separation of upper motor neuron lesions (i.e., located in the cerebral cortex, brainstem, or descending motor pathways of the spinal cord) from lower motor neuron lesions (i.e., located in the peripheral nerves and anterior horn cells of the spinal cord). William Gowers first distinguished the upper and lower motor segments in his 1888 *Manual of Diseases of the Nervous System*.[14] See Fig. 61.2 and the section on approach to weakness later in this chapter.

the anterior horn cell or proximal peripheral nerve. Tongue fasciculations occur in up to one-third of patients with amyotrophic lateral sclerosis.[18] (See the section on approach to weakness later.)

IV. Muscle Tone

Muscle tone refers to the involuntary muscle tension perceived by clinicians on repeatedly flexing and extending one of the patient's limbs. Such an assessment of muscle tone assumes that the patient is relaxed and that there are no bone or joint limitations to movement. Muscle tone may be increased (e.g., spasticity, rigidity, or paratonia) or diminished (flaccidity).

A. INCREASED MUSCLE TONE

1. Spasticity

a. Definition
Spasticity is increased muscle tone that develops in patients with upper motor neuron lesions.[19] The increased muscle tone of spasticity has three characteristics, as follows: **(1) Velocity-dependence**. The amount of muscle tone depends on the velocity of movement: the more rapid the movement, the greater the resistance; the slower the movement, the less the resistance; **(2) Differing tone in flexor and extensor muscles**. The tone in the flexors and extensors of a limb is not balanced, which commonly causes characteristic resting postures of that limb (see later); **(3) Associated weakness**. The muscle with spasticity is also weak. If left untreated, muscles shortened by spasticity may eventually develop fixed contractures.

b. Characteristic Postures
In spasticity, an imbalance in flexor and extensor tone commonly causes abnormal postures of the resting limb. In hemiplegia, for example, there is excess tone in the *flexors* of the arms and *extensors* of the legs, which causes the arm and hand to be fixed against the chest, flexed and internally rotated, and the leg to extend with the foot pointed (see Fig. 7.4 in Chapter 7).[20] In contrast, some patients with complete spinal cord lesions have excess tone in the *flexors* of the legs, which causes the legs to flex up on to the abdomen (**paraplegia-in-flexion**).[21]†

c. Clasp-Knife Phenomenon
Up to half of patients with spasticity have the **clasp-knife phenomenon**, a finding usually observed in the knee extensors, less often in the elbow flexors.[20,22] To elicit this phenomenon, the clinician extends the patient's knee using a constant velocity, but as the patient's knee nears full extension, the muscle tone of the quadriceps muscles increases dramatically and completes the movement, just as the blade of a pocket knife opens under the influence of its spring.[14] The clasp-knife phenomenon occurs because muscle tone is dependent on the muscle's length, the tone diminishing with stretching and increasing with shortening.

---

†These hemiplegic and paraplegic postures recall the neurologic development of normal infants. Paraplegia-in-flexion resembles the initial posture of babies, their legs flexed against their chest. After descending pathways from the brainstem mature enough to overcome the spinal reflexes responsible for the flexed position, the infant eventually is able to extend the leg and stand (resembling extensor tone of hemiplegia). After cerebral connections mature enough to provide fine motor control, the infant is able to walk. Damage to the cerebral hemispheres (e.g., stroke) disrupts this fine motor control and uncovers the extensor posture; damage to the spinal cord (e.g., severe multiple sclerosis or complete spinal cord transection) removes all supraspinal input, uncovering the original flexed posture of the legs.[19]

d. Relationship of Spasticity to Weakness

Although spasticity is a sign of upper motor neuron disease, its severity correlates poorly with the degree of weakness or hyperreflexia. Patients with slowly developing cerebral hemisphere lesions usually develop spasticity and weakness in concert.[23] Patients with strokes or spinal cord injury, in contrast, develop immediate weakness and flaccidity, spasticity appearing only days to weeks later.[20] Some elderly patients with large strokes have persistent **flaccid hemiplegia**, in which the paralyzed muscles never develop increased muscle tone despite being hyperreflexic.[23]

2. Rigidity

a. Definition

Rigidity is increased muscle tension with three characteristic features: **(1) No velocity-dependence**. The resistance to movement is the same with slow and rapid movements. **(2) Flexor and extensor tone are the same. (3) No associated weakness**. Patients with rigidity lack the clasp-knife phenomenon.[19] **Cogwheel rigidity** refers to rigidity that intermittently gives way as if the patient's limb were the lever pulling over a ratchet (see Chapter 66).

b. Distinguishing Spasticity from Rigidity

Most clinicians distinguish spasticity *from* rigidity by repeatedly extending and flexing the patient's limbs and observing the characteristics already noted. In the 1950s, Wartenberg[‡] introduced a simple bedside test to assess motor tone and to distinguish spasticity from rigidity.[24,25] In this test, the patient is seated on the edge of the examining table, which is open underneath to allow the legs to swing back and forth unobstructed. The clinician lifts both feet to extend the knees, instructs the patient to relax, and then releases the legs. The normal lower limb swings back and forth 6 or 7 times, smoothly and regularly in a perfect sagittal plane. In patients with spasticity, the limbs drop with normal velocity, but their movements are jerky and fall out of the sagittal plane, the great toe tracing zigzags or ellipses. In patients with rigidity, the swinging time and velocity are significantly reduced, resulting in a total of only one or two swings. Others have confirmed Wartenberg's findings.[26]

c. Clinical Significance

Rigidity is a common finding of extrapyramidal disease, the most common example of which is Parkinson disease (see Chapter 66).

3. Paratonia

a. Definition

Paratonia is excess muscle tension that is *not present at rest* but develops when the patient's limb *contacts* another object, as if such contact makes the patient unable to relax. There are two forms: **oppositional paratonia (gegenhalten)** and **facilitatory paratonia (mitgehen)**. In patients with oppositional paratonia, the clinician feels a stiffening of the limb with every applied movement, but unlike rigidity the stiffening depends entirely on contact and its force is proportional and opposite to the examiner's movements. Patients with facilitatory paratonia, in contrast, actively aid movements guided by the examiner.

b. Technique

One simple test of facilitatory paratonia is to take the arm of the seated patient and bend the elbow back and forth three times, from full flexion to 90° extension. The clinician then releases the

---

[‡]Robert Wartenberg, who wrote many popular neurology textbooks in the 1950s, was an ardent opponent of eponyms and called his test the *test for pendulousness of the legs*.

arm at the patient's lap and scores any further movement, 0 being no movement, 4 full flexion or more, and 1 to 3 intermediate movements.[27]

c. Clinical Significance

Both oppositional and facilitatory paratonia are associated with extensive frontal lobe disease and often appear in dementing illnesses.[27] Among patients with dementia, the severity of oppositional or facilitatory paratonia (including the score for the paratonia test described in the previous section) correlates inversely with the Folstein mini-mental status score ($r = -0.5$ to -0.7, $p < 0.05$).[27]

B. DECREASED MUSCLE TONE: HYPOTONIA (FLACCIDITY)

1. Definition

Hypotonia refers to reduced or absent muscle tension.

2. Technique

There are many ways to detect the flaccid muscle: the limb feels "like a rag doll," the muscles feel soft and flabby, the outstretched arm when tapped demonstrates wider than normal excursions, or the knee jerks are abnormally pendular. The original definition of abnormally pendular knee jerks—more than three back-and-forth swings of the patient's leg during testing of the knee jerk—should be revised, however, because many normal individuals have this finding.[28]

3. Clinical Significance

Hypotonia is a feature of lower motor neuron disease and cerebellar disease.

4. Pathogenesis

There is some evidence that "normal" muscle tone actually consists of tiny muscle contractions that assist the clinician in moving the extremity (even though the patient is trying to relax).[29] Clinicians perceive reduced muscle tension in hypotonic limbs because these contractions are absent.

V. Muscle Percussion

Striking the muscle with a reflex hammer may elicit two abnormal findings, percussion myotonia and myoedema.

A. PERCUSSION MYOTONIA

1. The Finding

Percussion myotonia is a prolonged muscle contraction that lasts several seconds and causes a sustained dimple to appear on the skin. Percussion myotonia of the thenar eminence may actually draw the thumb into sustained opposition with the fingers.

2. Clinical Significance

Percussion myotonia is a feature of some myotonic syndromes, such as myotonia congenita and myotonic dystrophy.[30]

B. MYOEDEMA

1. The Finding

Myoedema is a focal mounding of muscle lasting seconds at the point of percussion. Unlike myotonia, myoedema causes a lump instead of a dimple, and the lump may be oriented crosswise or diagonal to the direction of muscle fibers.[31] Instructive videos of the finding are available.[32,33]

Graves and Stokes originally described myoedema in 1830.

2. Clinical Significance

Myoedema is a normal physiologic response and does not necessarily indicate disease.[34] Its historical association with undernourished patients simply reflects the ease with which the response appears when there is no intervening subcutaneous fat.[31,34] Myoedema is frequently described in hypothyroidism, where the finding correlates with severity of disease. In one study, myoedema was elicited in 13% of patients with mild hypothyrodism (thyroid stimulating hormone [TSH] 50–100 mIU/L), 29% of those with moderate disease (TSH 100–150 mIU/L), and 62% of those with severe disease (TSH > 150 mIU/L).[35]

APPROACH TO WEAKNESS

I. Cause of Weakness

Neuromuscular weakness has four principal causes: (1) upper motor neuron disease (*pyramidal tract disease* or *central weakness*), (2) lower motor neuron disease (*denervation disease* or *peripheral weakness*), (3) neuromuscular junction disorders, and (4) muscle disease. Each disorder is associated with distinct physical signs (Table 61.2), neuroanatomy (Fig. 61.2), and etiologies (Table 61.3).

Most patients with weakness have disorders of the upper and lower motor neuron lesions. Clinicians should consider muscle disease in any patient with *symmetric* weakness of the *proximal* muscles of the arms and legs (sometimes associated with muscle pain, dysphagia, and weakness of the neck muscles). Disorders of the neuromuscular junction should be considered in patients whose weakness *varies* during the day or who have *ptosis* or *diplopia*. Associated abnormalities of sensation, tone, or reflexes of the weak limb exclude muscle or neuromuscular junction disease and argue instead for upper or lower motor neuron lesions.

TABLE 61.2 ■ Differential Diagnosis of Weakness*

Location of Lesion	Motor examination: Muscle Tone	Atrophy or Fasciculations?	Sensory Findings	Muscle Stretch Reflexes	Other Findings
Upper motor neuron	Spasticity	No	Sometimes	Increased	Babinski sign
Lower motor neuron	Hypotonia	Yes	Usually†	Decreased/absent	
Neuromuscular junction	Normal or hypotonia	No	No	Normal/decreased	Ptosis, diplopia
Muscle	Normal	No‡	No	Normal/decreased	Myotonia

*These characteristics are *specific* but not *sensitive*, and thus are helpful when *present*, not when absent. See the text.
†Sensory findings are in distribution of spinal segment, plexus, or peripheral nerve. See Chapter 64.
‡Atrophy may be a late finding.

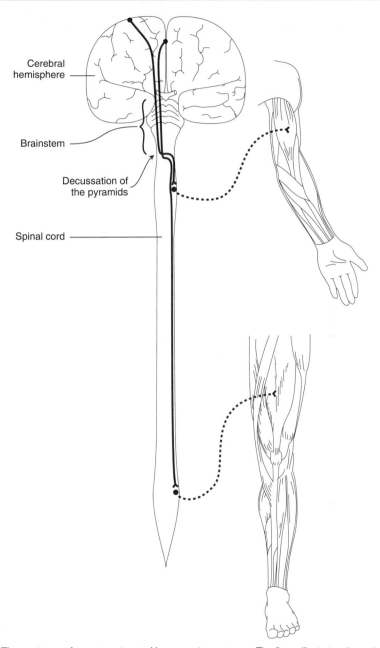

Fig. 61.2   The anatomy of upper motor and lower motor neurons. The figure illustrates the entire pathway of nerves responsible for movement, from cerebral cortex to muscle. Upper *motor neurons (solid line)* extend from the cerebral cortex through the brainstem to the spinal cord. *Lower motor neurons (dotted line)* originate in the spinal cord and travel to muscles within peripheral nerves. Because the upper motor neurons cross to the contralateral side at the border between the brainstem and spinal cord (decussation of the pyramids), weakness of the upper motor neuron type may result from lesions in the *ipsilateral* spinal cord, *contralateral* brainstem, or *contralateral* cerebral hemisphere. Lesions of the spinal cord, where both upper and lower motor neurons reside, may cause weakness of both types: of the *lower motor neuron* type *at* the level of the lesion and of the *upper motor neuron* type in muscles whose peripheral nerves originate *below* the level of the lesion.

TABLE 61.3 ▦ **Common Etiologies of Neuromuscular Weakness**

Location of Lesion	Common Etiology
Upper motor neuron	Cerebrovascular disease
	Multiple sclerosis
	Brain tumor
Lower motor neuron	Polyneuropathy (diabetes, alcoholism)
	Entrapment neuropathy (e.g., carpal tunnel syndrome)
	Trauma
Neuromuscular junction	Myasthenia gravis
Muscle	Drug-induced myopathy
	Thyroid disease
	Polymyositis

II. The Findings

A. UPPER VS. LOWER MOTOR NEURON LESIONS

Both upper motor neuron weakness and lower motor neuron weakness tend to affect *distal* muscles in either a symmetric or asymmetric pattern. The bedside findings that distinguish these two disorders are other neurologic findings in the weak limb, certain localizing signs of upper motor neuron disease, the Babinski sign, and the type of weakness produced.

1. Associated Findings in the Weak Limb (Table 61.2)

Spasticity and hyperreflexia indicate central weakness; hypotonia, atrophy, fasciculations, and absent muscle stretch reflexes indicate peripheral weakness. In patients with central weakness, sensory abnormalities vary from the isolated loss of cortical sensations in the distal limb to the dense loss of all sensation throughout the limb; if sensory abnormalities occur in peripheral weakness, they follow the distribution of spinal segments or peripheral nerves (see Chapter 64).

2. Localizing Signs of Upper Motor Neuron Weakness

The upper motor neuron pathway extends from the cerebral cortex down through the spinal cord (Fig. 61.2), traveling in tight quarters with central neurons innervating other structures. Consequently, in addition to producing central weakness, lesions along this pathway cause characteristic additional physical signs (Table 61.4) that confirm the weakness is of the central type and pinpoint its location.

3. Babinski Sign

The Babinski sign (see Chapter 63) indicates central weakness. In the positive response, the great toe moves upward after a scratching stimulus to the sole of the patient's foot.

4. Distribution of Weakness

a. Limbs Affected

The findings of monoparesis, paraparesis, and tetraparesis are, by themselves, unhelpful because they may occur in either central or peripheral weakness. Only hemiparesis is specific, indicating a central lesion.

b. Movement vs. Muscle

Central lesions paralyze *movements*; peripheral lesions paralyze *muscles*. This occurs because neurons from a single area of the cerebral cortex connect with many different spinal cord segments and muscles to accomplish a particular movement. A single muscle has many movements and thus receives information from many different upper segments, all of which converge on the single peripheral

TABLE 61.4 ■ Localizing Signs in Upper Motor Neuron Weakness

Anatomic location	Associated finding
Cerebral hemisphere	Seizures
	Hemianopia
	Aphasia (right hemiparesis)
	Inattention to left body, apraxia (left hemiparesis)
	Cortical sensory loss*
	Hyperactive jaw jerk
Brainstem	Crossed motor findings†
	Contralateral third nerve palsy (midbrain)
	Contralateral sixth nerve palsy (pons)
	Sensory loss on contralateral face*
Spinal cord	Sensory level*
	Pain and temperature sensory loss on contralateral arm and leg*
	No sensory or motor findings in face
	Additional lower motor neuron findings (atrophy, fasciculations)

*Chapter 62 describes the different sensory syndromes.
†Crossed motor findings refers to unilateral cranial nerve palsy opposite the side of weakness (an example is a *left* cranial nerve III palsy in a patient with *right* hemiparesis).

nerve travelling to the muscle. A lesion in that nerve, therefore, obliterates a muscle's entire repertoire of movement; a lesion in an upper segment eliminates only one of many possible movements.[25]

One example of this is the contrast between peripheral facial weakness (Bell palsy), which paralyzes all ipsilateral facial movements, and central facial weakness (e.g., strokes), which paralyzes voluntary movements but spares emotional ones (e.g., during laughing or crying; see Chapter 60).[36] Another example is the contrast between the peripheral paraparesis of Guillain-Barre syndrome, which paralyzes all leg movements, and the central paraparesis of spinal cord injury, which eliminates volitional movements of the legs but allows the powerful flexor spasms induced by a mild scratching of the patient's foot.[21]

B. THE DIAGNOSTIC PROCESS

1. Upper Motor Neuron Weakness

In patients with upper motor neuron weakness, associated neurologic findings indicate the *level* of the lesion (Table 61.4); the distribution of weakness indicates the *side* of the lesion. For example, bilateral weakness (paraparesis or tetraparesis) indicates *bilateral* lesions (in the thoracic cord or higher if paraparesis, and in the cervical cord or higher if tetraparesis). Monoparesis or hemiparesis indicates a *unilateral* lesion, either in the *contralateral* cerebral hemisphere or brainstem or the *ipsilateral* spinal cord.§

Fig. 61.3 illustrates this diagnostic process in the analysis of central weakness. In the first column is the distribution of central weakness for hypothetical patients, which narrows the diagnostic possibilities to a smaller region of the central motor pathway (second column). The associated findings (third column) identify the level of the lesion within that region, thus pinpointing the lesion's location (fourth column).

---

§It is the contralateral cerebral hemisphere and brainstem because the descending central motor pathways originate in the contralateral hemisphere, but it is the ipsilateral spinal cord because these pathways cross just below the brainstem (Fig. 61.2).

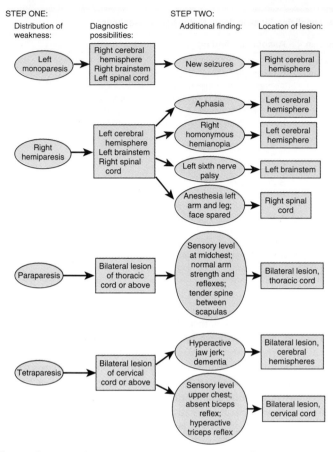

Fig. 61.3   The diagnostic approach to upper motor neuron weakness. The figure illustrates the sequential steps in identifying the location of an upper motor neuron lesion. See the text.

2. Lower Motor Neuron Weakness

In patients with monoparesis of the lower motor neuron type, the clinician should determine whether the muscles affected are supplied by a single spinal segment (**radiculopathy**), peripheral nerve (**peripheral neuropathy**) or combination of the two (**plexopathy**). Further evaluation of these patients is discussed in Chapter 64.

In lower motor neuron weakness, the lesion is always *ipsilateral* to the side of the weakness.

3. Combined Upper and Lower Motor Neuron Weakness

Combined upper and lower motor neuron findings indicate disease in the spinal cord, the only anatomic location where both segments reside. Common causes are myelopathy and amyotrophic lateral sclerosis.

a. Myelopathy

Myelopathy is a term describing a spinal cord lesion confined to a discrete level (e.g., trauma, tumor, disc disease). The lesion causes motor, sensory, and reflex abnormalities *at* the level of the lesion and *below* it. The weakness is of the peripheral type *at* the level of the lesion (from damage

TABLE 61.5 ■ **Segmental Innervation of Muscles***

Spinal level	Muscles
Arm	
C5	Elbow flexors (biceps, brachialis)
C6	Wrist extensors (extensor carpi radialis longus and brevis)
C7	Elbow extensors (triceps)
C8	Finger flexors (flexor digitorum profundus of middle finger)
T1	Little finger abductors (abductor digiti minimi)
Leg	
L2	Hip flexors (iliopsoas)
L3	Knee extensors (quadriceps)
L4	Ankle dorsiflexors (tibialis anterior)
L5	Long toe extensors (extensor hallucis longus)
S1	Ankle plantarflexors (gastrocnemius, soleus)

*Most muscles are innervated by nerves from more than one spinal root. This table, based upon references 38 and 39, simplifies this innervation to standardize the description of spinal cord injury. A more thorough description of segmental innervation of muscle appears in Figs 64.1 and 64.6.

to anterior horn cells and spinal roots)¶ and of the central type *below* the level of the lesion (from damage to the descending upper motor neuron paths).

Identifying the level of the lesion requires knowledge of which spinal segments innervate which muscle. Table 61.5 presents the standardized segmental innervation used internationally by spinal cord specialists (Chapter 64 discusses the derivation of this table). For example, in a patient with a lesion involving the C7 segment of the spinal cord, there is peripheral weakness in the C7 muscles (i.e., atrophy and weakness of the elbow extensors) but central weakness of all the muscles below this level (hyperreflexia and increased tone of the hands, legs, and feet, and a positive Babinski sign). The muscles from segments above C7, the biceps and wrist extensors, are normal.#

b. Amyotrophic Lateral Sclerosis

Amyotrophic lateral sclerosis is a degenerative disorder of descending motor tracts and motor nuclei of the spinal cord. The disorder causes both lower motor neuron findings (atrophy, fasciculations) and upper motor neuron findings (hyperreflexia). About half of patients have a Babinski response.[18] The disease may start in the arms (44%), legs (37%), or bulbar muscles (causing tongue fasciculations, change in voice, and difficulty swallowing, 19%).[18] There are no sensory findings.

Amyotrophic lateral sclerosis and cervical myelopathy are commonly confused at the bedside, even by experienced neurologists.[40] In patients with both upper and lower motor neuron signs, findings that increase probability of amyotrophic lateral sclerosis are (1) prominent fasciculations, (2) absence of sensory findings, and (3) signs of lower motor neuron degeneration affecting more than one level of the spinal cord simultaneously.[41,42] **

¶Exceptions to this are lesions at the foramen magnum and C3C4 level, which sometimes produce atrophy in the hands.[37]
#By convention, the neurologic level in spinal cord injury refers to the most caudal level with *normal* function, rather than the first level with abnormal function.[39] The motor level for this hypothetical patient is therefore C6.
**The four spinal cord levels are bulbar (jaw, face, tongue, larynx), cervical (neck, arm, hand, diaphragm), thoracic (back, abdomen), and lumbosacral (back, abdomen, leg, and foot).

III. Clinical Significance

The clinical significance of the motor examination cannot be tested in the conventional manner of this book, because bedside criteria alone are sufficient to diagnose many causes of weakness (e.g., cerebrovascular disease, amyotrophic lateral sclerosis, and peripheral nerve injuries are routinely diagnosed by bedside criteria; see Chapter 1).

Nonetheless, several investigations allow a few conclusions.

A. CLINICAL SYNDROMES ARE OFTEN INCOMPLETE

Most studies show that the full lower motor or upper motor neuron syndromes, as depicted in Table 61.2, are often incomplete. In upper motor neuron weakness, up to 25% of patients lack exaggerated reflexes[43,44] and the absence of spasticity is common, especially in acute lesions (see earlier discussion). Similarly, in many examples of lower motor weakness, the nerve affected does not even innervate a clinical reflex (e.g., median or ulnar neuropathy); the reflexes of these limbs are thus preserved. Therefore, in the evaluation of weak patients, the *absence* of spasticity or hyperreflexia does not argue against the presence of upper motor neuron disease, nor does the *absence* of hypotonicity or hyporeflexia argue against the presence lower motor neuron disease.

On the other hand, the *presence* of abnormal reflexes is very helpful: In one study of patients with weakness, 87% had abnormal reflexes, and in every case, areflexia correctly predicted lower motor neuron disease and hyperreflexia correctly predicted upper motor neuron disease.[44]

The fact that syndromes are often incomplete emphasizes the importance of the complete neurologic examination. For example, in a patient with weakness of the fingertips, in whom the absence of sensory or reflex changes prevents classifying the weakness as peripheral or central using the criteria of Table 61.2, the discovery of any additional neurologic finding from Table 61.4 indicates the lesion is central and pinpoints its location precisely.

B. PROXIMAL WEAKNESS INDICATES MUSCLE DISEASE

If *proximal weakness* is defined as strength of a limb's proximal muscles being one MRC grade less than the distal muscles, proximal weakness appears in 92% of patients with muscle disease.[44] The *absence* of proximal weakness, therefore, decreases probability of muscle disease.

C. THE SPECIAL TESTS FOR CEREBRAL HEMISPHERIC LESIONS ARE ACCURATE

EBM Box 61.1 presents the diagnostic accuracy of various physical signs for detecting unilateral cerebral hemispheric lesions in patients undergoing computed tomography or magnetic resonance imaging (MRI) of the head. Most of the patients in these studies lacked motor weakness by conventional power testing, and the neuroimaging was performed to assess headaches, seizures, or other neurologic symptoms. In these patients, the findings that increase probability of *contralateral* cerebral hemispheric lesions the most are a positive forearm rolling test (LR = 15.6), pronator drift (LR = 9.6), Babinski response (LR = 8.5), index finger rolling test (LR = 6), hyperreflexia (LR = 5.3), positive finger tapping test (LR = 4.7), and hemianopia (LR = 4.3). The *absence* of pronator drift (LR = 0.3) diminishes the probability of contralateral cerebral disease.

EBM BOX 61.1	**Unilateral Cerebral Hemispheric Disease***			
Finding (Reference)†	**Sensitivity (%)**	**Specificity (%)**	**Likelihood Ratio‡ if Finding Is**	
			Present	**Absent**
Cranial nerves				
Hemianopia[8,45]	22–30	93–98	4.3	0.8
Motor examination				
Pronator drift[8,10,12,45]	22–91	90–98	9.6	0.3
Arm rolling test[8,10,12,45]	17–87	97–98	15.6	0.6
Index finger rolling test[12,45]	33–42	92–98	6.0	0.7
Little finger rolling test[12]	7	95	NS	NS
Finger tapping test[8,10,12,45]	16–79	88–98	4.7	0.5
Foot tapping test[12,45]	11–23	89–93	NS	NS
Sensory examination				
Hemisensory disturbance[8]	29	98	NS	0.7
Reflex examination				
Hyperreflexia[10,45]	11–69	88–95	5.3	NS
Babinski response[8,12,45]	9–45	98	8.5	NS

*Diagnostic standard: for *unilateral cerebral hemispheric disease*, magnetic resonance imaging or computed tomography.
†Definition of findings: for *arm rolling test, pronator drift*, and *finger tapping test*, see Fig. 61.1.
‡Likelihood ratio (LR) if finding present = positive LR; LR if finding absent = negative LR.
NS, Not significant.

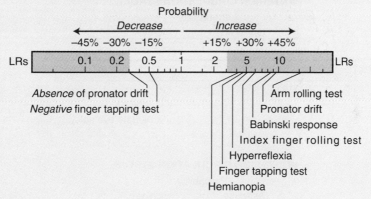

UNILATERAL CEREBRAL HEMISPHERIC DISEASE
Probability

Absence of pronator drift
Negative finger tapping test

Arm rolling test
Pronator drift
Babinski response
Index finger rolling test
Hyperreflexia
Finger tapping test
Hemianopia

D. ADDITIONAL SIGNS DISTINGUISH ANTERIOR FROM POSTERIOR CIRCULATION STROKES

Four arteries supply the brain: the right and left internal carotid arteries and the right and left vertebral arteries. The two internal carotid arteries supply most of the cerebral hemispheres (except the posterior occipital lobes) and collectively are called the **anterior circulation**. The two vertebral arteries unite to form the basilar artery; together, these arteries supply the brainstem, cerebellum, and posterior cerebrum (occipital cortex) and are called the **posterior circulation**. Strokes in the distribution of either circulation may produce hemiparesis, but because the anterior and posterior

EBM BOX 61.2 | **Stroke: Anterior vs Posterior Circulation[46,47]**

Finding (Reference)[†]	Sensitivity (%)	Specificity (%)	Likelihood Ratio[‡] if Finding Is Present	Absent
Detecting anterior circulation stroke				
Aphasia	22–44	95–99	**12.1**	0.7
Conjugate gaze palsy	11–23	92–97	**3.2**	NS
Detecting posterior circulation stroke				
Ataxia	32	95	**5.8**	0.7
Horner syndrome	4	100	**72.0**	NS
Heterotropia	7	99	**10.0**	NS
Nystagmus	12	99	**14.0**	0.9
Crossed motor paresis	4	100	**24.0**	NS
Crossed sensory findings	3	10	**54.7**	NS

*Diagnostic standard: for *posterior* or *anterior circulation stroke*, localization by magnetic resonance imaging.

[†]Definition of findings: for *ataxia*, see Chapters 7 and 65; for *Horner syndrome*, see Chapter 21; for *nystagmus*, see Chapter 65; for *crossed motor paresis* and *crossed sensory findings*, the facial motor or sensory finding is contralateral to the body motor or sensory finding; for *aphasia*, impaired production or comprehension of spoken or written language; for *conjugate gaze palsy*, deviation of both eyes to one side, usually (if cerebral hemispheric stroke) to the side of the lesion and contralateral to the side with weakness.

[‡]Likelihood ratio (LR) if finding present = positive LR.

NS, Not significant.

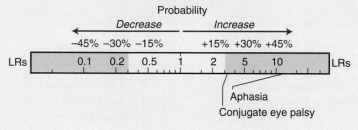

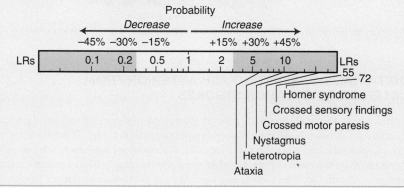

circulation also supply areas of the brain with unique functions, additional telltale findings localize the infarction more accurately. For example, the anterior circulation supplies the areas of the brain controlling language and conjugate eye movements (i.e., movement of both eyes in the same direction, such as to the right or left sides). The posterior circulation, in contrast, supplies areas essential to balance, pupillary function, and alignment of the eyes (i.e., keeping both eyes aligned in the same direction). Also, because descending motor tracts from the brain to the limbs *cross* just below the brainstem, an injury on one side of the *brainstem* (i.e., posterior circulation) may produce *ipsilateral* cranial nerve findings but *contralateral* limb findings (i.e., crossed motor or crossed sensory findings; see Fig. 61.2; Table 61.4; Fig. 62.2b).

These traditional teachings were confirmed in two studies of patients with strokes, all of whom underwent magnetic resonance imaging (MRI) to localize the injury to the anterior or posterior circulation.[46,47] In these patients, the following findings increased probability of *anterior* circulation stroke: aphasia (LR = 12.1, EBM Box 61.2) and conjugate gaze palsy (i.e., difficulty moving *both* eyes in an aligned fashion to the right or left; LR = 3.2). The probability of *posterior* circulation stroke was increased if the following findings were present: Horner syndrome (LR = 72), crossed sensory findings (LR = 54.7), crossed motor paresis (LR = 24), nystagmus (LR = 14), heterotropia (i.e., the eyes are not aligned; LR = 10), and ataxia (LR = 5.8). Some findings were diagnostically unhelpful, appearing just as often in anterior circulation stroke as in posterior circulation stroke: altered consciousness, hemiparesis, hemianopia, dysarthria, and seizures (LRs not significant or close to the value of 1).

Importantly, the negative LR for each of the above diagnostic findings is either not significant or close to the value of 1. This means that, even though the *presence* of a particular finding is helpful, its *absence* is not. For example, the *presence* of crossed motor findings is pathognomonic for a brainstem infarction (posterior circulation; LR = 24), but the *absence* of crossed motor findings in a patient with stroke does not change at all the probability of posterior (or anterior) circulation stroke (LR = NS).

E. DIAGNOSIS OF PERIPHERAL NERVE DISORDERS

Chapter 64 discusses the clinical significance of muscle weakness and its localizing value to the diagnosis of peripheral nerve disorders.

References may be accessed online at *Elsevier eBooks for Practicing Clinicians*.

Examination of the Sensory System

- For screening examinations, testing only the sensation of touch should suffice. Nonetheless, in patients with sensory complaints involving large portions of limbs or the trunk, testing all simple sensations (i.e., pain, temperature, vibration, touch) is necessary to uncover sensory dissociation (i.e., loss of one simple sensation but preservation of another), an important clue to disease of the spinal cord.
- Diseases of the peripheral nerves, spinal cord, brainstem, and cerebral hemispheres each produce distinct sensory syndromes. These syndromes are distinguished by the distribution of sensory loss and the presence or absence of a sensory level, sensory dissociation, facial involvement, Horner syndrome, and weakness.
- Testing cortical sensations (e.g., stereognosis, graphesthesia) requires preservation of the simple sensations. Abnormalities of cortical sensations indicate disease in the contralateral cerebral cortex.
- The lateral medullary stroke (Wallenberg syndrome) does not usually cause weakness but instead produces dramatic vertigo and loss of pain and temperature sensation on the ipsilateral face and contralateral body.

SIMPLE SENSATIONS

I. Definitions

There are four simple sensations: pain, temperature, touch, and vibration. These sensations are all called simple because their perception does not require a healthy contralateral cerebral cortex. Hypesthesia refers to diminished ability to perceive a simple sensation; anesthesia refers to the complete inability to perceive a simple sensation. Although both hypesthesia and anesthesia originally referred only to the sensation of touch, many clinicians use the terms when reporting any of the simple sensations. **Hypalgesia** means there is a decreased sensitivity to painful stimuli; **analgesia**, a complete insensitivity. **Hyperpathia, hyperesthesia,** and **allodynia** all refer to an increased sensitivity to sensory stimuli, often with unpleasant qualities, although some experts restrict hyperpathia to increased sensitivity from *painful* stimuli and allodynia to discomfort from *tactile* stimuli.

II. Technique

The choice of sensory tests to be included in the physical examination depends on the clinical setting. For screening examinations of patients without sensory complaints, testing only touch sensation on all four extremities should suffice. If there are sensory complaints confined to one limb, testing for touch and pain sensation is usually performed, although testing pain sensation has a better chance of detecting subtle radiculopathies and peripheral nerve disorders.[1,2] (See the section on dermatomes.) For screening diabetic feet and limbs at risk for neuropathic ulcers and arthropathy, clinicians should use Semmes-Weinstein monofilaments (see Chapter 55). Finally, for any patient with sensory complaints involving large portions of a limb or the trunk, testing for all simple sensations is necessary to uncover **sensory dissociation** (i.e., perception of one modality but not another), a finding suggesting spinal cord disease. (See the section on sensory syndromes).

During sensory testing, the patient's perceptions are compared with either a known standard of normal sensation (e.g., Semmes-Weinstein monofilaments for tactile sensation and tuning fork tests for vibratory sensation), to the contralateral companion part of the patient's body, or to the clinician's own sense of what is normal gathered from previous experience.

A. TOUCH

The sensation of touch is usually tested qualitatively by stimulating the patient's skin lightly with a cotton wisp, piece of tissue paper, or the clinician's finger, or quantitatively by using Semmes-Weinstein monofilaments (see Chapter 55).

B. PAIN AND TEMPERATURE

The usual techniques for testing pain sensation are a safety pin bent at right angles or the sharp edge of a broken wooden applicator stick, both of which must be discarded after use to prevent the transmission of infection.[3] It is no longer permissible to use the built-in pin of many reflex hammers or the traditional tailor's pinwheel, because of the risk of transmitting infection.

The traditional test for temperature sensation uses tubes of warm and cold water, although testing the patient's ability to distinguish the cold stem of the tuning fork from the warmer index finger is much simpler.[4]

C. VIBRATION

Vibratory sensation is tested with a tuning fork (usually 128 Hz; less often 256 Hz).[5] There is no compelling reason for using one tuning fork over the other, except that standards have been developed for the 128 Hz fork. Humans are most sensitive to vibration frequencies of 200 to 300 Hz and have difficulty consistently detecting frequencies below 100 Hz.[6,7] Traditionally, the tuning fork is applied against bony prominences, although this is based on the mistaken belief that bones contain the "vibration receptors"; vibratory sensation is just as good, or even better, over soft tissues without underlying bone (the clinician can easily demonstrate this by testing sensation on the abdominal wall).[8]

When a 128 Hz tuning fork is struck from a distance of 20 cm against the heel of the clinician's palm, a healthy 40 year-old person should perceive vibrations for at least 11 seconds when the stem of the fork is held against the lateral malleolus, and for at least 15 seconds when it is held against the ulnar styloid.[9] These values decrease two seconds for every decade of age greater than 40 years.

One disadvantage to vibratory testing is the conduction of the vibrating impulse away from the tuning fork, thus preventing precise definition of sensory boundaries in patients with peripheral nerve injuries.[8]

Rumpf introduced the tuning fork to bedside neurology in 1889.[10]

III. Clinical Significance

A. TOUCH, PAIN, AND TEMPERATURE SENSATION

Abnormalities of simple sensations define all important clinical sensory syndromes: peripheral nerve injury, radiculopathy, spinal cord syndromes, lateral medullary infarction, and thalamic and cerebral hemispheric syndromes. (See the section on sensory syndromes.) No diagnostic test has proved superior to bedside examination. The finding of diminished pain sensation (to safety pin stimulus) detects small nerve fiber loss on skin biopsies with a sensitivity of 88%, specificity of 81%, positive likelihood ratio (LR) = 4.6, and negative LR = 0.2,[11] and the clinician's bedside assessment of hypesthesia is a more specific predictor of nerve fiber loss than automated touch-pressure esthesiometers.[12] Physical examination may even be superior to nerve conduction testing, a test of only the large myelinated peripheral nerve fibers, not the smaller unmyelinated fibers that carry pain and temperature sensations and from which many uncomfortable sensory syndromes originate.[13]

Diabetic feet insensate to the 5.07 monofilament have increased risk of subsequent foot ulceration and amputation (see Chapter 55).

B. VIBRATORY SENSATION

Vibratory sensation is often diminished in peripheral neuropathy and spinal cord disease but spared in disease confined to the cerebral cortex.[8] Vibration is a highly developed sensation—Helen Keller could interpret speech by feeling the vibrations of the speaker's larynx, lips and nose.[8] Traditionally, it is associated with proprioception, because impulses from both sensations ascend in the posterior columns of the spinal cord,[5] but there are many clinical examples of dissociation of vibratory and proprioceptive loss, both in peripheral neuropathy and spinal cord disease.[8,14] (See the section on proprioception.)

C. HYPERPATHIA AND ALLODYNIA ARE NONSPECIFIC FINDINGS

Hyperpathia and allodynia occur in many different painful conditions, including peripheral neuropathy, brainstem infarction, and thalamic stroke; by themselves, they have no localizing value.[15,16]

PROPRIOCEPTION

I. Definition

Proprioception allows individuals to detect joint motion and limb position when their eyes are closed.[17] Like most of the simple sensations, proprioception has distinct sense organs and ascending pathways in the spinal cord. Unlike simple sensations, however, full perception requires a healthy contralateral cerebral cortex; in this way, it resembles cortical sensations.[18,19] (See the section on Cortical Sensations.)

Sir Charles Bell originally called proprioception the "sixth sense." In 1906, Sherrington introduced the term "proprioception" to describe this sensation.[17,20]

II. Technique

The conventional test of proprioception is to lightly hold the sides of the patient's finger or toe and bend it slowly up and down.[5] The patient is asked to indicate any sensation of movement and the movement's direction. Because normal persons perceive motion much more easily than direction, a normal person may accurately indicate the presence of motion all of the time but indicate the wrong direction up to 10% of the time.[21] Normal individuals can detect 1 to 2 degrees of movement in most joints, the hips being the most sensitive.[21,22]

Another test of proprioception tests the ability to direct a limb to a given point, again with eyes closed. In one version, the clinician positions the patient's outstretched index finger on the clinician's own index finger. The patient then drops the arm to the side and attempts to find the previous position. Normal individuals consistently come within 5 cm of the target.[20]

Patients with severe proprioceptive loss depend on vision for balance and thus become very unstable when they close their eyes or walk in darkness. This dependence on vision forms the basis for another test of proprioceptive loss, Romberg sign, which is discussed fully in Chapter 7.

III. Clinical Significance

Proprioceptive loss is common in peripheral neuropathy (e.g., diabetes mellitus), spinal cord disease (e.g., multiple sclerosis, vitamin B12 deficiency, tabes dorsalis), and severe hemispheric disease. In unilateral disease of the spinal cord (e.g., the Brown-Séquard syndrome), proprioception is lost on the side of weakness, opposite the side with pain and temperature loss. (See the section on sensory syndromes.) In patients with strokes, proprioceptive loss indicates extensive damage and correlates with a poorer functional recovery and higher mortality.[23]

According to traditional teachings, a disproportionate loss of vibration sensation and proprioception (compared with pain and temperature sensation) occurs in diseases of the dorsal columns of the spinal cord (e.g., tabes dorsalis, multiple sclerosis, vitamin B12 deficiency) and some peripheral neuropathies (e.g., diabetic polyneuropathy). Although this teaching is true, most patients with these disorders also have abnormalities of pain and temperature sensation.[8,24]

CORTICAL SENSATIONS

I. Definition

Cortical sensations are those sensations requiring higher integration and processing for them to be perceived properly. Consequently, perception of cortical sensations requires a healthy contralateral cerebral cortex. They may become abnormal in cerebral hemispheric disease, *even though* the simple sensations are preserved.

II. Technique

Testing for cortical sensations has three requirements: (1) the patient's eyes are closed; (2) the patient lacks dementia; and (3) most of the simple sensations, especially touch, are preserved. If the simple sensations are profoundly altered, as in severe peripheral neuropathy, no sensory information will reach the cerebral hemisphere and tests for cortical sensation become uninterpretable.

A. TWO-POINT DISCRIMINATION

Two-point discrimination is the ability to distinguish two compass points simultaneously applied to the skin. The normal minimal distance is 3 cm for the hand or foot and 0.6 cm for the fingertips.[14,18,25,26]

B. TACTILE RECOGNITION (STEREOGNOSIS)

Tactile recognition is the ability to recognize common objects like a key, paper clip, coin, tweezers, or rubber ball placed in the hand. Normal individuals can name more than 90% of objects within 5 seconds.[27,28]

C. GRAPHESTHESIA

Graphesthesia is the ability to identify letters or numbers traced on the hand or foot. Normal individuals can easily recognize symbols 1 cm in height on the fingertips and 6 cm tall elsewhere.[18]

D. LOCALIZATION

Localization is the ability to accurately point to a spot on the body just touched by the clinician.

E. BILATERAL SIMULTANEOUS TACTILE STIMULATION

This tests the patient's ability to recognize that both sides of the body are being touched simultaneously. The term **tactile extinction** refers to the patient's consistent failure to detect the stimulus on one side of the body.[29]

F. APPRECIATION OF WEIGHTS

Appreciation of weights is the ability to perceive differences in weight between two objects, placed sequentially in the patient's hand. This test was used more often several decades ago than it is now.[30]

III. Clinical Significance

Lesions of the posterior parietal lobe may preserve the simple sensations but eliminate proprioception and cortical sensations. The loss is typically confined to just the contralateral distal parts of the limbs, sparing the face and trunk.[19,30–32]

It is important to note that cortical disease also may eliminate any or all of the simple sensations, especially if the lesion involves the anterior parietal lobe (postcentral gyrus) or deeper white matter.[8,19,30,33] These lesions often cause a dense sensory loss on the opposite side of the body, involving the trunk, limbs, and face, sometimes referred to as the **pseudothalamic syndrome** because of its resemblance to the sensory loss of thalamic disease (see the section on sensory syndromes, later).[19]

DERMATOMES

I. Definition

A dermatome defines the area of skin innervated by a single nerve root or spinal segment. They are primarily used to determine whether the sensory loss on a limb corresponds to a single spinal segment, implying the lesion is of that nerve root (i.e., radiculopathy), and to assign the neurologic "level" to a spinal cord lesion.

II. Derivation of the Dermatomal Maps

The original human dermatomal maps emerged from Sherrington's experiments with monkeys and Head's observations of patients with herpes zoster infection.[2,34,35] These maps have been subsequently revised, based on several types of evidence collected over the last century, including neurosurgical observations (by Cushing, Foester, and Keegan), experiments injecting Novocaine next to the nerve roots of medical student volunteers, and electrical stimulation of the skin while recording potentials at the nerve roots.[1,2,34,36–38] Differences among dermatomal maps, which are minor and primarily deal with how far proximally some limb dermatomes extend, probably reflect biologic variation and differences in experimental method (i.e., sensory loss from a herniated disc or novocaine injection is not necessarily the same as that from root resection).

III. Technique

The dermatomal map in Fig. 62.1 is the international standard used for classifying patients with spinal cord injury (see also Table 62.1).[39] Two principles apply when evaluating the dermatomal pattern of sensory loss. First, contiguous dermatomes overlap, which means that damage to one nerve root may cause either no anesthesia or a sensory loss confined to a small area. These small areas, which are

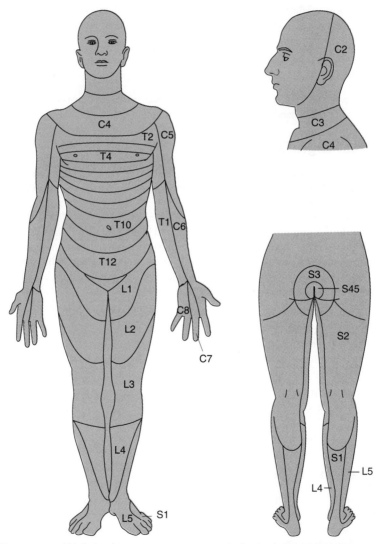

Fig. 62.1   Dermatomes. This is the dermatome map recommended by the American Spinal Injury Association,[39] which provides printable copies at their website. Note that the C2 dermatome includes the angle of the jaw and most of the ear. The precise boundaries of the S1 and S2 dermatomes are the most controversial.[36]

TABLE 62.1 ▦ **Dermatomes and Their Signature Zones**

Spinal level	Signature Zone
Cervical	
C3	Supraclavicular fossa
C4	Top of acromioclavicular joint
C5	Lateral side of antecubital fossa
C6	Thumb
C7	Middle finger
C8	Little finger
Thoracic (selected levels)	
T1	Medial (ulnar) side of the antecubital fossa
T2	Apex of axilla
T4	Fourth intercostal space (nipple line)
T10	Tenth intercostal space (umbilicus)
T12	Inguinal ligament at midpoint
Lumbar	
L1	Half the distance between T12 and L2
L2	Mid-anterior thigh
L3	Medial femoral condyle
L4	Medial malleolus
L5	Dorsum of the foot at the third metatarsal phalangeal joint
Sacral	
S1	Lateral heel
S2	Popliteal fossa in the mid-line
S3	Ischial tuberosity
S4–5	Perianal level

Based on reference 39 and original work cited in text.

referred to as **signature zones**, define the sensory level in patients with spinal cord disease.* Second, tactile dermatomes are larger than pain dermatomes. This suggests that when only one or two segments are affected, testing for pain sensibility is a more sensitive method of examination than testing for abnormal touch.[1,2]

IV. Clinical Significance

A. THE SENSORY LEVEL IN SPINAL CORD DISEASE

The patient's sensory level is often several segments *below* the actual level of the lesion in the spine (e.g., the patient with a T8 sensory level may have a lesion in the T3 segment of the spinal cord).[40–43,†] There are two explanations for this phenomenon: (1) The organization of the ascending spinothalamic pathway (carrying pain and temperature sensation) makes the more lateral fibers carrying lower body sensations more vulnerable to external injury. (2) Instead of directly damaging the contiguous cord, the spinal lesion causes injury at a more distant segment by compromising the cord's blood supply.[40,41]

When the sensory and motor levels disagree, the motor level is a more reliable indicator of level of injury and future disability.[44] In some patients with spinal cord disease, the most accurate

---

*In sensory testing, as in motor testing, the neurologic "level" refers to the most caudal level with normal function, rather than the first level with abnormal function. For example, a patient with sensation in the nipple line but none below it has a "T4 sensory level."

†In 1887, during the first successful operation to remove a spinal tumor, the surgeon's initial incision, which had been based on the patient's sensory level at T5, had to be revised upward twice before the tumor was found at the T2 level.[68]

indicator of the spinal segment affected is the site of the patient's vertebral pain and tenderness or the level of the patient's radicular pain.[42,45]

B. DERMATOMAL LOSS IN RADICULOPATHY

The clinical significance of dermatomal sensory loss in disorders of the nerve roots is discussed in Chapter 64.

SENSORY SYNDROMES

I. Technique

Fig. 62.2 depicts the sensory loss of the important sensory syndromes. Sensory loss confined to a *portion* of a limb suggests injury to a peripheral nerve, plexus, or spinal root, subjects discussed in Chapter 64. When sensory loss involves *most of a limb* or the *trunk*, a systematic approach using the following questions defines the syndrome:

A. DOES THE SENSORY LOSS INVOLVE BOTH SIDES OF THE BODY?

Involvement of *both* sides indicates polyneuropathy or spinal cord disease. Involvement of *one* side indicates contralateral disease of the brainstem, thalamus, or cerebral cortex. In patients with pure hemisection of the spinal cord (i.e., Brown-Séquard syndrome), there is sensory loss on both sides of the body, although pain and temperature sensation is lost on the side *opposite to* the lesion and tactile sensation is lost on the side *of* the lesion.

B. IS THERE A SENSORY LEVEL?

A sensory level is a distinct border on the trunk, below which sensory testing is abnormal and above which it is normal. A sensory level indicates spinal cord disease, although the finding sometimes also occurs in lateral medullary infarction.[15,46–49]

C. IS THERE SENSORY DISSOCIATION?

Sensory dissociation is a disproportionate loss of one or more simple sensations with preservation of others. Loss of pain and temperature sensation with preservation of touch and vibration sensation is a feature of some *incomplete* spinal cord syndromes (e.g., syringomyelia, spinal stroke, and Brown-Séquard syndrome).

D. IS THERE SENSORY LOSS ON THE FACE?

Sensory loss on the face indicates disease above the spinal cord—in the brainstem, thalamus, or cerebral hemispheres. In brainstem disease (e.g., lateral medullary syndrome), the sensory loss on the patient's face is *opposite* to the side of sensory loss on the body; in disease of the thalamus or cerebral hemisphere, the sensory loss on the face and body are on the *same* side.

E. ARE THERE ASSOCIATED NEUROLOGIC SIGNS?

Most disorders causing the sensory syndromes depicted in Fig. 62.2 also cause significant weakness (indicated by the arrows in Fig. 62.2), a major exception being the lateral medullary syndrome.

The presence of an associated **Horner syndrome** (see Chapter 21 for definition) indicates disease of the ipsilateral brainstem or cervical spinal cord.[50]

II. Definition of the Sensory Syndromes

Peripheral nerve and spinal root disorders are discussed in Chapter 64.

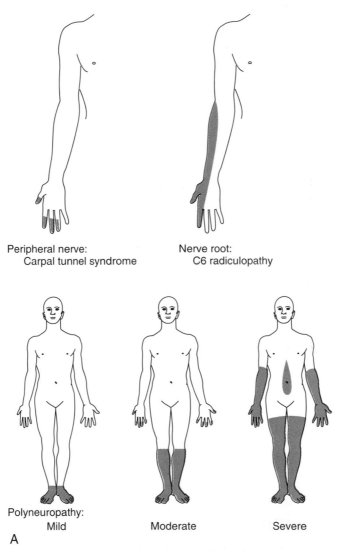

Fig. 62.2 **Sensory Syndromes.** In these figures (A and B), the *blue shading* indicates hypalgesia (loss of pain sensation) and the *arrows* indicate limbs with significant accompanying weakness. In the Brown-Séquard syndrome (hemisection of the cord, *top row*, Fig. 62.2B), there is often diminished tactile sensation on the side of weakness and opposite the side with hypalgesia.

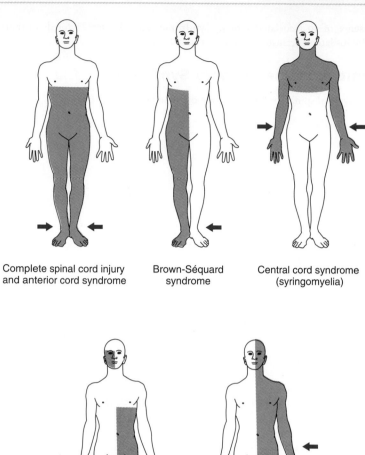

Complete spinal cord injury   Brown-Séquard   Central cord syndrome
and anterior cord syndrome   syndrome   (syringomyelia)

B   Brainstem injury   Thalamic or cerebral
                                      hemisphere injury

Fig. 62.2 cont'd

A. POLYNEUROPATHY

Polyneuropathy is a bilateral **stocking-glove** sensory loss that spares the face (the sensory loss resembles the pattern of a stocking or glove because polyneuropathy affects all nerves of the same length equally). Because the sensory loss of polyneuropathy affects the longest nerves first, hypesthesia initially appears in the feet, later in the fingertips, and—only after extensive involvement of the arms and legs—finally in the anterior trunk.[51] Atrophy of the small muscles of the feet and hands and absent ankle reflexes are common. Distal weakness may occur, but because the nerves to the foot dorsiflexors are longer than those to the plantarflexors, patients with polyneuropathy have more trouble walking on their heels than on their toes (the opposite finding, trouble walking on toes but not on heels, suggests an alternative diagnosis).[52]

Any of the simple sensations may be lost in polyneuropathy. In one study of 312 affected patients, vibration sensation was lost in 73%, pinprick in 72%, temperature in 60%, light touch in 45%, and proprioception in 36%.[53]

B. SPINAL CORD SYNDROMES

1. Complete Spinal Cord Lesion

A complete spinal cord lesion causes a sensory level with loss of all simple sensations below that level, weakness (tetraparesis or paraparesis), and urinary retention.

2. Incomplete Spinal Cord Lesions[54]

a. Anterior Cord Syndrome
Spinal stroke, which may follow prolonged hypotension or trauma to the aorta, resembles the complete spinal cord lesion, except there is a disproportionate loss of pain and temperature sensation and relative sparing of touch and vibration, owing to the more vulnerable blood supply of the ventral cord.[55]

b. Brown-Séquard Syndrome Syndrome
This describes injury to one-half of the cord, causing *contralateral* loss of pain and temperature sensation but *ipsilateral* paralysis and diminished touch sensation.[50] Unilateral disease of the cervicothoracic region may involve the ascending sympathetic fibers and cause an ipsilateral Horner syndrome.[50]

The pure Brown-Séquard syndrome is rare. Instead, most patients with unilateral disease of the spinal cord present with bilateral weakness and sensory loss, although the weakness is greatest on the side of the lesion and the hypalgesia is greatest opposite the lesion.[50]

c. Central Cord Syndrome
In syringomyelia, the sensory loss typically involves one or both arms. Seventy-five percent of patients have atrophy and weakness of one or both hands or sternocleidomastoid muscles.[56,57]

C. LATERAL MEDULLARY INFARCTION (WALLENBERG SYNDROME)

Wallenberg syndrome is a dramatic syndrome presenting with dizziness and sensory loss on opposite sides of face and body but no weakness (the lesion is ipsilateral to the facial analgesia). Common associated signs are diminished corneal reflex, ipsilateral limb ataxia, nystagmus, ipsilateral Horner syndrome, gait ataxia, and ipsilateral palate weakness (Table 62.2).

D. THALAMIC DISEASE

A lesion in the thalamus may cause loss of all simple sensations on the opposite side of the body, associated with hemiparesis, vertical gaze abnormalities, miosis, and aphasia.[33,66,67]

E. CEREBRAL HEMISPHERIC DISEASE

Cerebral hemispheral disease may cause a dense sensory loss and hemiparesis identical to thalamic disease (**pseudothalamic syndrome**),[19] or the selective loss of cortical sensations in the distal parts of the extremities. (See the section on cortical sensations.)

TABLE 62.2 ■ **Lateral Medullary Infarction (Wallenberg Syndrome)**

Physical Finding	Frequency (%)*
Cranial nerves	
Diminished corneal reflex (V and VII)	91
Ipsilateral Horner syndrome[†]	41–95
Ipsilateral face analgesia (V)	48–86
Nystagmus	56–100
Ipsilateral palate weakness (IX, X)	39–86
Ipsilateral facial weakness (VII)	18–43
Sensory	
Contralateral body analgesia	87
Coordination	
Ipsilateral limb ataxia	52–95
Gait ataxia	90

Data obtained from 531 patients from references 48,58–65.
*Results are overall mean frequency or, if statistically heterogeneous, the range of values.
[†]Strictly speaking, Horner syndrome does not involve cranial nerves, although it is discovered during examination of the pupils and eyelids.

References may be accessed online at *Elsevier eBooks for Practicing Clinicians.*

Examination of the Reflexes

- Abnormal muscle stretch reflexes *in isolation* do not necessarily indicate disease. Instead, an absent or exaggerated muscle stretch reflex is significant only in the following situations: hyporeflexia is associated with additional signs of lower motor neuron disease (weakness, atrophy, fasciculations); hyperreflexia is associated with signs of upper motor neuron disease (weakness, spasticity, Babinski sign); the reflex amplitude is asymmetric; or a reflex is unusually brisk when compared to a reflex from a higher spinal level.
- Criteria for the pathologic upgoing toe (Babinski response) include the following: the extensor hallucis longus muscle contracts; there are abnormal fine motor movements of the affected foot (e.g., abnormal foot tapping); other flexor muscles in the limb contract at least slightly during the test (e.g., hamstrings, tensor fascia lata); and the abnormal response is reproducible.
- Primitive reflexes (e.g., palmomental reflex, glabellar reflex, grasp reflex, snout reflex and suck reflex) are common findings in frontal lobe disease, parkinsonism, and dementing illnesses.

Reflexes are involuntary contractions of muscles, induced by specific stimuli. In the neurologic examination, there are three types of reflexes: (1) muscle-stretch reflexes (deep tendon or myotatic reflexes), (2) cutaneous reflexes, and (3) primitive reflexes (or release reflexes). This chapter also discusses the **Babinski response**, which is an abnormal cutaneous reflex of the foot that appears in upper motor neuron disease.

REFLEX HAMMERS

I. Types Of Reflex Hammers

Early in the history of reflex testing,* clinicians used various implements to elicit reflexes: The great British neurologist Gowers used the ulnar aspect of his hand or his rigid stethoscope. Other clinicians were less selective, using paper weights, laboratory stands, or even table lamps.[1–3] In the late 1800s and early 1900s, many different reflex hammers were produced, some of which remain popular today.

---

*Reflex testing became common after Erb and Westphal simultaneously discovered the value of muscle stretch reflexes in 1875.[105,106]

A. TAYLOR HAMMER

The Taylor hammer was developed in 1888 by J.M. Taylor, personal assistant to S. Weir Mitchell at the Philadelphia Orthopedic Hospital and Infirmary for Nervous Disease. This hammer has a tomahawk-shaped soft rubber hammer with a broad edge for percussing most tendons and a rounded point for reaching the biceps tendon or percussing muscles directly. The original handle ended in an open loop; the pointed end was added about 1920 for use in eliciting cutaneous reflexes.[3]

B. QUEEN SQUARE HAMMER

The Queen Square hammer was developed by a Miss Wintle, head nurse at the National Hospital for Nervous Diseases at Queen's Square, London, who for years made hammers from ring pessaries, solid brass wheels, and bamboo rods to sell to resident medical officers. This hammer has a rubber-lined disc attached to the end of a long rod, like a wheel on an axle.[1]

C. BABINSKI HAMMER (BABINSKI/RABINER HAMMER)

This hammer has a handle that can be removed and attached either perpendicular or parallel to the disc-shaped head. Babinski's name probably reflects marketing more than innovation.[3]

D. TROEMNER HAMMER

The Troemner hammer, the only one of the four that actually resembles a hammer, was made popular in this country by the Mayo Clinic, where the neurologist Woltman introduced it in 1927.[4,5]

II. Clinical Significance

No study has demonstrated any hammer to be superior to another, and selection depends more on personal preference and tradition. The Taylor is popular in America, the Queen Square in England, and the Troemner in continental Europe.[6] The built-in pins of some models (e.g., older Babinski hammers), designed for testing pain sensation and cutaneous reflexes, should not be used because they could transmit infections.[7]

MUSCLE STRETCH REFLEXES

I. Definition

Muscle stretch reflexes are involuntary contractions of muscles induced by a brisk stretch of the muscle. Muscle stretch reflexes are usually named after the muscle being tested (Table 63.1), the one notable exception being the Achilles or ankle jerk. Although these reflexes are often called **deep tendon reflexes**, this name is a misnomer because tendons have little to do with the response, other than being responsible for mechanically transmitting the sudden stretch from the reflex hammer to the muscle spindle. In addition, some muscles with stretch reflexes have no tendons (e.g., "jaw jerk" of the masseter muscle).

Most healthy persons have the muscle stretch reflexes listed in Table 63.1.

TABLE 63.1 ■ Common Muscle Stretch Reflexes[22,28,94-103]

Name of Reflex	Peripheral Nerve	Spinal Level
Brachioradialis	Radial	C5-C6
Biceps	Musculocutaneous	C5-C6
Triceps	Radial	C7-C8
Quadriceps (patellar)	Femoral	L2-L4
Medial hamstring*	Sciatic	L5, S1
Achilles (ankle)	Tibial	S1

*An online video demonstrating the medial hamstring reflex is available in reference 104.

TABLE 63.2 ■ NINDS* Muscle Stretch Reflex Scale

Grade	Finding
0	Reflex absent
1	Reflex small, less than normal; includes a trace response or a response brought out only with reinforcement
2	Reflex in lower half of normal range
3	Reflex in upper half of normal range
4	Reflex enhanced, more than normal; includes clonus if present, which optionally can be noted in an added verbal description of the reflex

NINDS, National Institute of Neurological Disorders and Stroke, from reference 13.

II. Technique

A. Method

The usual stimulus is a sharp tap with the reflex hammer on the muscle's tendon, near where the tendon inserts distally on bone. The Achilles reflex is also elicited sometimes by the plantar strike method, in which the reflex hammer strikes the clinician's hand, which is resting on the ball of the foot. In clinical studies of the Achilles reflex, both the plantar strike and tendon strike methods are equivalent.[8-11]

B. Grading Reflex Amplitude

The most important observation during reflex examination is the reflex's amplitude. Unlike examination of motor strength, examination of reflexes lacks a single universally accepted grading system. Proposed schemes range from S. Weir Mitchell's original four grades[3] to the Mayo Clinic's nine grades.[12] A five-point grading system (i.e., grades 0 through 4), reproduced in Table 63.2, is recommended by the National Institute of Neurological Disorders and Stroke (NINDS).[13]

C. Reinforcement: The Jendrassik Maneuver

According to the NINDS scale (see Table 63.2), grade 1 reflexes describe reflexes made conspicuous by reinforcement maneuvers, and grade 0 reflexes are those that are absent despite reinforcement. The most common method of reinforcing reflexes is the **Jendrassik maneuver**. In 1885, Erno Jendrassik reported that clinicians could enhance the reflexes of a normal patient by having him "hook together the flexed fingers of his right and left hands and pull them apart as strongly as possible" while the clinician taps on the tendon.[1] Reflex enhancement with this maneuver persists as long as the patient is pulling apart the arms, up to 10 seconds in some studies.[14,15] In one study of normal elderly patients, the absent ankle jerk was made to appear 70% of the time using reinforcing maneuvers.[16]

III. Clinical Significance

A. AMPLITUDE OF REFLEX

The amplitude of muscle stretch reflexes depends on the integrity of the lower and upper motor neurons innervating the reflex (see Fig. 61.2 in Chapter 61 for definition of lower and upper motor neurons). (1) The lower motor neurons of a reflex are its peripheral nerve (2nd column in Table 63.1) and its spinal segment (3rd column in Table 63.1): Disease at either of these locations *reduces* or *abolishes* the relevant reflex. (2) The upper motor neurons are the descending corticospinal pathways innervating the reflex: Disease anywhere along this pathway (e.g., cerebral hemisphere, brainstem) *exaggerates* the reflex. (3) Disease of the *spinal cord*, where both upper and lower motor neurons reside, abolishes the reflex *at* the level of the lesion (lower motor neuron response) and exaggerates all reflexes from spinal levels *below* the level of the lesion (upper motor neuron response).

Nonetheless, absent or exaggerated reflexes, by themselves, do not signify neurologic disease.[17–19] For example, 6% to 50% of elderly persons without neurologic disease lack the ankle jerk bilaterally, despite the Jendrassik maneuver,[16,20] and a small percentage of normal individuals have generalized hyperreflexia.[17–19,21] Instead, the absent or exaggerated reflex is significant only when it is associated with one of the following clinical settings:

- The absent reflex is associated with other findings of lower motor neuron disease (weakness, atrophy, fasciculations).
- The exaggerated reflex is associated with other findings of upper motor neuron disease (i.e., weakness, spasticity, Babinski sign).
- The reflex amplitude is asymmetric, which suggests either lower motor neuron disease of the side with the diminished reflex or upper motor neuron disease of the side with exaggerated reflex.
- The reflex is unusually brisk compared with reflexes from a higher spinal level, which raises the possibility of spinal cord disease at some level of the spinal cord between the segments with exaggerated reflexes and those with diminished ones.

B. LOCALIZING VALUE OF DIMINISHED REFLEXES

In patients with nerve complaints of the arm or leg suggesting disorders of the cervical or lumbosacral nerve roots, the diminished reflex has important localizing value that indicates a lesion of the reflex's respective spinal root (see Table 63.1). A diminished biceps or brachioradialis reflex indicates C6 radiculopathy (likelihood ratio [LR] = 14.2),[22] a diminished triceps reflex indicates C7 radiculopathy† (LR = 3),[22,23] a diminished quadriceps reflex indicates L3 or L4 radiculopathy (LR = 8.5),[24–27] a diminished medial hamstring reflex indicates L5 disease (LR = 6.2),[28] and a diminished Achilles reflex indicates S1 radiculopathy (though only modestly, LR = 2.7)[24–26,29–31] (see also Chapter 64).

C. ANKLE JERK AND DIABETIC PERIPHERAL NEUROPATHY

In one study of adult outpatients with type 2 diabetes mellitus, the absent Achilles reflex detected peripheral neuropathy (defined by nerve conduction testing) with a sensitivity of 92%, specificity

---

†C6 and C7 radiculopathies are much more common than C5 or C8 radiculopathies (see Chapter 64).

of 67%, positive LR = 2.8, and negative LR = 0.1.[32] This indicates that in diabetic patients, the *presence* of the ankle jerk greatly *decreases* probability of diabetic peripheral neuropathy (LR = 0.1). In this study, examination of the ankle jerk was more accurate in predicting neuropathy than the duration of diabetes or presence of neuropathic symptoms or retinopathy.

D. ADDITIONAL FINDINGS IN THE HYPERREFLEXIC PATIENT

The physical finding of hyperreflexia has generated more eponyms in physical diagnosis than any other physical finding,[‡] even though the basic pathophysiology for all exaggerated reflexes is the same (i.e., loss of corticospinal inhibition) and the reflexes differ only by which muscle is stretched and which method the clinician uses to stretch the muscle. Of the many findings that have been described in hyperreflexic patients, commonly recognized ones are finger flexion reflexes, jaw jerks, clonus, and irradiating reflexes.

1. Finger Flexion Reflexes

Finger flexion reflexes were introduced by Hoffman in approximately 1900. In a positive response, sudden stretching of the finger flexors causes the finger flexors to involuntarily contract (the finger flexion reflex, therefore, is no different from any other muscle stretch reflex). There are many ways to elicit this finding, each with its own eponym (e.g., **Hoffman sign**, **Finger Rossolimo** sign, **Troemner** sign, **von Bechterew reflex**). One of these methods is described in Fig. 63.1. Like other exaggerated reflexes, finger flexion reflexes by themselves have little diagnostic value (i.e., they are detectable in 3% of healthy college students),[21] and, to be significant, they must accompany one of the settings

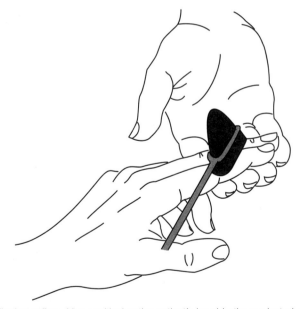

Fig. 63.1 Finger flexion reflex. After positioning the patient's hand in the supinated position with fingers slightly flexed, the clinician places his own index and middle fingers across the tips of the patient's fingers and taps them with the reflex hammer. Reflex contraction of the patient's finger flexor muscles is a positive response.

[‡]Dorland's Medical Dictionary lists 115 neurologic reflexes, 46 having eponyms.[107]

described previously in the section on amplitude of reflex." The diagnostic value of finger flexion reflexes in patients with neck pain appears later in the section on the Babinski response.

2. Jaw Jerk

The **jaw jerk** was originally described by Morris Lewis in 1882.[33,34] In a positive response, sudden stretching of the masseter muscle causes reflex contraction, moving the jaw briskly upward. With the patient's jaw slightly open, the clinician can elicit the reflex by tapping with a reflex hammer directly on the chin or on a tongue blade resting on the lower teeth or tongue. An exaggerated jaw jerk, sometimes appearing with clonus (see below), implies bilateral disease above the level of the pons (e.g., pseudobulbar palsy).[17] In patients with spastic tetraparesis, for example, an exaggerated jaw jerk excludes cervical cord disease and points to pyramidal tract disease above the pons.

3. Clonus

Clonus is a self-sustained, oscillating stretch reflex induced when the clinician briskly stretches a hyperreflexic muscle and then continues to apply stretching force to that muscle. Each time the muscle relaxes from the previous reflex contraction, the applied stretching force renews the reflex, setting up a rhythmic series of muscle contractions that continue as long as the tension is applied. These rhythmic oscillations (clonus) are most easily elicited in the foot (usually with oscillations of 5 to 8 Hz) by briskly dorsiflexing the patient's ankle. Clonus also may be elicited in the quadriceps, finger flexors, jaw, and other muscles.

As expected mathematically, the frequency of clonus varies inversely with the length of the reflex path ($r = -0.80$, $p < 0.001$). Clonus of the wrist has a higher frequency than that of the ankle, simply because the nerves to the forearm are shorter than those to the calf.[35]

Instructive videos are available of clonus at the ankle,[36] wrist,[37] and jaw.[38]

4. Irradiation of Reflexes

In some hyperreflexic patients, the blow of the reflex hammer is conducted mechanically through bone and tissues, where it may stretch hyperexcitable muscles at distant sites, thus producing additional, unexpected movements (e.g., crossed adductor reflex).[18,39] Also, if this distant irradiation of a reflex is combined with paralysis of the reflex of interest, paradoxical movements or *inverted* reflexes may appear.

a. Crossed Adductor Reflex

Tapping on the medial femoral condyle, patella, or patellar tendon causes the contralateral adductor muscle to contract, moving the contralateral knee medially.[40]

b. Inverted Supinator Reflex

The **inverted supinator reflex** (the supinator reflex is the brachioradialis reflex) was introduced by Babinski in 1910. This sign indicates spinal cord disease at the C5 to C6 level.[18,41,42] In a positive response, tapping on the brachioradialis muscle fails to flex the elbow but instead flexes the fingers. The lesion at C5 to C6 eliminates the brachioradialis reflex (lower motor neuron) but exaggerates all reflexes below that level (upper motor neuron), including the finger flexion reflexes (C8), which are stimulated by mechanical conduction of the blow on the brachioradialis.

The diagnostic value of the inverted supinator reflex in patients with neck pain appears later in the section on the Babinski response.

c. Inverted Knee Jerk

The **inverted knee jerk**[43] indicates spinal cord disease at the L2-L4 level. In the positive response, attempts to elicit the knee jerk instead cause paradoxical knee flexion. Its two components are denervation of L2 to L4 (thus paralyzing the quadriceps jerk) and conduction of the blow to the muscle spindles of the hamstrings (innervated by the L5 to S1 level and made hyperexcitable by the same lesion).

CUTANEOUS REFLEXES (SUPERFICIAL REFLEXES)

I. Definition

Cutaneous reflexes are involuntary muscle contractions that follow stimulation of the skin surface by scratching, stroking, or pinching.

II. Superficial Abdominal Reflex (T6 To T11)

A. TECHNIQUE

In the superficial abdominal reflexes, stroking the skin of the abdomen causes the underlying abdominal wall muscle to contract, sometimes pulling the umbilicus towards the stimulus (see the reference by Gosavi[44] for an online video). The clinician usually tests one abdominal quadrant at a time using a side-to-side motion with a wooden applicator stick or the pointed end of the reflex hammer handle. The abdominal reflexes appear just as often whether the direction is medial-to-lateral or lateral-to-medial.[45]

B. CLINICAL SIGNIFICANCE

According to traditional teachings, superficial abdominal reflexes disappear with both upper and lower motor neuron disease. Their clinical value is slight, however, because they are also absent in about 20% of normal individuals, more so in the elderly.[45,46] Moreover, the observation of asymmetric reflexes or ones preserved only in the upper quadrants, patterns traditionally associated with neurologic disease, also are a common finding in healthy persons.[45–47]

III. Bulbocavernosus Reflex (S2 To S4)

A. TECHNIQUE

After positioning the patient in the lithotomy position, sudden manual compression of the glans penis or clitoris causes reflex contraction of the bulbocavernosus muscle and external anal sphincter. The reflex is detected either by palpating the skin behind the scrotum (bulbocavernosus muscle) or, more commonly, placing the index finger in the anal canal (external anal sphincter). Other effective stimuli are percussing the suprapubic area[48] or pulling the retention balloon of an indwelling Foley catheter against the bladder neck.[49]

B. CLINICAL SIGNIFICANCE

The bulbocavernosus reflex is one of the few ways to test the conus medullaris (distal end of the spinal cord) and the S2 to S4 pelvic nerves (the only other bedside test of this region is testing sensation in the perineal, or "saddle," area).[49–51] This reflex is particularly important in patients with urinary retention, which may be caused by disease of the pelvic nerves or cauda equina. In one study of consecutive patients referred for urodynamic studies,[49] most of whom had difficulty with urination, an *absent* reflex predicted disease in the S2 to S4 segments only modestly in women

(LR = 2.7) but much better in men (LR = 13). The modest accuracy of the sign in women may reflect damage to the pudendal nerve from prior childbirth or pelvic surgery.[49] In this study, the *presence* of a bulbocavernosus reflex was unhelpful: although the positive response is expected in patients with urinary retention from common disorders like prostate hypertrophy, it also is commonly found in incomplete lesions of the sacral nerves.

In spinal cord injury above the S2 to S4 level (i.e., lesion of upper motor neurons innervating the S2 to S4 segment), the bulbocavernosus reflex also disappears, but only temporarily for a period of one to six weeks.[49]

BABINSKI RESPONSE

I. Definition

The Babinski response is an abnormal cutaneous reflex found in upper motor neuron disease affecting the muscles of the foot. In these patients, scratching the sole of the patient's foot causes an upward movement of the great toe, instead of the normal downward movement (Fig. 63.2). Much revered and researched, this reflex was originally described by Babinski in 1896.[52,53] It goes by various names, including Babinski response, Babinski sign, Babinski reflex, upgoing toe, and extensor response.

In some patients with bilateral corticospinal tract disease, scratching the foot may even cause the contralateral great toe to move upward, a response termed **crossed dorsiflexion** or **crossed extensor response.**[52]

II. Pathogenesis

In response to painful stimuli applied to the lower limbs, most mammals rapidly withdraw that limb by flexing the hips and knees and dorsiflexing the feet and toes. This primitive reflex, the **flexion response,** also occurs in human infants until the age of 1 or 2 years, after which the developing pyramidal tracts cause two important changes: (1) the flexion response becomes less brisk and (2) the toes no longer move upward but instead move downward because of the interval development of a normal plantar cutaneous reflex.[54] If pyramidal tract disease develops later in the person's life, the normal plantar cutaneous reflex disappears, and, instead, painful stimulation of the foot causes the great toe to again move upward.

The use of the term *extensor response* to describe the Babinski response is unfortunate and confusing: even though anatomists have always named the upward movement "extension" (e.g., great toe extensor muscle), physiologists have named the same upward movement "flexion" (e.g., the primitive flexion response discussed earlier).

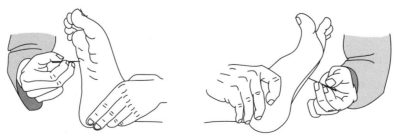

Fig. 63.2   Babinski response. Drawing of the normal plantar cutaneous reflex (*left*) and the Babinski response (*right*). Adapted from photographs taken by Babinski himself in 1900.[52]

III. Technique

A. ELICITING THE RESPONSE

Of the many ways to elicit this reflex,[55,56] a slow (i.e., 5 to 6 second) hockey-stick stroke beginning the lateral plantar surface is best, using a wooden applicator stick, key, or pointed handle of the reflex hammer (Fig. 63.2). This method is superior to other methods, including scratching the lateral sole, scratching below the lateral malleolus (**Chaddock method**), rubbing the anterior shin (**Oppenheim method**), or—the least effective stimulus—squeezing the calf (**Gordon method**).[57,58]

B. INTERPRETING THE RESPONSE

Helpful guidelines in assessing an equivocal toe response, based on careful electrodiagnostic studies and patient follow-up, are as follows: (1) The pathologic upgoing toe results from contraction of the extensor hallucis longus muscle, whose tendon is conspicuous under the skin on top of the great toe.[59,60] Movement of the toe per se is not critical and may be prevented by joint disease. Moreover, the toe may seem to be upgoing—without contraction of the extensor hallucis longus muscle—when the ankle dorsiflexes or when the toe returns from an initial downward movement. (2) More than 90% of the time, the foot with the pathologic upgoing toe is weak or has difficulty with fine motor movements. An excellent test of fine motor movement is rapid foot tapping against the examiner's hand: normal persons accomplish 20 to 40 taps per 10 seconds. (3) The pathologic upgoing toe coincides with a flexion response in the whole limb, which may be slight but is evident in the ipsilateral tensor fascia lata and hamstrings; and (4) The pathologic upgoing toe is reproducible.[54,61,62]

As Babinski himself pointed out, fanning of the toes is a normal phenomenon and not part of the pathologic response.[52,54]

Some ticklish patients have such dramatic withdrawal that interpreting the direction of the great toe's movement is difficult. Often, having these patients perform the test themselves by stroking their own sole reduces withdrawal and reveals a clear positive or negative response.[63]

IV. Clinical Significance

A. ASSOCIATED CONDITIONS

The Babinski response is found in both destructive lesions of the pyramidal tracts (see Chapter 61) and in many metabolic disorders affecting these tracts, most of which are associated with altered mental status, such as seizures, meningitis, drug overdose, renal and hepatic failure.[52] In patients with a variety of neurologic complaints who undergo neuroimaging, the Babinski response greatly increases probability of a lesion in the contralateral cerebral hemisphere (LR = 8.5, see Chapter 61).

B. FALSE-NEGATIVE RESPONSE

Patients may have pyramidal tract disease yet lack the upgoing toe (i.e., false negative response) because they have the following: (1) spinal shock,[59] (2) a peroneal palsy denervating the muscles that dorsiflex the great toe (a common problem in bedridden patients due to pressure against the head of the fibula),[59] or (3) pyramidal tract disease sparing the muscles of the foot (e.g., upper motor neuron weakness is confined to the arm of that side).[64]

C. BABINSKI RESPONSE AND NECK PAIN

In patients with neck or arm pain characteristic of cervical spine disease, a positive Babinski response suggests significant cervical cord compression (see the section myelopathy in Chapter 61). In support of this, studies of patients with neck or arm pain show that a positive Babinski response greatly increases probability of myelopathy on cervical magnetic resonance imaging (MRI) (sensitivity of 36%, specificity of 99%, positive LR = 24.8, negative LR = 0.6).[65] In this study and others of patients with neck pain, the Babinski response is more accurate than the findings of an inverted supinator reflex (LR = 1.7)[65] or abnormal finger flexion reflexes (LR = not significant).[65,66]

PRIMITIVE REFLEXES

I. Definition

Primitive reflexes (or **release reflexes**) are a hodgepodge of reflexes that are present normally in infants but disappear during normal development of the central nervous system, only to reappear sometimes later in life when neurologic disease or aging removes (or "releases") the inhibiting influences of the central nervous system.[67] Among many primitive reflexes,[68] the more common ones are the palmomental reflex, glabellar reflex, grasp reflex, snout reflex, and suck reflex.

II. Technique

A. PALMOMENTAL REFLEX

In this reflex, a key or other blunt object is used to apply an unpleasant stimulus to the patient's thenar eminence, stroking it briskly in a proximal to distal direction. A positive response is a brief contraction of the ipsilateral mentalis muscle, causing the ipsilateral lower lip to protrude, rise, or wrinkle.[69] An instructive video of the finding is available.[70]

The wrinkle response at the corner of the mouth is probably the beginnings of a wince that would develop with more painful stimuli.[71] Theoretically, the stimulus could be applied anywhere on the skin of the patient's body, and in fact, descriptions of similar response after stimulation of the patient's arm, chest, trunk, sole of the foot, and tongue have all appeared.[71] The most sensitive area, however, is the thenar eminence.[72]

In a study of 226 outpatients with symptoms suggestive of intracranial disease (e.g., headache, seizure, or known malignancy), the finding of a definite palmomental reflex detected frontal lobe lesions on MRI with a sensitivity of 19%, specificity of 97%, positive LR = 6.3, and negative LR = 0.8.[73]

Marinesco and Radovici discovered the palmomental reflex in 1920.[71]

B. GLABELLAR REFLEX

The stimulus for the glabellar reflex is light taps with the finger or soft rubber reflex hammer, about two times per second, over the patient's glabella. Although most normal persons respond to this by blinking bilaterally, the blinking stops after the first few taps in normal individuals. Persistent blinking is a positive response, although there is no consensus whether habituation should be indefinite or just beyond a certain number of blinks (e.g., more than 4 successive blinks).

The glabellar reflex is sometimes called the **blink reflex** or **Myerson reflex**, although the original description was by Overend in 1896.[74]

C. GRASP REFLEX

In the grasp reflex, the clinician places his index and middle fingers over the thenar aspect of the patient's wrist and exerts pressure on the skin while withdrawing the fingers between the patient's thumb and index finger. In a positive response, the patient grasps the clinician's fingers, and the grasp progressively increases as the clinician attempts to withdraw.[68]

III. Clinical Significance

A. GENERAL COMMENTS

Primitive reflexes are common findings in frontal lobe disease,[75] parkinsonism,[76–79] dementing illnesses,[80–84] and advanced human immunodeficiency virus infection.[85] Other than the grasp reflex (see below), the precise neuroanatomical cause of these reflexes is unknown.

B. PALMOMENTAL REFLEX

The palmomental reflex is bilateral 38% to 75% of the time and unilateral 25% to 62% of the time.[86,87] The side of the reflex does not correlate with the side of the lesion.[69,86] In one study of 39 patients with a unilateral palmomental reflex, 44% had an ipsilateral cerebral hemispheric lesion, 36% a contralateral lesion, 10% bilateral lesions, and 10% no lesions.[87] In patients with Parkinson disease, the palmomental reflex correlates with the degree of akinesia, and the reflex often disappears with the onset of levodopa-induced dyskinesias.[76]

C. GLABELLAR REFLEX

The afferent limb of the glabellar reflex is the trigeminal nerve, and the efferent limb is the facial nerve. Lesions of either nerve may interrupt the reflex (although in facial nerve palsy, the blinking continues on the sound side). This reflex is also a common finding in Parkinson disease, and in these patients, the positive response may reverse after administration of levodopa.[77]

D. GRASP REFLEX

A positive grasp reflex is common in frontal lobe disease and, if both arms can be tested (i.e., no paralysis), the grasp reflex when present is usually bilateral.[75] In patients with dementia, the sign correlates with more severe cognitive and functional impairment and greater loss of pyramidal cells in the frontal lobe.[80,81,84] Among patients admitted to a neurologic ward, a positive grasp reflex (defined as no habituation with three successive strokes) predicted discrete lesions in the frontal lobe or deep nuclei and subcortical white matter with a sensitivity of 13% to 50%, specificity 99%, and positive LR of 19.1.[75,88]

E. PRIMITIVE REFLEXES AND NORMAL AGING

The palmomental and glabellar reflexes, but not the grasp reflex, may appear in normal persons, although the reported frequencies from different studies vary widely.[82,83,85,89] The reported frequency for the palmomental sign in normal persons varies from 3% to 70%; that for the glabellar sign, from 3% to 33%.[76,83,85,89–92] A few of these "normal" persons with primitive reflexes undoubtedly have subclinical disease, as indicated by lesions in the basal ganglia or subcortical white matter on MRI.[90] Even so, others have no evidence of neurologic disease, although importantly, their findings differ from the pathologic response in two important ways: (1) the primitive reflex of patients without neurologic lesions is weak and fatigable, disappearing after the first few repetitive stimuli spaced evenly apart,[67] and (2) the primitive reflex of patients without neurologic lesions is an isolated finding. For example, less than 1% of normal persons have a positive palmomental reflex, if it is defined as persistence beyond 5 or more strokes of the thenar eminence.[72,76] In addition, even if the definition of a positive response includes fatigable primitive reflexes, less than 12% of normal persons have two primitive reflexes, and less than 2% have three or more primitive reflexes.[85,89,91–93]

Disorders of the Nerve Roots, Plexuses, and Peripheral Nerves

I. Introduction

Nerve roots destined to innervate the limbs exit through vertebral foramina and intermingle in plexuses (i.e., the brachial and lumbosacral plexuses) before emerging as peripheral nerves that extend to the fingers and toes. Lesions anywhere along this pathway—from spinal nerve roots to the final peripheral nerve branch—produce combinations of pain, *lower* motor neuron weakness, and sensory loss.

A lesion in the nerve root is called **radiculopathy**; one in the plexus, **plexopathy**; and one in the peripheral nerve, **peripheral neuropathy**. This chapter explains how to distinguish these lesions in patients with nerve complaints of the arms or legs. Because the neuroanatomy of these lesions is complex, accurate diagnosis requires systematic examination of all the limb's muscles, sensation, and reflexes.

II. The Arm

A. INTRODUCTION

In patients presenting with nerve complaints of the upper extremity, the most common neurologic diagnosis is carpal tunnel syndrome, followed by polyneuropathy, ulnar neuropathy, and cervical radiculopathy.[1-3] Other focal neuropathies and plexopathies are less common. Most cervical radiculopathies affect the C6 or C7 root.[4-7]

B. NEUROLOGIC FINDINGS

1. Motor

Most muscles of the arm are innervated by nerves from more than one spinal segment. Fig. 64.1 presents the relationship between the different peripheral nerves (grouped in rows) and their corresponding spinal roots (in columns). The spinal levels listed in Fig. 64.1 are based upon several lines of evidence, including Bolk's detailed dissection of a single human subject,[8,9] electrodiagnostic studies,[10,11] and bedside observations of patients with documented spinal root lesions.[5,12]

a. Radiculopathy

Even though most muscles receive innervation from more than one spinal nerve root, injury to one root is usually sufficient to cause significant loss of power. The motor examination of radiculopathy

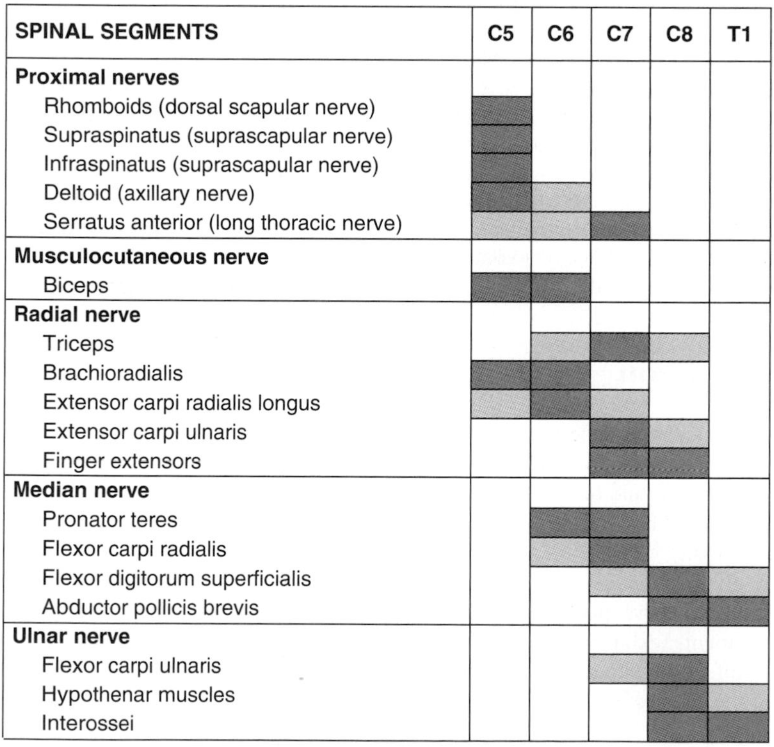

SPINAL SEGMENTS	C5	C6	C7	C8	T1
Proximal nerves					
Rhomboids (dorsal scapular nerve)					
Supraspinatus (suprascapular nerve)					
Infraspinatus (suprascapular nerve)					
Deltoid (axillary nerve)					
Serratus anterior (long thoracic nerve)					
Musculocutaneous nerve					
Biceps					
Radial nerve					
Triceps					
Brachioradialis					
Extensor carpi radialis longus					
Extensor carpi ulnaris					
Finger extensors					
Median nerve					
Pronator teres					
Flexor carpi radialis					
Flexor digitorum superficialis					
Abductor pollicis brevis					
Ulnar nerve					
Flexor carpi ulnaris					
Hypothenar muscles					
Interossei					

Fig. 64.1   Innervation of muscles of the arm. This figure indicates those spinal levels that usually (*dark blue shade*) and sometimes (*light blue shade*) contribute to the corresponding muscle; based on references.[4,5,8-14]

has two characteristics: (1) Weakness affects two or more muscles from the same spinal segment but different peripheral nerves (i.e., all of the weak muscles are in the same *column* in Fig. 64.1). For example, a C6 radiculopathy may simultaneously weaken the elbow flexion (biceps muscle, musculocutaneous nerve) and wrist extension (radial and ulnar wrist extensors, radial nerve).[5] (2) Weakness may involve muscles innervated by *proximal nerves*, which are listed in the top rows of Fig. 64.1. Proximal nerves originate from the nerve roots but then promptly innervate muscles of the shoulder, thus moving away from the course of the peripheral nerves of the arm. Therefore, if a muscle innervated by one of these nerves is weak in a patient with nerve complaints of the arm or hand, the lesion must be a proximal one near the nerve roots. A common example is the finding of scapular winging (i.e., weak serratus anterior muscle, long thoracic nerve) in a patient with arm pain and triceps weakness. Involvement of the serratus anterior points to the C7 root and away from the radial nerve or brachial plexus.[13]

b. Brachial Plexopathy
Lesions of the brachial plexus cause simultaneous weakness of muscles from two or more adjacent spinal segments (i.e., adjacent *columns* in Fig. 64.1) and from two or more peripheral nerves. Brachial plexus lesions usually affect either the upper plexus (C5 to C6) as a group, causing weakness of the shoulder and upper arm but sparing all muscles of the hand, or the lower plexus (C7 to T1) as a group, affecting all muscles of the hand but sparing those of the shoulder and upper arm.

c. Peripheral Nerve Disorders
These lesions weaken two or more muscles from a *single* peripheral nerve (which may have different spinal segments) and spare muscles from other nerves. For example, a complete radial nerve injury weakens the brachioradialis muscle (C5-C6),* elbow extension (triceps, C7), wrist extension (wrist extensors, C6-C7), and finger extension (finger extensors, C8).

In Fig. 64.1, the muscles belonging to each peripheral nerve are listed in the order that their branches diverge from the main trunk. Therefore, a proximal lesion of the radial nerve in the axilla would cause the findings described in the previous paragraph, but a lesion of the radial nerve at the elbow, after the branch to the brachioradialis muscle, spares the triceps and brachioradialis but weakens more distal muscles (i.e., wrist and finger extensors).

Some peripheral nerve lesions can be recognized at a glance, such as the wrist drop of radial neuropathy (Fig. 64.2) and the claw hand appearance of ulnar neuropathy (Fig. 64.3). A callus over the hypothenar eminence in a patient with ulnar muscle weakness suggests damage to the deep

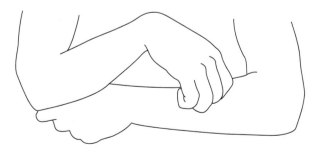

Fig. 64.2   Wrist drop of radial neuropathy. This patient has a right radial nerve palsy, thus eliminating the patient's wrist and finger extensor strength and causing the hand to droop downwards from its own weight.

---

*Testing elbow flexion with the forearm midway between supination and pronation reveals brachioradialis weakness.[14]

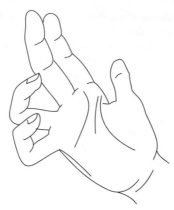

Fig. 64.3 **Claw hand of ulnar nerve palsy.** All metacarpophalangeal joints are hyperextended because of paralysis of all interossei and unopposed action of finger extensors (radial nerve). The hyperextension is less prominent in the index and middle fingers because the lumbricals of these digits, innervated by the median nerve, act to flex the joint. Tethering from the flexor tendons causes all interphalangeal joints to flex.

branch of the ulnar nerve, caused by chronic pressure on the heel of the hand from bicycling or using a walker.[15,16]

2. Sensory Findings

Radiculopathy causes sensory loss in a dermatomal pattern (see Table 62.1 and Fig. 62.1 in Chapter 62). Brachial plexus lesions cause sensory loss from adjacent dermatomes. Peripheral nerve lesions cause the sensory loss described in Fig. 64.4.

One pure sensory syndrome of the arm is **cheiralgia paresthetica**, from injury to the superficial branch of the radial nerve, usually because of too tight a wrist band or hand cuffs. Sensory findings are confined to the radial aspect of the dorsal hand.[17]

3. Reflexes

The three muscle stretch reflexes of the arm are the biceps (musculocutaneous nerve, C5-C6), brachioradialis (radial nerve, C5-C6), and triceps (radial nerve, C7-C8).[†] Therefore, the finding of abnormal reflexes *excludes* both median and ulnar neuropathies (nerves lacking reflexes) and instead *increases* probability of radiculopathy or plexopathy. Radial nerve lesions usually spare the brachioradialis and triceps reflex because the branches to these muscles diverge from the main trunk proximally in the axilla, and most injuries to this nerve occur at a more distal point (e.g., humeral fracture, or **Saturday night palsy**).

4. Provocative Tests

One traditional test for cervical radiculopathy is the **Spurling test** or **neck compression test**. In this test, the clinician turns and tilts the patient's head and neck toward the painful side and then adds a compressive force to the top of the head.[18] Aggravation of pain is a positive response. The **Tinel sign** and **Phalen sign** are provocative tests traditionally used to diagnose carpal tunnel syndrome. (See the section on diagnosis of carpal tunnel syndrome.) The Katz hand diagram (for carpal tunnel syndrome) appears in Fig. 64.5.

[†]Even though weakness of the triceps may follow lesions in the C6 or C7 roots (C7 is most common; see Fig. 64.1), the absent triceps jerk usually results from C7 or C8 lesions.[5]

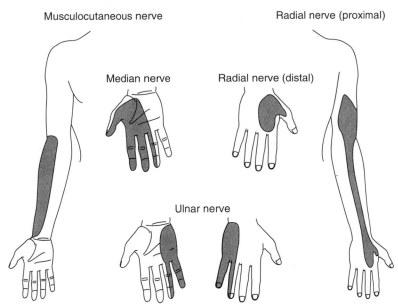

Fig. 64.4   Sensory branches of peripheral nerves of the arm. The three figures on the left depict the *volar* surface of the arm; the three on the right, the *dorsal* surface. Proximal lesions of the radial nerve (upper right), near the axilla (and above the origin of the posterior cutaneous nerves of the arm and forearm) affect sensation of the posterior arm, forearm, *and* hand; more distal lesions in the radial nerve (e.g., at the elbow) affect only the dorsal hand. Proximal lesions of the median nerve affect both palm and fingers; more distal ones (e.g., in the carpal tunnel) affect just the fingers. The sensory innervation of the medial arm and forearm derives from cutaneous nerves that branch directly off the brachial plexus.

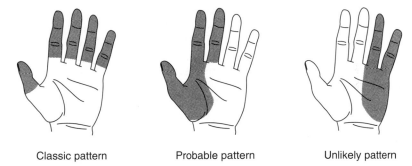

Fig. 64.5   Katz hand diagram. The Katz hand diagram is a self-administered diagram of the hand that depicts the patient's symptoms: the "classic" pattern (example, *left*) describes symptoms affecting at least two of digits 1, 2, or 3 but sparing the palm and dorsum of hand (digit 1 is thumb; digit 5 is little finger); the "probable" pattern is similar to the classic pattern although palm symptoms are allowed; the "unlikely" pattern depicts symptoms not involving digits 1, 2, or 3.[19] Palm symptoms are not part of the "classic" pattern because the palmar cutaneous branch of the median nerve does not travel through the carpal tunnel.[20]

C. ADDITIONAL DIAGNOSTIC CLUES

1. The Clavicle

The brachial plexus lies just behind the clavicle. Therefore, additional physical findings in the supraclavicular space, such as mass, adenopathy, hemorrhage, or other evidence of trauma, suggest injury to the brachial plexus. Trauma *above* the clavicle injures roots; that *below* the clavicle injures peripheral nerves.

2. Horner Syndrome (see Chapter 21)

An associated Horner syndrome (i.e., ipsilateral small pupil and ptosis) indicates radiculopathy (C8-T1) or a lesion of the lower brachial plexus.

D. CLINICAL SIGNIFICANCE

1. Diagnosing Cervical Radiculopathy

EBM Box 64.1 presents the diagnostic accuracy of bedside examination for cervical radiculopathy, as applied to patients presenting with neck pain, arm pain, or both. In these patients, the findings that *increase* probability of radiculopathy the most are reduced biceps reflex (likelihood ratio [LR] = 9.1, see EBM Box 64.1), a positive Spurling test (LR = 4.8), and reduction of any arm reflex (i.e., biceps, brachioradialis, or triceps reflex, LR = 3.6). Findings that *decrease* probability of radiculopathy are normal rotation of the neck (i.e., can rotate to affected side >60 degrees, LR = 0.2) and the absence of arm muscle weakness (LR = 0.4).

Despite its modest accuracy, however, the Spurling test should probably *not* be performed. In other studies of cervical radiculopathy, its sensitivity is only 9% to 16%,[27,28] and in patients with rheumatoid arthritis, cervical malformations, or metastatic disease, the test risks serious injury to the spine.

2. Localizing Cervical Radiculopathy

EBM Box 64.2 presents the diagnostic accuracy of the motor, sensory, and reflex examination in patients with known cervical radiculopathy, illustrating the accuracy of findings in predicting the exact level of the lesion. According to these LRs, the best indicator of C5 radiculopathy is weak elbow flexion (LR = 5.3). A diminished biceps or brachioradialis reflex (LR = 14.2), sensory loss affecting the thumb (LR = 8.5), and weak wrist extension (LR = 2.3) indicate C6 radiculopathy. Weak elbow extension (LR = 4) and a diminished triceps reflex (LR = 3) indicate C7 radiculopathy, whereas normal elbow extensor strength decreases probability modestly for this diagnosis (LR = 0.4). Sensory loss affecting the little finger (LR = 41.4) and weak finger flexion (LR = 3.8) indicate C8 radiculopathy.

These LRs show that each of the indicator muscles discussed in Chapter 61 (i.e., elbow flexion for C5, wrist extension for C6, elbow extension for C7, and finger flexion for C8) predict the level involved (LRs = 2.3–5.3). The weaker a muscle is, the more significant its localizing value.[5] Also, although certain sensory findings are diagnostic (e.g., sensory loss affecting little finger of C8 radiculopathy, LR = 41.4), fewer than one in three patients with cervical radiculopathy has any sensory loss, and therefore the finding of *normal* sensation is never a compelling argument *against* cervical radiculopathy (i.e., negative LRs for all sensory findings are not significant).

Importantly, the LRs in EBM Box 64.2 apply only to patients with cervical radiculopathy. Patients with carpal tunnel syndrome may also develop hypesthesia of the thumb and those with ulnar neuropathy may develop hypesthesia of the little finger, although in these patients, the arm reflexes and arm and wrist strength are normal.

3. Plexopathy in Cancer Patients

If brachial plexopathy develops in a patient with cancer who has received radiation near the shoulder, the question arises whether the plexopathy is due to metastatic disease or radiation injury. Findings increasing probability of *metastatic* involvement are motor and sensory findings confined to C7-T1 (LR = 30.9) and Horner syndrome (LR = 4.1). Findings increasing probability of *radiation* injury are motor and sensory findings confined to C5-C6 (LR = 8.8) and lymphedema of the ipsilateral arm (LR = 4.9).[29]

EBM BOX 64.1	Diagnosing Cervical Radiculopathy in Patients With Neck and Arm Pain*			

| Finding (Reference)† | Sensitivity (%) | Specificity (%) | Likelihood Ratio‡ if Finding Is | |
			Present	Absent
Motor examination				
Weakness of any arm muscle[6]	73	61	1.9	0.4
Sensory examination				
Reduced vibration or pinprick sensation in arm[6]	38	46	NS	NS
Reflex examination				
Reduced biceps reflex[6]	10	99	**9.1**	NS
Reduced brachioradialis reflex[6]	8	99	NS	NS
Reduced triceps reflex[6]	10	95	NS	NS
Reduced biceps, triceps, or brachioradialis reflex[6]	21	94	**3.6**	0.8
Other tests				
Spurling test[7,21–26]	12–92	83–98	**4.8**	0.6
Rotation of neck to involved side <60°[7]	89	48	1.7	**0.2**

*Diagnostic standard: for cervical radiculopathy, nerve conduction studies[7,21,25]; neuroimaging (computed tomography or magnetic resonance imaging),[23,24,26] or MRI and surgery.[22]
†Definition of findings: for *Spurling test*, see text.
‡Likelihood ratio (LR) if finding present = positive LR; LR if finding absent = negative LR.
MRI, Magnetic resonance imaging; *NS*, not significant.

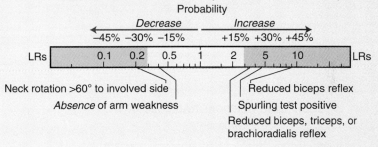

CERVICAL RADICULOPATHY (IF NECK AND ARM PAIN)
Probability

Neck rotation >60° to involved side
Absence of arm weakness

Reduced biceps reflex
Spurling test positive
Reduced biceps, triceps, or brachioradialis reflex

4. Peripheral Nerve Injury: Diagnosis of Carpal Tunnel Syndrome

EBM Box 64.3 summarizes the diagnostic accuracy of findings for the most common peripheral neuropathy of the arm, carpal tunnel syndrome. According to this EBM Box, three findings modestly increase probability of carpal tunnel syndrome: diminished pain sensation in the distribution of the median nerve (LR = 3.1), thenar atrophy (LR = 2.9), a square wrist ratio (defined in footnote of EBM Box 64.3, LR = 2.7), and a "classic" or "probable" hand diagram (LR = 2.4; see Fig. 64.5). The finding *decreasing* probability of carpal tunnel syndrome the most is an "unlikely" hand diagram (LR = 0.2). Several traditional tests such as the Tinel sign and Phalen sign and other novel ones such as the pressure provocation and flick signs (defined in a footnote in EBM Box 64.3) do not distinguish carpal tunnel syndrome from other common disorders causing hand dysesthesias (such as polyneuropathy, ulnar neuropathy, or radiculopathy, using electrodiagnosis as the diagnostic standard).[1,46]

| EBM BOX 64.2 | Localizing Cervical Radiculopathy* | | | |

Finding (Reference)	Sensitivity (%)	Specificity (%)	Likelihood Ratio† if Finding Is	
			Present	Absent
Motor examination				
Weak elbow flexion, detecting C5 radiculopathy[5]	83	84	**5.3**	NS
Weak wrist extension, detecting C6 radiculopathy[5]	37	84	2.3	NS
Weak elbow extension, detecting C7 radiculopathy[5]	65	84	**4.0**	0.4
Weak finger flexion, detecting C8 radiculopathy[5]	50	87	**3.8**	NS
Sensory examination				
Sensory loss affecting thumb, detecting C6 radiculopathy[5]	32	96	**8.5**	NS
Sensory loss affecting middle finger, detecting C7 radiculopathy[5]	5	98	NS	NS
Sensory loss affecting little finger, detecting C8 radiculopathy[5]	23	99	**41.4**	NS
Reflex examination				
Diminished biceps or brachioradialis reflex, detecting C6 radiculopathy[5]	53	96	**14.2**	0.5
Diminished triceps reflex, detecting C7 radiculopathy[5,6]	15–65	81–93	**3.0**	NS

*Diagnostic standard: for *level of radiculopathy*, surgical findings[5] or electrodiagnosis.[6]
†Likelihood ratio (LR) if finding present = positive LR; LR if finding absent = negative LR.
NS, Not significant.

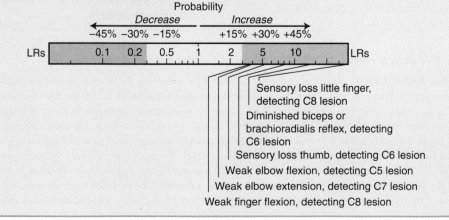

LOCALIZING CERVICAL RADICULOPATHY

EBM BOX 64.3	Diagnosing Carpal Tunnel Syndrome*

Finding (Reference)[†]	Sensitivity (%)	Specificity (%)	Likelihood Ratio[‡] if Finding Is	
			Present	Absent
Hand diagram				
"Classic" or "probable"[19]	64	73	2.4	0.5
"Unlikely"[19]	4	77	**0.2**	…
Motor examination				
Weak thumb abduction[30-32]	37–66	62–74	1.8	0.6
Thenar atrophy[31-35]	4–28	82–100	2.9	NS
Sensory examination (median distribution)				
Hypalgesia[30,33]	15–51	85–93	**3.1**	NS
Diminished 2 point discrimination[31,34-36]	6–63	64–99	NS	NS
Abnormal vibration sensation[31,36]	20–61	71–81	NS	NS
Diminished monofilament sensation[36,37]	59–98	15–59	NS	NS
Other tests				
Tinel sign[30-36,38,39]	23–89	41–91	1.4	0.8
Phalen sign[30-36,38-42]	10–91	33–86	1.4	0.6
Pressure provocation test[30,32,35,36,40,41,43]	28–96	17–74	NS	NS
Square wrist ratio[30,44]	47–69	73–83	2.7	0.5
Flick sign[39,45]	37–93	74–96	NS	NS

*Diagnostic standard: for *carpal tunnel syndrome*, abnormal motor or sensory conduction within the carpal tunnel, measured by nerve conduction testing.

[†]Definition of findings: for *hand diagram*, see Fig. 64.5; for all *sensory findings*, perception diminished in index finger compared with ipsilateral little finger (*2-point discrimination* used compass points separated by 4–6 mm, *vibratory* sensation used 126 or 256 Hz tuning fork, *monofilament* sensation abnormal if >2.83); for *Tinel sign*, *Phalen sign*, and *pressure provocation test*, the positive response is paresthesias in distribution of median nerve, although each test uses a different stimulus—tapping on the distal wrist crease over the median nerve (*Tinel sign*), maximal wrist flexion for 60 seconds (*Phalen sign*), and firm pressure with examiner's thumbs on palmar aspect of patient's distal wrist crease for 60 seconds (*pressure provocation test*)[46]; for *square wrist ratio*, anteroposterior dimension of wrist divided by mediolateral dimension, measured with calipers at distal wrist crease, is ≥0.7; and for *Flick sign*, upon asking the patient, "What do you actually do with your hand(s) when the symptoms are at their worst?", the patient demonstrates a flicking movement of the wrist and hand, similar to that employed in shaking down a thermometer.[45]

[‡]Likelihood ratio (LR) if finding present = positive LR; LR if finding absent = negative LR.

NS, Not significant.

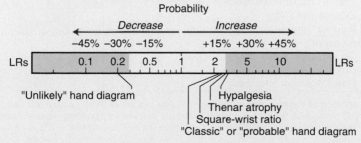

CARPAL TUNNEL SYNDROME
Probability

III. The Leg

A. INTRODUCTION

Among patients presenting with lower extremity nerve complaints, the most common neurologic diagnosis is by far lumbosacral radiculopathy, which usually affects the L5 or S1 roots (each are affected with about the same frequency).[4,47–52]

B. NEUROLOGIC FINDINGS

1. Motor

Fig. 64.6 presents the innervation of the muscles of the leg, showing the relationship between different spinal roots (in columns) and the different peripheral nerves (grouped in rows).

a. Radiculopathy

Like radiculopathy of the arm, radiculopathy of the leg has two characteristics: (1) Weakness affects two or more muscles from the same spinal segment but different peripheral nerves (i.e., all muscles innervated by same *column* in Fig. 64.6). For example, an L5 radiculopathy may affect both the dorsiflexors of the foot and toes (peroneal nerve) and inversion of the foot (tibial nerve). (2) Weakness may involve *proximal nerves* to the glutei muscles, which produces characteristic weakness and gait abnormalities (i.e., gluteus maximus gait and Trendelenburg gait; see Chapter 7).

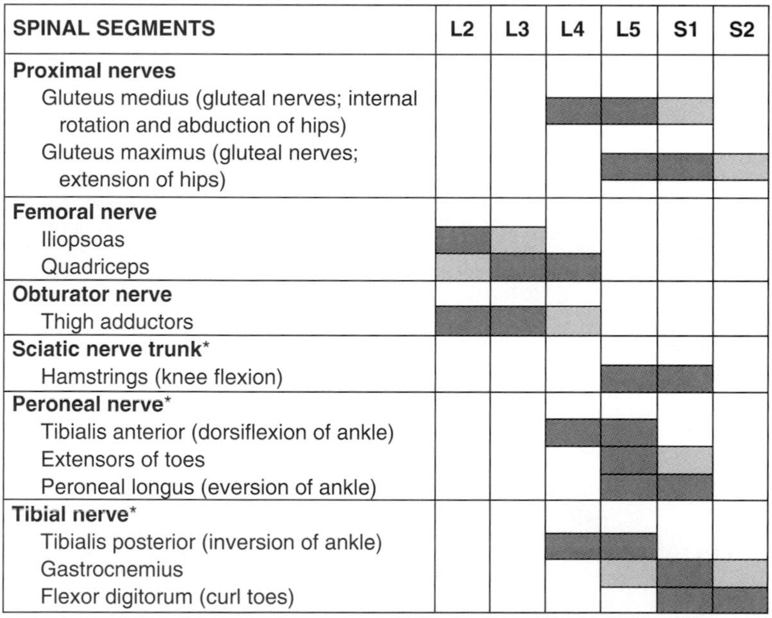

SPINAL SEGMENTS	L2	L3	L4	L5	S1	S2
Proximal nerves						
Gluteus medius (gluteal nerves; internal rotation and abduction of hips)				■	□	
Gluteus maximus (gluteal nerves; extension of hips)				■	■	□
Femoral nerve						
Iliopsoas	■	□				
Quadriceps	□	■	■			
Obturator nerve						
Thigh adductors	■	■	□			
Sciatic nerve trunk*						
Hamstrings (knee flexion)				■	■	
Peroneal nerve*						
Tibialis anterior (dorsiflexion of ankle)			■	■		
Extensors of toes				■	□	
Peroneal longus (eversion of ankle)				■	■	
Tibial nerve*						
Tibialis posterior (inversion of ankle)			■	■		
Gastrocnemius					■	■
Flexor digitorum (curl toes)				■	■	■

Fig. 64.6   Innervation of the muscles of the leg. This figure indicates those spinal levels that usually (*dark blue shade*) and sometimes (*light blue shade*) contribute to the corresponding muscle; based on references.[4,8,9,12,14,53,54] The sciatic nerve trunk divides above the knee into the peroneal and tibial nerves; therefore, lesions of the sciatic nerve trunk affect muscles of all three branches (indicated by the asterisk in the figure; see text).

b. Lumbosacral Plexopathy

Unlike brachial plexus lesions, lumbosacral plexopathies tend to affect the entire leg (L2-S1) simultaneously, and discrete upper and lower plexus syndromes are rare.[55,56]

c. Peripheral Nerve Disorders

Peripheral nerve lesions weaken two or more muscles from a *single* peripheral nerve (which may belong to different spinal segments) and spare muscles from other nerves. For example, over 85% of patients with foot drop due to peroneal nerve injury have weak ankle dorsiflexion (L4-L5) and eversion (L5-S1) but preservation of inversion (i.e., same spinal segments but different nerve, the tibial nerve).[57]

The sciatic trunk divides into the peroneal and tibial nerves just above the knee. Lesions of the sciatic trunk may therefore affect any of the muscles listed under the sciatic nerve trunk, peroneal nerve, and tibial nerve headings of Fig. 64.6. Most patients with sciatic neuropathy have either greater involvement of the peroneal division (75% of patients) or equal involvement of the peroneal and tibial divisions (20% of patients). A sciatic neuropathy with greater involvement of the tibial nerve muscles is uncommon.[58]

The finding of weakness predominantly of the proximal leg muscles is unlikely in sciatic, peroneal, or tibial neuropathy because all of these nerves innervate muscles below the knee. Therefore, proximal weakness suggests femoral or obturator neuropathy; lumbosacral plexopathy or radiculopathy; or, if sensory findings are absent, muscle disease.

2. Sensory Findings

Radiculopathy causes sensory loss in a dermatomal pattern (see Table 62.1; Fig. 62.1 in Chapter 62), peripheral nerve lesions causes the sensory loss described in Fig. 64.7, and lumbosacral plexopathies tend to affect the entire leg.

A pure sensory syndrome is **meralgia paresthetica**, which consists of hypesthesia of the anterior and lateral thigh, usually caused by mechanical compression of the lateral femoral cutaneous nerve (e.g., obesity, pregnancy, or carpenter's belts).[59]

3. Reflexes

The three muscle stretch reflexes of the leg are the quadriceps reflex (femoral nerve, L2 to L4), medial hamstring reflex (L5), and Achilles reflex (tibial nerve, S1). The peroneal nerve does not contribute to the Achilles reflex. Consequently, in patients with foot drop, the finding of an asymmetrically diminished or absent ankle jerk *decreases* probability peroneal palsy and *increases* probability of sciatic neuropathy (87% have abnormal ankle jerk)[58] or lumbosacral radiculopathy (14% to 48% have an abnormal ankle jerk).[12,47,51,60,61]

4. Provocative Tests

The **straight leg raising** test is a traditional maneuver used to diagnose lumbosacral radiculopathy, which is usually caused by disc herniation. In the maneuver, the clinician lifts the extended leg of the supine patient, flexing the leg at the hip. In a positive response, the patient develops pain down the ipsilateral leg (if pain develops just in the hip or back, the test is considered negative). The **crossed straight leg raising** maneuver consists of pain in the affected leg when the clinician lifts the contralateral healthy limb. The pathogenesis of the sign is believed to be stretching of the sciatic nerve and its nerve roots.[62]

A positive straight leg raising test is sometimes called the **Lasègue sign**, after the French clinician Charles Lasègue (1816 to 1883), although Lasègue never published a description of the sign. His student Forst described the maneuver in his 1881 doctoral thesis, crediting Lasègue. An earlier description of the sign was published by Yugoslavian physician Lazarevic in 1880.[63–65]

The **femoral nerve stretch test** was designed to confirm an upper lumbar radiculopathy (i.e., L2 to L4 roots). In this test, the patient is positioned prone and the clinician passively flexes the

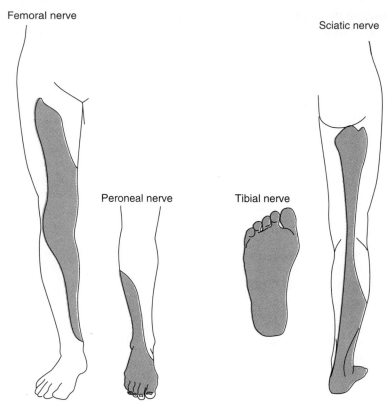

Fig. 64.7   Sensory branches of peripheral nerves of the leg. The two figures on the left depict the *front*
surface of the leg; the two on the right, the sole of foot and back of the leg. The sciatic nerve trunk divides
above the knee into the peroneal and tibial nerves; therefore, lesions of the sciatic nerve trunk affect sensation
from all three branches (i.e., *posterior thigh*, posterior cutaneous nerve of the thigh; *lateral calf and top of foot*,
peroneal nerve; and *sole of foot*, tibial nerve).

knee of the patient's affective limb. The positive response is pain in the patient's back and anterior
thigh, presumably from stretching of the irritated upper lumbar roots.[66,67]

C. CLINICAL SIGNIFICANCE

1. Lumbosacral Radiculopathy

EBM Boxes 64.4 and 64.5 review the diagnostic accuracy of the bedside examination in patients
with nerve pain of one leg (i.e., sciatica). EBM Box 64.4 applies to all patients with sciatica. EBM
Box 64.5 applies only to patients with known lumbosacral radiculopathy and addresses how accurately findings localize the level of the lesion.

In patients with sciatica, the findings that *increase* probability of disc herniation and lumbosacral radiculopathy[‡] are calf wasting (LR = 5.2), weak ankle dorsiflexion (LR = 4.9), the *crossed*
straight leg raising maneuver (LR = 3.4), and the absent ankle jerk (LR = 2.1). A *negative* straight
leg raising maneuver modestly *decreases* probability of disc herniation (LR = 0.4).

[‡]A L4-L5 disc compresses the L5 root and a L5-S1 disc compresses the S1 root.

EBM BOX 64.4	Diagnosing Lumbosacral Radiculopathy in Patients with Sciatica*

Finding (Reference)†	Sensitivity (%)	Specificity (%)	Likelihood Ratio‡ if Finding Is	
			Present	Absent
Motor examination				
Weak ankle dorsiflexion[51]	54	89	**4.9**	0.5
Ipsilateral calf wasting[51]	29	94	**5.2**	0.8
Sensory examination				
Leg sensation abnormal[51,60,61,68]	16–50	62–86	NS	NS
Reflex examination				
Abnormal ankle jerk[51,60,61,68]	14–48	73–93	2.1	0.8
Other tests				
Straight leg raising maneuver[48,51,61,68–72]	53–98	11–89	1.5	0.4
Crossed straight leg raising maneuver[51,69–71,73]	22–43	88–98	**3.4**	0.8

*Diagnostic standard: for *lumbosacral radiculopathy*, surgical findings,[48,51,69,70] electrodiagnosis,[60] or magnetic resonance imaging or computed tomography[61,68,71,72] indicating lumbosacral nerve root compression.
†Definition of findings: for *ipsilateral calf wasting*, maximum calf circumference at least 1 cm smaller than contralateral side[51]; for *straight leg raising maneuvers*, flexion at hip of supine patient's leg, extended at the knee, causes radiating pain in affected leg (pain confined to back or hip is negative response); for *crossed straight leg raising maneuver*, raising contralateral leg provokes pain in affected leg.
‡Likelihood ratio (LR) if finding present = positive LR; LR if finding absent = negative LR.
NS, Not significant.

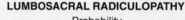

LUMBOSACRAL RADICULOPATHY
Probability

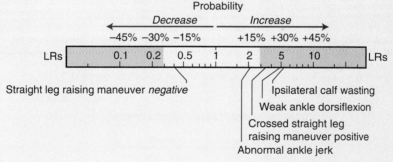

Some clinicians propose performing the straight leg raising maneuver in the seated patient whose hip is already flexed at 90°; the maneuver then consists of simply extending the knee. Two studies,[79,80] however, have demonstrated that this maneuver has diminished sensitivity compared to the traditional maneuver performed in the supine patient.

In patients with sciatica and lumbosacral radiculopathy (EBM Box 64.5), an abnormal quadriceps reflex (LR = 8.5) or weak knee extension (LR = 4) indicate the L3 or L4 level. A positive femoral stretch test also localizes the lesion to the upper lumbar level (L2 to L4; LR = 31.2). The best test for L5 radiculopathy is an asymmetric medial hamstring reflex (LR = 6.2) or L5 sensory

| EBM BOX 64.5 | Localizing Lumbosacral Radiculopathy* | | | |

Finding (Reference)[†]	Sensitivity (%)	Specificity (%)	Likelihood Ratio[‡] if Finding Is	
			Present	Absent
Motor Examination				
Weak knee extension, detecting L3 or L4 radiculopathy[60,66,74]	38–48	89–90	**4.0**	0.6
Weak hallux extension, detecting L5 radiculopathy[47,51,60,66]	12–62	54–91	1.7	0.7
Weak ankle dorsiflexion, detecting L5 radiculopathy[51,75]	37–62	51–77	NS	NS
Weak ankle plantarflexion, detecting S1 radiculopathy[51,60]	26–45	75–99	NS	0.7
Ipsilateral calf wasting, detecting S1 radiculopathy[51]	43	82	2.4	0.7
Sensory Examination				
Sensory loss L5 distribution, detecting L5 radiculopathy[47,51,75]	20–53	77–98	**3.1**	0.8
Sensory loss S1 distribution, detecting S1 radiculopathy[47,51,75]	32–49	70–90	2.4	0.7
Reflex Examination				
Asymmetric quadriceps reflex, detecting L3 or L4 radiculopathy[47,60,66,76]	29–56	93–96	**8.5**	0.7
Asymmetric medial hamstring reflex, detecting L5 radiculopathy[77]	57	91	**6.2**	0.5
Asymmetric Achilles reflex, detecting S1 radiculopathy[47,51,60,75,76,78]	45–91	53–94	2.7	0.5
Other Tests				
Femoral stretch test, detecting L2-L4 radiculopathy[66]	52	98	**31.2**	0.5

*Diagnostic standard: for *level of radiculopathy*, surgical findings and preoperative myelography,[47,51,75,76,78] myelography, magnetic resonance imaging,[66,74] or electrodiagnosis.[60]

[†]Definition of findings: for *weak knee extension*, manual muscle testing[60,74] or the *sit-to-stand test* (with the clinician holding the seated patient's hands as a balance aid only, the patient is *unable* to stand using the affected leg)[66]; for *ipsilateral calf wasting*, maximum calf circumference at least 1 cm smaller than contralateral side.[51]

[‡]Likelihood ratio (LR) if finding present = positive LR; LR if finding absent = negative LR.

NS, Not significant.

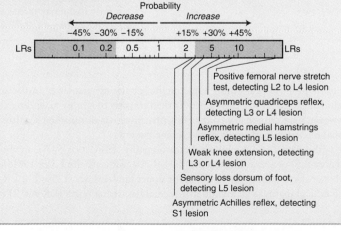

LOCALIZING LUMBOSACRAL RADICULOPATHY

loss (dorsum of the foot; LR = 3.1). The best predictors for the S1 level are sensory loss in the S1 distribution (lateral heel, LR = 2.4), reduced Achilles reflex (LR = 2.7), and ipsilateral calf wasting (LR = 2.4).

As discussed earlier, the finding of *proximal* muscle weakness (top row of Fig. 64.6) in a patient with distal limb symptoms convincingly argues for radiculopathy and against peripheral neuropathy. As an example, in one study of patients with foot drop from various causes, the finding of ipsilateral hip abductor weakness (i.e., gluteus medius weakness) accurately detected lumbosacral radiculopathy (sensitivity of 86%; specificity of 96%; positive LR = 24; negative LR = 0.1).[81]

2. Lumbosacral Plexopathy

a. Cancer Patients

In patients with known cancer and prior pelvic irradiation who present with lumbosacral plexopathy, findings confined to one leg increase probability of *recurrent tumor* (LR = 4.5) whereas findings in both legs increase probability of *radiation plexopathy* (LR = 7.5).[55]

b. Diabetic Amyotrophy.[82–87]

Diabetic amyotrophy (or **diabetic proximal neuropathy**) is a lumbosacral plexopathy of diabetic patients with presenting symptoms of weak thigh muscles and severe pain in the thighs or back, or both. The quadriceps, adductor, and iliopsoas muscles are weak 100% of the time, and the glutei and hamstrings 50% of the time (all are proximal muscles). The weakness may be unilateral or bilateral, but it is always asymmetric. Sensation is normal (70% of the time) or diminished over the thigh (30% of the time). The quadriceps reflex is absent in 80% of patients.

Although patients with diabetes also develop femoral neuropathy,[88] femoral neuropathy affects only thigh flexion and knee extension and spares other proximal leg muscles.

References may be accessed online at *Elsevier eBooks for Practicing Clinicians.*

Coordination and Cerebellar Testing

I. Introduction

In the 1920s, after closely observing patients with cerebellar tumors and World War I soldiers with gunshot wounds to the posterior fossa, the British neurologist Gordon Holmes concluded that four physical signs were fundamental to cerebellar disease: ataxia, nystagmus, hypotonia, and dysarthria.[1-5]

II. The Findings

A. ATAXIA

Ataxia refers to incoordinated voluntary movements that lack the speed, smoothness, and appropriate direction seen in normal persons. Because the cerebellum's role is to organize and administer movement, testing for ataxia is only possible in patients with adequate motor strength (i.e., 4 or 5 on the MRC scale; see Chapter 61). Tests of ataxia include observation of the patient's gait (see Chapter 7), the finger-nose-finger test, heel-knee-shin test, and rapid alternating movements.

1. Finger-Nose-Finger Test

In this test, the seated patient takes the index finger of his outstretched hand and alternately touches his or her own nose and the clinician's index finger being held a couple of feet away. The patient with cerebellar disease may misjudge the range of movement (i.e., **dysmetria**), overshooting the target (i.e., **hypermetria**, as in missing the nose and slapping the hand into his or her own face) or undershooting the target (i.e., **hypometria**, as in stopping before reaching the clinician's finger). The patient's finger also may deviate from a smooth course, especially if clinician shifts the target during the test. As the patient's finger approaches the target, an increasing side-to-side tremor may appear (i.e., **intention tremor** or kinetic tremor). Nonetheless, the term *intention tremor* can be confusing because it is applied to two distinct tremors, one of cerebellar disease and another of any action tremor that worsens as the hand approaches a target (e.g., the essential tremor that worsens as a soup spoon or cup approaches the patient's mouth; see Chapter 66). The intention tremor of cerebellar disease, however, is markedly *irregular*, large amplitude, low frequency (i.e., less than 5 Hz) and associated with dysmetria; whereas the intention tremor of essential tremor is *regular*, fine, rapid (8 to 12 Hz), and unassociated with dysmetria.[6]

2. Heel-Knee-Shin Test

In this test, the supine patient places the heel of one leg on the opposite knee and then slides it down the shin. Like the finger-to-nose test, a positive response may reveal any combination of ataxia, dysmetria, and intention tremor.

Decomposition of movement denotes an abnormal sequence of actions. For example, during the heel-knee-shin test, the patient may completely flex the hip before beginning to bend the knee, thus lifting the heel abnormally high in the air before lowering to complete the movement.[2]

3. Rapid Alternating Movements

Difficulty with rapid alternating movements is called **dysdiadochokinesia** (Babinski coined the original term *adiadochokinesis*).[3] The usual test is rapid pronation and supination of the forearm, but other tasks such as clapping hands, tapping a table, or stamping the foot are just as adequate.[3] In all these tests, the movements of patients with cerebellar disease are slower and significantly more irregular in rhythm, range, and accuracy.

B. NYSTAGMUS

1. Definition

Nystagmus is an involuntary to-and-fro oscillation of the eyes.[7] Nystagmus may be congenital or acquired, and the movements may affect both eyes (*bilateral*) or just one eye (*unilateral*). Bilateral nystagmus may be *conjugate*, which means both eyes have identical movements, or *dissociated*, which implies separate movements. Nystagmus may be *pendular*, which means the to- and fro-movements have the same velocity, or *rhythmic*, which means the movement is slow in one direction and quick in the other (rhythmic nystagmus is usually called jerk nystagmus). **Jerk nystagmus** is named after the direction of the quick component (e.g., right conjugate jerk nystagmus). Finally, the direction of the nystagmus may be horizontal, vertical, or rotatory.

2. Patterns of Nystagmus

Although nystagmus is a complicated subject that sometimes defies general principles*, several well recognized patterns are described next.

a. Cerebellar Nystagmus

The most common nystagmus of cerebellar disease is a conjugate horizontal jerk nystagmus on lateral gaze. (See the section on clinical significance.)

One rare type of nystagmus, **rebound nystagmus**, has been described only in patients with cerebellar disease.[8-10] To test for this nystagmus, the patient first looks to one direction (say, to the right). In patients with a positive response, a brisk nystagmus with its fast component to the right appears. If the patient continues looking in this direction for about 20 seconds, the nystagmus fatigues and disappears (sometimes even reversing direction). The patient then returns his eyes to

---

*One famous neuro-ophthalmologist once advised his students "never write on nystagmus, it will lead you nowhere."[25]

the primary position (i.e., straight ahead), and nystagmus to the left, not present initially, appears, although it fatigues over time. In these patients, the direction of the nystagmus in primary gaze can be reversed at will, depending on whether the patient looks first to the left or right.[8]

b. Nystagmus and Non-Cerebellar Disorders

Other useful patterns of nystagmus (not features of cerebellar disease) are optokinetic nystagmus (see Chapter 58), the nystagmus of internuclear ophthalmoplegia (see Chapter 59), and the nystagmus of vestibular disease (see Chapter 68).

3. Effect of Retinal Fixation

Retinal fixation means the patient is focusing his or her eyes on an object. Spontaneous nystagmus that diminishes during retinal fixation argues that the responsible lesion is located in the peripheral vestibular system; nystagmus that increases or remains unchanged during fixation argues that the lesion is in the central nervous system (i.e. brainstem or cerebellum). Neuro-ophthalmologists usually use electronystagmography to detect the effects of fixation (by comparing eye movements with eyes open with those with eyes closed), but general clinicians can accomplish the same during direct ophthalmoscopy: In a dimly lit room, the clinician examines the optic disc of one eye and compares its movements as the patient fixes the opposite eye on a distant target with those when the patient's opposite eye is covered. If rhythmic movements of the optic disc first appear or worsen when the fixating eye is occluded, a peripheral vestibular disturbance is likely.[11] A simpler version of this test, using just a penlight without ophthalmoscopy, has been proposed.[12]

C. HYPOTONIA (SEE CHAPTER 61)

The limbs of patients with cerebellar disease offer no resistance to passive displacement, sometimes resembling (in the words of Gordon Holmes) the "muscles of a person deeply under an anaesthetic, or of a corpse recently dead."[1] Holding the forearms vertically causes the wrist to bend to an angle much more acute than normal. Displacing the patient's outstretched arm downwards causes abnormally wide and prolonged up-and-down oscillations, even when the patient is requested to resist such movements. Striking the patellar tendon causes pendular knee jerks, traditionally defined as three or more swings,[13] although, as already stated in Chapter 61, this threshold will have to be revised upward because many normal persons also demonstrate three or more swings.[14]

D. DYSARTHRIA

The speech of patients with cerebellar disease is slow, slurred, and irregular in volume and rhythm, findings that are collectively referred to as **dysarthria**. In contrast to patients with aphasia, however, patients with dysarthria can name objects, repeat words, comprehend language, and speak sentences with words whose order makes sense.

III. Clinical Significance

A. INDIVIDUAL FINDINGS

1. Ataxia

Ataxia of gait is the most common finding in all cerebellar syndromes (see Table 65.1); therefore, examination of the gait should be part of the evaluation of any patient with suspected cerebellar disease. Many patients with cerebellar disease have difficulty walking despite the absence of all other findings of limb ataxia.

TABLE 65.1 ■ Unilateral Cerebellar Lesions*

Physical Finding[†]	Frequency (%)[‡]
Ataxia	
Gait ataxia	80–93
Limb ataxia	
Dysmetria	71–86
Intention tremor	29
Dysdiadochokinesia	47–69
Nystagmus	54–84
Hypotonia	76
Pendular knee jerks	37
Dysarthria	10–25

Diagnostic standard: clinical imaging, surgical findings, or postmortem examination.
[†]*Definition of findings*: see the text.
[‡]Results are overall mean frequency or, if statistically heterogenous, the range of values.
Data from 444 patients from references 13,17

Simple measurements of the patient's dysdiadochokinesia—such as how quickly and accurately the patient can alternately tap two buttons spaced about 12 inches apart[†]—are accurate measures of ataxia that correlate well with other measures of disability.[15]

2. Nystagmus

Seventy-five percent of cerebellar nystagmus is a conjugate horizontal jerk nystagmus that appears on lateral gaze (15% is a rotatory nystagmus and 10% a vertical nystagmus). Nonetheless, a horizontal jerk nystagmus is not specific for cerebellar disease and also occurs in peripheral vestibular disease and other central nervous system disorders. The direction of the jerk nystagmus has less localizing value than tests of ataxia. (See the section on cerebellar hemisphere syndrome.)

The clinical utility of rebound nystagmus is limited because it is a late finding, and all patients described with the finding have had many other obvious cerebellar signs.[8,9]

3. Dysarthria

Dysarthria, the least common of the fundamental cerebellar signs (see Table 65.1), appears more often with lesions of the left cerebellar hemisphere than with those of the right hemisphere.[16]

B. CEREBELLAR SYNDROMES

Most patients with cerebellar disease present with difficulty walking or headache, or both.[13,17] In adults, there are four common cerebellar syndromes, each of which is characterized by a different distribution of the principal cerebellar signs.

1. Cerebellar Hemisphere Syndrome

a. Cerebellar Findings

Table 65.1 presents the physical findings of 444 patients with focal lesions (mostly tumors) confined to one hemisphere.[13,17] According to traditional teachings, cerebellar signs appear on the side of the body *ipsilateral* to the lesion. This teaching proved generally correct in the patients of

---

[†]Ninety percent of normal persons can accomplish at least 32 taps within 15 seconds, whereas 90% of patients with cerebellar ataxia cannot.[15]

Table 65.1, in whom signs of limb ataxia (i.e., dysmetria, intention tremor, dysdiadochokinesia) were unilateral 85% of the time, and, if unilateral, were on the side ipsilateral to the lesion 80% to 90% of the time. These patients also had more hypotonia on the side of the lesion and tended to fall toward the side of the lesion when walking.

Nystagmus has less localizing value. When present, nystagmus is unilateral in only 65% of patients, and in these patients the direction of nystagmus points to the side of the lesion only 70% of the time.

b. Associated Findings

Despite having a lesion confined to the cerebellum, patients with structural cerebellar lesions may also have (1) cranial nerve findings (10% to 20% of patients; usually of cranial nerves V, VI, VII, or VIII, ipsilateral to the side of the lesion 75% of the time[13,17]; (2) altered mental status (38% of patients, from compression of the brainstem or complicating hydrocephalus); (3) upper motor neuron signs such as hyperactive reflexes and the Babinski sign (28% of patients); and (4) papilledema (68% of patients).

In contrast, severe weakness and sensory disturbance are both uncommon, affecting only 4%.

2. Anterior Cerebellar Degeneration (Rostral Vermis Syndrome)[18]

In contrast to the cerebellar hemisphere syndrome, these patients have ataxia of gait (100%) and of both legs (88%) with relative sparing of the arms (only 16% of patients). Nystagmus and dysarthria also are much less frequent (9%, for both findings). This syndrome most often results from chronic alcohol ingestion.

3. Pancerebellar Syndrome

This syndrome causes the same signs listed in Table 65.1, but instead of being on one side of the body, the cerebellar signs are symmetric. Causes include drug intoxication (e.g., phenytoin), inherited disorders, and paraneoplastic syndromes.

4. Cerebellar Infarction

The physical signs of cerebellar infarction resemble those of the cerebellar hemisphere syndrome described above, with three exceptions: In infarction, (1) all the signs appear *abruptly*, (2) dysarthria is more prominent (44% of patients), and (3) weakness occurs more often (22% have hemiparesis; 24% have tetraparesis).[19–22] The three main arteries supplying the cerebellum are the superior cerebellar artery, anterior inferior cerebellar artery, and posterior inferior cerebellar artery.[23] An associated lateral medullary syndrome (see Table 62.2 in Chapter 62) suggests an infarct in the distribution of the posterior inferior cerebellar artery.[21,24]

The **acute vestibular syndrome**—the abrupt onset of sustained vertigo, nausea and vomiting, and imbalance—raises the possibility of cerebellar infarction as well as peripheral vestibular disease. This subject is fully discussed in Chapter 68.

References may be accessed online at *Elsevier eBooks for Practicing Clinicians.*

PART 13

Selected Neurologic Disorders

Tremor and Parkinson Disease

- The diagnosis of Parkinson disease is based on bedside findings.
- The three cardinal findings of Parkinson disease are bradykinesia, rest tremor, and rigidity. *Parkinsonism* is defined as bradykinesia in combination with either rest tremor, rigidity, or both.
- Some patients with parkinsonism have Parkinson disease. Others have mimicking neurodegenerative disorders collectively called Parkinson-plus or atypical parkinsonian disorders.
- In patients with parkinsonism, the following findings *increase* probability of Parkinson disease: asymmetric onset, absence of atypical features, positive response to levodopa, and asymmetric arm swing when walking.
- In patients with parkinsonism, the following findings *decrease* probability of Parkinson disease: inability to perform a 10-step tandem walk, positive applause sign, and presence of atypical features (i.e., marked autonomic dysfunction, early dementia, pyramidal tract or cerebellar findings, difficulty looking down, use of neuroleptic medications).

I. Introduction

In a remarkably concise essay published in 1817, the British physician James Parkinson described in nine pages most of the features we now associate with Parkinson disease—insidious onset, asymmetric rest tremor, bradykinesia, postural instability, sialorrhea, flexed posture, shuffling steps, and festinating gait.[1] One sign Parkinson failed to describe was rigidity, an oversight leading many historians to believe Parkinson never actually touched a patient and instead based his conclusions solely on observation.[2] In 1877, Charcot provided the first full account of Parkinson disease that included rigidity.[2]

II. The Finding

The three cardinal findings in Parkinson disease are rest tremor, bradykinesia, and cogwheel rigidity (rigidity is discussed fully in Chapter 61). A patient with bradykinesia in combination with either rest tremor, rigidity, or both is said to have **parkinsonism**.[3]

A. TREMOR

A **tremor** is a rhythmic involuntary oscillation of a body part. There are two basic tremors: (1) **rest tremor** and (2) **action tremor**.[4-6]

Rest tremors occur when muscles are inactive and the body part is completed supported against gravity. Action tremors occur during voluntary contraction of muscle and are further subdivided into **postural tremors** (e.g., when holding the arms outstretched), **intention tremors** (e.g., when a limb approaches a visually-guided target such as finger-nose-finger testing), **task-related tremors** (e.g., when pouring water from cup to cup), and **isometric tremors** (e.g., when making a fist or gripping the examiner's fingers).* One confusing tremor is a postural tremor (i.e., action tremor) that continues after the examiner supports the outstretched arms (thus mimicking a rest tremor): if such patients are given a glass of water to drink, the amplitude of true postural tremor increases or remains the same as the glass approaches the patient's mouth, whereas that of the genuine rest tremor diminishes in amplitude.

Movement disorder specialists have identified at least a dozen types of tremor, the most common being essential tremor and parkinsonian rest tremor.[4-6] **Essential tremor** is a 4- to 12 Hz[†] bilateral postural tremor that usually involves the hands or forearms. It may be asymmetric and have an associated kinetic component (i.e., associated intention or task-related component). In contrast, the **parkinsonian rest tremor** (which is only one of the different tremors that may appear in Parkinson disease) is a 4- to 6 Hz "pill-rolling" tremor of the fingertips, hand, or forearm. It begins *asymmetrically*, initially in one hand, followed years later by involvement of the contralateral hand. Essential tremor may involve the jaw, tongue, or head (producing a characteristic rhythmic "nodding yes" or "shaking no" motion); the Parkinsonian tremor may involve jaw, lips, or tongue but spares the head.

B. BRADYKINESIA

Bradykinesia describes movements with two characteristics: abnormal slowness and diminished amplitude. Clinicians detect bradykinesia by simple observation during the interview or by various tests, such as finger tapping, pronation-supination movements, or foot tapping.[3] One additional test for bradykinesia is to observe the patient's blink rate. Normal persons blink about 24 ± 15 times per minute, whereas patients with Parkinson disease blink more slowly, about 12 ± 10 times per minute. Severely symptomatic patients blink only 5 to 6 times per minute.[7,8] The contrast between the reduced spontaneous blink rate but exaggerated reflex blink rate (during glabellar reflex testing, see Chapter 63) is striking in Parkinson disease. During treatment with levodopa, the spontaneous blink rate increases as the reflex rate during glabellar testing diminishes.[9,10]

C. ATYPICAL FEATURES OF PARKINSON DISEASE

Confirming the diagnosis of Parkinson disease during life is difficult because the disorder still lacks biochemical, genetic, or imaging diagnostic standards. In patients diagnosed during life with Parkinson disease, 10% to 25% have an alternative diagnosis discovered at postmortem examination.[11-16] These alternative mimicking conditions consist of a variety of neurodegenerative disorders collectively referred to as **Parkinson-plus syndromes** (or atypical parkinsonian syndromes), disorders that tend to progress more rapidly, present more symmetrically, and respond less well to levodopa than does Parkinson disease.[17] Several clinical clues, called **atypical features**, suggest one of these mimicking Parkinson-plus disorders: (1) marked autonomic dysfunction (e.g., postural hypotension, neurogenic bladder or bowel), (2) early severe dementia, (3) pyramidal tract findings

---

Intention tremor and *task-related tremor* are sometimes collectively called *kinetic tremors*, i.e., action tremors appearing during movement.

[†]"Hz" indicates "hertz," a unit of frequency equal to one cycle per second. A Parkinsonian tremor of 5 Hz, therefore, has 300 oscillations per minute (i.e., 5×60), thus explaining why this tremor sometimes produces electrocardiographic artifacts mimicking tachyarrhythmias (e.g., atrial flutter or ventricular tachycardia).

(i.e., hyperreflexia, spasticity, or Babinski sign; see Chapter 61), (4) cerebellar findings (i.e., limb ataxia, gait ataxia, or nystagmus; see Chapter 65), (5) supranuclear gaze palsy (i.e., difficulty looking down), (6) use of neuroleptic medications, (7) multiple prior strokes, and (8) encephalitis at the time of onset of symptoms.[3,11]

The most common Parkinson-plus syndromes are multiple system atrophy, progressive supranuclear palsy, and vascular parkinsonism.[‡]

D. TANDEM GAIT TESTING (SEE ALSO CHAPTER 7)

The gait of patients with Parkinson disease has a much narrower base than that of most Parkinson-plus patients, leading neurologists to wonder whether tandem gait testing might more easily provoke imbalance in patients with Parkinson-plus disorders, thus distinguishing them from Parkinson disease. According to this hypothesis, inability to complete 10 tandem steps would suggest a Parkinson-plus disorder, not Parkinson disease.

A similar sign addressing balance is the **bicycle sign**.[18] This sign, which reflects the better balance of patients with Parkinson disease, should be applied only to patients with parkinsonism who were bicycle riders just before the onset of their symptoms. According to this sign, the *ability* to continue riding a bicycle after onset of their symptoms favors Parkinson disease, whereas the *inability* to continue riding favors Parkinson-plus disorders.

E. APPLAUSE SIGN (CLAPPING TEST)

The **applause sign** refers to the tendency of some patients to continue clapping their hands in response to instructions to clap three times. Initially, the sign was proposed as a way to distinguish progressive supranuclear palsy (more than three claps, i.e., a positive applause sign) from Parkinson disease (only three claps),[19] although subsequently a positive applause sign has been noticed in many other neurodegenerative disorders, especially those causing frontal lobe dysfunction.[20] To perform the sign, the clinician asks the patient to clap three times as quickly as possible and then demonstrates the clapping. The patient's response is normal if he or she claps just three times and abnormal if there are more than three claps. The exact cause of the abnormal applause sign is unknown, although many believe it could be related to frontal disinhibition.[21,22]

III. Clinical Significance: Diagnosing Parkinson Disease

In patients with combinations of tremor, bradykinesia, and rigidity (i.e., patients with parkinsonism), the following symptoms increase probability of Parkinson disease: the complaint of feet suddenly freezing in doorways (likelihood ratio [LR] = 4.4), voice progressively becoming softer (LR = 3.2), or handwriting becoming progressively smaller (i.e., micrographia, LR = 2.7).[23,24]

The following physical findings also increase probability of pathologic Parkinson disease: the combined presence of all three cardinal features, asymmetric onset, and no atypical features (LR = 4.1, see EBM Box 66.1), a good response to levodopa (LR = 4.1), and asymmetric arm swing when walking (LR = 2.7). Inability to perform 10 tandem steps (LR = 0.2), absence of good response to levodopa (LR = 0.2), and positive applause sign (LR = 0.3) decrease probability of Parkinson disease.

[‡]**Multiple system atrophy** has three phenotypes: *Shy-Drager syndrome* (early autonomic insufficiency is prominent), *olivopontocerebellar atrophy* (cerebellar signs are prominent), and *striatonigral degeneration* (both cerebellar and pyramidal tract signs are prominent). **Vascular parkinsonism** refers to parkinsonism that appears abruptly after a stroke; neuroimaging reveals subcortical or deep brain infarction.

Two studies examining the bicycle sign in patients with parkinsonism (who were bicycle riders at onset of symptoms) showed that the *ability* to continue riding the bicycle favored Parkinson disease (LR = 2.4).[18,27]

In patients with parkinsonism, the presence of cerebellar signs (LR = 6.6, EBM Box 66.1), autonomic dysfunction (LR = 4.3), or speech/bulbar signs (LR = 4.1) increase the probability of multiple system atrophy. The combination of a downgaze palsy and early postural instability from axial rigidity increases probability of progressive supranuclear palsy (LR = 9.5). The presence of

EBM BOX 66.1	Suspected Parkinson Disease*			
			Likelihood Ratio‡ if Finding Is	
Finding (Reference)†	Sensitivity (%)	Specificity (%)	Present	Absent
Diagnosing parkinson disease				
Unable to perform 10 tandem steps[25–27]	8–33	9–23	0.2	4.6
Asymmetric arm swing[28]	59	79	2.7	0.5
Positive applause sign[19–21,29]	3–30	27–42	0.3	2.4
Tremor, bradykinesia, rigidity[11]				
3 of 3 present	64	71	2.2	0.5
3 of 3 present, asymmetry, no atypical features	68	83	4.1	0.4
Good response to levodopa[30,31]	86–98	53–90	4.1	0.2
Diagnosing multiple system atrophy				
Rapid progression[32,33]	54–64	78	2.5	0.6
Absence of tremor[32–34]	39–91	39–76	NS	NS
Speech and/or bulbar signs[32]	87	79	4.1	0.2
Autonomic dysfunction[32–34]	73–84	74–90	4.3	0.3
Cerebellar signs[32,34,35]	32–63	90–99	6.6	0.6
Pyramidal signs[32,34,35]	31–50	82–93	3.0	0.7
Dementia[32,34]	17–25	36–45	0.3	1.9
Diagnosing progressive supranuclear palsy				
Downgaze palsy and postural instability within first year of symptoms[36–38]	35–50	93–99	9.5	0.6
Diagnosing vascular parkinsonism				
Pyramidal tract signs[39–43]	26–72	92–99	16.2	0.5
Lower body parkinsonism[39–41]	59–69	88–91	6.1	0.4

All LRs apply only to patients with suspected Parkinson disease (i.e., combinations of tremor, bradykinesia, and rigidity).

*Diagnostic standard: for *Parkinson disease*, careful clinical observation[19–21,25,26,28,29] or postmortem examination of brain revealing depletion of nigral pigmented neurons with Lewy bodies in remaining nerve cells (all other studies); for *progressive supranuclear palsy*, pathologic examination; for *vascular parkinsonism*, infarction on neuroimaging or postmortem examination revealing cerebrovascular disease and absence of depigmentation and Lewy bodies.[42]

†Definition of findings: for *atypical features*, see text; for *rapid progression*, the appearance of unsteadiness and tendency to fall at initial visit[32] or within 3 years of onset of first symptom[33]; for *speech or bulbar findings*, dysarthria, dysphagia, and excessive sialorrhoea; for *autonomic dysfunction*, symptomatic postural hypotension, urinary urge or fecal incontinence, or neurogenic bladder[32] or abnormalities on formal testing of cardiovascular reflexes[33]; for *cerebellar findings, applause sign*, and *pyramidal tract findings*, see text.

‡Likelihood ratio (LR) if finding present = positive LR; LR if finding absent = negative LR.

NS, Not significant.

continued

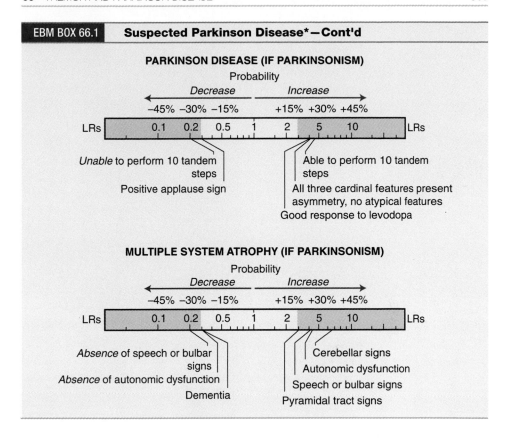

| EBM BOX 66.1 | **Suspected Parkinson Disease*—Cont'd** |

PARKINSON DISEASE (IF PARKINSONISM)

Probability

Decrease　　　　*Increase*

−45% −30% −15%　　　+15% +30% +45%

LRs　　0.1　0.2　0.5　1　2　5　10　LRs

Unable to perform 10 tandem steps
Positive applause sign

Able to perform 10 tandem steps
All three cardinal features present asymmetry, no atypical features
Good response to levodopa

MULTIPLE SYSTEM ATROPHY (IF PARKINSONISM)

Probability

Decrease　　　　*Increase*

−45% −30% −15%　　　+15% +30% +45%

LRs　　0.1　0.2　0.5　1　2　5　10　LRs

Absence of speech or bulbar signs
Absence of autonomic dysfunction
Dementia

Cerebellar signs
Autonomic dysfunction
Speech or bulbar signs
Pyramidal tract signs

pyramidal tract signs increases probability of vascular parkinsonism (LR = 16.2) and multiple system atrophy (LR = 3). Parkinsonian findings confined to the legs suggests vascular parkinsonism (LR = 6.1), as does abrupt onset of parkinsonian findings (LR = 21.9).[40,41]

References may be accessed online at *Elsevier eBooks for Practicing Clinicians.*

Hemorrhagic Versus Ischemic Stroke

I. Introduction

Stroke is the fifth leading cause of death in the United States.[1] The two fundamental subtypes of strokes are **hemorrhagic stroke** (intracerebral hemorrhage or subarachnoid hemorrhage) and **ischemic stroke** (infarction from thrombosis or embolism). In the United States, 87% of strokes are ischemic and 13% are hemorrhagic (10% are intracerebral and 3% are subarachnoid),[1] but in some developing nations more than 50% of strokes are hemorrhagic.[2,3] All patients with stroke require prompt neuroimaging to distinguish these subtypes and direct management, although bedside examination is still helpful when neuroimaging is unavailable and while monitoring patients during treatment.[4]

Since the times of ancient Babylonia, Greece, and Rome, clinicians have recognized stroke, calling it *apoplexy*.[5,6] Although ancient physicians understood that damage to one cerebral hemisphere produced weakness on the opposite side of the body, modern concepts of cerebrovascular disease were lacking until 1655, when Johann Jakob Wepfer, a Swiss physician, first described intracranial hemorrhage, both its clinical features and postmortem findings.[7]

II. Findings

Both cerebral hemorrhage and infarction cause abrupt *deficits* of neurologic function, such as hemiparesis, aphasia, hemisensory disturbance, ophthalmoplegia, visual field defects, and ataxia. Nonetheless, cerebral hemorrhage differs from infarction by the presence of an *expanding* hemorrhage within the brain, which may produce *additional* symptoms beyond neurologic deficits (Fig. 67.1). Examples of

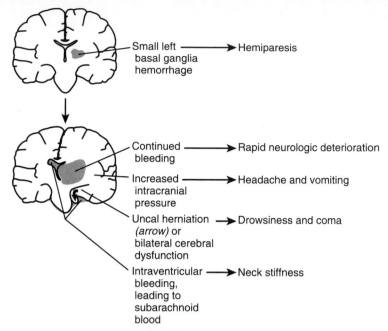

Fig. 67.1 "Additional" findings of hemorrhagic stroke (coronal section of brain). *Top half*: There is a small hemorrhage in the left basal ganglia, causing hemiparesis and clinical findings indistinguishable from ischemic stroke. *Bottom half*: Progressive intracranial hemorrhage causes the "additional" findings of hemorrhage, including rapid neurologic deterioration, headache, vomiting, coma, and neck stiffness. Intraventricular blood follows the normal path of cerebrospinal circulation through the median and lateral apertures of the fourth ventricle to reach the subarachnoid space at the base of the brain (only rarely does intracerebral hemorrhage directly rupture in the subarachnoid space).

additional symptoms are prominent vomiting (from increased intracranial pressure), severe headache (from meningeal irrigation or increased intracranial pressure), rapid progression of neurologic deficits (from expansion of the hematoma), coma (from bilateral cerebral dysfunction, uncal herniation, or posterior fossa mass effect), and bilateral Babinski signs (from bilateral dysfunction).

Over the last several decades, clinicians have developed several different stroke scores to distinguish hemorrhagic from ischemic infarction,[4] but the most widely used is the Siriraj Stroke Score, developed by Poungvarin[8] in 1991 (Table 67.1).

III. Clinical Significance

The data in EBM Boxes 67.1 and 67.2 stem from analysis of 40 studies enrolling more than 11,000 patients with stroke from across the globe. The diagnosis of hemorrhagic stroke in these studies includes both intracranial and subarachnoid hemorrhage, although relatively few patients had subarachnoid hemorrhage. Diagnostic accuracy of bedside findings is the same if patients with subarachnoid hemorrhage are excluded.[4]

A. SYMPTOMS

According to a systematic review,[4] the following symptoms increase probability of hemorrhagic stroke: seizures accompanying the neurologic deficit (likelihood ratio [LR] = 4.7), vomiting

(LR = 3), headache (LR = 2.9), and loss of consciousness (LR = 2.6). A history of prior transient ischemic attack decreases probability of hemorrhagic stroke (LR = 0.3).

B. INDIVIDUAL PHYSICAL FINDINGS

According to the LRs in EBM Box 67.1, the physical findings that increase probability of hemorrhagic stroke the most are coma (LR = 6.3), neurologic deterioration during the first 3 hours (LR = 5.8), neck stiffness (LR = 5.4), systolic blood pressure greater than 220 mm Hg (LR = 4), and Babinski response in both toes (LR = 2.4).

TABLE 67.1 ■ **Siriraj Stroke Score***

Characteristic	Points
Mental status[†]	
Coma	+ 5
Semicoma	+ 2.5
Vomiting	+ 2
Headache within 2 hours	+ 2
Diastolic blood pressure	+ 0.1 × DBP in mm Hg
Diabetes, angina, or intermittent claudication	−3
Correction factor	−12

*From reference 8. Interpretation of total score: >1 hemorrhage; −1 to 1 uncertain; < −1 infarction.
†Alert *mental status* receives 0 points.
DBP, Diastolic blood pressure.

EBM BOX 67.1   **Hemorrhagic Stroke***

Finding (Reference)[†]	Sensitivity (%)	Specificity (%)	Likelihood Ratio[‡] if Finding Is Present	Likelihood Ratio[‡] if Finding Is Absent
Vital signs				
Systolic BP >220 mm Hg[9]	17	96	**4.0**	NS
Systolic BP <160 mm Hg[10,11]	13–29	30–55	0.4	1.9
Additional findings				
Mental status[8,10,12–15]				
Coma	18–51	90–99	**6.3**	...
Drowsy	17–59	...	1.7	...
Alert	21–54	21–41	0.5	...
Neurologic deterioration during first 3 hours[16]	77–81	85–88	**5.8**	0.2
Kernig or Brudzinski sign[16,17]	3–15	98	NS	NS
Neck stiffness[3,8,10,16–18]	16–48	81–98	**5.4**	0.7
Babinski response[8,18,19]				
Both toes extensor	12–22	90–95	2.4	...
Single toe extensor	30–73	....	NS	...
Both toes flexor	8–48	40–75	0.5	...
Neurologic deficits				
Deviation of eyes[13,18,19]	27–62	64–81	1.9	0.7
Hemiparesis[12,13,18–21]	17–87	12–73	NS	NS
Aphasia[13,18,22]	12–35	62–92	NS	NS

(continued)

| EBM BOX 67.1 | Hemorrhagic Stroke*—Cont'd | | | | |

| Finding (Reference)[†] | Sensitivity (%) | Specificity (%) | Likelihood Ratio[‡] if Finding Is | |
			Present	Absent
Hemisensory disturbance[12,13,18,19]	0–80	40–98	1.3	NS
Hemianopia[13]	35	73	1.3	NS
Ataxia[13]	15	80	NS	NS
Other findings				
Cervical bruit[10,13]	1	81–93	**0.1**	NS
Atrial fibrillation on ECG[12,16,18,19,23]	1–21	60–91	**0.3**	1.3

*Diagnostic standard: for *hemorrhagic stroke*, computed tomography (all studies), sometimes with magnetic resonance imaging[15] or autopsy.[15,24]

[†]Definition of findings: for *both toes extensor,* the Babinski response is *present* in both feet; for *both toes flexor,* the Babinski response is *absent* in both feet.

[‡]Likelihood ratio (LR) if finding present = positive LR; LR if finding absent = negative LR.

BP, Blood pressure; *ECG,* electrocardiogram; *NS,* not significant.

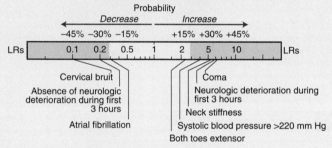

HEMORRHAGIC STROKE

| EBM BOX 67.2 | Siriraj Score for Hemorrhagic Stroke* | | | | |

| Finding (Reference)[†] | Sensitivity (%) | Specificity (%) | Likelihood Ratio[‡] if Finding Is | |
			Present	Absent
Siriraj score "hemorrhage" (>1)	23–87	65–99	**5.7**	…
Siriraj score "uncertain (−1 to 1)	1–51	…	NS	…
Siriraj score "infarction (<−1)	3–53	13–60	**0.3**	…

*Diagnostic standard: for *hemorrhagic stroke*, see EBM Box 67.1. Based on references 3,8,11,16–18,20,24–41.

[†]For calculation of *Siriraj score*, see Table 67.1.

[‡]Likelihood ratio (LR) if finding present = positive LR; LR if finding absent = negative LR.

NS, Not significant.

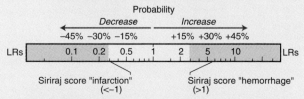

HEMORRHAGIC STROKE - SIRIRAJ SCORE

The findings that decrease probability of hemorrhagic stroke the most are cervical bruit (LR = 0.1), absence of neurologic deterioration during the first 3 hours (LR = 0.2), and presence of atrial fibrillation (LR = 0.3).

As expected (see the section on findings) the presence or absence of neurologic *deficits*—hemiparesis, hemisensory disturbance, deviation of eyes, aphasia, hemianopia, and ataxia—fail to distinguish hemorrhagic from ischemic stroke.

C. COMBINED FINDINGS (SIRIRAJ STROKE SCORE)

A Siriraj score of greater than 1 (hemorrhage) increases probability of hemorrhagic stroke (LR = 5.7, EBM Box 67.2), while a score less than −1 (infarction) decreases probability (LR = 0.3). Nonetheless, in these studies an average of 19% of patients with stroke (range 8% to 48%) were classified as "uncertain" by the Siriraj score, a score lacking diagnostic value (LR is not significant).

References may be accessed online at *Elsevier eBooks for Practicing Clinicians.*

Acute Vertigo and Imbalance

I. Introduction

Acute sustained vertigo and imbalance, often associated with nausea and vomiting, is collectively called the **acute vestibular syndrome** (or **acute vestibulopathy**). Most affected patients have benign disorders of the peripheral vestibular system, either dysfunction of the vestibular nerve (**vestibular neuritis**) or labyrinth (**labyrinthitis**). A few affected patients, however, are experiencing serious strokes of the cerebellum or brainstem, problems that may rapidly cause coma and death from acute hydrocephalus or brainstem compression.[1-3]

The full syndrome of brainstem stroke causing vertigo is described in Chapter 62 (see lateral medullary, or Wallenberg, stroke) and that of cerebellar infarction appears in Chapter 65. Nonetheless, 5% to 17% of strokes causing dizziness present as *isolated* dizziness or vertigo without other telltale cerebellar and brainstem findings.[4,5] This chapter focuses on these patients and discusses additional bedside findings that help distinguish stroke from peripheral vestibular disease.

II. The Findings

The additional findings that suggest stroke in acutely dizzy patients are *normal* bilateral vestibuloocular reflexes (detected by the head-impulse test), skew deviation, abnormal visual tracking (saccadic pursuit), and direction-changing nystagmus.

A. THE VESTIBULOOCULAR REFLEX

In healthy humans, any head movement is involuntarily matched by opposing conjugate movements of the eyes through the actions of the **vestibuloocular reflex**. Without this reflex, it would be impossible to focus on objects when walking, riding, or even breathing.* The accuracy and efficiency of this reflex can be easily demonstrated by holding a pencil vertically in front of the face and moving it side to side through a 10-degree arc, 5 times per second. The pencil will appear blurred because the retina cannot compensate quickly enough for the shifting image. If the experiment is repeated with the pencil stationary and the head moved back and forth through the same arc and with the same frequency, the pencil remains sharply defined. The eye movements are *identical* in the two examples, yet only in the second experiment is the vestibuloocular reflex employed to keep the pencil in focus.[7]

The vestibuloocular reflex stabilizes retinal images by specific connections between the semicircular canals and eye muscles (Fig. 68.1). When there is unilateral damage to the neural pathways of this reflex, two consequences follow: (1) unopposed stimulation of six eye muscles, three on each side, causes prominent vertigo and nystagmus and (2) a deficient vestibuloocular reflex is conspicuous when the head is turned to the affected side, a disorder best identified by the head impulse test.

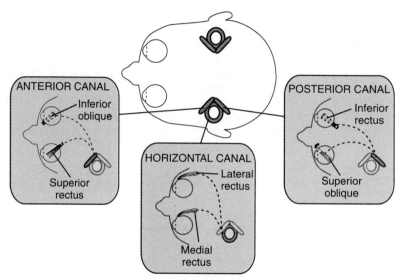

Fig. 68.1 Connections between semicircular canals and eye muscles. Each of the *blue-shaded boxes* illustrates the orientation and specific connections between the semicircular canals —the anterior canal on *left*, the horizontal canal in *middle*, and the posterior canal on *right*—and specific eye muscles (in these drawings, the semicircular canals are greatly magnified). Importantly, there are six semicircular canals (three on each side) and twelve eye muscles (six on each side). Therefore, each semicircular canal is yoked to two eye muscles, one on each side, muscles that pull the eyes conjugately *in the same plane* as the paired canal. The anterior canal is linked to the ipsilateral superior rectus and contralateral inferior oblique (both muscles are oriented in the same plane as the canal); the horizontal canal, to the ipsilateral medial rectus and contralateral lateral rectus; and the posterior semicircular canal, to the ipsilateral superior oblique and contralateral inferior rectus. When a person's head rotates in a plane perpendicular to the left posterior semicircular canal, for example, movements of the left superior oblique muscle and right inferior rectus muscle (muscles in the same plane of the left posterior semicircular canal) move the eyes in the exact opposite direction, thus stabilizing the retinal image. From information in reference 8.

---

*A dramatic description of life without the vestibuloocular reflex appears in the story "Living without a balancing mechanism,"[6] written by a physician with bilateral vestibular damage after long-term streptomycin treatment. He describes difficulty reading in bed and having to brace his "head between two metal bars at the head of the bed (to) minimize the effect of the pulse beat, which made the letters on the page jump and blur."

B. HEAD IMPULSE TEST (FIG. 68.2)

First described by Halmagyi in 1988,[10] the head impulse test demonstrates the integrity of the vestibuloocular reflex. The clinician sits in front of the patient and places his or her hands on each side of the patient's head. Throughout the test, the patient is asked to focus on the clinician's nose while the clinician focuses on the patient's eyes. If the vestibuloocular reflex is intact, the patient can maintain gaze on the clinician's nose during rapid head movements to both sides, and no corrective saccades are observed at the end of the head movement. If the peripheral vestibular system (and vestibuloocular reflex) is abnormal, however, the eyes move away with the rotating head when turned to the abnormal side and, at the end of rotation, the patient's eyes quickly move back to pick up the image of the clinician's nose (i.e., the clinician observes a **corrective saccade**). When compared to asymmetric caloric responses (the traditional definition of the unilateral peripheral

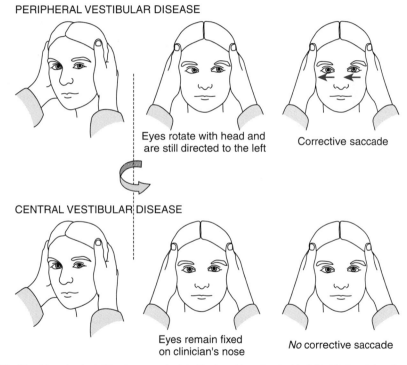

PERIPHERAL VESTIBULAR DISEASE

Eyes rotate with head and are still directed to the left

Corrective saccade

CENTRAL VESTIBULAR DISEASE

Eyes remain fixed on clinician's nose

No corrective saccade

Fig. 68.2 Head-impulse test. The *top row* depicts the head impulse test in left-sided *peripheral* vestibular disease; the *bottom row*, in *central* vestibular disease (e.g., stroke). In this example, the clinician is testing the patient's left ear (and left vestibuloocular reflex) by first positioning the patient's head 20 degrees to the *patient's* right (*left* column) and then rapidly rotating the head to the straight-ahead position (*middle* column). Throughout the test, the patient is asked to focus on the clinician's nose. The most important observation is what the clinician observes immediately following head rotation (*right* column). In peripheral vestibular disease (*top row*), there is a *corrective saccade (arrows)* revealing a deficient vestibuloocular reflex and the patient's attempt to focus again on the clinician's nose. In central vestibular disease (*bottom row*), the intact vestibuloocular reflex allows the patient's eyes to track the clinician's nose throughout the rotation and no corrective saccade appears. When performing the test, neuro-otologists usually start with a warm up period of slow movements back and forth to help the patient relax, thus permitting the more rapid movements necessary for the test. Most experts perform many trials, randomly to one side or the other; the test is abnormal if most trials to one side (e.g., two out of three) reveal the corrective saccade. In patients with peripheral disease, the more rapid the initial head movement, the greater the amplitude of the corrective saccade.[9]

vestibular disease), the abnormal head impulse test (i.e., corrective saccade present) has a sensitivity of 34% to 57%, specificity of 90% to 99%, positive likelihood ratio [LR] = 6.7, and negative LR = 0.6.[11-13]

In patients with acute vertigo or dizziness, a *normal* vestibuloocular reflex bilaterally (i.e., *no* corrective saccades observed) *decreases* the probability of the peripheral vestibular system and suggests the cause of the dizziness is central (e.g., stroke).

An excellent online video of the abnormal head impulse test (with corrective saccades) appears in the supplementary material of reference by Edlow.[14] The only reported complication of the test is complete heart block, observed in a single patient, presumably induced by vasovagal reaction.[15] †

C. SKEW DEVIATION

Skew deviation refers to an acquired hypertropia, which means one eye is aligned higher than the other, a sign of cerebellar or brainstem disease. It is best revealed by the alternate cover test, a test discussed in Chapter 59.

D. ABNORMAL VISUAL TRACKING: SACCADIC PURSUIT

The patient is asked to follow a slowly moving small target (e.g., clinician's finger) both horizontally and vertically (the patient's head is still). Most patients have no difficulty following the target (i.e., the pursuit is smooth), but some patients with cerebellar or brainstem disease instead reveal conspicuous quick "catch-up" movements, called **saccadic pursuit**.

E. DIRECTION-CHANGING NYSTAGMUS (FIG. 68.3)

Many patients with acute vertigo have a spontaneous conjugate jerk nystagmus when looking straight ahead (Chapter 65 defines the terms used to describe nystagmus).‡ In most patients, whether the disorder is peripheral or central, the nystagmus will persist or worsen when they look *in the direction* of the quick component of the nystagmus. The distinguishing finding appears when the patient looks in the *opposite* direction, i.e., contralateral to the quick component of the nystagmus. In patients with peripheral disease, the nystagmus diminishes or disappears. In 20% to 57% of patients with stroke, however, it *reverses directions*, a finding called **direction-changing nystagmus**.

A second distinguishing feature of nystagmus is whether the nystagmus is suppressed during retinal fixation (i.e., when the patient is focusing on an object; see Chapter 65). In peripheral disease, the nystagmus diminishes in intensity during retinal fixation; in central disease, it is unchanged.

III. Clinical Significance

Most patients presenting to emergency departments with dizziness, vertigo, or imbalance have benign peripheral disease. Only 2% to 5% are ultimately are diagnosed with stroke and most of these patients present with obvious focal neurologic findings. For example, diagnostic findings of stroke in patients with dizziness include ophthalmoparesis (LR = 70), limb ataxia (LR = 23.9), dysarthria (LR = 20.6), facial droop (LR = 18.8), visual field cut (LR = 17.5), focal weakness (LR = 8.6), focal sensory disturbance (LR = 7), and gait abnormality (LR = 4.5).[4,5,16-19]

---

†The authors of this report confirmed the heart block was not due to carotid sinus hypersensitivity

‡In peripheral vestibular disease, the direction of the nystagmus (i.e., its quick component) is *away* from the abnormal side.

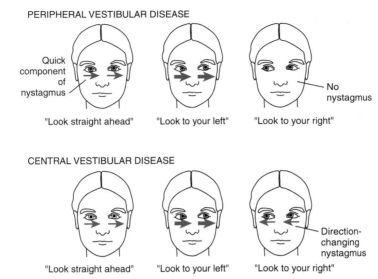

PERIPHERAL VESTIBULAR DISEASE

Quick
component
of
nystagmus

"Look straight ahead"   "Look to your left"   "Look to your right"

No
nystagmus

CENTRAL VESTIBULAR DISEASE

"Look straight ahead"   "Look to your left"   "Look to your right"

Direction-
changing
nystagmus

Fig. 68.3 Direction-changing nystagmus. In this example, the patient has a spontaneous conjugate left-beat-ing jerk nystagmus (*left*, "look straight ahead"; in each example, the arrows indicate the direction of the *quick* component of the nystagmus). The patient is asked to "look to your left" (i.e., the direction of the nystagmus, *middle*) and then "to your right" (the contralateral direction, *right*). In both peripheral (*top row*) and central nys-tagmus (*bottom row*), the nystagmus increases when looking in the direction of the nystagmus ("to your left", *middle*). The distinguishing feature appears when the patient looks in the direction contralateral to the nystag-mus ("to your right", *right*). In peripheral disease, nystagmus diminishes or disappears; in central disease, it may *change* directions (direction-changing nystagmus). Importantly, the direction-changing nystagmus must appear before extreme lateral gaze to be regarded pathologic, because many normal persons have a small amplitude jerk nystagmus on *extreme* lateral gaze.

In patients with isolated dizziness, additional neuro-ophthalmologic findings help identify patients with strokes.

A. INDIVIDUAL FINDINGS

EBM Box 68.1 presents the accuracy of additional bedside findings in 358 patients with acute vertigo and imbalance, all of whom underwent neuroimaging. The findings that increase prob-ability of stroke the most are severe truncal ataxia (unable to sit unassisted, LR = 17.9), *normal* vestibuloocular reflex during the head impulse test (i.e., *no* corrective saccades, LR = 10.8), direc-tion-changing nystagmus (LR = 8.4), skew deviation (LR = 7.1), and saccadic pursuit (LR = 4.6). The presence of smooth pursuit (i.e., absence of saccadic pursuit) and an *abnormal* head impulse test (i.e., corrective saccade observed, indicating peripheral vestibular disease) both decrease prob-ability of stroke (LRs = 0.2).

B. COMBINED FINDINGS

Three oculomotor signs—normal vestibuloocular reflex on head impulse test (i.e., no corrective saccades), direction-changing nystagmus, and skew deviation—are all characteristic of stroke. In studies of acutely dizzy patients, the presence of *any* of these findings increased probability of stroke (LR = 13.6, EBM Box 68.1). More importantly, the *absence of all three* findings mark-edly decreased probability of stroke (LR = 0.02). This LR (0.02) is less than the LR for a *normal*

EBM BOX 68.1   Acute Vertigo, Detecting Ischemic Stroke*

Finding (Reference)[†]	Sensitivity (%)	Specificity (%)	Likelihood Ratio[‡] if Finding Is Present	Likelihood Ratio[‡] if Finding Is Absent
Individual findings				
Severe truncal ataxia[20]	34	98	17.9	0.7
Skew deviation present[20-23]	24–55	86–99	7.1	0.6
Saccadic pursuit[21,22]	70–88	80–90	4.6	0.2
Direction-changing nystagmus[20-23]	20–57	82–99	8.4	0.6
Normal head impulse test (i.e., no corrective saccade)[20-24]	60–97	82–99	10.8	0.2
Combined findings: (1) normal head impulse test (no corrective saccades); (2) direction-changing nystagmus; (3) skew deviation.[20,22,23]				
1 or more finding	95–99	86–94	13.6	0.02

*Diagnostic standard: for *ischemic stroke*, magnetic resonance imaging of cerebellum and brainstem.
†Definition of findings: see text.
‡Likelihood ratio (LR) if finding present = positive LR; LR if finding absent = negative LR.

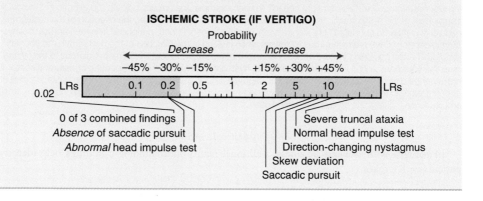

(diffusion-weighted) magnetic resonance (MRI) image (LR = 0.2; i.e., the probability of stroke decreases *more* with the absence of these three findings than it does with a normal MRI result)[§] [20]

References may be accessed online at *Elsevier eBooks for Practicing Clinicians*.

---

§In this study, the diagnostic accuracy of the initial magnetic resonance/diffusion weight imaging for stroke was sensitivity of 85%, specificity of 98%, positive LR = 44.2 and negative LR = 0.2. The 8 patients with falsely negative MRIs (5 lateral medullary, 1 lateral pontomedullary, and 2 middle cerebellar peduncle infarctions) all had positive repeat MRIs an average of 3 days later.[20]

CHAPTER 69

Examination of Nonorganic Neurologic Disorders

I. Traditional Physical Findings of Nonorganic Disease

Nonorganic neurologic disorders (also called hysterical, psychogenic, or functional disorders) occur commonly, accounting for up to 9% of admissions to a neurologic service[1] and 30% of outpatient referrals to neurologists.[2] Of the many proposed findings of nonorganic neurologic disease,* the most prominent are findings whose severity fluctuates during the examination, findings that defy neuroanatomic explanation, bizarre movements not normally seen in organic disease, and findings elicited during special tests.

A. FINDINGS WHOSE SEVERITY FLUCTUATES DURING THE EXAMINATION

Examples are the patient who falls suddenly while walking but catches himself with knees and hips flexed, a position that requires considerable strength, or the patient whose stance is unstable until distracted by asking him to perform the finger-nose test.[6]

Two examples of formal bedside tests designed to demonstrate fluctuating findings are the **knee-lift test** (Fig. 69.1) and **chair test**. The chair test is used in patients with gait disorders: The clinician first asks the patient to walk 20 to 30 feet and back again and then places the patient in a

---

*Review articles by Stone[3]; Lanska[4] and Daum[5] exhaustively review nonorganic neurologic signs.

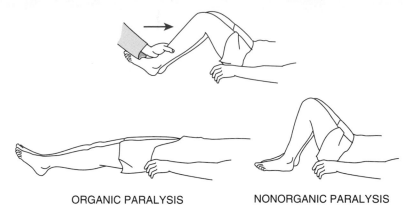

ORGANIC PARALYSIS　　　　　NONORGANIC PARALYSIS

Fig. 69.1　Knee-lift test for nonorganic paraparesis. The knee-lift test is designed to test patients with leg weakness from suspected spinal cord lesions; it is interpretable only if the supine patient cannot lift his or her knees off the examination table. The clinician raises both of the patient's knees (*top*) and then gently releases the patient's legs. Patients with organic paralysis cannot hold the knees upright (negative test, *lower left*). If the patient maintains the knees upright, the test is positive (for nonorganic paralysis, *lower right*).[7]

wheeled swivel chair (with back) and asks him or her to propel themselves over the same distance in the chair with their legs. Marked improvement when using the chair (compared with walking) is a positive test.

B. FINDINGS THAT DEFY NEUROANATOMICAL EXPLANATION

Findings that defy neuroanatomic explanation[8,9] include the following: **(1) hysterical hemianopia**, as in the patient who has a right hemianopia with both eyes open or just the right eye open, but normal visual fields when just the left eye is open,[10,11] **(2) wrong-way tongue deviation**, which describes a tongue deviating *away* from the hemiparetic side (in cerebral hemispheric disease, the tongue deviates toward the hemiparetic side, see Chapter 60),[12] and **(3) peripheral facial palsy and ipsilateral hemiparesis** (if a single lesion causes peripheral facial weakness and hemiparesis, the lesion is in the brainstem and the findings should be on opposite sides of the body).[13]

C. BIZARRE MOVEMENTS NOT NORMALLY SEEN IN ORGANIC DISEASE

Examples are the patient who drags a hemiparetic leg after him as if it were an inanimate object[6,14] or the ataxic patient who sways dramatically without falling.[11]

D. FINDINGS ELICITED DURING SPECIAL TESTS

Findings elicited during special tests include the following: **(1) optokinetic nystagmus** (for functional blindness): Because patients with intact vision cannot suppress this nystagmus (see Chapter 58), the presence of optokinetic nystagmus uncovers that the blindness is functional, **(2) procedures that confuse the patient of sidedness**, such as a maneuver that mixes up the fingers to uncover hysterical hemianalgesia (Fig. 69.2),[15] **(3) upper limb drift *without* pronation test**. When patients with organic unilateral arm weakness are asked to stretch the supinated arms in front of them (palms up) and then close the eyes, the weak arm will slowly drift down *and pronate* (i.e., the

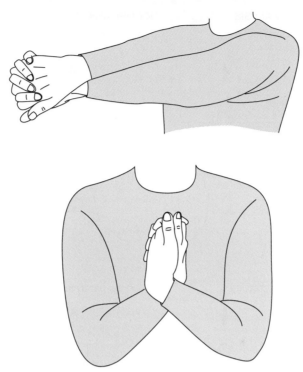

Fig. 69.2 Test for hysterical hemianalgesia. This test simply mixes up the fingers and confuses the body image. In the first step (*top*), the patient's hands are pronated with the little fingers on top, the palms are outward, and fingers are interlocked. In the second step (*bottom*), the hands are rotated downward, inward, and upward, so the interlocked fingers are positioned in front of the chest. The clinician then repeats the sensory examination to determine if the patient is consistent in describing his sensory loss. In the final position, the fingertips end up on the same side of the body as their respective arms, and the thumbs (which are not interlocked) end up on the side opposite the fingers.

palm slowly turns to face downwards; see Fig. 61.1 in Chapter 61). In patients with nonorganic weakness, in contrast, the weak arm may drift down *without* pronation. This is the positive test. **(4) The Hoover sign of nonorganic weakness** (Fig. 69.3), first described by the American physician Charles Hoover in 1908.[16]

II. Clinical Significance

A. DIAGNOSTIC ACCURACY

According to the LRs in EBM Box 69.1, tests of nonorganic weakness are quite accurate: The chair test identifies functional gait disorder (positive likelihood ratio [LR] = 17, negative LR = 0.2); the knee-lift test identifies nonorganic paraparesis (positive LR = 7.1, negative LR = 0.04)†; the drift-without-pronation test identifies nonorganic arm weakness (positive LR = 11.4, negative LR = 0.02), and the Hoover sign identifies nonorganic leg weakness (positive LR = 42, negative LR = 0.3).

---

†The knee-lift test has also been used in the immediate postoperative period after spinal surgery to identify new-onset organic paralysis in patients (sensitivity of 89%, specificity of 100%, positive LR = 462, and negative LR = 0.1).[21]

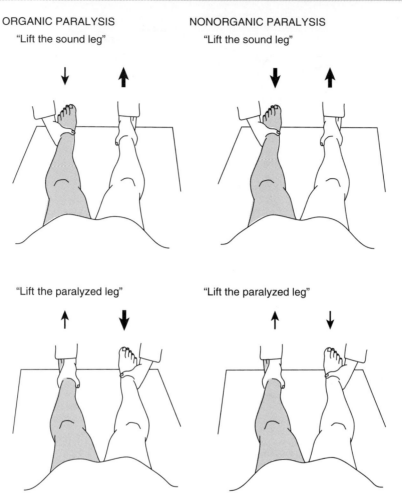

Fig. 69.3   Hoover sign of nonorganic paralysis. The left half of the figure depicts *organic* paralysis and the right half, *nonorganic* paralysis; in each drawing, the patient's right leg is the sound leg and the left leg (*shaded blue*) is the paretic leg. In the *top rows*, the clinician stands at the foot of the bed and, with his or her hands around the patient's ankles, asks the patient to *lift the sound leg* as strongly as possible while the clinician resists the movement (the *size of arrows* indicates the power perceived by the clinician). In organic paralysis, the *downward* force of the paretic leg is weak; in nonorganic weakness the downward force is paretic leg is *strong*. Then (in the *bottom rows*), the patient is asked to lift the *paretic* leg as strongly as possible. In organic weakness, the downward force of the strong leg is strong, whereas in nonorganic weakness the downward force is *weak*. The Hoover test relies on the principle that strong muscular contractions of healthy persons are involuntarily matched by opposing movements of the opposite limb, unless organic weakness intervenes. The appeal of the Hoover test is its interpretation relies on observation of the leg *opposite* of the one being tested (i.e., in the first test—*top row*—the patient is focused on the sound leg, but the clinician observes the paretic leg; in the second test—*bottom row*—the patient is focused on the paretic leg, but the clinician observes the sound leg).

Other investigators have adapted Hoover sign to develop an analogous test for arm weakness, which has similar diagnostic accuracy.[22] Nonetheless, these impressive LRs likely overestimate diagnostic accuracy because the clinician performing the tests are also probably familiar with the final diagnosis, a diagnosis that in turn was probably determined by the same clinician using clinical criteria (see footnote to EBM Box 69.1).

EBM BOX 69.1　　**Nonorganic Neurologic Disease***

Finding (Reference)[†]	Sensitivity (%)	Specificity (%)	Likelihood Ratio[‡] if Finding Is Present	Absent
Diagnosing nonorganic gait disorder				
Chair test positive[17]	85	95	17.0	0.2
Diagnosing nonorganic paraparesis				
Knee-lift test positive[7]	97	86	7.1	0.04
Diagnosing nonorganic arm weakness				
Arm drift without pronation[18]	98	91	11.4	0.02
Diagnosing nonorganic leg weakness				
Hoover sign positive[5,19,20]	39–85	97–100	42.0	0.3

*Diagnostic standard: for *nonorganic gait disorder*, Haye's criteria[17]; for *nonorganic paraparesis*, disproportionate motor paralysis, nonanatomic sensory loss, and normal neuroimaging; for *nonorganic weakness*, neurologic examination and observation over time.

[†]Definition of findings: for *Chair test*, see text; for *Knee-lift test*, see Fig. 69.1; for Hoover sign, see Fig. 69.3.

[‡]Likelihood ratio (LR) if finding present = positive LR; LR if finding absent = negative LR.

NONORGANIC NEUROLOGIC DISEASE

Probability

Decrease　　　　　*Increase*

−45% −30% −15%　　　+15% +30% +45%

LRs　0.1　0.2　0.5　1　2　5　10　LRs

0.02

Drift *with* pronation, *arguing against* nonorganic weakness

Negative knee-lift test, *arguing against* nonorganic paraparesis

Negative chair test, *arguing against* nonorganic gait disorder

Negative Hoover sign, *arguing against* nonorganic leg weakness

Hoover sign, detecting nonorganic leg weakness

Chair test, detecting nonorganic gait

Drift without pronation, detecting nonorganic arm weakness

Knee-lift test, detecting nonorganic paraparesis

B. CAVEATS TO THE DIAGNOSIS OF NONORGANIC DISORDERS

Clinicians should be reluctant to diagnose nonorganic disease, primarily because many "nonorganic" findings, when subjected to serious study, also appear in patients with organic disease. For example, in studies of patients with known organic disorders, 8% to 15% "split" their sensory findings precisely at the midline, up to 85% feel vibration less in numb areas, 48% have sensory findings that change between examinations or make no sense neuroanatomically, and 3% to 33% have "give-away" weakness.[23–26] All of these findings, at one point in time, have been presented as reliable markers of psychogenic disease.[27]

Rare disorders also will trip up the unwary clinician. For example, patients with the medial medullary syndrome also may point their tongue to the "wrong" side, patients with advanced Huntington's disease are often regarded as having a nonorganic gait when it is viewed in isolation,[14]

and patients with Marchiafava-Bignami disease (damage to the corpus callosum) may present with a hemianopia that switches sides during examination, depending on the method of testing.[28]

In clinical studies conducted over the last several decades, an average of 8% of patients given a diagnosis of nonorganic neurologic disease are subsequently found to have a genuine organic neurologic disease that accounts for their findings.[29] The diagnosis of nonorganic illness, therefore, is a diagnostic snare, best left to neurologic specialists.

References may be accessed online at *Elsevier eBooks for Practicing Clinicians.*

PART 14

Examination in the Intensive Care Unit

CHAPTER 70

Examination of Patients in the Intensive Care Unit

I. Introduction

The traditional physical examination meets many challenges in the ICU. First, it must compete with legions of additional sensory information, including continuous telemetry of vital signs, heart rhythm displays, ventilator parameters, and flow sheets of urine output, mental status, and intravenous medications. Second, there are many barriers to traditional inspection, palpation, percussion, and auscultation: central lines and dressings conceal the neck veins, anasarca limits normal palpation, and cardiac leads and ventilator noise obscure heart and lung sounds. Even so, the careful examination retains value in the ICU patient because it is the only way, among many examples, to detect the purulence around intravenous lines, the warmth of an infected joint, the purpuric skin lesions of septic emboli, the wheezing of bronchospasm, the neck stiffness of meningitis, or the absent doll's-eyes of cerebellar stroke.

This chapter brings together those aspects of the physical examination that are relevant to critically ill patients already discussed in previous chapters of this book and presents several findings not previously reviewed.

II. The Findings

Other chapters in this book discuss vital signs (Chapters 15 to 20), asynchronous breathing (Chapter 19), anisocoria (Chapter 21), assessments of peripheral perfusion (Chapter 54), and neck stiffness (Chapters 26 and 67). This chapter reviews these findings and introduces additional findings: the modified early warning score, passive leg elevation in assessments of hypovolemia, and the diagnosis of septic and cardiogenic shock.

A. MODIFIED EARLY WARNING SCORE (TABLE 70.1)

Developed in 2001 by Subbe[1] who simplified previous scores used in critically ill surgical patients, the **Modified Early Warning Score** relies on measurements of four vital signs (systolic blood pressure, heart rate, respiratory rate, and temperature) and mental status (using the acronym AVPU, which stands for **A**lert, responsive to **V**oice, responsive to **P**ain, or **U**nresponsive). In Table 70.1, normal parameters are shaded grey. The greater the deviation from these normal measurements, in either direction, the greater the score and presumed risk of hospital death. Patients at highest risk may benefit from observation in an ICU.

B. ASSESSMENT OF PERIPHERAL PERFUSION IN THE ICU

There are three findings of peripheral perfusion in ICU patients[2]: (1) temperature of limbs, which should reflect the volume of blood circulating in the most superficial vessels of the skin[3]; (2) capillary refill time (see Chapter 54); and (3) mottled skin, especially of the knees. Mottling describes a lacy purplish net-like discoloration of the skin, a sign indicating sluggish blood flow in dilated superficial postcapillary venules.[3,4]

C. PULSE PRESSURE CHANGES WITH PASSIVE LEG ELEVATION (HYPOVOLEMIA)

Critical care physicians have long sought ways to anticipate which patients with hypotension would benefit from intravascular saline infusions. Based on the hypothesis that pulse pressure reflects stroke volume (see Chapter 17) and the idea that passive elevation of the patient's legs reversibly transfers blood from the legs to the thorax, clinicians have investigated whether changes in pulse pressure after passive leg elevation might predict volume responsiveness.

The methods of this test are not standardized, but the procedures used in the studies from EBM Box 70.1 are as follows: The clinician measures baseline blood pressure with the patient's

TABLE 70.1 ■ **Modified Early Warning Score***

Points	3	2	1	0	1	2	3
Systolic blood pressure (mm Hg)	<70	71–80	81–100	101–199	—	≥200	—
Heart rate (beats/min)	—	<40	41–50	51–100	101–110	111–129	≥130
Respiratory rate (breaths/min)	—	<9	—	9–14	15–20	21–29	≥30
Temperature (°C)	—	<35	—	35.0–38.4	—	≥38.5	—
Neurologic score	—	—	—	Alert	Voice	Pain	Unresponsive

*From reference 1.

legs horizontal on the bed.* After baseline measurements, the clinician lifts the patient's legs to a 45 degree angle (the trunk is now supine). Both the baseline and post-elevation blood pressure measurements are measured (4 of 5 studies used intra-arterial catheters) and multiple readings over 1 to 4 minutes in both positions are averaged (after leg elevation, changes in blood pressure usually appear within one minute). An increase in mean pulse pressure of at least 9% to 12% after elevating the legs is *test positive*. For example, if a patient's average blood pressure is 100/54 at baseline and 114/61 after leg elevation, the pulse pressure has increased from 46 to 53, an increase of 7/46 or 15%.

Patients with deep venous thrombosis of either leg were excluded from these trials.

III. Clinical Significance

A. MODIFIED EARLY WARNING SCORE

In eight studies of 5700 with acute medical illness (i.e., trauma excluded), a modified early warning score of 5 or more predicts increased risk of hospital death (likelihood ratio [LR] = 4.8, EBM Box 70.1; in these studies, overall mortality was 1% to 15%): Patients with a score of 5 or more may benefit from more intensive monitoring. A score of 0 (i.e., all parameters within the gray-shaded area of Table 70.1) predicts a reduced risk of death (LR = 0.3).

EBM BOX 70.1	**Examination of Patients in the ICU***			
Finding (Reference)[†]	Sensitivity (%)	Specificity (%)	Likelihood Ratio[‡] if Finding Is	
			Present	Absent
Vital signs				
Modified early warning score, predicting hospital mortality[5–12]				
0 points	1–18	39–94	0.3	...
≥5 points	22–86	79–97	4.8	...
Shock				
Detecting septic shock[13]				
Hands warm	88	67	2.7	0.2
Bounding pulses	64	73	2.4	0.5
Detecting cardiogenic shock[13]				
CVP >8 cm H_2O	82	79	4.0	0.2
Lung crackles	55	72	1.9	NS
CVP >8 cm H_2O and crackles	55	99	56.4	0.5
Detecting hypovolemic shock				
Pulse pressure increase ≥12% with passive leg elevation[14–18]	48–79	80–92	3.9	0.5
Lungs				
Asynchronous breathing during COPD exacerbation, predicting intubation or death[19]	64	80	3.2	NS
Asymmetric breath sounds after intubation, detecting right mainstem bronchus intubation[20–23]	28–83	88–98	12.8	0.5

(continued)

*The position of the trunk during baseline measurements was supine in three studies[15,17,18] and elevated at a 45-degree angle in two others.[14,16]

EBM BOX 70.1	Examination of Patients in the ICU*—Cont'd			
			Likelihood Ratio‡ if Finding Is	
Finding (Reference)†	Sensitivity (%)	Specificity (%)	Present	Absent
Diminished breath sounds, detecting underlying pleural effusion in mechanically ventilated patients.[24,25]	34–42	84–90	**3.0**	0.7
Neurologic				
Anisocoria in patients with coma, detecting structural intracranial lesion[26]	39	96	**9.0**	0.6
Neck stiffness[27–32]	16–48	81–98	**5.4**	0.7

*Diagnostic standard: for *septic shock*, blinded consensus diagnosis based on microbiologic and radiographic data acquired after onset of shock; for *cardiogenic shock*, evidence of acute ventricular dysfunction on echocardiography; for *hypovolemic shock*, 500 cc intravenous saline challenge produces ≥15% increase in aortic blood flow,[14,15] cardiac index,[16,18] or echocardiographic stroke volume[17]; for *structural lesion*, supratentorial and subtentorial lesions with gross anatomical abnormality, including cerebrovascular disease, intracranial hematoma, tumor, and contusion.
†Definition of findings: for *Modified Early Warning Score*, see Table 70.1; for *hands warm* and *bounding pulses* (septic shock), hands are warmer and pulses more bounding in the patient than in the examiner; for *pulse pressure increase* (after passive leg elevation), increase in pulse pressure of at least 9%,[17,18] 11%,[16] or 12%[14,15]; for *asynchronous breathing*, see Chapter 19 and Fig. 19.2.
‡Likelihood ratio (LR) if finding present = positive LR; LR if finding absent = negative LR.
ARDS, Acute respiratory distress syndrome; *COPD*, chronic obstructive pulmonary disease; *CVP*, central venous pressure; *NS*, not significant.

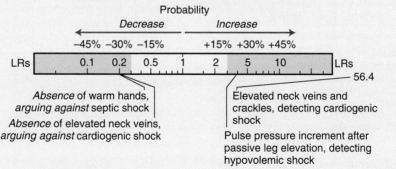

EXAMINATION OF PATIENTS WITH SHOCK

B. SEPTIC SHOCK AND CARDIOGENIC SHOCK

In one study of 68 hospitalized patients with acute shock (systolic blood pressure less than 90 mm Hg), the presence of warm hands and bounding pulses modestly increased probability of septic shock (LRs 2.4 to 2.7). More importantly, the *absence* of warm hands in this study decreased probability of septic shock (LR = 0.2). In this same study, cardiogenic shock was the likely cause of hypotension if the patient had elevated venous pressure (central venous pressure [CVP] >8 cm

H_2O) *and* lung crackles (LR = 56.4). The absence of elevated neck veins decreased probability of cardiogenic shock (LR = 0.2). In this study, the diagnostic standard for septic and cardiogenic shock was a blinded post hoc review of the patient's clinical course, based in part on subsequent microbiologic and radiographic evidence of infection (septic shock) and echocardiographic evidence of ventricular dysfunction (cardiogenic shock).

C. PULSE PRESSURE CHANGES WITH PASSIVE LEG ELEVATION (HYPOVOLEMIA)

In five studies of 263 critically ill hypotensive patients (most mechanically ventilated), a pulse pressure increase (variably defined as at least 9% to 12%) after passive leg elevation increased the probability of hypovolemic shock, which was defined as subsequent response to infusion of 500 cc of intravenous saline (or equivalent fluid, LR = 3.9). The absence of such an increment in pulse pressure was unhelpful (LR = 0.5).

One cause of a false negative result (i.e., the patient is hypovolemic yet lacks a pulse pressure increment of at least 9% to 12%) is intraabdominal hypertension (i.e., bladder pressure more than 16 mm Hg).[33] Presumably, the high pressures within the abdomen of these patients interfere with the normal increment of central blood volume after leg elevation, thus producing the negative test result even if the patient is truly hypovolemic. To address the possibility that leg elevation fails to increase central volume, one investigator suggests restricting interpretation of the test to just those patients whose CVP increases 2 mm or more during passive leg elevation. In these patients, the positive pulse pressure increment with leg elevation is more accurate (positive LR = 9.3, negative LR = 0.1).[18]

D. ASSESSMENT OF PERIPHERAL PERFUSION IN THE ICU

In patients with critical illness, all three signs of poor peripheral perfusion (cool limbs, prolonged capillary refill times, and mottling of the limbs), alone or in combination, identify patients with reduced cardiac output, worse prognosis, or both. For example, the finding of cool legs in ICU patients increases the probability of low cardiac output (LR = 3.7, EBM Box 70.2), even in the subset of patients with sepsis (LR = 5.2). A capillary refill time of 5 seconds or more predicts major postoperative complications after intraabdominal surgery (LR = 12.1) and predicts 14-day mortality in patients with sepsis (LR = 4.6). In patients with sepsis, testing capillary refill time *after* initial fluid resuscitation is more accurate than testing before it (LRs = 10.5 vs. not significant, predicting mortality).[42] Mottling of the skin over the knees and extending to the upper thigh also predicts mortality in patients with sepsis (LR = 10.2), independent of the use of vasopressor medications,[41] and its course over time heralds the patient's outcome (i.e., patients whose mottling diminishes over time have better survival than those whose mottling persists).[39] Studies of mottling excluded patients with dark skin.

Other investigators have focused on combinations of findings. For example, in one study of intubated patients with acute lung injury, the simultaneous presence of capillary refill time more than 2 sec[†], mottling over the knees, and cool limbs increased the probability of low cardiac output (LR = 7.5; EBM Box 70.2). In another series of ICU patients, the findings of *either* cool limbs or capillary refill time of 5 second or more increased probability of an elevated lactate levels (LR = 2.2) and predicted future progressive multiorgan dysfunction (LR = 2.6).

[†]This study contrasts with other studies of capillary refill by applying only *mild* pressure on the patient's fingertip to elicit the finding, not firm pressure, and by defining the abnormal test as just 2 seconds or more.

| EBM BOX 70.2 | Peripheral Perfusion of ICU Patients* | | | |

Finding (Reference)†	Sensitivity (%)	Specificity (%)	Likelihood Ratio‡ if Finding Is	
			Present	Absent
Detecting low cardiac output				
Both legs cool (all patients)[34]	23	94	**3.7**	0.8
Both legs cool (patients with sepsis)[34]	30	94	**5.2**	0.7
Combinations of hypoperfusion findings[2]				
0 of 3 findings present	36	24	0.5	…
1 of 3 findings present	52	…	2.3	…
3 or 3 findings present	12	98	**7.5**	…
Capillary refill time ≥5 s[35]	25	85	1.6	NS
Detecting elevated arterial lactate level				
Limb is cool *or* capillary refill time ≥5 s[36]	67	69	2.2	0.5
Predicting multiorgan dysfunction				
Limb is cool *or* capillary refill time ≥5 s[36]	77	70	2.6	**0.3**
Predicting major postoperative complications after intraabdominal surgery				
Capillary refill time ≥5 s[37]	79	93	**12.1**	0.2
Predicting mortality if septic shock				
Capillary refill time ≥5 s[38]	50	89	**4.6**	0.6
Mottling of skin extending to upper thigh[39–41]	9–41	96–97	**10.2**	NS

*Diagnostic standard: for *low cardiac output*, cardiac index <2.2 L/min/M[2],[35] <2.5 L/min/M[2],[2] or <3 L/min/M[2].[34] for *elevated lactate level*, blood lactate >2 mmol/L; for *multiorgan dysfunction*, SOFA score that increases during the first 48 hours of hospitalization (SOFA score is the Sequential Organ Failure Assessment, a score tabulating the following variables: P_aO_2/F_iO_2, number of vasoactive pressors being administered, bilirubin, platelet count, Glasgow coma scale, and creatinine or urine output); for *major postoperative complication*, one requiring endoscopy, repeat surgery, general anesthesia, or ICU transfer[37]; for *mortality*, 14 day[39] or 28 day[40,41] mortality.
†Definition of findings: for *both legs cool*, either all 4 limbs have cool temperature or legs cool despite warm arms (patients with known peripheral vascular disease were excluded)[34]; for *combinations of hypoperfusion findings*, there are 3: (1) capillary refill time >2 sec, (2) skin mottling over the knees, and (3) cool limbs[2]; for all *capillary refill times*, testing performed on the patient's finger or nailbeds, and; for *mottling of skin over knees*, mottling extending at least to the level of mid-thigh (only light-skinned patients were tested)[39].
‡Likelihood ratio (LR) if finding present = positive LR; LR if finding absent = negative LR.
ICU, Intensive care unit; *NS*, not significant.

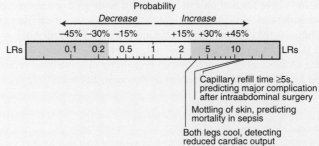

HYPOPERFUSION IN THE ICU
Probability

| Decrease | Increase |

−45% −30% −15%   +15% +30% +45%

LRs   0.1   0.2   0.5   1   2   5   10   LRs

Capillary refill time ≥5s, predicting major complication after intraabdominal surgery

Mottling of skin, predicting mortality in sepsis

Both legs cool, detecting reduced cardiac output

E. LUNG FINDINGS

In patients hospitalized with exacerbations of chronic obstructive pulmonary disease, the finding of asynchronous breathing (see Chapter 19) accurately predicts subsequent need for intubation or hospital mortality (LR = 3.2). In patients examined after intubation, asymmetric breath sounds are pathognomonic for endobronchial intubation (LR = 12.8), although physical examination *never excludes* this important complication (i.e., symmetric breath sounds do not significantly decrease the probability of endobronchial intubation; LR = 0.5). Confirmation of appropriate tube placement by means other than physical examination is always indicated. In patients mechanically ventilated for acute respiratory distress syndrome, the finding of absent vesicular breath sounds increases the probability of underlying pleural effusion (LR = 3).

F. NEUROLOGIC FINDINGS

The finding of anisocoria in an unresponsive patient raises concern for the Hutchinson pupil (see Chapter 21), the abnormal larger pupil representing an early sign of an ipsilateral expanding cerebral mass (LR = 9). A common mimic of this finding in the ICU is the pharmacologic pupil, from nebulized bronchodilators, which can be distinguished from the Hutchinson pupil by its lack of response to topical pilocarpine (see Chapter 21).

Neck stiffness raises concern for meningeal irritation, from either purulent secretions (meningitis) or blood (intracranial or subarachnoid hemorrhage). In patients with stroke, the finding of neck stiffness markedly increases probability of intracranial or subarachnoid hemorrhage (LR = 5.4).

References may be accessed online at *Elsevier eBooks for Practicing Clinicians*.

Appendix

Appendix A

CHAPTER 71

Appendix: Likelihood Ratios, Confidence Intervals, and Pretest Probability

The following Table displays the point estimates and 95% confidence intervals for all of the likelihood ratios (LRs) presented in this book. Also, the Table presents the range of disease prevalences observed in the studies used to calculate the LRs (i.e., *pretest probability of disease*, see Chapter 2). Chapter 3 presents the methods used to obtain the point estimates of LRs and their confidence intervals, and individual chapters define each physical finding and further discuss its significance.

APPENDIX TABLE 1 ■ Likelihood Ratios, Confidence Intervals, and Pretest Probability

Finding	Positive LR (95% CI)	Negative LR (95% CI)	Pre-test Probability (Range)
EBM Box 6.1 Dementia and delirium			
Abnormal clock drawing test	4 (2.7, 5.9)	0.5 (0.4, 0.6)	22–73
Mini-Cog score 2 or less	4.5 (2.7, 7.4)	0.1 (0.1, 0.3)	3–52
Mini-mental status 23 or less	7.8 (6, 10.2)	0.2 (0.2, 0.3)	4–77
Mini-mental status 20 or less	14.4 (8, 26.1)	...	9–35
Mini-mental status 21–25	2.1 (1.7, 2.6)	...	14–35
Mini-mental status 26 or more	0.1 (0.1, 0.2)	...	14–77
Confusion assessment method	11.5 (7.2, 18.4)	0.2 (0.1, 0.3)	14–64
Chapter 7 Stance and gait			
Positive Trendelenburg sign and gait, detecting gluteus medius tear	3.2 (1.1, 9.1)	0.4 (0.1, 1)	46
Hip abductor weakness, detecting lumbosacral radiculopathy if foot drop	24 (3.5, 165.8)	0.1 (0.1, 0.4)	43
Asymmetric arm swing, detecting focal cerebral lesion	2.1 (0.5, 8.6)	0.9 (0.7,1.1)	71
Inability to tandem walk, detecting Parkinson-plus disorder if parkinsonism	4.9 (2, 11.9)	0.2 (0.1, 0.3)	37–72
Positive Romberg test, detecting spinal stenosis	4.3 (1.6, 11.8)	0.7 (0.5, 0.9)	48
Prior fall in last year, predicting future fall	2.4 (2, 2.9)	0.6 (0.4, 0.9)	19–53
Timed-up-and-go test >16 s, detecting Parkinson-plus disorder	5.6 (1.5, 21)	0.4 (0.2, 0.6)	72
Timed-up-and-go test >16 s, detecting Parkinson disease	0.2 (0, 0.7)	2.6 (1.7, 4)	28
EBM BOX 7.1 Gait abnormalities			
Able to tandem walk, detecting Parkinson disease if parkinsonism	4.6 (3.1, 6.8)	0.2 (0.1, 0.5)	28–63

(continued)

APPENDIX TABLE 1 ▪ Likelihood Ratios, Confidence Intervals, and Pretest Probability—Cont'd

Finding	Positive LR (95% CI)	Negative LR (95% CI)	Pre-test Probability (Range)
Any gait or balance disorder, detecting Alzheimer dementia	0.2 (0.1, 0.3)	3.4 (1.9, 5.8)	75
Parkinsonian gait, detecting Lewy body dementia or Parkinson disease with dementia	8.8 (4.3, 18.1)	0.2 (0.2, 0.4)	50
Frontal gait, detecting vascular dementia	6.1 (3.2, 11.3)	0.5 (0.3, 0.7)	25
EBM Box 7.2 Predicting falls			
Palmomental reflex present	2.8 (1.7, 4.4)	0.8 (0.7, 0.9)	32
Failure to stand with feet together and eyes open for 10 seconds	4.5 (2.1, 9.8)	1 (0.9, 1)	19
Failure in tandem walk (>2 errors)	1.7 (1.5, 2)	0.7 (0.6, 0.8)	19
Stops walking when talking	3 (1.3, 6.8)	0.8 (0.7, 1)	36–48
Timed up and go <15 sec	0.1 (0, 0.3)	...	53
Timed up and go 15–35 sec	1.1 (0.9, 1.4)	...	53
Timed up and go ≥35 sec	2.6 (1.4, 4.7)	...	53
Chapter 8 Jaundice			
Caput medusa, detecting varices	1.5 (0.1, 15.7)	1 (0.9, 1.1)	58
Spider angiomas, detecting varices	1.2 (0.9, 1.6)	0.9 (0.8, 1.1)	13–46
Jaundice, detecting varices	1.1 (0.5, 2.4)	1 (0.8, 1.2)	13
Hepatomegaly, detecting varices	0.5 (0.1, 1.9)	1.1 (1, 1.3)	13
Palpable spleen, detecting varices	1.4 (1, 1.8)	0.8 (0.6, 1)	13–46
Ascites, detecting varices	1.5 (1.2, 2)	0.7 (0.6, 0.8)	13–58
Encephalopathy, detecting varices	1.3 (1.1, 1.6)	0.9 (0.8, 1)	13–58
Dyspnea, detecting hepatopulmonary syndrome	3.3 (2.1, 5.1)	0.5 (0.4, 0.7)	14–37
Platypnea, detecting hepatopulmonary syndrome	10.6 (4.4, 25.8)	0.4 (0.2, 0.6)	26
Child class C cirrhosis, detecting hepatopulmonary syndrome	2.2 (1.2, 4.1)	0.5 (0.3, 0.7)	14–34
EBM Box 8.1 Hepatocellular jaundice			
Weight loss	0.8 (0.2, 3.2)	1.3 (0.5, 3.3)	65–67
Spider angiomas	4.7 (1, 22.4)	0.6 (0.5, 0.9)	65–67
Palmar erythema	9.8 (1.4, 67.6)	0.5 (0.4, 0.7)	67
Dilated abdominal veins	17.5 (1.1, 277)	0.6 (0.5, 0.8)	67
Ascites	4.4 (1.1, 17.1)	0.6 (0.5, 0.8)	67
Palpable spleen	2.9 (1.2, 6.8)	0.7 (0.6, 0.9)	65–67
Palpable gallbladder	0.04 (0, 0.7)	1.4 (1.1, 1.9)	67
Palpable liver	0.9 (0.8, 1.1)	1.4 (0.6, 3.4)	65–67
Liver tenderness	1.4 (0.8, 2.6)	0.8 (0.7, 1.1)	65–67
EBM Box 8.2 Cirrhosis			
Spider angiomas	4.2 (2.3, 7.6)	0.6 (0.5, 0.7)	7–67
Palmar erythema	3.7 (1.4, 9.8)	0.6 (0.4, 0.9)	11–67
Gynecomastia	7 (5.2, 9.4)	0.6 (0.3, 1.1)	11–16
Reduction of body or pubic hair	8.8 (6.3, 12.5)	0.6 (0.4, 1)	11–16
Jaundice	3.8 (2, 7.2)	0.8 (0.8, 0.9)	11–53
Dilated abdominal wall veins	9.5 (1.8, 49.2)	0.8 (0.6, 1)	11–55
Hepatomegaly	2.3 (1.6, 3.3)	0.6 (0.4, 0.7)	7–67
Palpable liver in epigastrium	2.7 (1.9, 3.9)	0.3 (0.1, 0.9)	7–37
Liver edge firm to palpation	3.3 (2.2, 4.9)	0.4 (0.3, 0.4)	27–67
Splenomegaly	2.5 (1.6, 3.8)	0.8 (0.7, 0.9)	18–67
Ascites	6.6 (3.6, 12.1)	0.8 (0.7, 0.8)	16–55
Peripheral edema	3 (1.9, 4.8)	0.7 (0.6, 0.9)	16–55
Encephalopathy	8.8 (3.3, 23.7)	0.9 (0.8, 1)	16–39

APPENDIX TABLE 1 ■ **Likelihood Ratios, Confidence Intervals, and Pretest Probability—Cont'd**

Finding	Positive LR (95% CI)	Negative LR (95% CI)	Pre-test Probability (Range)
EBM Box 8.3 Hepatopulmonary syndrome			
Clubbing	4.3 (2.7, 6.7)	0.6 (0.5, 0.8)	14–37
Cyanosis	4.4 (2, 9.8)	0.7 (0.5, 0.8)	19–51
Palmar erythema	1.7 (1.01, 2.8)	0.8 (0.5, 1.2)	14–26
Spider angiomas	2.1 (1.4, 3)	0.4 (0.3, 0.7)	14–34
Ascites	1.1 (1, 1.2)	0.9 (0.7, 1.1)	14–33
Jaundice	1 (0.8, 1.5)	1 (0.8, 1.1)	26–33
EBM Box 8.4 Portal-pulmonary hypertension			
Blood pressure ≥140/90	7.3 (2.5, 21.6)	0.4 (0.2, 1)	15
O_2 sat <92%	2.4 (0.5, 10.1)	0.8 (0.6, 1.3)	15
Elevated neck veins	2 (0.2, 16.6)	0.9 (0.7, 1.2)	15
Right ventricular heave	8.8 (1.7, 44.7)	0.7 (0.4, 1.1)	15
Loud P_2	17.6 (2.1, 149)	0.6 (0.4, 1.1)	15
Ascites, edema	1.2 (0.7, 1.9)	0.7 (0.2, 2.4)	15
Chapter 9 Cyanosis			
Cyanosis, detecting hepatopulmonary syndrome	4.4 (2, 9.8)	0.7 (0.5, 0.8)	19–51
EBM Box 9.1 Cyanosis			
Central cyanosis	7.4 (1.5, 36.8)	0.2 (0.1, 0.5)	9–12
EBM Box 10.1 Anemia			
Pallor at any site	3.8 (2.7, 5.3)	0.5 (0.4, 0.6)	2–71
Facial pallor	3.8 (2.5, 5.8)	0.6 (0.5, 0.7)	39
Nailbed pallor	4.3 (1.4, 13.8)	0.5 (0.4, 0.7)	39–71
Palmar pallor	5.6 (1.1, 29.1)	0.4 (0.4, 0.5)	39–71
Palmar crease pallor	7.9 (1.8, 35.3)	0.9 (0.9, 1)	39
Conjunctival pallor	4.7 (1.9, 11.5)	0.6 (0.4, 0.9)	39–71
Tongue pallor	3.7 (2.5, 5.4)	0.6 (0.5, 0.7)	21
Conjunctival rim pallor present	16.7 (2.2, 125)	…	47
Conjunctival rim pallor borderline	2.3 (1.5, 3.5)	…	47
Conjunctival rim pallor absent	0.6 (0.5, 0.8)	…	47
EBM Box 11.1 Hypovolemia			
Dry axilla	3.8 (2.4, 6.2)	0.5 (0.4, 0.7)	23–52
Dry mucous membranes of mouth and nose	2.8 (1.8, 4.3)	0.4 (0.2, 0.7)	33–77
Dry tongue	3.6 (1.6, 7.9)	0.4 (0.2, 0.7)	47–79
Longitudinal furrows on tongue	2 (1, 4)	0.3 (0.1, 0.6)	77
Sunken eyes	3.7 (1.3, 11)	0.6 (0.4, 0.9)	52–79
Abnormal skin turgor	3.5 (2.7, 4.4)	0.3 (0.3, 0.4)	33
Confusion	10 (0.5, 223)	0.5 (0.4, 0.6)	33–77
Weakness	2.3 (0.6, 8.6)	0.7 (0.5, 1)	78
Speech unclear or rambling	3.1 (0.9, 11.1)	0.5 (0.3, 0.8)	80
Chapter 12 Malnutrition and weight loss			
Alcoholism, detecting organic disease	4.5 (1.1, 18.9)	0.8 (0.7, 1)	55
Cigarette smoking, detecting organic cause	2.2 (1.1, 4.4)	0.6 (0.4, 0.9)	55
Prior psychiatric disease, detecting organic cause	0.2 (0.1, 0.5)	1.8 (1.3, 2.5)	55
Normal physical examination, detecting organic cause	0.4 (0.3, 0.6)	20.3 (2.9, 143)	55
Underestimation, predicting organic cause	5.4 (2, 14.5)	0.6 (0.5, 0.8)	50
Overestimation, predicting nonorganic cause	3.6 (2, 6.5)	0.4 (0.2, 0.6)	50
EBM Box 12.1 Malnutrition and complications			
Weight loss >10%	1.4 (1.1, 1.8)	0.9 (0.9, 1)	13–51
Low body weight	2 (1.4, 2.9)	0.9 (0.8, 1)	13–40

(continued)

APPENDIX TABLE 1 ■ Likelihood Ratios, Confidence Intervals, and Pretest Probability—Cont'd

Finding	Positive LR (95% CI)	Negative LR (95% CI)	Pre-test Probability (Range)
Upper arm muscle circumference <85% predicted	2.5 (1.7, 3.6)	0.8 (0.7, 0.9)	13–40
Forearm muscle circumference <85% predicted	3.2 (2, 5.1)	0.8 (0.6, 0.9)	14–40
Reduced grip strength	2.6 (1.9, 3.4)	0.4 (0.3, 0.6)	13–59
Chapter 14 Cushing syndrome			
Osteoporosis, detecting Cushing syndrome	8.6 (2.3, 32.6)	0.5 (0.3, 0.8)	25–69
Weight loss, detecting ectopic ACTH syndrome	20 (1.2, 341)	0.5 (0.2, 1.1)	24
Symptom duration <18 mo, detecting ectopic ACTH syndrome	15 (3.2, 71.4)	0.1 (0, 1)	23
Male sex, detecting ectopic ACTH syndrome	2.9 (1.7, 4.8)	0.7 (0.5, 0.9)	5–24
EBM Box 14.1 Cushing syndrome			
Hypertension	2.3 (1.5, 3.7)	0.8 (0.6, 0.9)	25–56
Moon facies	1.6 (1.1, 2.5)	0.1 (0, 0.9)	58
Dorsal cervical fat pad	2.3 (1.5, 3.6)	0.6 (0.4, 0.9)	7
Central obesity	3 (2, 4.4)	0.2 (0.1, 0.3)	25–56
Generalized obesity	0.1 (0, 0.2)	2.5 (2.1, 3.1)	25
BMI >30 kg/M^2	0.6 (0.3, 1.3)	3.1 (1.7, 5.6)	7–58
Skin fold thickness <1.8 mm	115.6 (7, 1854)	0.2 (0.1, 0.6)	17
Plethora	2.7 (2.1, 3.5)	0.3 (0.1, 0.5)	25
Hirsutism, in women	1.4 (1.02, 1.9)	0.8 (0.6, 1)	7–65
Ecchymoses	4.5 (1.8, 11.3)	0.6 (0.4, 0.7)	25–58
Red or blue striae	1.7 (1.2, 2.4)	0.8 (0.7, 1)	7–58
Acne	1.2 (0.4, 4.1)	0.9 (0.5, 1.7)	25–58
Proximal muscle weakness	3.8 (1.1, 12.5)	0.7 (0.4, 1)	7–58
Edema	1.8 (1.1, 3.1)	0.7 (0.6, 0.9)	25–57
Chapter 15 Pulse rate and contour			
Heart rate ≤50/min, predicting mortality if severe trauma	20.7 (17, 25.2)	0.8 (0.8, 0.9)	5
Heart rate ≤40/min in acute illness, predicting hospital mortality	39.1 (22.6, 68)	0.9 (0.9, 0.9)	5
Pulsus paradoxus >12 mm Hg, detecting cardiac tamponade	5.9 (2.4, 14.3)	0.03 (0, 0.2)	63
Oximetry paradoxus <1.2, detecting cardiac tamponade	0.05 (0, 0.7)	2.1 (1.5, 2.7)	26
Carotid upstroke delayed, detecting severe aortic stenosis	3.5 (2.6, 4.6)	0.4 (0.2, 0.7)	5–69
Hyperkinetic pulse in patients with mitral stenosis, detecting additional valvular disease	14.2 (7.4, 27.2)	0.3 (0.2, 0.4)	35
EBM Box 15.1 Tachycardia			
Heart rate >85/min, predicting postoperative complications if lung cancer surgery	3.8 (2.6, 5.6)	0.4 (0.2, 0.6)	23
Heart rate >90/min, predicting hospital mortality in trauma patients with hypotension	1.5 (1.4, 1.7)	0.2 (0.1, 0.5)	10
Heart rate >95 /min, predicting hospital mortality in patients with septic shock	2 (1.3, 3.3)	0.1 (0, 0.5)	60
Heart rate >100/min, predicting hospital mortality in patients with myocardial infarction	3 (2.4, 3.7)	0.9 (0.8, 0.9)	2–10
Heart rate >100/min, predicting active UGI hemorrhage	4.9 (3.2, 7.6)	0.3 (0.2, 0.5)	27
Heart rate >100/min, predicting postoperative complications if hernia surgery	5.6 (3.4, 9)	0.5 (0.3, 0.8)	7
Heart rate >100/min, predicting complications in patients with gallstone pancreatitis	6.8 (3.7, 12.5)	0.2 (0, 1)	7

APPENDIX TABLE 1 ■ **Likelihood Ratios, Confidence Intervals, and Pretest Probability—Cont'd**

Finding	Positive LR (95% CI)	Negative LR (95% CI)	Pre-test Probability (Range)
Heart rate >110/min, predicting hospital mortality in patients with pontine hemorrhage	25.4 (1.6, 395)	0.3 (0.2, 0.6)	55
Heart rate >125/min, predicting mortality in patients with pneumonia	2.6 (2.2, 3.1)	0.9 (0.8, 1)	7–16
EBM Box 15.2 Pulsus paradoxus and asthma			
Pulsus paradoxus >10 mm Hg, detecting severe asthma	2.7 (1.7, 4.3)	0.5 (0.4, 0.7)	36–77
Pulsus paradoxus >20 mm Hg, detecting severe asthma	8.2 (1.7, 40.3)	0.8 (0.7, 0.9)	36–67
Pulsus paradoxus >25 mm Hg, detecting severe asthma	22.6 (1.4, 363)	0.8 (0.8, 0.9)	77
EBM Box 15.3 Pulses and hypovolemic shock			
Carotid pulse present, detecting systolic blood pressure ≥60 mm Hg	1.2 (0.9, 1.8)	0.2 (0, 2.1)	70
Femoral pulse present, detecting systolic blood pressure ≥60 mm Hg	2.9 (1.1, 7.2)	0.1 (0, 0.5)	70
Radial pulse present, detecting systolic blood pressure ≥60 mm Hg	4.7 (0.7, 31.3)	0.5 (0.3, 0.9)	70
Chapter 16 Abnormalities of pulse rhythm			
Rapid regular pounding in neck, detecting atrioventricular nodal reentrant tachycardia	7.7 (1.9, 31.8)	0.6 (0.5, 0.9)	22–71
EBM Box 16.1 AV dissociation and ventricular tachycardia			
Varying arterial pulse, detecting AV dissociation of ventricular tachycardia	2.1 (1, 4.4)	0.5 (0.3, 1)	55
Intermittent cannon a waves in neck veins, detecting AV dissociation of ventricular tachycardia	3.8 (1.8, 8.2)	0.1 (0, 0.4)	55
Changing intensity S_1, detecting AV dissociation of ventricular tachycardia	24.4 (1.5, 385)	0.4 (0.3, 0.7)	55
EBM Box 16.2 Atrial fibrillation			
Radial pulse not regular	6.4 (4, 10)	0.1 (0.1, 0.2)	3–30
Chaotic pulse	24.1 (15.2, 38)	0.5 (0.4, 0.6)	6
Chapter 17 Blood pressure			
Blood pressure <90 mm Hg, detecting future adverse events if syncope	4.2 (3, 5.8)	0.9 (0.9, 0.9)	8–12
Interarm blood pressure difference >20 mm Hg, detecting subclavian stenosis	89.1 (12.3, 643)	0.2 (0.1, 0.8)	7
Mediastinal widening on CXR, detecting aortic dissection	2 (1.2, 3.4)	0.3 (0.2, 0.4)	45–51
Systolic blood pressure <100 mm Hg, detecting type a dissection	5 (1.8, 14)	0.9 (0.9, 1)	61
Murmur of aortic regurgitation, detecting type a dissection	5 (2.6, 9.8)	0.6 (0.5, 0.8)	43–91
Pulse deficit, detecting type a dissection	1.9 (1.5, 2.3)	0.9 (0.8, 0.9)	43–91
Findings of aortic coarctation, detecting coarctation	242 (89.3, 657)	0.2 (0.1, 0.4)	2
Proportional pulse pressure <0.25, detecting low cardiac index	6.9 (3, 15.8)	0.2 (0.1, 0.6)	50–64
Pulse pressure ≥80 mm Hg, detecting moderate-to-severe aortic regurgitation	10.9 (1.5, 77.1)	0.5 (0.2, 0.8)	42
Positive tourniquet test, detecting dengue infection	6.8 (2.4, 19.1)	0.6 (0.4, 0.7)	41–89

(continued)

APPENDIX TABLE 1 ■ **Likelihood Ratios, Confidence Intervals, and Pretest Probability—Cont'd**

Finding	Positive LR (95% CI)	Negative LR (95% CI)	Pre-test Probability (Range)
EBM Box 17.1 Hypotension and prognosis			
Systolic blood pressure <90 mm Hg, predicting mortality in intensive care patients	3.1 (1.9, 5.1)	0.5 (0.2, 1.3)	21–37
Systolic blood pressure <90 mm Hg, predicting mortality in patients with bacteremia	4.9 (4.2, 5.7)	0.6 (0.2, 1.4)	5–13
Systolic blood pressure <90 mm Hg, predicting mortality in patients with pneumonia	5.3 (3.6, 7.8)	0.7 (0.6, 0.9)	1–10
Systolic blood pressure <90 mm Hg, predicting mortality in emergency department patients with acute illness	15.3 (13.3, 17.4)	0.9 (0.9, 0.9)	2
Systolic blood pressure <80 mm Hg, predicting mortality in patients with acute myocardial infarction	15.5 (12.2, 20)	0.7 (0.7, 0.7)	18
Systolic blood pressure ≤90 mm Hg, detecting adverse outcomes in hospitalized patients	4.7 (3.4, 6.5)	0.7 (0.7, 0.8)	49
Systolic blood pressure ≤85 mm Hg, detecting adverse outcomes in hospitalized patients	9 (5.3, 15.2)	0.8 (0.7, 0.8)	49
Systolic blood pressure ≤80 mm Hg, detecting adverse outcomes in hospitalized patients	16.7 (7.6, 36.4)	0.8 (0.8, 0.8)	49
EBM Box 17.2 Aortic dissection			
Pulse deficit	4.3 (2.4, 7.6)	0.8 (0.7, 0.9)	13–76
Aortic regurgitation murmur	1.6 (1.02, 2.5)	1 (0.9, 1)	23–76
Focal neurologic signs	13.8 (1.3, 152)	0.9 (0.8, 0.9)	23–51
Systolic blood pressure <90 mm Hg	5.6 (3.8, 8.3)	0.9 (0.8, 1)	23
0 predictors	0.1 (0, 0.2)	…	51
1 predictor	0.5 (0.4, 0.8)	…	51
2 predictors	5.3 (3, 9.4)	…	51
3 predictors	65.8 (4.1, 1062)	…	51
EBM Box 17.3 Systolic blood pressure and impaired consciousness			
Systolic blood pressure ≥160 mm Hg in patients with impaired consciousness, detecting structural brain lesions	7.3 (3.6, 14.6)	0.6 (0.4, 0.8)	46–59
Chapter 18 Temperature			
WBC >15,000, detecting bacteremia	1.6 (1.2, 2.2)	0.8 (0.8, 0.9)	9–37
Band count >1,500, detecting bacteremia	2.6 (1.3, 5.1)	0.7 (0.6, 0.9)	8–19
Low food consumption, detecting bacteremia	1.9 (1.4, 2.7)	0.3 (0.2, 0.5)	9–12
High food consumption, detecting bacteremia	0.2 (0.1, 0.3)	1.5 (1.3, 1.8)	9–12
Chills, detecting bacteremia	2 (1.8, 2.3)	0.7 (0.6, 0.8)	7–37
Shaking chills, detecting bacteremia	4.1 (3.2, 5.2)	0.5 (0.3, 0.8)	8–15
Stepladder pattern of fever, detecting enteric fever	177 (11, 2842)	0.5 (0.4, 0.6)	38
Pulse ≤90/min, detecting dengue infection	3.3 (1.8, 5.9)	0.4 (0.3, 0.6)	50
Pulse ≤80/min, detecting dengue infection	5.3 (1.7, 17.2)	0.7 (0.6, 0.9)	50
Relative bradycardia, detecting enteric fever	1.7 (1.4, 2.1)	0.3 (0.1, 0.6)	25
Splenomegaly in FUO, predicting diagnostic bone marrow examination	2.9 (1.9, 4.4)	0.7 (0.5, 0.8)	24–45
Lymphadenopathy in FUO, predicting diagnostic bone marrow examination	1.9 (1.1, 3.2)	0.9 (0.8, 1)	24–45
EBM Box 18.1 Temperature, detecting infection			
Rectal temperature >37.8°C	6.1 (3.9, 9.6)	0.6 (0.5, 0.7)	25
Forehead temperature >37.9°C	4.2 (2.8, 6.5)	0.7 (0.6, 0.8)	25
Tympanic temperature >37.5°C	8.5 (4.7, 15.4)	0.7 (0.6, 0.8)	25

APPENDIX TABLE 1 ▦ **Likelihood Ratios, Confidence Intervals, and Pretest Probability—Cont'd**

Finding	Positive LR (95% CI)	Negative LR (95% CI)	Pre-test Probability (Range)
EBM Box 18.2 Detection of fever			
Patient's report of fever	5.3 (1.4, 19.2)	0.2 (0.1, 0.5)	6–45
Patient's forehead abnormally warm	2.8 (2.4, 3.3)	0.3 (0.2, 0.5)	24–49
EBM Box 18.3 Detection of bacteremia			
Age 50 years or more	1.4 (1.2, 1.6)	0.3 (0.1, 0.8)	16–19
Renal failure	4.6 (2.6, 8.1)	0.8 (0.7, 0.9)	14–21
Hospitalization for trauma	3 (2.4, 3.8)	0.7 (0.3, 1.3)	16–18
Intravenous drug use	1.8 (0.8, 4.1)	1.0 (1.0, 1.0)	7
Previous stroke	1.5 (0.5, 4.4)	1 (0.8, 1.1)	16–21
Diabetes mellitus	1.4 (1.2, 1.7)	0.9 (0.9, 1)	6–37
Poor functional performance	3.6 (2.2, 5.9)	0.6 (0.4, 0.8)	14–21
Rapidly fatal disease (<1 mo)	2.7 (1.4, 5.2)	0.9 (0.9, 1)	7–19
Indwelling urinary catheter present	2.7 (1.7, 4.3)	1 (0.9, 1)	7–37
Central intravenous line present	2.4 (1.7, 3.4)	0.9 (0.9, 0.9)	7–32
Temperature $\geq$38.5 °C	1.2 (1.1, 1.4)	0.7 (0.6, 0.9)	8–19
Tachycardia	1.2 (1.2, 1.3)	0.8 (0.7, 0.9)	9–37
Respiratory rate >20/min	1 (0.9, 1.2)	0.9 (0.8, 1.1)	14–37
Hypotension	2.3 (1.9, 2.9)	0.9 (0.8, 0.9)	7–37
Acute abdomen	1.9 (1.5, 2.3)	0.9 (0.9, 1)	7–32
Confusion or depressed sensorium	1.5 (1.3, 1.7)	0.9 (0.9, 1)	8–37
EBM Box 18.4 Extremes of temperature			
Hyperthermia, predicting death if pontine hemorrhage	23.7 (1.5, 371)	0.4 (0.2, 0.6)	55
Hypothermia, predicting death if congestive heart failure	5.3 (2.7, 10.3)	0.8 (0.7, 1)	5–6
Hypothermia, predicting death if pneumonia	3.5 (1.1, 10.9)	0.8 (0.5, 1.2)	4–9
Hypothermia, predicting death if sepsis	3.6 (2.5, 5.1)	0.9 (0.9, 1)	10–43
Chapter 19 Respiratory rate and patterns			
Portal venous gas on CT, detecting bowel ischemia	3.2 (1.9, 5.4)	0.8 (0.7, 0.9)	51–52
Dilated bowel on CT, detecting bowel ischemia	1.3 (1.1, 1.6)	0.6 (0.5, 0.8)	51–52
Pneumoperitoneum on CT, detecting bowel ischemia	1.4 (0.6, 3.4)	0.9 (0.8, 1.1)	52
Respirations $\leq$12/min if altered mental status, predicting response to naloxone	15.5 (9.6, 25.1)	0.2 (0.1, 0.5)	6
Kussmaul respirations, detecting severe metabolic acidosis in patients with malaria	5.3 (3.2, 8.6)	0.6 (0.5, 0.7)	3–51
Asynchronous breathing, predicting need for intubation or hospital mortality in hospitalized patients with COPD	3.2 (1.3, 7.8)	0.5 (0.2, 1)	31
Paradoxical abdominal movements, detecting diaphragmatic weakness	3.2 (1.7, 5.9)	0.1 (0, 1.1)	27
Orthopnea, detecting ejection fraction <50%	2.7 (1.5, 4.9)	0.04 (0, 0.7)	46
Platypnea, detecting hepatopulmonary syndrome	10.6 (4.4, 25.8)	0.4 (0.2, 0.6)	26
Bendopnea test, detecting pulmonary capillary wedge pressure $\geq$22 mm Hg	3.2 (1.6, 8.5)	0.6 (0.5, 0.8)	45
EBM Box 19.1 Tachypnea			
Respirations >20/min, predicting ischemic bowel or obstruction if pneumatosis	5.9 (1.6, 20.9)	0.8 (0.7, 0.8)	51–52
Respirations >24/min, predicting failure of weaning from mechanical ventilation	2.9 (1.2, 7.1)	0.1 (0, 1.4)	41
Respirations >27/min, predicting cardiopulmonary arrest, in medical inpatients	4.3 (2.1, 8.6)	0.7 (0.5, 0.9)	20–39

(continued)

APPENDIX TABLE 1 ■ **Likelihood Ratios, Confidence Intervals, and Pretest Probability—Cont'd**

Finding	Positive LR (95% CI)	Negative LR (95% CI)	Pre-test Probability (Range)
Respirations >28/min, detecting pneumonia in outpatients with cough and fever	2.7 (1.4, 5.1)	0.9 (0.8, 0.9)	9–38
Respirations >30/min, predicting hospital mortality in patients with pneumonia	2.4 (2.1, 2.8)	0.9 (0.8, 0.9)	2–17
EBM Box 19.2 Cheyne-Stokes respirations			
Cheyne-Stokes respirations, detecting EF <40% (all patients)	5.4 (3.2, 9.2)	0.7 (0.6, 0.8)	20
Cheyne-Stokes respirations, detecting EF <40% (≤80 years old)	8.1 (4, 16.3)	0.7 (0.6, 0.8)	21
Cheyne-Stokes respirations, detecting EF <40% (>80 years old)	2.7 (1.1, 6.6)	0.7 (0.4, 1.1)	17
EBM Box 20.1 Pulse oximetry			
O_2 sat <90%, predicting hospital mortality	4.5 (1.9, 10.5)	0.8 (0.7, 0.9)	6–15
O_2 sat <96%, detecting hepatopulmonary syndrome in patients with chronic liver disease	4.3 (2.2, 8.7)	0.7 (0.6, 0.9)	32–36
O_2 sat <95%, detecting pneumonia in outpatients with cough and fever	3 (2.2, 4.2)	0.7 (0.6, 0.8)	11–51
Chapter 21 The pupils			
Marcus Gunn pupil, detecting abnormal retinal fiber layer in glaucoma	4.2 (2.2, 7.8)	0.1 (0, 0.7)	27
Marcus Gunn pupil, detecting abnormal retinal fiber layer in multiple sclerosis	3.6 (2.1, 6)	0.6 (0.4, 0.9)	9
Positive swinging flashlight test, detecting pathologic cup-to-disc ratio	4.8 (2.2, 10.4)	0.3 (0.1, 1.6)	5
Marcus Gunn pupil, detecting optic nerve or retinal disease if unilateral visual loss	16.8 (4.2, 67.8)	0.3 (0.1, 0.7)	23
Marcus Gunn pupil, detecting macular or media disease if unilateral visual loss	0.1 (0, 0.2)	3.4 (1.5, 7.7)	77
Both pupils nonreactive to light, detecting unfavorable outcome after craniotomy for subdural hematoma	3.4 (1.5, 7.6)	0.4 (0.4, 0.5)	45–53
Pinpoint pupils, detecting response to naloxone if abnormal mental status (opiate intoxication)	8.5 (6.1, 11.9)	0.1 (0, 0.4)	6
EBM Box 21.1 Pupils and anisocoria			
Anisocoria >1 mm, detecting intracranial structural lesion in patients with coma	9 (2.8, 28.8)	0.6 (0.5, 0.8)	40
Absent light reflex in at least one eye, detecting intracranial structural lesion in patients with coma	3.6 (2.3, 5.6)	0.2 (0.1, 0.4)	40
Anisocoria and 3rd nerve palsy, detecting intracranial hemorrhage in patients with stroke	3.2 (1.5, 7.1)	0.7 (0.6, 0.9)	48
Horner syndrome, detecting posterior circulation disease if stroke	72 (4.3, 1213)	1 (0.9, 1)	26
Anisocoria or abnormal light reaction, detecting intracranial aneurysm in patients with 3rd nerve palsy	2.4 (1.9, 3.1)	0.2 (0.1, 0.4)	17–38
Anisocoria (≥1 mm difference) in red eye, with smaller pupil in red eye, detecting serious disease	6.5 (2.6, 16.3)	0.8 (0.8, 0.9)	47
Anisocoria in red eye, with larger pupil in red eye, detecting acute angle closure glaucoma	57.6 (3.6, 915)	0.1 (0, 1.4)	11

APPENDIX TABLE 1 ■ Likelihood Ratios, Confidence Intervals, and Pretest Probability—Cont'd

Finding	Positive LR (95% CI)	Negative LR (95% CI)	Pre-test Probability (Range)
EBM Box 21.2 Horner syndrome, eyedrop tests			
Post topical cocaine anisocoria >1 mm, detecting Horner syndrome	96.8 (6.1, 1527)	0.1 (0, 0.1)	68
Reversal of anisocoria after apraclonidine, detecting Horner syndrome	14 (2.1, 92.3)	0.1 (0, 0.4)	50–69
Small pupil dilates with hydroxyamphetamine, detecting 1st/2nd neuron lesion in patients with Horner syndrome	9.2 (2, 43.6)	0.2 (0.1, 0.3)	45–52
Small pupil fails to dilate with topical phenylephrine, detecting 1st/2nd neuron lesion in patients with Horner syndrome	4.2 (1.3, 13.4)	0.2 (0, 2.1)	21
Asymmetric facial sweating, detecting 1st/2nd neuron lesion in patients with Horner syndrome	2.4 (0.9, 6.1)	0.6 (0.4, 0.9)	63
Chapter 22 Diabetic retinopathy			
Nonmydriatic imaging (>2 F), detecting diabetic retinopathy	24.5 (7.0, 85.8)	0.1 (0.1, 0.2)	
EBM Box 22.1 Diabetic retinopathy			
Abnormal visual acuity 20/40 or worse	1.5 (1.3, 1.7)	0.9 (0.9, 1)	2–24
Direct ophthalmoscopy, nondilated pupils	6.2 (2.5, 14.9)	0.5 (0.3, 0.8)	21
Direct ophthalmoscopy, dilated pupils, general providers	9.4 (6.2, 14.3)	0.4 (0.3, 0.5)	5–15
Direct ophthalmoscopy, dilated pupils, specialists	25.5 (8.2, 79.1)	0.3 (0.2, 0.5)	5–15
Chapter 23 The red eye			
Matting of both eyes, detecting bacterial conjunctivitis	2.6 (1.8, 3.7)	0.7 (0.6, 0.8)	36
Absence of eye matting, detecting bacterial conjunctivitis	0.3 (0.2, 0.7)	1.2 (1.1, 1.3)	36
Itching, detecting bacterial conjunctivitis	0.9 (0.7, 1.1)	1.1 (0.9, 1.3)	36–40
Burning sensation, detecting bacterial conjunctivitis	0.9 (0.5, 1.7)	1.1 (0.9, 1.3)	36–40
Report of "purulent" secretions, detecting bacterial conjunctivitis	0.8 (0.3, 2.1)	1.1 (0.7, 1.6)	40
Clinical diagnosis bacterial conjunctivitis	5.3 (4.2, 6.8)	0.2 (0.1, 0.2)	43
Clinical diagnosis viral conjunctivitis	3.5 (2.8, 4.4)	0.4 (0.3, 0.5)	42
Clinical diagnosis allergic conjunctivitis	16.4 (11.8, 23)	0.01 (0, 0.2)	8
EBM Box 23.1 Serious eye disease			
Direct photophobia	8.3 (2.7, 25.9)	0.4 (0.3, 0.5)	28–59
Indirect photophobia	28.8 (1.8, 459)	0.6 (0.4, 0.7)	59
Finger-to-nose convergence test	21.4 (12, 38.3)	0.3 (0.1, 0.6)	4
Anisocoria (smaller pupil in red eye), serious eye disease	6.5 (2.6, 16.3)	0.8 (0.8, 0.9)	47
Anisocoria (larger pupil in red eye), acute glaucoma	57.6 (3.6, 915)	0.1 (0, 1.4)	11
EBM Box 23.2 Bacterial conjunctivitis			
Redness, periphery only	0.7 (0.5, 1)	1.2 (1, 1.4)	36
Redness observed at 20 feet	1.5 (1.1, 1.9)	0.2 (0, 0.8)	42
Redness obscures tarsal vessels completely	4.6 (1.2, 17.1)	0.7 (0.5, 1)	42
No discharge	0.4 (0.2, 0.8)	…	40–42
Watery discharge	0.4 (0.2, 1.2)	…	40–42
Mucous discharge	1.8 (0.9, 3.8)	…	40–42
Purulent discharge	3.9 (1.7, 9.1)		40–42

(continued)

APPENDIX TABLE 1 ▪ **Likelihood Ratios, Confidence Intervals, and Pretest Probability—Cont'd**

Finding	Positive LR (95% CI)	Negative LR (95% CI)	Pre-test Probability (Range)
Follicular conjunctivitis	1 (0.5, 1.7)	1 (0.6, 1.9)	40
Papillary conjunctivitis	4.4 (0.8, 25.5)	0.8 (0.6, 1.1)	40
Preauricular adenopathy	0.6 (0.1, 4)	1.1 (0.8, 1.6)	40–42
Chapter 24 Hearing			
Patient's perceptions of hearing difficulty	2.5 (0.9, 7)	0.4 (0.2, 0.6)	34–73
EBM Box 24.1 Hearing tests			
Abnormal whispered voice test	6.7 (5, 8.9)	0.1 (0.1, 0.2)	43–73
Cannot hear strong finger rub	355 (22, 5685)	0.4 (0.3, 0.5)	34
Cannot hear faint finger rub	3.9 (3.2, 4.8)	0.02 (0, 0.1)	34
Cannot hear ticking watch	106 (6.6, 1696)	0.6 (0.5, 0.7)	44
Rinne test	27.6 (11.2, 68)	0.3 (0.2, 0.4)	4–72
Weber test lateralizes to good ear, detecting neurosensory loss	2.5 (1.2, 5.6)	0.8 (0.5, 1.4)	30–77
Weber test lateralizes to bad ear, detecting conductive loss	17.1 (0.9, 333)	0.5 (0.3, 0.6)	23–70
Chapter 25 Thyroid disease			
Half relaxation time >380 ms, detecting hypothyroidism	18.7 (13.3, 26)	0.1 (0, 0.2)	9–15
EBM Box 25.1 Goiter			
No goiter by palpation or inspection	0.4 (0.3, 0.5)	...	37–79
Goiter by palpation, visible only after neck extension	0.9 (0.4, 2.1)	...	52
Goiter by palpation and inspection with neck in normal position	26.3 (5.2, 132)	...	37–65
EBM Box 25.2 Goiter and thyroid nodules, predicting carcinoma			
Goiter, cervical adenopathy	15.4 (4.8, 49)	0.6 (0.4, 0.7)	32
Goiter, vocal cord paralysis	11.3 (2.2, 59.3)	0.7 (0.6, 0.9)	12–27
Goiter, fixation to tissues	10.5 (4.7, 23.5)	0.4 (0.3, 0.6)	32
Goiter nodular (vs diffuse)	1.5 (1.2, 1.9)	0.4 (0.2, 0.8)	31
Goiter, pyramidal lobe present	0.2 (0, 1.7)	1.1 (1, 1.2)	31
Thyroid nodule, vocal cord paralysis	17.9 (3.9, 81.1)	0.9 (0.9, 1)	15–23
Thyroid nodule, fixation to surrounding tissues	7.8 (3.3, 18.3)	0.8 (0.6, 1)	23–46
Thyroid nodule, cervical adenopathy	7.2 (4.3, 12)	0.8 (0.7, 0.9)	15–23
Thyroid nodule, ≥4 cm diameter	1.9 (1.4, 2.7)	0.5 (0.4, 0.7)	46
Thyroid nodule, very firm nodule	3.3 (0.2, 52.1)	1 (0.9, 1)	23
EBM Box 25.3 Hypothyroidism			
Cool and dry skin	4.7 (3.1, 7.1)	0.9 (0.8, 0.9)	12
Coarse skin	3.4 (1.4, 8)	0.7 (0.5, 0.9)	18
Cold palms	1.6 (1, 2.7)	0.8 (0.6, 1.1)	18
Dry palms	1.5 (1, 2.4)	0.8 (0.6, 1.1)	18
Puffiness of face	1.7 (0.7, 4.2)	0.6 (0.4, 0.8)	18
Puffiness of wrists	2.9 (1.7, 4.9)	0.7 (0.5, 0.9)	18
Hair loss of eyebrows	1.9 (1.1, 3.6)	0.8 (0.7, 1)	18
Pretibial edema	1.1 (0.9, 1.5)	0.7 (0.3, 1.6)	18
Hypothyroid speech	5.4 (2.7, 10.7)	0.7 (0.5, 0.9)	18
Slow pulse rate	4.2 (3.2, 5.4)	0.7 (0.7, 0.8)	12–20
Enlarged thyroid	2.8 (2.3, 3.4)	0.6 (0.6, 0.7)	12
Delayed ankle reflex	3.4 (1.8, 6.4)	0.6 (0.4, 0.9)	18
Slow movements	1 (0.8, 1.2)	1 (0.3, 3.2)	18
Billewicz score <−15 points	0.1 (0, 0.2)	...	30–37
Billewicz score −15 to +29 points	0.9 (0.4, 2.1)	...	30–37
Billewicz score +30 points or more	18.8 (1.2, 301)	...	30–37

APPENDIX TABLE 1 ■ Likelihood Ratios, Confidence Intervals, and Pretest Probability—Cont'd

Finding	Positive LR (95% CI)	Negative LR (95% CI)	Pre-test Probability (Range)
EBM Box 25.4 Hyperthyroidism			
Pulse rate ≥90/min	4.5 (3.9, 5.2)	0.2 (0.2, 0.3)	50
Skin moist and warm	6.8 (5, 9.2)	0.7 (0.7, 0.7)	50
Thyroid enlargement	2.3 (2.1, 2.5)	0.1 (0.1, 0.2)	50
Eyelid retraction	33.2 (17.2, 64)	0.7 (0.6, 0.7)	50
Eyelid lag	18.6 (9.6, 36.1)	0.8 (0.8, 0.8)	50
Fine finger tremor	11.5 (8.8, 14.9)	0.3 (0.3, 0.4)	50
Wayne index <11 points	0.04 (0, 0.3)	…	32–43
Wayne index 11 to 19 points	1.2 (0.7, 2)	…	32–43
Wayne index ≥20 points	18.2 (2.9, 114)	…	32–43
Chapter 26 Meninges			
Nuchal rigidity, detecting CSF WBC >100/uL	1.5 (1.1, 1.9)	0.9 (0.7, 1)	7–35
Kernig sig, detecting CSF WBC >100/uL	2.5 (1.3, 4.9)	0.9 (0.9, 1)	7–35
Brudzinski sign, detecting CSF WBC >100/uL	2.2 (1.1, 4.6)	0.9 (0.9, 1)	7–35
Lack of focal neurologic findings, detecting subarachnoid hemorrhage in stroke	5.9 (3.5, 9.9)	0.4 (0.2, 0.7)	11
EBM Box 26.1 Meningitis			
Nuchal rigidity, detecting CSF WBC >5/uL	1.5 (1.2, 1.9)	0.7 (0.6, 0.9)	21–69
Kernig sig, detecting CSF WBC >5/uL	2.1 (1.02, 4.3)	0.9 (0.8, 1)	21–69
Brudzinski sign, detecting CSF WBC >5/uL	2.4 (1.5, 3.8)	0.8 (0.7, 1)	21–69
Jolt accentuation headache	1.8 (1.2, 2.7)	0.7 (0.5, 0.9)	20–69
EBM Box 26.2 Intracranial hemorrhage			
Neck stiffness, detecting subarachnoid hemorrhage, if sudden headache	6.7 (5.5, 8.2)	0.7 (0.5, 0.8)	6–46
Neck stiffness, detecting intracranial hemorrhage if stroke	5.4 (2.5, 11.3)	0.7 (0.7, 0.9)	18–59
Chapter 27 Lymphadenopathy			
Generalized pruritus, detecting serious disease	4.9 (1.8, 13.1)	0.9 (0.9, 1)	26
Throat soreness, detecting serious disease	0.2 (0.1, 0.4)	1.4 (1.2, 1.6)	26–71
Posterior cervical adenopathy, detecting infectious mononucleosis	3.1 (1.6, 5.9)	0.7 (0.5, 1)	3
Posterior auricular adenopathy, detecting infectious mononucleosis	11 (4.8, 25.3)	0.7 (0.5, 1)	2
Axillary adenopathy, detecting infectious mononucleosis	3 (1.2, 7.1)	0.8 (0.6, 1.1)	2
Inguinal adenopathy, detecting infectious mononucleosis	3 (1.8, 4.9)	0.6 (0.3, 1)	2
Marked axillary adenopathy, detecting infectious mononucleosis	19.8 (5.7, 69.4)	0.8 (0.6, 1)	2
Epitrochlear nodes >0.5 cm, detecting HIV infection	4.5 (3.1, 6.7)	0.2 (0.1, 0.3)	56
Axillary adenopathy if tuberculosis, detecting HIV infection	4.9 (2.2, 11.2)	0.7 (0.5, 0.9)	9–56
Lymphadenopathy, indicating bone marrow examination diagnostic if FUO	1.9 (1.1, 3.2)	0.9 (0.8, 1)	24–45
Axillary adenopathy, detecting metastases if breast cancer	9.3 (2.3, 37.6)	0.7 (0.7, 0.8)	25–40
EBM Box 27.1 Lymphadenopathy			
Male sex	1.3 (1.1, 1.6)	0.8 (0.7, 0.9)	26–60
Age ≥40 years	2.4 (1.7, 3.5)	0.4 (0.3, 0.6)	26–63
Weight loss	2.8 (1.7, 4.8)	0.8 (0.8, 0.9)	26–53
Fever	0.7 (0.5, 0.9)	1.1 (1.1, 1.2)	26–57

(continued)

APPENDIX TABLE 1 ■ Likelihood Ratios, Confidence Intervals, and Pretest Probability—Cont'd

Finding	Positive LR (95% CI)	Negative LR (95% CI)	Pre-test Probability (Range)
Head and neck nodes (not supraclavicular)	0.9 (0.8, 1.03)	1.1 (1, 1.2)	14–70
Supraclavicular nodes	2.9 (2.4, 3.6)	0.8 (0.8, 0.9)	14–70
Axillary nodes	0.8 (0.7, 0.9)	1.1 (1, 1.1)	14–70
Inguinal nodes	0.6 (0.4, 0.9)	1.1 (1, 1.1)	14–70
Epitrochlear nodes	0.7 (0.1, 7.6)	1 (1, 1.1)	41
Generalized lymphadenopathy	1.3 (0.8, 2.1)	0.9 (0.8, 1.1)	14–60
Node size <4 cm^2	0.4 (0.3, 0.7)	...	26
Node size 4–8.99 cm^2	2 (0.4, 9.2)	...	26
Node size ≥9 cm^2	8.4 (2.1, 32.8)	...	26
Hard texture	3.2 (2.4, 4.3)	0.6 (0.4, 0.7)	26
Lymph node tenderness	0.4 (0.3, 0.6)	1.3 (1.1, 1.5)	26–53
Fixed lymph node	10.9 (2, 59.2)	0.7 (0.3, 1.3)	26–53
Rash	0.6 (0.3, 1.4)	1 (1, 1.1)	26–41
Palpable spleen	1.2 (0.6, 2.5)	1 (0.9, 1)	26–41
Palpable liver	1.2 (0.7, 1.9)	1 (0.9, 1.1)	26–41
Score –3 or less	0.04 (0, 0.2)	...	24–26
Score –2 or –1	0.1 (0, 0.3)	...	24–26
Score 0 to 4	1.1 (0.5, 2.3)	...	24–26
Score 5 or 6	5.1 (2.9, 8.8)	...	24–26
Score 7 or more	21.9 (2.7, 179)	...	24–26
Chapter 28 Inspection of the chest			
Schamroth sign positive, detecting interphalangeal ratio >1	8 (5.1, 12.5)	0.2 (0.1, 0.3)	38
EBM Box 28.1 Clubbing			
Finger clubbing, detecting hypoxemia	3.2 (1.7, 6.1)	0.1 (0.1, 0.3)	75
Finger clubbing, detecting endocarditis	5.1 (2.9, 9.2)	0.9 (0.9, 1)	20
Finger clubbing, detecting hepatopulmonary syndrome	4.3 (2.7, 6.7)	0.6 (0.5, 0.8)	14–37
EBM Box 28.2 Inspection of the chest			
Barrel chest, detecting chronic obstructive disease	1.5 (1.2, 2)	0.6 (0.4, 0.8)	49
AP/L chest diameter ratio ≥0.9, detecting chronic obstructive disease	2 (1.1, 3.3)	0.8 (0.7, 1)	49
Pursed-lip breathing, detecting chronic obstructive disease	2.7 (1.8, 4)	0.5 (0.4, 0.7)	49
Scalene/sternomastoid muscle use, detecting chronic obstructive disease	3.3 (1.8, 5.9)	0.7 (0.6, 0.8)	49
Accessory muscle use in patients with ALS detecting respiratory neuromuscular weakness	4.9 (0.4, 61.7)	0.2 (0.1, 0.6)	92
Accessory muscle use, detecting pulmonary embolism	1.5 (0.6, 3.6)	0.9 (0.8, 1.1)	21
Intercostal retractions, detecting acidosis	2.2 (1.5, 3.1)	0.6 (0.4, 0.8)	21
Suprasternal retractions, detecting acidosis	4 (2.1, 7.6)	0.7 (0.6, 0.9)	21
Nasal flaring, detecting acidosis	4.6 (2.9, 7.4)	0.5 (0.3, 0.7)	21
EBM Box 29.1 Palpation of the chest			
Asymmetric chest expansion, detecting pneumonia	44.1 (2.1, 905)	1 (0.9, 1)	10
Asymmetric chest expansion, detecting pleural effusion	8.1 (5.2, 12.7)	0.3 (0.2, 0.4)	21
Asymmetric chest expansion, detecting right mainstem bronchus intubation	15.8 (5, 49.6)	0.6 (0.4, 0.8)	5–50

APPENDIX TABLE 1 ■ **Likelihood Ratios, Confidence Intervals, and Pretest Probability—Cont'd**

Finding	Positive LR (95% CI)	Negative LR (95% CI)	Pre-test Probability (Range)
Diminished tactile fremitus, detecting pleural effusion	5.7 (4, 8)	0.2 (0.1, 0.4)	20
Chest wall tenderness, detecting pneumonia	1.2 (0.3, 5.3)	1 (0.9, 1.1)	16
Chest wall tenderness, detecting pulmonary embolism	0.8 (0.6, 1.1)	1.1 (1, 1.1)	21–23
Chest wall tenderness, detecting coronary artery disease	0.8 (0.7, 0.9)	1.1 (1, 1.3)	44–62
Chest wall tenderness, detecting myocardial infarction	0.3 (0.2, 0.5)	1.2 (1.2, 1.3)	12–21
EBM Box 29.2 Percussion of the chest			
Percussion dullness, detecting pneumonia	3.6 (2.4, 5.4)	0.9 (0.9, 1)	3–38
Percussion dullness, detecting chest radiograph abnormality	3 (1.4, 6.3)	0.9 (0.9, 1)	26–46
Percussion dullness, detecting pleural effusion	4.8 (3.6, 6.4)	0.1 (0.1, 0.3)	21
Hyperresonance upper right anterior chest, detecting chronic obstructive disease	7.3 (3.6, 14.9)	0.8 (0.7, 0.9)	16–40
Reduced diaphragm excursion, detecting chronic airflow obstruction	5.3 (0.8, 35)	0.9 (0.7, 1.1)	16
Auscultatory percussion abnormal, detecting chest radiograph abnormality	1.7 (1, 3)	0.8 (0.6, 1.1)	26–46
Auscultatory percussion abnormal, detecting pleural effusion	8.3 (1.8, 38.7)	0.2 (0, 1.6)	21–40
Chapter 30 Auscultation of the Lungs			
Any crackles, predicting 30 day mortality in myocardial infarction	4.5 (3.9, 5.3)	0.7 (0.6, 0.8)	4
EBM Box 30.1 Breath sounds and vocal resonance			
Breath sound score ≤9	10.2 (4.6, 22.7)	…	19–56
Breath sound score 10–12	3.6 (1.4, 9.5)	…	19–56
Breath sound score 13–15	0.7 (0.3, 1.5)	…	19–56
Breath sound score ≥16	0.1 (0, 0.3)	…	19–56
Diminished breath sounds, detecting obstructive lung disease	3.5 (2.1, 5.6)	0.5 (0.4, 0.7)	15–49
Diminished or absent breath sounds, detecting pleural effusion in hospitalized patients	5.2 (3.8, 7.1)	0.1 (0.1, 0.3)	21
Diminished breath sounds, detecting underlying pleural effusion in mechanically ventilated patients	3 (1.5, 6)	0.7 (0.6, 0.9)	26–48
Diminished breath sounds, detecting asthma during methacholine challenge	4.2 (1.9, 9.5)	0.3 (0.1, 0.6)	50
Diminished breath sounds, detecting pneumonia in patients with cough and fever	2.4 (1.9, 3)	0.8 (0.8, 0.9)	5–41
Asymmetric breath sounds, detecting endobronchial intubation	12.8 (5.8, 28.4)	0.5 (0.3, 0.8)	5–62
Bronchial breath sounds, detecting pneumonia in patients with cough and fever	3.3 (2.3, 4.8)	0.9 (0.8, 0.9)	14–20
Egophony, detecting pneumonia in patients with cough and fever	4.1 (2.1, 7.8)	0.9 (0.9, 1)	3–38
Reduced vocal fremitus, detecting pleural effusion in hospitalized patients	6.5 (4.4, 9.6)	0.3 (0.2, 0.4)	20
EBM Box 30.2 Crackles			
Crackles, detecting pulmonary fibrosis in asbestos workers	5.9 (2, 17.2)	0.2 (0.1, 0.5)	58
Crackles, detecting "honeycombing" on CT	1.8 (1.5, 2.1)	0.04 (0, 0.7)	18

(continued)

APPENDIX TABLE 1 ▦ Likelihood Ratios, Confidence Intervals, and Pretest Probability—Cont'd

Finding	Positive LR (95% CI)	Negative LR (95% CI)	Pre-test Probability (Range)
Crackles, detecting elevated left atrial pressure in patients with cardiomyopathy	2.1 (1.2, 3.8)	0.8 (0.7, 1)	54–86
Crackles, detecting myocardial infarction in patients with chest pain	2.1 (1.6, 2.8)	0.8 (0.7, 1)	6–12
Crackles, detecting pneumonia in patients with cough and fever	2.8 (1.8, 4.4)	0.8 (0.7, 0.8)	3–41
Early inspiratory crackles, detecting airway obstruction in patients with crackles	14.6 (3, 70)	0.4 (0.1, 1.4)	15–55
Early inspiratory crackles, detecting severe disease in patients with chronic airflow obstruction	20.8 (3, 142.2)	0.1 (0, 0.4)	48
EBM Box 30.3 Wheezes, rubs, and squawks			
Unforced wheezing, detecting chronic airflow obstruction	2.6 (1.7, 3.9)	0.8 (0.7, 0.9)	13–83
Wheezing, detecting pneumonia in patients with cough and fever	0.8 (0.7, 0.9)	1.1 (1, 1.1)	5–41
Wheezing, detecting pulmonary embolism	0.4 (0.1, 0.97)	1.1 (1, 1.2)	23–40
Wheezing during methacholine challenge testing, detecting asthma	6 (1.5, 24.3)	0.6 (0.4, 0.9)	50
Pleural rub, detecting pulmonary embolism	1.4 (0.6, 3.1)	1 (1, 1)	21–23
Pleural rub, detecting pleural effusion	3.9 (0.8, 18.7)	1 (0.9, 1)	21
Inspiratory squawk, detecting hypersensitivity pneumonitis	3.2 (1.9, 5.5)	0.9 (0.9, 1)	22
EBM Box 31.1 Ancillary tests			
Forced expiratory time 9 or more seconds, detecting chronic obstruction	3.9 (2.7, 5.7)	...	50–71
Forced expiratory time 3–9 seconds, detecting chronic obstruction	1.1 (0.8, 1.4)	...	50–71
Forced expiratory time <3 seconds, detecting chronic obstruction	0.2 (0.1, 0.3)	...	50–71
Unable to blow out the match, detecting $FEV_1 \leq 1.6L$	9.6 (5.5, 16.6)	0.2 (0.1, 0.8)	37–56
Chapter 32 Pneumonia			
CRB-65 0, predicting mortality	0.3 (0.2, 0.4)	...	2–13
CRB-65 1, predicting mortality	0.7 (0.6, 0.8)	...	2–14
CRB-65 2, predicting mortality	1.9 (1.6, 2.3)	...	2–14
CRB-65 3, predicting mortality	4.7 (3.8, 5.8)	...	2–14
CRB-65 4, predicting mortality	10.1 (7.7, 13.2)	...	2–14
EBM Box 32.1 Pneumonia			
Cachexia	4 (1.7, 9.6)	0.9 (0.8, 1)	3
Abnormal mental status	1.9 (1.2, 3)	0.9 (0.9, 1)	14–38
Pulse >100/min	2.1 (1.8, 2.5)	0.8 (0.7, 0.8)	3–41
Temperature >37.8°C	2.5 (2, 3.1)	0.7 (0.6, 0.8)	3–51
Respiratory rate >28/min	2.7 (1.4, 5.1)	0.9 (0.8, 0.9)	9–38
Oxygen saturation <95%	3 (2.2, 4.2)	0.7 (0.6, 0.8)	11–51
All vital signs normal	0.3 (0.2, 0.5)	2.3 (1.5, 3.4)	7–38
Asymmetric chest expansion	44.1 (2.1, 905)	1 (0.9, 1)	10
Chest wall tenderness	1.2 (0.3, 5.3)	1 (0.9, 1.1)	16
Percussion dullness	3.6 (2.4, 5.4)	0.9 (0.9, 1)	3–38
Diminished breath sounds	2.4 (1.9, 3)	0.8 (0.8, 0.9)	5–41
Bronchial breath sounds	3.3 (2.3, 4.8)	0.9 (0.8, 0.9)	14–20
Egophony	4.1 (2.1, 7.8)	0.9 (0.9, 1)	3–38
Crackles	2.8 (1.8, 4.4)	0.8 (0.7, 0.8)	3–41

APPENDIX TABLE 1 ■ Likelihood Ratios, Confidence Intervals, and Pretest Probability—Cont'd

Finding	Positive LR (95% CI)	Negative LR (95% CI)	Pre-test Probability (Range)
Wheezing	0.8 (0.7, 0.9)	1.1 (1, 1.1)	5–41
0 or 1 findings	0.3 (0.2, 0.4)	...	7–35
2 or 3 findings	1 (0.9, 1.2)	...	15–35
4 or 5 findings	8.2 (5.8, 11.5)	...	15–35
EBM Box 32.2: Pneumonia and mortality			
Abnormal mental status	3.9 (3.1, 5)	0.8 (0.8, 0.9)	1–31
Heart rate >125/min	2.6 (2.2, 3.1)	0.9 (0.8, 1)	7–16
Systolic blood pressure <90 mm Hg	5.3 (3.6, 7.8)	0.7 (0.6, 0.9)	1–10
Hypothermia	3.5 (1.1, 10.9)	0.8 (0.5, 1.2)	4–9
Respiratory rate ≥30/min	2.4 (2.1, 2.8)	0.9 (0.8, 0.9)	2–17
Oxygen saturation <90%	2.8 (1.4, 5.8)	0.8 (0.6, 1)	1–10
CURB-65 0	0.2 (0.2, 0.3)	...	1–20
CURB-65 1	0.6 (0.5, 0.6)	...	1–20
CURB-65 2	1.3 (1.1, 1.6)	...	1–20
CURB-65 3	2.5 (2.1, 3)	...	1–20
CURB-65 4	5.4 (4.2, 7)	...	1–20
CURB-65 5	8.4 (5.6, 12.5)	...	4–20
Chapter 33 Chronic obstructive lung disease			
Early inspiratory crackles, detecting severe disease	20.8 (3, 142.2)	0.1 (0, 0.4)	48
Any crackles, detecting chronic obstructive pulmonary disease	0.9 (0.5, 1.6)	1 (1, 1)	40–44
EBM Box 33.1 Chronic obstructive pulmonary disease			
Barrel chest	1.5 (1.2, 2)	0.6 (0.4, 0.8)	49
AP/L chest diameter ratio ≥0.9	2 (1.1, 3.3)	0.8 (0.7, 1)	49
Pursed lip breathing	2.7 (1.8, 4)	0.5 (0.4, 0.7)	49
Scalene/sternomastoid muscle use	3.3 (1.8, 5.9)	0.7 (0.6, 0.8)	49
Maximum laryngeal height ≤4 cm	3.6 (2.1, 6)	0.7 (0.6, 0.8)	52
Laryngeal descent, >3 cm	0.9 (0.5, 1.4)	1 (0.9, 1.1)	52
Hoover sign	4.2 (2.5, 7)	0.5 (0.4, 0.7)	37
Subxiphoid cardiac impulse	7.4 (2, 27.1)	0.9 (0.7, 1.1)	16–44
Absent cardiac dullness left lower sternum	11.8 (1.2, 121)	0.9 (0.7, 1.1)	14
Hyperresonance upper right anterior chest	7.3 (3.6, 14.9)	0.8 (0.7, 0.9)	16–40
Diaphragm excursion <2 cm	5.3 (0.8, 35)	0.9 (0.7, 1.1)	16
Reduced breath sounds	3.5 (2.1, 5.6)	0.5 (0.4, 0.7)	15–49
Breath sound score ≤9	10.2 (4.6, 22.7)	...	19–56
Breath sound score 10–12	3.6 (1.4, 9.5)	...	19–56
Breath sound score 13–15	0.7 (0.3, 1.5)	...	19–56
Breath sound score ≥16	0.1 (0, 0.3)	...	19–56
Early inspiratory crackles	14.6 (3, 70)	0.4 (0.1, 1.4)	15–55
Any unforced wheeze	2.6 (1.7, 3.9)	0.8 (0.7, 0.9)	13–83
Forced expiratory time 9 or more seconds	3.9 (2.7, 5.7)	...	50–71
Forced expiratory time 3–9 seconds	1.1 (0.8, 1.4)	...	50–71
Forced expiratory time <3 seconds	0.2 (0.1, 0.3)	...	50–71
≥2 combined findings	25.7 (6.2, 106)	0.3 (0.2, 0.7)	16
EBM Box 33.2 Prognosis of COPD			
BAP-65 class 1	0.3 (0.2, 0.4)	...	3–11
BAP-65 class 2	0.4 (0.3, 0.6)	...	3–11
BAP-65 class 3	1 (0.9, 1.2)	...	3–11
BAP-65 class 4	3.7 (3.2, 4.3)	...	3–11
BAP-65 class 5	9 (6.2, 13.2)	...	3–11
Chapter 34 Pulmonary embolism			
Sudden dyspnea	2.4 (2, 2.9)	0.3 (0.2, 0.3)	40–43

(continued)

APPENDIX TABLE 1 ▪ Likelihood Ratios, Confidence Intervals, and Pretest Probability—Cont'd

Finding	Positive LR (95% CI)	Negative LR (95% CI)	Pre-test Probability (Range)
Syncope	2 (1.6, 2.5)	0.9 (0.8, 1)	19–40
Hemoptysis	1.9 (1.5, 2.5)	1 (0.9, 1)	12–43
Pulse <90/min	0.3 (0.1, 0.8)	1.8 (1.3, 2.5)	33
PaO_2 <80 mm Hg	1.1 (1, 1.3)	0.7 (0.4, 1.1)	28–36
A-a gradient ≤20 mm Hg	0.6 (0.4, 1.01)	1.2 (0.9, 1.5)	27–36
PERC negative and low clinical probability	0.1 (0.1, 0.2)	1.2 (1.2, 1.3)	2–12
EBM Box 34.1 Pulmonary embolism			
Diaphoresis	0.6 (0.3, 1.4)	1 (1, 1.1)	23
Cyanosis	2.3 (0.4, 15.6)	1 (1, 1)	21–23
Pulse rate >100/min	1.4 (1.1, 1.7)	0.9 (0.8, 1)	12–43
Systolic blood pressure ≤100 mm Hg	1.9 (1.1, 3)	1 (0.9, 1)	27
Temperature >38°C	0.5 (0.3, 0.9)	1.1 (1, 1.1)	21–43
Respiratory rate >30/min	2 (1.5, 2.8)	0.9 (0.8, 0.9)	28
Accessory muscle use	1.5 (0.6, 3.6)	0.9 (0.8, 1.1)	21
Crackles	0.8 (0.4, 1.6)	1.1 (0.7, 1.8)	23–38
Wheezes	0.4 (0.1, 0.97)	1.1 (1, 1.2)	23–40
Pleural friction rub	1.4 (0.6, 3.1)	1 (1, 1)	21–23
Elevated neck veins	1.7 (1.1, 2.6)	1 (0.9, 1)	21–38
Left parasternal heave	2.4 (1.03, 5.5)	1 (1, 1)	21–23
Loud P_2	2 (0.8, 5.1)	0.9 (0.8, 1)	22–33
New gallop (S_3 or S_4)	2.7 (1, 7)	0.8 (0.6, 1)	33
Chest wall tenderness	0.8 (0.6, 1.1)	1.1 (1, 1.1)	21–23
Unilateral calf pain or swelling	2.9 (2.2, 4)	0.8 (0.7, 0.8)	12–43
Wells score low probability	0.3 (0.2, 0.4)	…	9–43
Wells moderate probability	1.6 (1.4, 1.8)	…	9–43
Wells high probability	8.2 (5, 13.5)	…	9–43
Revised Geneva low probability	0.4 (0.3, 0.5)	…	15–32
Revised Geneva moderate probability	1.1 (1, 1.3)	…	15–32
Revised Geneva high probability	5.9 (4.5, 7.6)	…	15–32
Chapter 35 Pleural effusion			
Diminished breath sounds, detecting underlying pleural effusion in mechanically ventilated patients	3 (1.5, 6)	0.7 (0.6, 0.9)	26–48
EBM Box 35.1 Pleural effusion			
Asymmetric chest expansion	8.1 (5.2, 12.7)	0.3 (0.2, 0.4)	21
Reduced tactile fremitus	5.7 (4, 8)	0.2 (0.1, 0.4)	20
Dullness by conventional percussion	4.8 (3.6, 6.4)	0.1 (0.1, 0.3)	21
Auscultatory percussion (Guarino method)	8.3 (1.8, 38.7)	0.2 (0, 1.6)	21–40
Decreased or absent breath sounds	5.2 (3.8, 7.1)	0.1 (0.1, 0.3)	21
Diminished vocal resonance	6.5 (4.4, 9.6)	0.3 (0.2, 0.4)	20
Crackles	0.7 (0.5, 1)	1.5 (1.1, 2)	21
Pleural rub	3.9 (0.8, 18.7)	1 (0.9, 1)	21
Chapter 36 Inspection of neck veins			
Measured RA pressure ≥10 mm Hg, detecting pulmonary capillary wedge pressure ≥22 Hg	3.5 (2.2, 5.7)	0.3 (0.2, 0.5)	51–62
Hand vein measure of venous pressure, detecting CVP >12 mm Hg	4.9 (1.6, 14.3)	0.8 (0.6, 0.9)	34
Hand vein measure of venous, detecting CVP <7 mm Hg	2.3 (1.7, 3.2)	0.1 (0, 0.8)	14
Kussmaul sign, predicting mortality	3.5 (1.5, 8.1)	0.7 (0.5, 0.9)	43
Intermittent cannon a waves, detecting atrioventricular dissociation	3.8 (1.8, 8.2)	0.1 (0, 0.4)	55

APPENDIX TABLE 1 ■ **Likelihood Ratios, Confidence Intervals, and Pretest Probability—Cont'd**

Finding	Positive LR (95% CI)	Negative LR (95% CI)	Pre-test Probability (Range)
EBM Box 36.1 Inspection of neck veins			
Elevated venous pressure, detecting CVP >8 cm water	8.9 (4.6, 17.3)	0.3 (0.2, 0.5)	30–70
Elevated venous pressure, detecting CVP >12 cm water	6.6 (2.7, 16.1)	0.2 (0.1, 0.4)	17–55
Elevated venous pressure, detecting elevated left heart diastolic pressures	3.9 (1.6, 9.4)	0.7 (0.5, 1)	19–75
Elevated venous pressure, detecting low left ventricular ejection fraction	6.3 (3.5, 11.3)	0.9 (0.8, 1)	8–69
Elevated venous pressure, detecting pulmonary hypertension	2.5 (1.2, 5.4)	0.4 (0.3, 0.6)	84
Elevated venous pressure, detecting myocardial infarction in patients with chest pain	2.4 (1.4, 4.2)	0.9 (0.9, 1)	6
Elevated venous pressure, predicting postoperative pulmonary edema	11.3 (5, 25.8)	0.8 (0.7, 1)	4
Elevated venous pressure, predicting postoperative myocardial infarction or CHF	9.4 (4, 22.4)	0.8 (0.7, 1)	4
Estimated venous pressure ≤5 cm water, detecting measured venous pressure ≤5 cm water	8.4 (2.8, 25)	0.1 (0, 0.7)	26
Positive abdominojugular test, detecting elevated left heart diastolic pressures	8 (2.1, 31.2)	0.3 (0.2, 0.6)	17–75
Early systolic outward movement, detecting moderate-to-severe tricuspid regurgitation	10.9 (5.5, 21.7)	0.7 (0.5, 0.8)	18
EBM Box 37.1 Percussion of the heart			
Cardiac dullness >10.5 cm from midsternal line (patient supine), detecting cardiothoracic ratio >0.5	2.5 (1.8, 3.4)	0.05 (0, 0.3)	36
Cardiac dullness extending >10.5 cm from midsternal line (patient supine), detecting increased left ventricular end-diastolic volume	1.4 (1.1, 1.7)	0.2 (0, 1.3)	17
Cardiac dullness extending beyond midclavicular line (patient upright), detecting cardiothoracic ratio >0.5	2.4 (1.1, 5.2)	0.1 (0, 0.4)	76
Chapter 38 Palpation of the heart			
RV heave, detecting PA pressure ≥25 mm Hg in pulmonary hypertension clinic	2.7 (0.9, 7.8)	0.7 (0.5, 0.9)	84
Palpable P_2, detecting PA pressure ≥25 mm Hg in pulmonary hypertension clinic	0.9 (0.5, 1.7)	1.1 (0.7, 1.5)	84
EBM Box 38.1 Size and position of apical impulse			
Supine apical impulse lateral to MCL, detecting cardiothoracic ratio >0.5	3.4 (1.6, 7.3)	0.6 (0.5, 0.8)	25–28
Supine apical impulse lateral to MCL, detecting low ejection fraction	10.3 (5, 21.1)	0.7 (0.6, 0.9)	8–69
Supine apical impulse lateral to MCL, detecting increased left ventricular end-diastolic volume	5.1 (2.7, 9.7)	0.7 (0.6, 0.8)	15–48
Supine apical impulse lateral to MCL, detecting pulmonary capillary wedge pressure >12 mm Hg	5.8 (1.3, 26)	0.6 (0.4, 1)	30
Supine apical impulse >10 cm from midsternal line, detecting cardiothoracic ratio >0.5	4.3 (0.3, 70.8)	0.5 (0.3, 0.8)	25–36
Apical beat diameter ≥4 cm in left lateral decubitus position at 45°, detecting increased left ventricular end diastolic volume	4.7 (2.1, 10.2)	0.4 (0.2, 1)	32–50

(continued)

APPENDIX TABLE 1 ▦ Likelihood Ratios, Confidence Intervals, and Pretest Probability—Cont'd

Finding	Positive LR (95% CI)	Negative LR (95% CI)	Pre-test Probability (Range)
EBM Box 38.2 Abnormal palpable movements			
Hyperkinetic apical movement, detecting associated mitral regurgitation or aortic valve disease in patients with mitral stenosis	11.2 (6.4, 19.5)	0.3 (0.2, 0.4)	39
Sustained or double supine apical impulse, detecting left ventricular hypertrophy	5.6 (3.3, 9.5)	0.5 (0.3, 0.7)	27
Sustained apical movement detecting aortic stenosis in patients with aortic flow murmurs	4.1 (1.7, 10.1)	0.3 (0.1, 0.5)	69
Sustained apical movement, detecting moderate-to-severe aortic regurgitation in patients with basal early diastolic murmurs	2.4 (1.4, 4)	0.1 (0, 0.9)	41
Lower sternal movements, detecting moderate-to-severe tricuspid regurgitation	12.5 (4.1, 38)	0.8 (0.8, 0.9)	18
Sustained left lower parasternal movement, detecting right ventricular peak pressure ≥50 mm Hg	3.6 (1.4, 8.9)	0.4 (0.2, 0.7)	51
RV rock, detecting moderate-to-severe tricuspid regurgitation	31.4 (1.6, 601)	0.9 (0.9, 1)	18
Pulsatile liver, detecting moderate-to-severe tricuspid regurgitation	6.5 (2.2, 19.3)	0.8 (0.7, 1)	18–41
Palpable S_2, detecting pulmonary hypertension in patients with mitral stenosis	3.6 (1.5, 8.8)	0.05 (0, 0.8)	52
EBM Box 40.1 First and second heart sounds			
Varying intensity of S_1, detecting atrioventricular dissociation	24.4 (1.5, 385)	0.4 (0.3, 0.7)	55
Fixed wide splitting of S_2, detecting atrial septal defect	2.6 (1.6, 4.3)	0.1 (0, 0.8)	30
Paradoxical splitting of S_2, detecting significant aortic stenosis	2.4 (0.8, 7)	0.6 (0.2, 1.7)	5
Loud P_2, detecting pulmonary hypertension if mitral stenosis	1.2 (0.9, 1.5)	0.8 (0.3, 1.9)	32–52
Loud P_2, detecting pulmonary hypertension if cirrhosis	17.6 (2.1, 149)	0.6 (0.4, 1.1)	15
Palpable P_2, detecting pulmonary hypertension	3.6 (1.5, 8.8)	0.05 (0, 0.8)	52
Absent or soft S_2, detecting severe aortic stenosis in patients with aortic flow murmurs	3.8 (2.4, 6)	0.4 (0.4, 0.5)	5–60
Chapter 41 Third and fourth heart sounds			
S_3 in mitral regurgitation, detecting elevated filling pressure	1.7 (1,3)	0.7 (0.5, 0.9)	76
S_3 in mitral regurgitation, detecting low ejection fraction	1.9 (1.2, 2.9)	0.6 (0.4, 0.9)	34
S_3 in aortic stenosis, detecting pulmonary capillary wedge pressure >12 mm Hg	2.3 (1.3, 4)	0.9 (0.8, 1)	46
S_3 in aortic stenosis, detecting ejection fraction <0.5	5.7 (2.7, 12)	0.8 (0.7, 0.9)	41
S_3 in aortic regurgitation, detecting severe regurgitation	5.9 (1.4, 25.3)	0.8 (0.7, 0.9)	50
S_3 in aortic regurgitation, detecting ejection fraction <0.5	8.3 (3.6, 19.2)	0.4 (0.2, 0.9)	8
EBM Box 41.1 Third and fourth heart sounds			
S_3, detecting ejection fraction <0.5	3.4 (2.6, 4.4)	0.7 (0.5, 0.8)	30–80
S_3, detecting ejection fraction <0.3	4.1 (2.3, 7.3)	0.3 (0.2, 0.5)	19–47
S_3, detecting elevated left heart filling pressure	3.9 (2.1, 7.1)	0.8 (0.7, 0.9)	19–68

APPENDIX TABLE 1 ■ Likelihood Ratios, Confidence Intervals, and Pretest Probability—Cont'd

Finding	Positive LR (95% CI)	Negative LR (95% CI)	Pre-test Probability (Range)
S_3, detecting elevated BNP level	10.1 (4.2, 23.9)	0.5 (0.3, 0.8)	50–61
S_3, detecting myocardial infarction in patients with acute chest pain	3.2 (1.6, 6.5)	0.9 (0.8, 1)	12
S_3, predicting postoperative pulmonary edema	14.6 (5.7, 37.3)	0.8 (0.7, 1)	4
S_3, predicting postoperative myocardial infarction or cardiac death	8 (2.7, 23.4)	0.9 (0.8, 1)	4
S_4, detecting elevated left heart filling pressures	1.3 (0.8, 1.9)	0.9 (0.7, 1.2)	46–67
S_4, detecting severe aortic stenosis	0.9 (0.5, 1.9)	1.1 (0.6, 1.9)	5–90
S_4, predicting 5-year mortality in patients after myocardial infarction	3.2 (1.3, 7.8)	0.8 (0.6, 1.1)	9
EBM Box 43.1 Murmurs and valvular heart disease			
Functional murmur, detecting normal echocardiogram	5.4 (2.9, 10.2)	0.1 (0.1, 0.4)	21–88
Characteristic murmur, detecting mild or worse aortic stenosis	10.5 (2.8, 40)	0.1 (0.1, 0.3)	13–20
Characteristic murmur, detecting severe aortic stenosis	3.5 (3.1, 4)	0.1 (0, 0.2)	2–26
Characteristic murmur, detecting pulmonic stenosis	55.4 (7.1, 432)	0.4 (0.2, 1)	7
Characteristic murmur, detecting mild or worse mitral regurgitation	5.5 (3.8, 7.8)	0.5 (0.4, 0.6)	38–57
Characteristic murmur, detecting moderate or severe mitral regurgitation	3.8 (2, 7)	0.4 (0.3, 0.5)	8–20
Characteristic murmur, detecting mild or worse tricuspid regurgitation	10.1 (5.1, 19.8)	0.6 (0.3, 1.1)	23–39
Characteristic murmur detecting moderate or severe tricuspid regurgitation	10.3 (6.7, 16)	0.7 (0.5, 0.9)	7–18
Characteristic murmur, detecting ventricular septal defect	28.1 (12.5, 63)	0.1 (0, 0.4)	4–13
Characteristic murmur, detecting mitral valve prolapse	12.1 (4, 36.4)	0.5 (0.2, 0.9)	11
Characteristic murmur, detecting mild aortic regurgitation or worse	10.1 (5.3, 19.2)	0.3 (0.3, 0.4)	23–88
Characteristic murmur, detecting moderate or severe aortic regurgitation	4.3 (2.1, 8.6)	0.1 (0.1, 0.2)	8–35
Characteristic murmur, detecting pulmonic regurgitation	17.4 (3.6, 83.2)	0.9 (0.8, 1)	15
Characteristic murmur, detecting mitral stenosis	31.2 (7.9, 123)	0.1 (0, 0.3)	32
EBM Box 43.2 Differential diagnosis of systolic murmurs in adults			
Detecting aortic stenosis			
Broad apical-base murmur pattern	9.7 (6.7, 14)	0.1 (0.1, 0.2)	20
Broad apical murmur pattern	0.2 (0.1, 0.9)	1.1 (1.1, 1.2)	20
LLSB murmur pattern	0.7 (0.2, 2.4)	1 (1, 1.1)	20
S_1 inaudible	5.1 (3.5, 7.4)	0.5 (0.4, 0.6)	20
S_2 inaudible	12.7 (5.3, 30.4)	0.7 (0.6, 0.8)	21
S_2 loud	1.7 (0.9, 3.1)	0.9 (0.8, 1)	21
Radiation to neck	2.4 (1.9, 3)	0.2 (0.1, 0.3)	33
Timing mid-systolic or early systolic	0.4 (0.3, 0.6)	2 (1.5, 2.5)	33
Timing long systolic or holosystolic	2.2 (1.7, 2.8)	0.4 (0.3, 0.6)	33
Coarse quality murmur	3.3 (2.4, 4.5)	0.3 (0.2, 0.4)	33
Murmur same intensity in beat after pause	0.4 (0.2, 0.7)	1.9 (1.3, 2.8)	36
Detecting moderate or severe mitral regurgitation			
Broad apical-base murmur pattern	1.1 (0.7, 1.7)	1 (0.8, 1.1)	20

(continued)

APPENDIX TABLE 1 ■ Likelihood Ratios, Confidence Intervals, and Pretest Probability—Cont'd

Finding	Positive LR (95% CI)	Negative LR (95% CI)	Pre-test Probability (Range)
Broad apical murmur pattern	6.8 (3.9, 11.9)	0.7 (0.6, 0.8)	20
LLSB murmur pattern	1.1 (0.4, 3.4)	1 (0.9, 1.1)	20
S_1 inaudible	1.4 (0.9, 2.2)	0.9 (0.8, 1.1)	20
S_2 inaudible	0.5 (0.2, 1.6)	1.1 (1, 1.1)	20
S_2 loud	4.7 (2.7, 8.3)	0.7 (0.6, 0.9)	20
Radiation to neck	0.6 (0.4, 0.9)	1.6 (1.2, 2.1)	28
Timing mid-systolic or early systolic	0.4 (0.2, 0.6)	1.9 (1.5, 2.5)	28
Timing long systolic or holosystolic	1.9 (1.5, 2.4)	0.5 (0.3, 0.7)	28
Coarse quality murmur	0.5 (0.3, 0.8)	1.5 (1.2, 1.8)	28
Murmur same intensity in beat after pause	2.5 (1.5, 4.3)	0.4 (0.3, 0.7)	44
Detecting moderate or severe tricuspid regurgitation			
Broad apical-base murmur pattern	0.8 (0.4, 1.3)	1.1 (0.9, 1.3)	18
Broad apical murmur pattern	2.5 (1.4, 4.5)	0.8 (0.7, 1)	18
LLSB murmur pattern	8.4 (3.5, 20.3)	0.8 (0.7, 0.9)	18
S_1 inaudible	1 (0.6, 1.7)	1 (0.9, 1.1)	18
S_2 inaudible	1.4 (0.6, 3.3)	1 (0.9, 1.1)	18
S_2 loud	3.6 (2.1, 6.3)	0.7 (0.6, 0.9)	18
Radiation to neck	0.6 (0.4, 0.9)	1.5 (1.2, 2)	22
Timing mid-systolic or early systolic	0.5 (0.3, 0.8)	1.7 (1.3, 2.1)	22
Timing long systolic or holosystolic	1.7 (1.3, 2.2)	0.5 (0.3, 0.8)	22
Coarse quality murmur	0.5 (0.3, 0.9)	1.4 (1.2, 1.8)	22
Murmur same intensity in beat after pause	2.3 (1.4, 3.6)	0.4 (0.2, 0.8)	35
EBM Box 43.3 Systolic murmurs and maneuvers			
Murmur louder with inspiration, detecting right-sided murmur	7.8 (3.7, 16.7)	0.2 (0.1, 0.5)	20–50
Murmur louder with Valsalva strain, detecting hypertrophic cardiomyopathy	14 (3.4, 57.4)	0.3 (0.1, 0.8)	20
Murmur louder with squatting-to-standing, detecting hypertrophic cardiomyopathy	6 (2.9, 12.3)	0.1 (0, 0.8)	20
Murmur softer with standing-to-squatting, detecting hypertrophic cardiomyopathy	7.6 (2.5, 22.7)	0.1 (0, 0.4)	20–41
Murmur softer with passive leg elevation, detecting hypertrophic cardiomyopathy	9 (3.5, 23.3)	0.1 (0, 0.7)	20
Murmur softer with hand grip, detecting hypertrophic cardiomyopathy	3.6 (2, 6.4)	0.1 (0, 0.9)	20
Murmur louder with hand grip, detecting mitral regurgitation or ventricular septal defect	5.8 (1.9, 17.3)	0.3 (0.2, 0.5)	40–65
Murmur louder with transient arterial occlusion, detecting mitral regurgitation or ventricular septal defect	48.7 (3.1, 769)	0.2 (0.1, 0.5)	40
Murmur softer with amyl nitrite inhalation, detecting mitral regurgitation or ventricular septal defect	10.5 (5.1, 21.5)	0.2 (0.1, 0.6)	40–71
Chapter 44 Aortic stenosis			
Effort syncope and aortic murmur, detecting severe aortic stenosis	3.1 (1.3, 7.3)	0.9 (0.8, 1)	70–75
Angina and aortic murmur, detecting severe aortic stenosis	0.9 (0.7, 1)	1.3 (0.9, 1.9)	70
Dyspnea and aortic murmur, detecting severe aortic stenosis	1.4 (0.6, 3.1)	0.8 (0.4, 1.5)	70
Calcification of aortic valve on CXR, detecting severe aortic stenosis	3.9 (2.1, 7.3)	0.5 (0.4, 0.7)	49–70
ECG LVH, detecting severe aortic stenosis	2.1 (1.7, 2.7)	0.5 (0.4, 0.6)	13–70

APPENDIX TABLE 1 ■ **Likelihood Ratios, Confidence Intervals, and Pretest Probability—Cont'd**

Finding	Positive LR (95% CI)	Negative LR (95% CI)	Pre-test Probability (Range)
Delayed carotid artery upstroke, detecting moderate-to-severe aortic stenosis	7.6 (3.8, 15.1)	0.5 (0.4, 0.7)	13–57
Absent or diminished S_2, detecting moderate-to-severe aortic stenosis	7.4 (2.8, 19.2)	0.5 (0.4, 0.7)	13–57
Prolonged duration of murmur, detecting moderate-to-severe aortic stenosis	11.4 (1.3, 97.2)	0.3 (0.2, 0.4)	24–57
Murmur late peaking, detecting moderate-to-severe aortic stenosis	13.7 (2.9, 65.7)	0.3 (0.2, 0.4)	24–49
0 to 6 points, detecting moderate-to-severe aortic stenosis	0.2 (0.1, 0.4)	4.7 (1.9, 11.4)	73
7 to 9 points, detecting moderate-to-severe aortic stenosis	2.7 (0.9, 8.1)	…	73
10 to 14 points, detecting moderate-to-severe aortic stenosis	10.6 (1.5, 73.3)	0.6 (0.4, 0.7)	73
EBM Box 44.1 Aortic stenosis murmur			
Aortic systolic murmur, detecting mild or worse aortic stenosis	10.5 (2.8, 40)	0.1 (0.1, 0.3)	13–20
Aortic systolic murmur, detecting severe aortic stenosis	3.5 (3.1, 4)	0.1 (0, 0.2)	2–26
EBM Box 44.2 Severe aortic stenosis			
Delayed carotid artery upstroke	3.5 (2.6, 4.6)	0.4 (0.2, 0.7)	5–69
Reduced carotid artery volume	2.3 (1.8, 2.9)	0.4 (0.3, 0.7)	28–69
Brachioradial delay	2.5 (1.4, 4.7)	0.04 (0, 0.7)	52
Sustained apical impulse	4.1 (1.7, 10.1)	0.3 (0.1, 0.5)	69
Apical-carotid delay	2.6 (1.4, 5.2)	0.05 (0, 0.7)	53
Absent or soft S_2	3.8 (2.4, 6)	0.4 (0.4, 0.5)	5–60
S_4 gallop	0.9 (0.5, 1.9)	1.1 (0.6, 1.9)	5–90
Murmur grade ≥3/6	1.2 (1, 1.4)	0.8 (0.5, 1.3)	29–70
Murmur early systolic	0.1 (0, 0.7)	1.6 (1.3, 2)	28
Murmur prolonged duration	3 (1.7, 5.2)	0.2 (0.1, 0.4)	5–28
Murmur late peaking	3.7 (2.6, 5.2)	0.2 (0.1, 0.2)	5–75
Murmur loudest over aortic area	1.8 (1.1, 2.9)	0.6 (0.4, 0.7)	5–49
Murmur radiates to neck	1.4 (1.1, 1.8)	0.1 (0.1, 0.3)	5–49
Murmur radiates to both sides of neck	1.9 (1.1, 3.4)	0.7 (0.4, 1)	28
Murmur quality blowing	0.1 (0, 0.8)	1.4 (1.2, 1.7)	28
Murmur with humming quality	2.1 (1.3, 3.5)	0.5 (0.3, 0.9)	28
EBM Box 45.1 Aortic regurgitation			
Characteristic diastolic murmur, detecting mild aortic regurgitation or worse	10.1 (5.3, 19.2)	0.3 (0.3, 0.4)	23–88
Characteristic diastolic murmur, detecting moderate or severe aortic regurgitation	4.3 (2.1, 8.6)	0.1 (0.1, 0.2)	8–35
Murmur loudest on right side of sternum, detecting dilated aortic root or endocarditis	8.2 (5, 13.3)	0.7 (0.7, 0.8)	14
Murmur softer with amyl nitrite, detecting aortic regurgitation (vs. Graham Steell murmur)	5.7 (0.5, 71.4)	0.1 (0, 0.3)	93
EBM Box 45.2 Moderate-to-severe aortic regurgitation			
Murmur grade 3 or louder	8.2 (2.2, 31.1)	0.6 (0.4, 0.9)	24–45
Diastolic blood pressure >70 mm Hg	0.2 (0.1, 0.9)	…	41–56
Diastolic blood pressure 51–70 mm Hg	1.1 (0.7, 1.7)	…	41–56
Diastolic blood pressure ≤50 mm Hg	19.3 (2.7, 141)	…	41–56
Pulse pressure <60 mm Hg	0.3 (0.1, 0.9)	…	42
Pulse pressure 60–79 mm Hg	0.8 (0.2, 2.9)	…	42
Pulse pressure ≥80 mm Hg	10.9 (1.5, 77.1)	…	42

(continued)

APPENDIX TABLE 1 ▓ **Likelihood Ratios, Confidence Intervals, and Pretest Probability—Cont'd**

Finding	Positive LR (95% CI)	Negative LR (95% CI)	Pre-test Probability (Range)
Hill's test, difference >40 mm Hg	6 (2, 17.9)	0.5 (0.3, 0.8)	42–90
Enlarged or sustained apical impulse	2.4 (1.4, 4)	0.1 (0, 0.9)	41
S_3 gallop	5.9 (1.4, 25.3)	0.8 (0.7, 0.9)	50
Duroziez's sign, femoral pistol shot, water hammer pulse	3.4 (0.4, 31)	0.7 (0.5, 0.9)	41–75
Chapter 46 Miscellaneous heart murmurs			
Apical mid-diastolic rumble, detecting mitral annular calcification	7.5 (2.3, 24.4)	0.9 (0.9, 1)	55
EBM Box 46.1 Moderate-to-severe mitral or tricuspid regurgitation			
MR murmur grade 3 or louder	4.4 (2.9, 6.7)	0.2 (0.1, 0.3)	42
S_3 gallop (MR)	4.4 (0.6, 31.8)	0.8 (0.7, 0.8)	49–62
CV wave, neck veins (TR)	10.9 (5.5, 21.7)	0.7 (0.5, 0.8)	18
Lower sternal precordial pulsation (TR)	12.5 (4.1, 38)	0.8 (0.8, 0.9)	18
RV rock (TR)	31.4 (1.6, 601)	0.9 (0.9, 1)	18
Pulsatile liver (TR)	6.5 (2.2, 19.3)	0.8 (0.7, 1)	18–41
EBM Box 46.2 Other findings in mitral stenosis			
Graham Steell murmur, detecting pulmonary hypertension	4.2 (1.1, 15.5)	0.4 (0.2, 0.9)	52
Hyperkinetic apical movement, detecting associated mitral regurgitation or aortic valve disease	11.2 (6.4, 19.5)	0.3 (0.2, 0.4)	39
Hyperkinetic arterial pulse, detecting associated mitral regurgitation	14.2 (7.4, 27.2)	0.3 (0.2, 0.4)	35
Chapter 47 Disorders of the pericardium			
Fever, detecting specific diagnosis (e.g., neoplasia, autoimmune, bacterial infection)	4.3 (2.9, 6.4)	0.6 (0.5, 0.8)	17
Fever, detecting idiopathic or viral pericarditis	0.2 (0.2, 0.3)	1.6 (1.3, 1.9)	83
Pericardial rub in patient with cancer and pericarditis, detecting idiopathic or radiation-induced pericarditis (not neoplastic)	5.5 (1.4, 21.9)	0.4 (0.2, 0.9)	42
Pericardial rub and inflammatory signs in patient with pericarditis, detecting non-neoplastic pericarditis	2.3 (1.1, 4.6)	0.7 (0.6, 0.9)	87
Pulsus paradoxus >12 mm Hg, detecting cardiac tamponade	5.9 (2.4, 14.3)	0.03 (0, 0.2)	63
Oximetry paradoxus <1.2, detecting cardiac tamponade	0.05 (0, 0.7)	2.1 (1.5, 2.7)	26
Tamponade, predicting a specific etiology will be found	21.5 (6.3, 73.6)	0.8 (0.8, 0.9)	17
Chapter 48 Congestive heart failure			
Crackles, detecting elevated filling pressure in patients with known cardiomyopathy	2.1 (1.2, 3.8)	0.8 (0.7, 1)	54–86
Pulse-amplitude ratio >0.7, detecting wedge pressure >15 mm Hg	5.2 (1.7, 16.6)	0.5 (0.3, 1)	39–55
Cheyne-Stokes respirations, detecting ejection fraction <0.40 (age 80 years or less)	8.1 (4, 16.3)	0.7 (0.6, 0.8)	21
Cheyne-Stokes respirations, detecting ejection fraction <0.40 (age >80 years)	2.7 (1.1, 6.6)	0.7 (0.4, 1.1)	17
S_3 gallop, detecting ejection fraction <30%	4.1 (2.3, 7.3)	0.3 (0.2, 0.5)	19–47
Proportional pulse pressure ≤25%, detecting low cardiac index	6.9 (3, 15.8)	0.2 (0.1, 0.6)	50–64
S_3, detecting consensus diagnosis of heart failure	7.7 (5.6, 10.6)	0.9 (0.9, 0.9)	29–55

APPENDIX TABLE 1 ■ **Likelihood Ratios, Confidence Intervals, and Pretest Probability—Cont'd**

Finding	Positive LR (95% CI)	Negative LR (95% CI)	Pre-test Probability (Range)
Displaced apical impulse, detecting consensus diagnosis of heart failure	6.7 (4, 11)	0.8 (0.7, 0.8)	29
Elevated neck veins, detecting consensus diagnosis of heart failure	4 (3.2, 5)	0.7 (0.7, 0.8)	29–71
BNP ≥100, detecting consensus diagnosis of heart failure	2.7 (2, 3.7)	0.1 (0.1, 0.2)	35–62
Cold profile if heart failure, predicting early mortality	3 (2, 4.5)	0.7 (0.6, 0.8)	5–18
EBM Box 48.1 Detecting elevated left heart filling pressure			
Heart rate >100/min at rest	5.5 (1.3, 24.1)	0.9 (0.9, 1)	19
Abnormal Valsalva response	7.6 (1.7, 34.3)	0.1 (0, 0.8)	48
Pulse increase of 10% during Valsalva strain	0.2 (0.1, 0.9)	1.7 (1.3, 2.2)	25
Crackles	1.6 (0.8, 2.9)	0.9 (0.9, 1)	19–77
Elevated jugular venous pressure	3.9 (1.6, 9.4)	0.7 (0.5, 1)	19–75
Positive abdominojugular test	8 (2.1, 31.2)	0.3 (0.2, 0.6)	17–75
Supine apical impulse lateral to MCL	5.8 (1.3, 26)	0.6 (0.4, 1)	30
S_3 gallop	3.9 (2.1, 7.1)	0.8 (0.7, 0.9)	19–68
S_4 gallop	1.3 (0.8, 1.9)	0.9 (0.7, 1.2)	46–67
Edema	1.4 (0.6, 3.2)	1 (0.9, 1)	19–68
Bendopnea test	3.2 (1.6, 6.5)	0.6 (0.5, 0.8)	45
EBM Box 48.2 Detecting low ejection fraction			
Heart rate >100 beats/min at rest	2.8 (1.3, 5.9)	0.8 (0.7, 1)	16
Cheyne-Stokes respirations	5.4 (3.2, 9.2)	0.7 (0.6, 0.8)	20
Abnormal Valsalva response	7.6 (4.9, 11.8)	0.3 (0.2, 0.4)	41–46
Crackles	1.5 (0.9, 2.4)	0.9 (0.8, 1)	8–69
Elevated jugular venous pressure	6.3 (3.5, 11.3)	0.9 (0.8, 1)	8–69
Supine apical impulse lateral to MCL	10.3 (5, 21.1)	0.7 (0.6, 0.9)	8–69
S_3 gallop	3.4 (2.6, 4.4)	0.7 (0.5, 0.8)	30–80
S_4 gallop	1.2 (0.8, 1.9)	0.9 (0.5, 1.4)	30–60
Murmur of mitral regurgitation	2.2 (0.9, 5.7)	0.8 (0.7, 1)	56
Hepatomegaly	0.9 (0.1, 9.4)	1 (0.9, 1.1)	69
Edema	1.2 (0.8, 1.8)	0.9 (0.9, 1)	8–69
Chapter 49 Coronary artery disease			
Cholesterol >300 mg/dL, detecting coronary artery disease	4 (2.5, 6.3)	...	24–50
Cholesterol <200 mg/dL, detecting coronary artery disease	0.3 (0.2, 0.4)	...	24–50
Right arm radiation, detecting myocardial infarction	2.7 (1.9, 3.9)	0.9 (0.8, 0.9)	12–49
Left arm radiation, detecting myocardial infarction	1.5 (1.3, 1.6)	0.8 (0.7, 0.9)	6–49
Chest wall tenderness, predicting acute coronary syndrome in next 30 days	0.1 (0, 0.4)	1.1 (1, 1.1)	20
EBM Box 49.1 Coronary artery disease			
Typical angina	5.8 (4.2, 7.8)	...	44–65
Atypical angina	1.2 (1.1, 1.3)	...	44–58
Non-anginal chest pain	0.1 (0.1, 0.2)	...	44–58
Pain duration >30 minutes	0.1 (0, 0.9)	1.2 (1, 1.3)	50
Associated dysphagia	0.2 (0.1, 0.8)	1.2 (1, 1.4)	50
Male sex	1.6 (1.5, 1.8)	0.4 (0.3, 0.5)	44–83
Age <30 years	0.1 (0, 1.1)	...	51–68
Age 30–49 years	0.6 (0.5, 0.7)	...	51–83
Age 50–70 years	1.3 (1.3, 1.4)	...	51–83
Age >70 years	2.6 (1.8, 4)	...	51–90

(continued)

APPENDIX TABLE 1 ■ Likelihood Ratios, Confidence Intervals, and Pretest Probability —Cont'd

Finding	Positive LR (95% CI)	Negative LR (95% CI)	Pre-test Probability (Range)
Prior myocardial infarction	3.8 (2.1, 6.8)	0.6 (0.5, 0.6)	58–83
Ear lobe crease	2.1 (1.6, 2.8)	0.5 (0.4, 0.7)	29–85
Arcus senilis	3 (1.02, 8.6)	0.7 (0.6, 0.8)	89
Chest wall tenderness	0.8 (0.7, 0.9)	1.1 (1, 1.3)	44–62
Ankle-to-arm pressure index <0.9	3.6 (2.3, 5.7)	0.9 (0.8, 1)	75–82
Laterally displaced apical impulse	13 (0.7, 228)	1 (0.9, 1)	50
ECG normal	0.6 (0.3, 1.1)	1.2 (1, 1.6)	44–58
ECG with ST/T wave abnormalities	1.4 (1, 1.9)	0.9 (0.9, 1)	44–76
EBM Box 49.2 Myocardial infarction			
Male sex	1.3 (1.2, 1.3)	0.7 (0.7, 0.7)	6–36
Age, <40 years	0.2 (0.1, 0.5)	...	17
Age, 40–59 years	0.8 (0.6, 1.1)	...	17
Age, ≥60 years	1.5 (1.4, 1.6)	...	14–36
Sharp pain	0.5 (0.3, 0.9)	1.2 (1.1, 1.4)	12–21
Pleuritic pain	0.3 (0.2, 0.6)	1.2 (1.1, 1.2)	12–21
Positional pain	0.6 (0.3, 1.01)	1.1 (1.1, 1.1)	12–21
Relief of pain with nitroglycerin	1 (0.9, 1.1)	1 (0.9, 1.2)	18–34
Levine sign	0.5 (0.2, 1.6)	1.1 (1, 1.2)	22
Palm sign	0.9 (0.5, 1.4)	1.1 (0.9, 1.4)	22
Arm sign	1.1 (0.5, 2.2)	1 (0.8, 1.2)	22
Pointing sign	0.4 (0.1, 3.5)	1 (1, 1.1)	22
Chest wall tenderness	0.3 (0.2, 0.5)	1.2 (1.2, 1.3)	12–21
Diaphoretic appearance	2.2 (1.7, 2.9)	0.7 (0.6, 0.8)	12–29
Pallor	1.4 (1.2, 1.6)	0.6 (0.5, 0.8)	29
Systolic blood pressure <100 mm Hg	3.6 (2, 6.5)	1 (0.9, 1)	18
Jugular venous distension	2.4 (1.4, 4.2)	0.9 (0.9, 1)	6
Pulmonary crackles	2.1 (1.6, 2.8)	0.8 (0.7, 1)	6–12
Third heart sound	3.2 (1.6, 6.5)	0.9 (0.8, 1)	12
ECG normal	0.2 (0.1, 0.3)	...	14–42
ECG non-specific ST changes	0.2 (0.1, 0.4)	...	14–29
ECG T wave inversion	2 (1.7, 2.4)	...	12–29
ECG ST depression	3.8 (3, 4.8)	...	12–29
ECG ST elevation	18.4 (11.3, 30)	...	12–29
Chapter 51 Palpation and percussion of the abdomen			
Pulsatile liver, detecting moderate or worse TR	6.5 (2.2, 19.3)	0.8 (0.7, 1)	18–41
Lymphadenopathy, detecting hepatic cause of splenomegaly	0.1 (0, 0.1)	1.5 (1.1, 2)	11–42
Massive splenomegaly, detecting hematologic cause of splenomegaly	2.8 (2.4, 3.2)	0.7 (0.6, 0.8)	27–57
EBM Box 51.1 Detecting enlarged liver and spleen			
Percussion span ≥10 cm, detecting enlarged liver	1.2 (1, 1.5)	0.5 (0.2, 1.7)	20–74
Palpable liver, detecting liver edge	234 (15, 3737)	0.5 (0.5, 0.6)	51
Palpable liver, detecting enlarged liver	1.9 (1.6, 2.3)	0.6 (0.5, 0.8)	20–44
Palpable spleen, detecting enlarged spleen	8.5 (6.2, 11.7)	0.6 (0.5, 0.7)	7–84
Spleen percussion sign, detecting enlarged spleen	1.7 (1.3, 2.2)	0.7 (0.5, 0.8)	26–63
Nixon method, detecting enlarged spleen	2 (1.2, 3.5)	0.7 (0.6, 0.9)	26–61
Traube space dullness, detecting enlarged spleen	2.1 (1.7, 2.6)	0.8 (0.6, 0.9)	36–61
EBM Box 51.2 Palpation of liver and spleen			
Palpable enlarged liver, detecting cirrhosis	2.3 (1.6, 3.3)	0.6 (0.4, 0.7)	7–67
Palpable liver in epigastrium, detecting cirrhosis	2.7 (1.9, 3.9)	0.3 (0.1, 0.9)	7–37

APPENDIX TABLE 1 ■ **Likelihood Ratios, Confidence Intervals, and Pretest Probability—Cont'd**

Finding	Positive LR (95% CI)	Negative LR (95% CI)	Pre-test Probability (Range)
Liver edge firm, detecting cirrhosis	3.3 (2.2, 4.9)	0.4 (0.3, 0.4)	27–67
Palpable liver (if jaundice), detecting hepatocellular disease	0.9 (0.8, 1.1)	1.4 (0.6, 3.4)	65–67
Liver tenderness (if jaundice), detecting hepatocellular disease	1.4 (0.8, 2.6)	0.8 (0.7, 1.1)	65–67
Palpable liver (if lymphadenopathy), detecting serious disease	1.2 (0.7, 1.9)	1 (0.9, 1.1)	26–41
Palpable spleen in returning travelers with fever, detecting malaria	6.5 (3.9, 10.7)	0.8 (0.8, 0.8)	27–29
Palpable spleen (if jaundice), detecting hepatocellular disease	2.9 (1.2, 6.8)	0.7 (0.6, 0.9)	65–67
Palpable spleen, detecting cirrhosis	2.5 (1.6, 3.8)	0.8 (0.7, 0.9)	18–67
Palpable spleen (if lymphadenopathy), detecting serious disease	1.2 (0.6, 2.5)	1 (0.9, 1)	26–41
Palpable spleen (if prolonged fever), predicting that bone marrow examination will be diagnostic	2.9 (1.9, 4.4)	0.7 (0.5, 0.8)	24–45
EBM Box 51.3 Palpation of gallbladder, bladder, and aorta			
Palpable gallbladder (in jaundiced patients), detecting extrahepatic obstruction	26 (1.5, 439.9)	0.7 (0.5, 0.9)	33
Palpable gallbladder, detecting malignant extrahepatic obstruction	2.6 (1.5, 4.6)	0.7 (0.6, 0.9)	32–80
Palpable bladder, detecting ≥400 mL urine	1.9 (1.4, 2.6)	0.3 (0.1, 0.7)	29
Expansile pulsating epigastric mass, detecting abdominal aortic aneurysm	8.4 (4.6, 15.6)	0.6 (0.5, 0.7)	2–50
EBM Box 51.4 Ascites			
Bulging flanks	1.9 (1.4, 2.6)	0.4 (0.2, 0.6)	24–33
Edema	3.8 (2.2, 6.6)	0.2 (0, 0.6)	24
Flank dullness	1.8 (0.9, 3.4)	0.3 (0.1, 0.7)	24–29
Shifting dullness	2.3 (1.5, 3.5)	0.4 (0.2, 0.6)	24–33
Fluid wave	5 (2.5, 9.9)	0.5 (0.3, 0.7)	24–33
Chapter 52 Abdominal pain and tenderness			
Sonographic McBurney point tenderness, detecting appendicitis	8.4 (2.9, 24.6)	0.1 (0.1, 0.3)	67
Sonographic Murphy sign, detecting cholecystitis	15.7 (5.6, 43.9)	0.5 (0.3, 0.7)	21–47
Murphy sign in patients with liver abscess, detecting biliary tract sepsis	2.8 (1.1, 6.9)	0.8 (0.6, 1)	40
Left lower quadrant tenderness, detecting diverticulitis (surgical finding)	13.8 (6.3, 30)	0.8 (0.7, 0.9)	17
Left lower quadrant tenderness, detecting diverticulitis (CT scan)	2.2 (1.7, 2.7)	0.4 (0.3, 0.5)	43
Guarding, detecting complicated diverticulitis	8.4 (2.5, 28)	0.9 (0.9, 1)	17
Loin tenderness, detecting ureterolithiasis	27.7 (10.7, 72)	0.9 (0.8, 0.9)	4
Renal tenderness, detecting ureterolithiasis	3.6 (3.1, 4.1)	0.2 (0.1, 0.3)	4
Microscopic hematuria, detecting ureterolithiasis	73.1 (41.7, 128)	0.3 (0.2, 0.4)	4
Positive abdominal wall tenderness test in chronic abdominal pain, predicting improvement with local analgesic injection	7 (3.4, 14.3)	0.2 (0.1, 0.5)	35
EBM Box 52.1 Acute abdominal pain, detecting peritonitis			
Fever	1.4 (1.2, 1.7)	0.7 (0.6, 0.8)	31–88
Guarding	2.3 (1.9, 2.8)	0.6 (0.5, 0.7)	11–88

(continued)

APPENDIX TABLE 1 ■ **Likelihood Ratios, Confidence Intervals, and Pretest Probability—Cont'd**

Finding	Positive LR (95% CI)	Negative LR (95% CI)	Pre-test Probability (Range)
Rigidity	3.6 (2.7, 4.8)	0.8 (0.7, 0.9)	11–75
Rebound tenderness	2 (1.7, 2.3)	0.4 (0.4, 0.5)	11–88
Percussion tenderness	2.4 (1.5, 3.8)	0.5 (0.4, 0.6)	30–50
Abnormal bowel sounds	2.2 (0.5, 9.7)	0.8 (0.7, 0.9)	13–82
Rectal tenderness	1.4 (1, 1.8)	0.8 (0.7, 1)	11–82
Positive abdominal wall tenderness test	0.1 (0, 0.7)	1.9 (0.9, 4.4)	58–72
Positive cough test	1.9 (1.5, 2.4)	0.5 (0.3, 0.6)	11–46
EBM Box 52.2 Acute abdominal pain, detecting appendicitis			
Right lower quadrant tenderness	1.9 (1.6, 2.4)	0.3 (0.2, 0.4)	11–85
McBurney point tenderness	3.4 (1.6, 7.2)	0.4 (0.2, 0.7)	39–65
Rovsing sign	2.1 (1.4, 3.2)	0.8 (0.7, 0.9)	36–58
Psoas sign	1.7 (1.3, 2.3)	0.9 (0.8, 1)	36–82
Obturator sign	1.5 (0.97, 2.2)	0.9 (0.9, 1)	57–82
Alvarado score 7 or more	3 (2.4, 3.7)	…	17–82
Alvarado score 5–6	0.7 (0.4, 1.2)	…	17–82
Alvarado score, 4 or less	0.1 (0.1, 0.2)	…	17–82
EBM Box 52.3 Right upper quadrant tenderness			
Fever	1.1 (0.8, 1.7)	0.9 (0.8, 1.1)	26–78
Right upper quadrant tenderness	2.4 (1.7, 3.4)	0.4 (0.2, 0.5)	10–80
Murphy sign (inspiratory arrest)	3.9 (1.9, 7.9)	0.5 (0.4, 0.7)	10–52
Right upper quadrant mass	0.8 (0.5, 1.2)	1 (1, 1)	26–80
EBM Box 52.4 Acute abdominal pain, detecting obstruction			
Visible peristalsis	18.8 (4.3, 81.9)	0.9 (0.9, 1)	4
Distended abdomen	9.6 (5, 18.6)	0.4 (0.3, 0.5)	4–8
Guarding	1 (0.6, 1.7)	1 (0.7, 1.4)	4–8
Rigidity	1.2 (0.4, 3.6)	1 (0.9, 1.2)	4–8
Rebound tenderness	0.9 (0.7, 1.1)	1.1 (1, 1.2)	4–8
Hyperactive bowel sounds	5 (2.4, 10.6)	0.6 (0.5, 0.8)	4–8
Abnormal bowel sounds	3.2 (1.7, 6.1)	0.4 (0.3, 0.5)	4–8
Rectal tenderness	0.9 (0.6, 1.5)	1 (1, 1.1)	4–8
EBM Box 52-5 Chronic upper abdominal pain			
Positive abdominal wall tenderness test, detecting visceral pain	0.1 (0.1, 0.3)	4.9 (3, 8)	60–65
Right upper quadrant tenderness, detecting cholelithiasis	1.1 (0.9, 1.4)	0.9 (0.7, 1.2)	41
Lower abdominal tenderness, detecting cholelithiasis	0.5 (0.3, 0.7)	1.4 (1.2, 1.6)	41
Epigastric tenderness, detecting positive upper endoscopy	0.9 (0.7, 1.3)	1.2 (0.6, 2.3)	61
Chapter 53 Auscultation of abdomen			
Abnormal bowel sounds, detecting bowel obstruction	3.2 (1.7, 6.1)	0.4 (0.3, 0.5)	4–8
EBM Box 53.1 Auscultation of abdomen			
Any abdominal bruit, detecting renovascular hypertension	5.6 (4, 7.7)	0.6 (0.5, 0.8)	18–36
Any abdominal bruit, detecting abdominal aortic aneurysm	2 (0.5, 8.6)	0.9 (0.8, 1.1)	9
Systolic/diastolic abdominal bruit, detecting renovascular hypertension	38.9 (9.5, 160)	0.6 (0.5, 0.7)	24
Chapter 54 Peripheral vascular disease			
ABI <0.9 by palpation, detecting ABI <0.9 by Doppler	4 (3, 5.2)	0.2 (0.1, 0.3)	4–23

APPENDIX TABLE 1 ■ Likelihood Ratios, Confidence Intervals, and Pretest Probability—Cont'd

Finding	Positive LR (95% CI)	Negative LR (95% CI)	Pre-test Probability (Range)
Pulse oximetry test positive (finger minus toe O_2 sat ≥2% [supine patient] *or* toe O_2 sat decreases ≥2% after elevating foot 12 inches	30.5 (7.7, 121)	0.2 (0.1, 0.4)	31
Absent or severely diminished femoral pulse, detecting aortoiliac disease	31 (1.9, 500.6)	0.6 (0.5, 0.8)	50
Limb bruit (with preserved popliteal pulse), detecting limb stenosis	3.2 (1.2, 8.7)	0.3 (0.1, 0.6)	68
Continuous femoral bruit, detecting arteriovenous fistula	80.8 (5.1, 1273)	0.04 (0, 0.6)	23
Expansile femoral pulsation, detecting false aneurysm	13.8 (3.6, 52.7)	0.1 (0, 0.3)	44
Prolonged capillary refill time (*after* fluid resuscitation), predicting hospital mortality	10.5 (2.8, 38.8)	0.6 (0.4, 1)	14
Prolonged capillary refill time (*before* fluid resuscitation), predicting hospital mortality	1.6 (0.8, 3.3)	0.7 (0.4, 1.3)	14
Mottling diminishes during hospitalization, predicting hospital mortality	0.2 (0.1, 0.5)	3.8 (1.4, 10.4)	66

EBM Box 54.1 Peripheral vascular disease

Finding	Positive LR (95% CI)	Negative LR (95% CI)	Pre-test Probability (Range)
Wounds or sores on foot	7 (3.2, 15.6)	1 (1, 1)	11
Foot color abnormally pale, red, or blue	2.8 (2.4, 3.2)	0.7 (0.7, 0.8)	9
Atrophic skin	1.7 (1.2, 2.3)	0.7 (0.5, 1)	8
Absent lower limb hair	1.7 (1.2, 2.3)	0.7 (0.6, 1)	8
Foot asymmetrically cooler	6.1 (4.2, 8.9)	0.9 (0.9, 0.9)	8
Absent femoral pulse	6.1 (3.8, 10)	0.9 (0.9, 1)	9
Both pedal pulses absent (PT and DP)	9.9 (7.4, 13.2)	0.4 (0.3, 0.4)	7–71
Limb bruit present	5.4 (3.9, 7.3)	0.7 (0.6, 0.8)	9–67
Capillary refill time ≥5 seconds	1.9 (1.2, 3.2)	0.8 (0.7, 1)	8
Venous filling time >20 seconds	3.6 (1.9, 6.8)	0.8 (0.7, 1)	8

EBM Box 54.2 Hypoperfusion in ICU patients

Finding	Positive LR (95% CI)	Negative LR (95% CI)	Pre-test Probability (Range)
Cool extremities in ICU patients, detecting low cardiac index	3.7 (2.1, 6.5)	0.8 (0.8, 0.9)	55
Cool extremities in septic ICU patients, detecting low cardiac index	5.2 (2.3, 12.1)	0.7 (0.6, 0.9)	47
0 of 3 findings present, detecting low cardiac index	0.5 (0.3, 0.8)	...	8
1 of 3 findings present, detecting low cardiac index	2.3 (1.6, 3.4)	...	8
All 3 findings present, detecting low cardiac index	7.5 (2.2, 25.3)	...	8
Capillary refill time ≥5 seconds, detecting low cardiac output	1.6 (1.2, 2.2)	0.9 (0.8, 1)	36
Limb is cool or capillary refill time >5 sec, detecting elevated lactate	2.2 (1.6, 3)	0.5 (0.4, 0.7)	50
Limb is cool or capillary refill time >5 sec, predicting multiorgan dysfunction	2.6 (1.9, 3.5)	0.3 (0.2, 0.5)	50
Capillary refill time ≥5 seconds, predicting major postoperative complications	12.1 (5.4, 27.1)	0.2 (0.1, 0.5)	17
Capillary refill time ≥5 seconds, predicting mortality if septic shock	4.6 (1.7, 12.8)	0.6 (0.4, 0.9)	37
Knee mottling, predicting mortality if septic shock	10.2 (3.2, 32)	0.8 (0.6, 1)	11–52

Chapter 55 The diabetic foot

Finding	Positive LR (95% CI)	Negative LR (95% CI)	Pre-test Probability (Range)
Insensate to 5.07 monofilament, predicting amputation during 3–4 y f/u	2.6 (1.5, 4.6)	0.4 (0.3, 0.7)	1–4
Positive Ipswich touch test, detecting positive monofilament testing	9.9 (5.9, 16.7)	0.3 (0.2, 0.3)	25–47

(continued)

APPENDIX TABLE 1 ■ Likelihood Ratios, Confidence Intervals, and Pretest Probability—Cont'd

Finding	Positive LR (95% CI)	Negative LR (95% CI)	Pre-test Probability (Range)
EBM Box 55.1 The diabetic foot			
Insensate to the 5.07 monofilament, predicting future foot ulceration	2.7 (2, 3.6)	0.5 (0.4, 0.6)	2–29
Ulcer area ≥2 cm^2, detecting osteomyelitis	2.2 (0.4, 11.4)	0.6 (0.2, 2.4)	52–68
Ulcer area ≥3 cm^2, detecting osteomyelitis	3.5 (1.6, 7.7)	0.3 (0.1, 0.6)	52
Ulcer area ≥4 cm^2, detecting osteomyelitis	7.3 (1.9, 28.3)	0.4 (0.2, 0.7)	52
Ulcer area ≥5 cm^2, detecting osteomyelitis	11 (1.6, 77.8)	0.5 (0.3, 0.8)	52
Probe-to-bone positive, detecting osteomyelitis	6 (4, 8.9)	0.2 (0.1, 0.4)	12–80
Ulcer depth >3 mm or bone exposed, detecting osteomyelitis	3.9 (1.9, 8.1)	0.3 (0.2, 0.6)	63–68
Erythema, swelling, purulence, detecting osteomyelitis	1.8 (0.9, 3.8)	0.8 (0.6, 1)	63–68
0 findings, predicting nonhealing wound	0.5 (0.4, 0.5)	...	53
1 findings, predicting nonhealing wound	0.8 (0.8, 0.8)	...	53
2 findings, predicting nonhealing wound	1.8 (1.7, 1.8)	...	53
3 findings, predicting nonhealing wound	3.5 (3.2, 3.8)	...	53
Chapter 56 - Edema and deep vein thrombosis			
Active cancer, detecting proximal leg DVT	2.9 (2.4, 3.6)	0.9 (0.8, 0.9)	13–34
Recent immobilization, detecting proximal leg DVT	1.6 (1.3, 2.1)	0.9 (0.8, 0.9)	13–34
Recent surgery, detecting proximal leg DVT	1.6 (1.3, 1.9)	0.9 (0.9, 1)	13–29
Modified Wells ≤0, detecting proximal DVT	0.3 (0.1, 0.6)	...	15–18
Modified Wells 1–2, detecting proximal DVT	1 (0.9, 1.2)	...	15–18
Modified Wells ≥3, detecting proximal DVT	3.9 (3.2, 4.8)	...	15–18
Modified Wells ≥2, detecting proximal DVT	1.8 (1.4, 2.5)	0.3 (0.2, 0.4)	15–36
EBM Box 56.1 Leg DVT			
Any calf or ankle swelling	1.2 (1.1, 1.3)	0.7 (0.6, 0.8)	25–54
Asymmetric calf swelling, ≥2 cm difference	2.1 (1.8, 2.5)	0.5 (0.4, 0.7)	13–16
Swelling of entire leg	1.5 (1.2, 1.8)	0.8 (0.6, 0.9)	22–34
Superficial venous dilation	1.6 (1.4, 1.9)	0.9 (0.8, 0.9)	22–44
Erythema	1 (0.6, 1.7)	1 (0.8, 1.2)	27–45
Superficial thrombophlebitis	0.9 (0.2, 5.1)	1 (0.9, 1.1)	43
Tenderness	1 (1, 1.1)	1 (0.9, 1.1)	22–54
Asymmetric skin coolness	1.2 (0.6, 2.2)	0.9 (0.6, 1.4)	46
Asymmetric skin warmth	1.4 (1.2, 1.7)	0.7 (0.5, 1.2)	27–45
Palpable cord	1.1 (0.7, 1.6)	1 (0.9, 1.1)	27–34
Homans sign	1.1 (0.9, 1.3)	1 (0.9, 1.1)	27–58
EBM Box 56.2 Leg DVT			
Wells low probability	0.2 (0.2, 0.3)	...	6–43
Wells moderate probability	1 (0.7, 1.3)	...	6–39
Wells high probability	6.3 (4, 10.1)	...	6–39
EBM Box 56.3 Arm DVT			
Constans score, 0 or 1	0.3 (0.1, 0.8)	...	25–35
Constans score, 2 or 3	3 (1.9, 4.8)	...	25–35
Chapter 57 Examination of the musculoskeletal system			
Constant pain in low back and buttock, detecting hip osteoarthritis	6.7 (2.4, 18.6)	0.5 (0.3, 0.8)	29
Pain in ipsilateral groin, detecting hip osteoarthritis	3.6 (1.1, 11.6)	0.8 (0.6, 1)	29
Knee flexion <120 degrees, detecting knee arthritis	3.4 (1.5, 8)	0.9 (0.8, 1)	8

APPENDIX TABLE 1 ■ **Likelihood Ratios, Confidence Intervals, and Pretest Probability—Cont'd**

Finding	Positive LR (95% CI)	Negative LR (95% CI)	Pre-test Probability (Range)
Overall clinical impression, detecting ACL tear	49.6 (29.1, 85)	0.1 (0, 0.2)	11–43
Clinical impression medial meniscal injury, detecting medial meniscal injury	3.6 (2.4, 5.4)	0.1 (0.1, 0.2)	19–69
Clinical impression lateral meniscal injury, detecting lateral meniscal injury	8.6 (4.9, 15.4)	0.5 (0.4, 0.6)	7–68
EBM Box 57.1 Shoulder pain			
Detecting acromioclavicular joint pain			
Acromioclavicular joint tenderness	1.1 (0.9, 1.3)	0.4 (0, 5.2)	74
Tenderness with AC joint compression	1.6 (0.8, 3)	0.4 (0.2, 1.1)	74
Crossed body adduction causes pain	3.7 (2.9, 4.7)	0.3 (0.2, 0.5)	6
Detecting rotator cuff tendinitis			
Neer impingement sign	1.6 (1.2, 2.3)	0.5 (0.4, 0.5)	28–90
Hawkins impingement sign	1.7 (1.2, 2.3)	0.3 (0.2, 0.5)	28–90
Neer or Hawkins impingement sign	1.6 (1.3, 2)	0.1 (0, 0.7)	28
Yergason sign	2.8 (1.2, 6.6)	0.7 (0.6, 0.9)	70
Speed test	1.9 (1.3, 2.8)	0.7 (0.6, 0.9)	65–70
Painful arc	2.9 (1.6, 5.3)	0.5 (0.3, 1.1)	65–90
Detecting rotator cuff tear			
Age ≤39 years	0.1 (0.1, 0.2)	...	50
Age 40–59 years	0.9 (0.7, 1.1)	...	50
Age ≥60 years	3.2 (2.4, 4.3)	...	50
Supraspinatus atrophy	2 (1.5, 2.7)	0.6 (0.5, 0.7)	67
Infraspinatus atrophy	2 (1.5, 2.7)	0.6 (0.5, 0.7)	67
Painful arc	1.6 (0.97, 2.8)	0.5 (0.3, 0.8)	38–67
Neer impingement sign	2.1 (1.3, 3.7)	0.5 (0.3, 0.8)	28–77
Hawkins impingement sign	1.7 (1.3, 2.3)	0.7 (0.6, 0.8)	28–77
Supraspinatus test causes pain	1.5 (1.1, 2)	0.5 (0.3, 0.8)	24–86
Supraspinatus weakness	2.1 (1.6, 2.7)	0.4 (0.3, 0.6)	23–86
Infraspinatus weakness	2.6 (1.5, 4.6)	0.6 (0.4, 0.9)	38–67
Dropped arm test	2.9 (2.1, 4)	0.9 (0.8, 1)	38–50
Palpable tear	10.2 (1.3, 80.9)	0.1 (0, 0.2)	42–81
EBM Box 57.2 Rotator cuff tear			
3 findings (Murrell)	48 (6.7, 344)	...	50
2 findings (Murrell)	4.9 (2.9, 8.3)	...	50
1 finding (Murrell)	0.9 (0.7, 1.1)	...	50
0 findings (Murrell)	0.02 (0, 0.1)	...	50
3 findings (Park)	15.9 (5.9, 43.1)	...	44
2 findings (Park)	3.6 (2.2, 5.7)	...	44
1 finding (Park)	0.8 (0.6, 1.1)	...	44
0 findings (Park)	0.2 (0.1, 0.3)	...	44
EBM Box 57.3 Hip osteoarthritis			
Squat causes pain in posterior hip	6.1 (1.3, 28.9)	0.8 (0.6, 1)	29
Abduction or adduction causes groin pain	5.7 (1.6, 19.8)	0.7 (0.5, 1)	29
Active hip flexion causes lateral hip pain	3.6 (1.5, 9)	0.6 (0.4, 1)	29
Active hip extension causes hip pain	2.7 (1.3, 5.3)	0.6 (0.4, 0.9)	29
Passive internal rotation ≤25 degrees	1.9 (1.3, 2.9)	0.4 (0.2, 0.9)	29
Passive internal rotation ≤15 degrees	9.9 (5.5, 17.7)	0.6 (0.5, 0.8)	6
EBM Box 57.4 Knee osteoarthritis			
Stiffness <30 minutes	3 (2.1, 4.4)	0.2 (0.1, 0.3)	55
Crepitus, passive motion	2.1 (1.7, 2.7)	0.2 (0.1, 0.3)	52
Bony enlargement	11.8 (4.9, 28.2)	0.5 (0.4, 0.6)	52
Palpable increase in temperature	0.3 (0.2, 0.5)	1.6 (1.4, 2)	52

(continued)

APPENDIX TABLE 1 ■ Likelihood Ratios, Confidence Intervals, and Pretest Probability—Cont'd

Finding	Positive LR (95% CI)	Negative LR (95% CI)	Pre-test Probability (Range)
Valgus deformity	1.4 (0.8, 2.4)	0.9 (0.8, 1)	52
Varus deformity	3.4 (1.6, 7.6)	0.8 (0.7, 0.9)	52
At least 3 out of 6 findings	3.1 (2.3, 4.1)	0.1 (0, 0.1)	55
EBM Box 57.5 Knee fracture			
Age ≥55 years	3 (1.6, 5.3)	0.7 (0.5, 1)	6–9
Joint effusion	2.5 (2, 3)	0.5 (0.3, 0.7)	6–9
Ecchymosis	2.2 (0.9, 5.3)	0.9 (0.7, 1.1)	9
Cannot flex beyond 90°	2.9 (2.5, 3.4)	0.5 (0.4, 0.7)	6–9
Cannot flex beyond 60°	4.7 (3.8, 5.9)	0.6 (0.5, 0.7)	6
Isolated tenderness of patella	2.2 (1.6, 2.9)	0.8 (0.8, 0.9)	6–9
Tenderness at head of fibula	3.4 (2.5, 4.7)	0.9 (0.8, 1)	6–9
Inability to bear weight, immediately and in emergency department	3.6 (3, 4.3)	0.6 (0.5, 0.7)	6–9
Ottawa knee rule positive	1.7 (1.4, 2)	0.1 (0, 0.2)	6–12
EBM Box 57.6 Ligament and meniscal injuries			
Anterior drawer sign, detecting ACL tear	12.2 (6.1, 24.2)	0.4 (0.3, 0.5)	26–76
Lachman sign, detecting ACL tear	20.5 (7.4, 56.3)	0.2 (0.1, 0.3)	26–76
Pivot shift sign, detecting ACL tear	8.2 (4.2, 16)	0.7 (0.6, 0.9)	26–76
Posterior drawer sign, detecting pcl tear	97.8 (24.2, 396)	0.1 (0, 0.5)	3–13
McMurray sign, detecting meniscal injury	3.6 (2.5, 5.1)	0.6 (0.5, 0.7)	25–85
Joint line tenderness, detecting meniscal injury	1.9 (1.4, 2.6)	0.4 (0.3, 0.6)	21–81
Block to full extension, detecting meniscal injury	3.2 (1.8, 5.9)	0.7 (0.5, 0.8)	50
Pain on forced extension, detecting meniscal injury	1.6 (1.2, 2.2)	0.7 (0.6, 0.9)	50–81
Valgus laxity, detecting medial collateral ligament injury	7.7 (1.6, 37)	0.2 (0.1, 0.3)	22–44
Varus laxity, detecting lateral collateral ligament injury	16.2 (2.4, 109)	0.8 (0.4, 1.3)	1
EBM Box 57.7 Ankle and midfoot fracture			
Detecting ankle fracture			
Tenderness over posterior lateral malleolus	2.4 (1.9, 2.8)	0.4 (0.3, 0.5)	10–14
Tenderness over posterior medial malleolus	4.8 (2.6, 9)	0.6 (0.6, 0.7)	10–14
Inability to bear weight immediately after injury	2.6 (2.2, 3.1)	0.5 (0.4, 0.6)	10–14
Inability to bear weight 4 steps in the emergency room	2.5 (2.2, 2.8)	0.3 (0.2, 0.4)	10–14
Ottawa ankle rule	1.5 (1.3, 1.7)	0.1 (0, 0.2)	9–34
Detecting midfoot fracture			
Tenderness at the base of the 5th metatarsal	2.9 (2.5, 3.3)	0.1 (0.1, 0.2)	12–14
Tenderness of navicular bone	0.4 (0.2, 0.9)	1.1 (1, 1.2)	12–14
Inability to bear weight immediately after injury	1 (0.5, 2.3)	1 (0.8, 1.3)	12–14
Inability to bear weight 4 steps in the emergency room	1.1 (0.8, 1.4)	0.9 (0.8, 1.1)	12–14
Ottawa foot rule	2.1 (1.3, 3.3)	0.1 (0, 0.2)	2–23
EBM Box 57.8 Achilles tendon tear			
Palpable gap in Achilles tendon	6.8 (2.3, 19.9)	0.3 (0.2, 0.4)	83
Calf squeeze test	13.5 (3.5, 51.2)	0.05 (0, 0.1)	83
Knee flexion test	6.2 (2.5, 15.4)	0.1 (0.1, 0.3)	73
Chapter 58 Visual field testing			
Visual field defect, detecting focal cerebral defect	4.3 (1.1, 17.6)	0.8 (0.7, 0.9)	71–75

APPENDIX TABLE 1 ■ Likelihood Ratios, Confidence Intervals, and Pretest Probability—Cont'd

Finding	Positive LR (95% CI)	Negative LR (95% CI)	Pre-test Probability (Range)
EBM Box 58.1 Visual field defects			
Confrontation technique, detecting anterior visual field defects	5.7 (3.7, 8.7)	0.7 (0.6, 0.8)	26–85
Confrontation technique, detecting posterior visual field defects	9.5 (4.5, 19.9)	0.4 (0.3, 0.6)	6–53
Asymmetric optokinetic nystagmus, detecting parietal lobe disease	5.7 (3.2, 10.1)	0.1 (0, 0.3)	33
Associated hemiparesis or aphasia, detecting parietal lobe disease	18.3 (6, 56.2)	0.1 (0, 0.7)	14
EBM Box 58.2 Visual field defects			
Finger counting	54.4 (7.6, 388)	0.7 (0.6, 0.8)	45–64
Kinetic finger boundary	13.3 (5.9, 29.8)	0.6 (0.6, 0.7)	45–64
Description of face	26.4 (8.5, 82.6)	0.6 (0.5, 0.7)	45–64
Kinetic red boundary testing	13.6 (3.6, 50.7)	0.4 (0.2, 0.6)	45–64
Laser target testing	6.3 (3.4, 12)	0.3 (0.2, 0.5)	47
Red target comparison	6.2 (0.1, 314)	0.6 (0.3, 1.2)	45–64
Chapter 59 Nerves of the eye muscles			
Periorbital emphysema (if face trauma), detecting orbital fracture	4.9 (2.7, 8.8)	0.8 (0.7, 0.8)	77
Inferior orbital hypoesthesia (if face trauma), detecting orbital fracture	3.5 (2.2, 5.4)	0.8 (0.7, 0.8)	77
Diplopia (if face trauma), detecting orbital fracture	2.6 (1.9, 3.7)	0.7 (0.7, 0.8)	77
Positive upright-supine test, detecting skew deviation	73.8 (4.4, 1227)	0.6 (0.5, 0.9)	20
Horizontal diplopia and esotropia, detecting VI palsy	19.2 (4, 91.8)	0.04 (0, 0.6)	29
Horizontal diplopia and exotropia, detecting internuclear ophthalmoplegia	68.4 (4.3, 1091)	0.1 (0, 1.4)	10
Vertical diplopia, anisocoria, and ptosis, detecting III palsy	7.4 (3.1, 18.1)	0.1 (0, 1.2)	15
Vertical diplopia and signs of orbitopathy, detecting orbital disease	68.4 (4.3, 1091)	0.1 (0, 1.4)	10
Isolated vertical diplopia, detecting IV palsy	11.3 (3.3, 38.7)	0.2 (0, 0.8)	20
EBM Box 59.1 Ice pack test for myasthenia			
Improvement in ptosis after application of ice	8.1 (5.3, 12.4)	0.1 (0.1, 0.3)	32–75
Improvement in diplopia and ophthalmoplegia after application of ice	30.6 (7.7, 123)	0.1 (0, 0.9)	18–50
Chapter 60 Miscellaneous cranial nerves			
Hutchinson sign in VZV, detecting ocular complications	4 (2.7, 5.7)	0.4 (0.3, 0.7)	28–86
EBM Box 60.1 Aspiration after stroke			
Abnormal voluntary cough	2.1 (1.5, 3)	0.7 (0.6, 0.8)	12–71
Dysphonia	1.5 (1.2, 1.9)	0.5 (0.4, 0.8)	12–71
Dysarthria	2 (1.4, 2.9)	0.5 (0.3, 0.7)	12–68
Drowsiness	3.6 (1.5, 8.7)	0.6 (0.4, 1.1)	12–42
Abnormal sensation face and tongue	0.5 (0.2, 1.2)	1.5 (0.9, 2.4)	46
Absent pharyngeal sensation	2.4 (1.6, 3.6)	0.03 (0, 0.5)	42
Tongue weakness	1.8 (1, 3.2)	0.6 (0.5, 0.9)	18–30
Bilateral cranial nerve signs	1.1 (0.8, 1.6)	0.8 (0.4, 1.6)	51–52
Abnormal gag reflex	1.4 (1.2, 1.7)	0.6 (0.5, 0.8)	19–71
Water swallow test	2.6 (1.9, 3.5)	0.4 (0.3, 0.6)	12–68
Oxygen desaturation 0–2 min after swallowing	3.5 (1.4, 9.2)	0.4 (0.3, 0.5)	28–64

(continued)

APPENDIX TABLE 1 ■ Likelihood Ratios, Confidence Intervals, and Pretest Probability—Cont'd

Finding	Positive LR (95% CI)	Negative LR (95% CI)	Pre-test Probability (Range)
Chapter 61 examination of motor system			
Ipsilateral calf wasting, diagnosing lumbosacral radiculopathy	5.2 (1.3, 20.8)	0.8 (0.6, 0.9)	74
EBM Box 61.1 Unilateral cerebral hemispheric disease			
Hemianopia	4.3 (1.1, 17.6)	0.8 (0.7, 0.9)	71–75
Pronator drift	9.6 (5.4, 16.9)	0.3 (0.2, 0.7)	51–76
Arm rolling test	15.6 (5.8, 41.5)	0.6 (0.4, 0.8)	51–76
Index finger rolling test	6 (2, 18.5)	0.7 (0.6, 0.8)	67–71
Little finger rolling test	1.5 (0.1, 15.2)	1 (0.9, 1.1)	58
Finger tapping test	4.7 (2.1, 10.3)	0.5 (0.3, 0.8)	51–76
Foot tapping test	2 (0.6, 6.5)	0.9 (0.7, 1.1)	67–71
Hemisensory disturbance	12.3 (0.8, 196)	0.7 (0.6, 0.9)	76
Hyperreflexia	5.3 (3, 9.5)	0.6 (0.2, 1.5)	51–71
Babinski response	8.5 (1.7, 43.3)	0.8 (0.6, 1)	67–76
EBM Box 61.2 Localization of stroke			
Aphasia, detecting anterior stroke	12.1 (5.5, 26.7)	0.7 (0.5, 0.9)	68–74
Conjugate gaze palsy, detecting anterior stroke	3.2 (2.3, 4.3)	0.9 (0.8, 1)	68–74
Ataxia, detecting posterior stroke	5.8 (4.2, 8)	0.7 (0.7, 0.8)	26
Horner syndrome, detecting posterior stroke	72 (4.3, 1213)	1 (0.9, 1)	26
Heterotropia, detecting posterior stroke	10 (4.2, 23.6)	0.9 (0.9, 1)	26
Nystagmus, detecting posterior stroke	14 (6.5, 30.4)	0.9 (0.9, 0.9)	26
Crossed motor paresis, detecting posterior stroke	24 (4.4, 129.9)	1 (0.9, 1)	26
Crossed sensory findings, detecting posterior stroke	54.7 (3.2, 938)	1 (0.9, 1)	26
Chapter 62 Examination of the sensory system			
Diminished pinprick sensation, detecting nerve fiber density <8 epidermal nerve fibers/mm	4.6 (2.4, 8.6)	0.2 (0.1, 0.3)	60
Chapter 63 Examination of the reflexes			
Diminished biceps or brachioradialis reflex, detecting C6 radiculopathy	14.2 (4.3, 46.7)	0.5 (0.3, 0.8)	19
Diminished triceps reflex, detecting C7 radiculopathy	3 (1.6, 5.6)	0.6 (0.3, 1.4)	54–69
Asymmetric quadriceps reflex, detecting L3 or L4 radiculopathy	8.5 (5, 14.5)	0.7 (0.6, 0.8)	2–46
Abnormal medial hamstring reflex, detecting L5 root disease	6.2 (1.6, 24.2)	0.5 (0.3, 0.7)	58
Asymmetric Achilles reflex, detecting S_1 radiculopathy	2.7 (1.9, 3.8)	0.5 (0.4, 0.6)	20–66
Asymmetric Achilles reflex, detecting diabetic neuropathy	2.8 (2.1, 3.8)	0.1 (0.1, 0.3)	39
Bulbocavernosus reflex in men, detecting S_2-S_4 lesion	13 (5.9, 28.9)	0.3 (0.2, 0.5)	27
Bulbocavernosus reflex in women, detecting S_2-S_4 lesion	2.7 (1.6, 4.6)	0.6 (0.5, 0.9)	22
Babinski sign, detecting cervical myelopathy	24.8 (1.5, 402)	0.6 (0.5, 0.8)	52
Inverted supinator reflex, detecting cervical myelopathy	1.7 (1.1, 2.5)	0.5 (0.2, 0.9)	52
Hoffman sign, detecting cervical myelopathy	1.7 (0.8, 3.3)	0.6 (0.3, 1.2)	31–52
Palmomental reflex, detecting frontal lobe lesion on MRI	6.3 (2.2, 18.3)	0.8 (0.7, 1)	14

APPENDIX TABLE 1 ■ Likelihood Ratios, Confidence Intervals, and Pretest Probability—Cont'd

Finding	Positive LR (95% CI)	Negative LR (95% CI)	Pre-test Probability (Range)
Positive grasp reflex, detecting discrete lesion in the frontal lobe, deep nuclei, or subcortical white matter	19.1 (5.9, 61.7)	0.7 (0.4, 1.2)	21–37
Chapter 64 Disorders of nerve roots, plexuses, and peripheral nerves			
Motor and sensory findings confined to C7-T1, detecting malignant plexopathy	30.9 (2, 483.8)	0.3 (0.2, 0.5)	61
Horner syndrome, detecting malignant plexopathy	4.1 (1.4, 12.2)	0.5 (0.3, 0.8)	61
Motor and sensory findings confined to C5C6, detecting radiation plexopathy	8.8 (2.9, 26.4)	0.2 (0.1, 0.5)	39
Lymphedema of arm, detecting radiation plexopathy	4.9 (2.1, 11.6)	0.3 (0.2, 0.6)	39
Weak hip abduction if foot drop, detecting lumbosacral radiculopathy	24 (3.5, 165.8)	0.1 (0.1, 0.4)	43
Unilateral involvement, detecting malignant lumbosacral plexopathy	4.5 (1.8, 10.8)	0.1 (0, 0.4)	58
Bilateral involvement, detecting radiation lumbosacral plexopathy	7.5 (2.5, 22.2)	0.2 (0.1, 0.5)	42
EBM Box 64.1 Diagnosing cervical radiculopathy			
Weakness of any arm muscle	1.9 (1.4, 2.5)	0.4 (0.3, 0.6)	52
Reduced sensation in arm	0.7 (0.5, 1)	1.4 (1, 1.8)	52
Reduced biceps reflex	9.1 (1.2, 69.4)	0.9 (0.8, 1)	52
Reduced brachioradialis reflex	7.3 (0.9, 56.8)	0.9 (0.9, 1)	52
Reduced triceps reflex	2.3 (0.7, 7)	0.9 (0.9, 1)	52
Reduced biceps, triceps, or brachioradialis reflex	3.6 (1.4, 9.2)	0.8 (0.7, 0.9)	52
Spurling test	4.8 (2.8, 8.2)	0.6 (0.4, 0.8)	10–79
Rotation of neck to involved side <60 degrees	1.7 (1.3, 2.3)	0.2 (0.1, 0.9)	22
EBM Box 64.2 Localizing cervical radiculopathy			
Weak elbow flexion, detecting C5 radiculopathy	5.3 (2.7, 10.5)	0.2 (0, 2.5)	2
Weak wrist extension, detecting C6 radiculopathy	2.3 (1.1, 5)	0.8 (0.5, 1.1)	19
Weak elbow extension, detecting C7 radiculopathy	4 (1.8, 9.2)	0.4 (0.3, 0.6)	69
Weak finger flexion, detecting C8 radiculopathy	3.8 (1.7, 8.5)	0.6 (0.3, 1.1)	10
Sensory loss of thumb, detecting C6 radiculopathy	8.5 (2.3, 31.1)	0.7 (0.5, 1)	19
Sensory loss of middle finger, detecting C7 radiculopathy	3.2 (0.2, 60.1)	1 (0.9, 1)	69
Sensory loss of little finger, detecting C8 radiculopathy	41.4 (2.1, 807)	0.8 (0.6, 1.1)	10
Diminished biceps or brachioradialis reflex, detecting C6 radiculopathy	14.2 (4.3, 46.7)	0.5 (0.3, 0.8)	19
Diminished triceps reflex, detecting C7 radiculopathy	3 (1.6, 5.6)	0.6 (0.3, 1.4)	54–69
EBM Box 64.3 Carpal tunnel syndrome			
"Classic" or "probable" Katz hand diagram	2.4 (1.6, 3.5)	…	37
"Unlikely" Katz hand diagram	0.2 (0, 0.7)	…	37
Weak thumb abduction	1.8 (1.4, 2.3)	0.6 (0.4, 0.9)	50–74
Thenar atrophy	2.9 (1.1, 7.9)	0.9 (0.8, 1)	35–74
Hypalgesia	3.1 (2, 5.1)	0.7 (0.5, 1.1)	35–62
Diminished 2-point discrimination	2 (0.7, 5.3)	0.8 (0.5, 1.2)	40–57
Abnormal vibration sensation	1.6 (0.8, 3)	0.8 (0.4, 1.3)	50–57
Diminished monofilament sensation	1.2 (1, 1.5)	0.4 (0.1, 2)	53–56

(continued)

APPENDIX TABLE 1 ▦ **Likelihood Ratios, Confidence Intervals, and Pretest Probability—Cont'd**

Finding	Positive LR (95% CI)	Negative LR (95% CI)	Pre-test Probability (Range)
Tinel sign	1.4 (1.2, 1.8)	0.8 (0.6, 0.9)	35–75
Phalen sign	1.4 (1.2, 1.7)	0.6 (0.5, 0.8)	35–88
Pressure provocation test	1.2 (0.8, 1.9)	0.7 (0.4, 1.2)	49–88
Square wrist ratio	2.7 (2.2, 3.4)	0.5 (0.4, 0.8)	60–62
Flick sign	5.5 (0.4, 77.4)	0.3 (0, 2.8)	54–67
EBM Box 64.4 Diagnosing lumbosacral radiculopathy			
Weak ankle dorsiflexion	4.9 (1.9, 12.5)	0.5 (0.4, 0.7)	74
Ipsilateral calf wasting	5.2 (1.3, 20.8)	0.8 (0.6, 0.9)	74
Leg sensation abnormal	1.1 (0.9, 1.5)	0.9 (0.8, 1.1)	47–74
Abnormal ankle jerk	2.1 (1.4, 3.1)	0.8 (0.7, 0.9)	47–74
Straight-leg raising maneuver	1.5 (1.2, 1.9)	0.4 (0.3, 0.6)	47–87
Crossed straight-leg raising maneuver	3.4 (1.8, 6.4)	0.8 (0.7, 0.9)	55–87
EBM Box 64.5 Localizing lumbosacral radiculopathy			
Weak knee extension, detecting L3 or L4 radiculopathy	4 (2.2, 7.2)	0.6 (0.5, 0.8)	25–63
Weak hallux extension, detecting L5 radiculopathy	1.7 (1.2, 2.6)	0.7 (0.5, 0.9)	52–57
Weak ankle dorsiflexion, detecting L5 radiculopathy	1.3 (0.9, 1.8)	0.8 (0.6, 1)	52–58
Weak ankle plantarflexion, detecting S_1 radiculopathy	4.8 (0.4, 60.4)	0.7 (0.6, 0.9)	20–48
Ipsilateral calf wasting, detecting S_1 radiculopathy	2.4 (1.2, 4.7)	0.7 (0.5, 0.9)	48
Sensory loss L5 distribution, detecting L5 radiculopathy	3.1 (1.8, 5.6)	0.8 (0.7, 0.9)	52–58
Sensory loss S_1 distribution, detecting S_1 radiculopathy	2.4 (1.3, 4.2)	0.7 (0.6, 0.9)	41–48
Asymmetric quadriceps reflex, detecting L3 or L4 radiculopathy	8.5 (5, 14.5)	0.7 (0.6, 0.8)	2–46
Asymmetric medial hamstring reflex, detecting L5 radiculopathy	6.2 (1.6, 24.2)	0.5 (0.3, 0.7)	58
Asymmetric Achilles reflex, detecting S_1 radiculopathy	2.7 (1.9, 3.8)	0.5 (0.4, 0.6)	20–66
Femoral stretch test, detecting L2–4 radiculopathy	31.2 (1.9, 499)	0.5 (0.3, 0.7)	46
Chapter 66 Tremor and Parkinson disease			
Feet suddenly freezing in doorway, detecting Parkinson disease	4.4 (1.5, 12.4)	0.7 (0.5, 1)	28–32
Voice becoming softer, detecting Parkinson disease	3.2 (1.8, 5.8)	0.5 (0.1, 1.9)	28–32
Micrographia, detecting Parkinson disease	2.7 (1.8, 4)	0.7 (0.3, 1.3)	28–32
Able to continue riding bicycle after symptom onset, detecting Parkinson disease	2.4 (1.3, 4.5)	0.2 (0, 1.6)	29–41
Acute onset parkinsonism, detecting vascular parkinsonism	21.9 (3, 161.8)	0.7 (0.6, 0.9)	24–58
EBM Box 66.1 Suspected Parkinson disease **Diagnosing Parkinson disease**			
Unable to perform perfect 10 tandem steps	0.2 (0.1, 0.5)	4.6 (3.1, 6.8)	28–63
Asymmetric arm swing	2.7 (1.2, 6.4)	0.5 (0.4, 0.8)	74
Positive applause sign	0.3 (0.2, 0.5)	2.4 (1.8, 3.1)	29–82
3 of 3 cardinal features present	2.2 (1.2, 4.2)	0.5 (0.3, 0.7)	76
3 of 3 cardinal features, asymmetry	4.1 (1.7, 10.2)	0.4 (0.3, 0.6)	76
Good response to levodopa	4.1 (1.1, 15.7)	0.2 (0.1, 0.2)	38–40

APPENDIX TABLE 1 ▪ **Likelihood Ratios, Confidence Intervals, and Pretest Probability—Cont'd**

Finding	Positive LR (95% CI)	Negative LR (95% CI)	Pre-test Probability (Range)
Detecting multisystem atrophy			
Rapid progression	2.5 (1.6, 4.1)	0.6 (0.4, 0.8)	20–55
Absence of tremor	1.4 (1, 2)	0.7 (0.5, 1.1)	15–55
Speech and/or bulbar signs	4.1 (2.7, 6.1)	0.2 (0.1, 0.4)	28
Autonomic dysfunction	4.3 (2.3, 7.8)	0.3 (0.2, 0.4)	15–55
Cerebellar signs	6.6 (2.9, 15)	0.6 (0.4, 0.8)	15–80
Pyramidal tract signs	3 (1.3, 7.1)	0.7 (0.6, 0.9)	15–80
Dementia	0.3 (0.2, 0.6)	1.9 (1.5, 2.4)	15–27
Diagnosing progressive supranuclear palsy			
Downgaze palsy and early postural instability	9.5 (3, 29.8)	0.6 (0.6, 0.7)	29–68
Detecting vascular parkinsonism			
Pyramidal tract signs	16.2 (8.2, 32.2)	0.5 (0.4, 0.7)	20–58
Lower body parkinsonism	6.1 (4.3, 8.7)	0.4 (0.3, 0.5)	20–58
Chapter 67 Hemorrhagic vs. ischemic stroke			
Seizures at onset	4.7 (1.6, 14.1)	0.9 (0.9, 1)	12–39
Vomiting	3 (1.7, 5.5)	0.7 (0.6, 0.9)	16–46
Severe headache	2.9 (1.7, 4.8)	0.7 (0.6, 0.8)	12–46
Loss of consciousness	2.6 (1.6, 4.2)	0.7 (0.5, 0.8)	43
Previous TIA	0.3 (0.2, 0.7)	1.2 (1.1, 1.3)	12–17
EBM Box 67.1 Hemorrhagic stroke			
Systolic BP >220 mm Hg	4 (1.1, 15.4)	0.9 (0.7, 1.1)	13
Systolic BP <160 mm Hg	0.4 (0.3, 0.6)	1.9 (1.3, 2.8)	35–43
Mental status coma	6.3 (3.4, 11.7)	...	12–48
Mental status drowsy	1.7 (1.2, 2.4)	...	12–48
Mental status alert	0.5 (0.3, 0.7)	...	16–48
Neurologic deterioration during first 3 hours	5.8 (4.3, 7.8)	0.2 (0.2, 0.4)	18
Kernig or Brudzinski sign	2.9 (0.6, 14.1)	1 (0.9, 1.1)	18–46
Neck stiffness	5.4 (2.5, 11.3)	0.7 (0.7, 0.9)	18–59
Babinski present, bilateral toes	2.4 (1.6, 3.6)	...	17–43
Babinski present, single toe	1 (0.9, 1.2)	...	17–43
Babinski absent both toes	0.5 (0.3, 0.9)	...	17–43
Deviation of eyes	1.9 (1.6, 2.3)	0.7 (0.5, 0.9)	15–17
Hemiparesis	0.9 (0.8, 1.1)	1.3 (1, 1.7)	12–31
Aphasia	1.1 (0.9, 1.3)	1 (0.9, 1)	14–53
Hemisensory disturbance	1.3 (1.2, 1.4)	0.8 (0.7, 1.1)	12–17
Hemianopia	1.3 (1.1, 1.6)	0.9 (0.8, 1)	16
Ataxia	0.7 (0.5, 1)	1.1 (1, 1.1)	16
Cervical bruit	0.1 (0, 0.4)	1.1 (1, 1.3)	16–43
Atrial fibrillation, ECG	0.3 (0.1, 0.5)	1.3 (1.1, 1.4)	12–44
EBM Box 67.2 Hemorrhagic stroke			
Siriraj score "hemorrhage" (>1)	5.7 (4.5, 7.2)	...	13–69
Siriraj score "uncertain (–1 to 1)	1 (0.9, 1.2)	...	13–69
Siriraj score "infarction (<–1)	0.3 (0.2, 0.4)	...	13–69
Chapter 68 Acute vertigo			
Head impulse test positive (corrective saccades), detecting abnormal caloric testing	6.7 (3.7, 12.1)	0.6 (0.5, 0.8)	19–52
Ophthalmoparesis, detecting stroke if dizzy	70 (8, 615)	0.9 (0.8, 1)	5
Limb ataxia, detecting stroke if dizzy	23.9 (2, 286)	0.8 (0.7, 0.9)	5–11
Dysarthria, detecting stroke if dizzy	20.6 (6.5, 65.8)	0.7 (0.5, 1.2)	5–8
Facial droop, detecting stroke if dizzy	18.8 (2, 174.8)	0.6 (0.3, 1.3)	5–8
Visual field defect, detecting stroke if dizzy	17.5 (1.1, 276)	1 (0.9, 1)	5
Focal weakness, detecting stroke if dizzy	8.6 (3.5, 21.3)	0.7 (0.6, 0.8)	3–30

(continued)

APPENDIX TABLE 1 ■ Likelihood Ratios, Confidence Intervals, and Pretest Probability—Cont'd

Finding	Positive LR (95% CI)	Negative LR (95% CI)	Pre-test Probability (Range)
Focal sensory disturbance, detecting stroke if dizzy	7 (2.4, 20.1)	0.8 (0.7, 1.1)	3–5
Gait abnormality, detecting stroke if dizziness	4.5 (2.7, 7.5)	0.4 (0.1, 1.8)	3–5
Acute infarct on MRI DWI, detecting ischemic stroke	44.2 (2.8, 690)	0.2 (0.1, 0.3)	75
EBM Box 68.1 Acute vertigo, detecting ischemic stroke			
Severe truncal ataxia	17.9 (1.1, 283)	0.7 (0.6, 0.8)	75
Skew deviation present	7.1 (3.5, 14.2)	0.6 (0.5, 0.8)	37–73
Saccadic "smooth" pursuit	4.6 (2.5, 8.4)	0.2 (0.1, 0.5)	50–52
Direction-changing nystagmus	8.4 (1.9, 36.9)	0.6 (0.4, 0.8)	37–75
Normal head impulse test (i.e., no corrective saccade)	10.8 (4.3, 27.2)	0.2 (0.1, 0.4)	37–75
Combined findings, 1 or more	13.6 (6.8, 27.1)	0.02 (0, 0.1)	37–75
Chapter 69 Nonorganic neurologic disorders			
Knee-up test positive, detecting postoperative motor deficit	462 (65, 3298)	0.1 (0, 0.4)	3
EBM Box 69.1 Nonorganic neurologic disease			
Chair test positive	17 (1.1, 257)	0.2 (0, 0.7)	50
Knee-lift test positive	7.1 (1.6, 31.5)	0.04 (0, 0.6)	58
Drift without pronation	11.4 (3.5, 37.3)	0.02 (0, 0.3)	48
Hoover sign positive	42 (8.4, 210)	0.3 (0.1, 0.7)	6–49
Chapter 70 Examination of patients in the ICU			
Pulse pressure increase ≥9%–12% (only patients with CVP increment after leg elevation), detecting patients who respond to fluid challenge	9.3 (3.1, 27.8)	0.1 (0, 0.5)	33
Prolonged capillary refill time (*after* fluid resuscitation), predicting hospital mortality	10.5 (2.8, 38.8)	0.6 (0.4, 1)	14
Prolonged capillary refill time (*before* fluid resuscitation), predicting hospital mortality	1.6 (0.8, 3.3)	0.7 (0.4, 1.3)	14
Mottling diminishes during hospitalization, predicting hospital mortality	0.2 (0.1, 0.5)	3.8 (1.4, 10.4)	66
EBM Box 70.1 Examination in the ICU			
MEWS = 0, predicting hospital death	0.3 (0.2, 0.4)	1.4 (1, 1.9)	9–14
MEWS ≥5, predicting hospital death	4.8 (3.2, 7.2)	0.6 (0.5, 0.7)	1–15
Warms hands, detecting septic shock if hypotension	2.7 (1.6, 4.5)	0.2 (0.1, 0.4)	54
Bounding pulses, detecting septic shock if hypotension	2.4 (1.3, 4.5)	0.5 (0.3, 0.8)	54
Elevated neck veins, detecting cardiogenic shock if hypotension	4 (2.2, 7.1)	0.2 (0.1, 0.6)	26
Lung crackles, detecting cardiogenic shock if hypotension	1.9 (1.1, 3.5)	0.6 (0.4, 1.1)	26
Elevated neck veins *and* crackles, detecting cardiogenic shock if hypotension	56.4 (3.5, 916)	0.5 (0.3, 0.7)	26
Pulse pressure increase ≥9%–12%, detecting patients who respond to fluid challenge	3.9 (2.6, 5.8)	0.5 (0.4, 0.6)	41–68
Asynchronous breathing during COPD exacerbation, predicting intubation or death	3.2 (1.3, 7.8)	0.5 (0.2, 1)	31
Asymmetric breath sounds, detecting endobronchial intubation	12.8 (5.8, 28.4)	0.5 (0.3, 0.8)	5–62
Diminished breath sounds in patients with ARDS, detecting underlying pleural effusion	3 (1.5, 6)	0.7 (0.6, 0.9)	26–48

APPENDIX TABLE 1 ■ Likelihood Ratios, Confidence Intervals, and Pretest Probability—Cont'd

Finding	Positive LR (95% CI)	Negative LR (95% CI)	Pre-test Probability (Range)
Anisocoria in patients with coma, detecting structural intracranial lesion	9 (2.8, 28.8)	0.6 (0.5, 0.8)	40
Neck stiffness in patients with stroke, detecting hemorrhagic stroke	5.4 (2.5, 11.3)	0.7 (0.7, 0.9)	18–59
EBM Box 70.2 Hypoperfusion in ICU patients			
Cool extremities in ICU patients, detecting low cardiac index	3.7 (2.1, 6.5)	0.8 (0.8, 0.9)	55
Cool extremities in septic ICU patients, detecting low cardiac index	5.2 (2.3, 12.1)	0.7 (0.6, 0.9)	47
0 of 3 findings present, detecting low cardiac index	0.5 (0.3, 0.8)	…	8
1 of 3 findings present, detecting low cardiac index	2.3 (1.6, 3.4)	…	8
All 3 findings present, detecting low cardiac index	7.5 (2.2, 25.3)	…	8
Capillary refill time ≥5 sec, detecting low cardiac output	1.6 (1.2, 2.2)	0.9 (0.8, 1)	36
Limb is cool or capillary refill time >4.5 sec, detecting elevated lactate	2.2 (1.6, 3)	0.5 (0.4, 0.7)	50
Limb is cool or capillary refill time >4.5 sec, predicting multiorgan dysfunction	2.6 (1.9, 3.5)	0.3 (0.2, 0.5)	50
Capillary refill time ≥5 sec, predicting major postoperative complications	12.1 (5.4, 27.1)	0.2 (0.1, 0.5)	17
Capillary refill time ≥5 sec, predicting mortality if septic shock	4.6 (1.7, 12.8)	0.6 (0.4, 0.9)	37
Knee mottling, predicting mortality if septic shock	10.2 (3.2, 32)	0.8 (0.6, 1)	11–52

AAI, Ankle/arm index; *ACL*, anterior cruciate ligament; *ACTH*, adrenocorticotropic hormone; *ALS*, amyotrophic lateral sclerosis; *ARDS*, acute respiratory distress syndrome; *AV*, atrioventricular; *BMI*, body mass index; *BNP*, brain-type natriuretic peptide; *BP*, blood pressure; *CHF*, congestive heart failure; *COPD*, chronic obstructive pulmonary disease; *CSF*, cerebrospinal fluid; *CT*, computed tomography; *CVP*, central venous pressure; *CXR*, chest radiograph; *DP*, dorsalis pedis; *DVT*, deep vein thrombosis; *DWI*, diffusion-weighted image; *ECG*, electrocardiogram; *EF*, ejection fraction; *FUO*, fever of unknown origin; *HIV*, human immunodeficiency virus; *ICU*, intensive care unit; *LLSB*, left lower sternal border; *LVH*, left ventricular hypertrophy; *MCL*, midclavicular line; *MEWS*, modified early warning system; *MRI*, magnetic resonance imaging; *MVP*, mitral valve prolapse; *PCL*, posterior cruciate ligament; *PR*, pulmonic regurgitation; *PT*, posterior tibialis; *RV*, right ventricular; *TIA*, transient ischemic attack; *UGI*, upper gastrointestinal; *VZV*, varicella-zoster virus; *WBC*, white blood cells.

INDEX

Page numbers followed by *f* indicate figures; *t*, tables; *b*, boxes.